MW01088950

Healing
Chronic
Candida

A Holistic, Comprehensive, and Natural Approach

Cynthia Perkins, M.Ed.

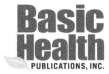

**Basic
Health**
PUBLICATIONS, INC.

The information contained in this book is based upon the research and personal and professional experiences of the author. It is not intended as a substitute for consulting with your physician or other health-care provider. Any attempt to diagnose and treat an illness should be done under the direction of a health-care professional.

The publisher does not advocate the use of any particular health-care protocol but believes the information in this book should be available to the public. The publisher and author are not responsible for any adverse effects or consequences resulting from the use of the suggestions, preparations, or procedures discussed in this book. Should the reader have any questions concerning the appropriateness of any procedures or preparation mentioned, the author and the publisher strongly suggest consulting a professional health-care advisor.

Turner Publishing Company
Nashville, TN
www.turnerpublishing.com

Library of Congress Cataloging-in-Publication Data is available through the Library of Congress.

Copyright © 2018 by Cynthia Perkins

All rights reserved. No part of this publication may be reproduced, stored in a retrieval system, or transmitted, in any form or by any means, electronic, mechanical, photocopying, recording, or otherwise, without the prior written consent of the copyright owner.

Interior design: Gary A. Rosenberg
Cover design: Maddie Cothren

Printed in the United States of America

10 9 8 7 6 5 4 3 2 1

In memory and honor of Dr. Orian C. Truss for his outstanding and groundbreaking work on the topic of candida, which first brought this issue to light and completely altered the course of my life. I would not be the person I am today if he and his work had not come before me.

A special thanks to all the other brave pioneers in the field who have brought awareness to the issue of candida, and to all the practitioners I have worked with, and to the clients who have graciously shared their experiences with me, all of which I have learned from and grown both personally and professionally.

Contents

Foreword

Healing is a journey. For too many, however, the path is long, arduous, and often frustrating, as our medical model doesn't always provide the clear path required for this journey. Over the past fifty years, there has been a growing movement to examine health disorders from a holistic point of view, incorporating factors from an individual's environment, nutritional intake, and lifestyle choices. There has also been an equally expansive body of evidence to suggest that there is a connection between the gut microbiome and a wide range of physical and psychological health problems. To this end, Cynthia Perkins's *Healing Chronic Candida: A Holistic, Comprehensive, and Natural Approach* offers a rich and succinct causality between the all-too-overlooked issue of candida overgrowth and human health.

As a clinician with over thirty years of medical practice, I have found candida to be a cofactor in a wide range of psychiatric disorders. As an integrative psychiatrist in the 1990s, my understanding of candida was based on the work of Crook and Truss. At that time, doctors, myself included, made dietary changes and used nutritional, herbal, and pharmacological antifungals to treat candida. Many patients got better; however, many also relapsed. It wasn't until I began the process of understanding the complex interplay of genetics, biochemical individuality, nutritional deficiencies, dysbiosis, and biofilms that I recognized that a personalized treatment program for each patient would begin to support patients in their journey to maintain health.

Healing Chronic Candida provides a detailed, well-organized, and easy-to-read overview of candida's biology and pathology. Cynthia Perkins places a particular emphasis on external factors that can lead to overgrowth, including poor diet, chronic stress, and antibiotic use. The second half of Perkins's book provides guidance in the design and implementation of candida treatments, first by covering the clinical effectiveness behind natural and pharmaceutical supplements, then by discussing lifestyle choices that can reduce the risk of overgrowth. Cynthia explains that the goal is not to eliminate all floras from the gastrointestinal tract, but instead to allow for the *restoration of* microbial balance.

In this groundbreaking book *Healing Chronic Candida*, Cynthia Perkins has explained and explored the scientific literature to help clinicians and patients understand the complex path of treating candida. This book is both comprehensive and concise in presenting a holistic model for the treatment of candida.

For most cases of health issues, patients and practitioners alike search for the singular underlying cause, with the hopes of uncovering a standardized treatment process. We have found this to rarely be the case—treatments always need to be personalized to individual needs and typically incorporate lifestyle changes for the better. Throughout the closing chapters of this book, the effects of diet and stress on controlling candida overgrowth are described in detail. This book provides a unique perspective on sympathetic dominance and methods to regulate activity within the sympathetic nervous system. In recent years, there has been a dramatic increase in publications demonstrating the efficacy of stress reduction interventions for cases of addiction, anxiety, chronic pain, depression, and disorders of the immune system. *Healing Chronic Candida* includes a comprehensive overview of lifestyle factors in addition to nutritional supports.

As an integrative psychiatrist, my days are saddened by many patients unable to find relief by using traditional psychiatric models or oversimplified alternative models. *Healing Chronic Candida* is the most innovative, inclusive treatment model for candida I have encountered. Cynthia Perkins weaves clinical experience, scientific literature, and simplifies complex medical information into relevant, clinically astute treatment models that are easy to understand for both clinicians and patients.

This book provides readers with the science to understand candida, the strength to commit to a journey toward healing, but, most importantly, hope. This hope is required for a clear, guided path on the journey towards wellness and health.

James M. Greenblatt, Chief Medical Officer, Walden Behavioral Care
Author of *Finally Focused: The Breakthrough Natural Treatment Plan for ADHD*

INTRODUCTION

The Healing Journey

The first and most important principle to understand about healing chronic candida is that healing is a lifelong journey, not a one-time event, and it is not always defined as a total cure. By *cure* I mean the complete eradication of overgrowth and a return to the lifestyle and diet one enjoyed prior to developing candida. Individuals who are fortunate enough to get a diagnosis shortly after acquiring candida and who have an exceptionally competent physician may achieve a total cure, but these people are rare. Because there are so few practitioners who recognize candida or have the expertise that is needed to treat it effectively, most people who have candida have it for decades, or even a lifetime, before receiving a diagnosis or finding a health-care provider who has enough knowledge to address all the critical aspects involved in healing.

Candida is among the most complicated, resilient, cunning, enigmatic, multifaceted, and adaptive organisms to be found. Chronic candida is exceptionally difficult to treat and very poorly understood. Even many doctors, practitioners, and remedy manufacturers who specialize in candida do not possess a deep understanding of the organism's complexity, depth, adaptable nature, and uncanny ability to survive. I've been researching and analyzing it for nearly three decades and I regularly discover new eye-opening and jaw-dropping information and find myself astonished by its unique yet frightening characteristics.

When one has housed candida overgrowth for an extended period of time, it becomes deeply ingrained in the body and very difficult, if not impossible, to eradicate completely. The longer the organisms have been present the more well-established and hardy their society becomes. Furthermore, candida possesses a wide array of abilities that enable it to evade detection and eradication, outwit even the most well thought out treatment plan, and continue to thrive. It is relentless and determined. On top of that, once candida is in place, numerous other conditions can develop—including sympathetic dominance, impaired detoxification, adrenal fatigue, parasite and bacterial overgrowth, hormone imbalances, inhibited immunity, nutritional deficiencies, leaky gut, and others—creating a vicious circle that fuels more overgrowth of candida, which only further perpetuates the conditions. Sometimes the individual's biochemistry gets so messed up that it becomes extremely difficult to unravel completely, even when he or she does everything right.

Taking the appropriate steps to address candida overgrowth, which will be presented in great detail throughout this book, can help a person alleviate many of the symptoms associated with yeast overgrowth, significantly improve the quality of his or her life, and help him or her reach a higher level of health. In some cases, the afflicted may be able to overcome a variety of conditions, syndromes, and disorders. In my case, the changes in diet and lifestyle that I made due to candida enabled me to overcome chronic drug and alcohol addiction (as of summer 2017 I've achieved twenty-nine years of craving-free and uninterrupted sobriety), compulsive overeating, clinical depression, disabling anxiety attacks, and fibromyalgia. By employing the same changes in diet and lifestyle, I helped my son, who was a child at the time, improve his ADHD by about 90 percent. Many other people report dramatic improvements in numerous other conditions such as hyperactivity, attention deficit, autism, multiple sclerosis, psoriasis, acne, arthritis, bowel and gastrointestinal disorders, depression, anxiety disorders, autoimmune conditions, and many others by following an anticandida regimen.

However, if one discontinues following strict dietary controls and engaging in the other treatment remedies presented in this book, candida overgrowth and its symptoms typically return. In most cases, chronic candida is not "cured"; it is managed, and lifelong vigilance is required for management. If one returns to eating a diet and living a lifestyle that encourage candida overgrowth, then candida is going to proliferate once again. We don't want to eliminate candida completely, because it affords a variety of beneficial effects in the body. Not only that, it's impossible to do so as candida is a natural inhabitant of the gastrointestinal tract. The organism is always hanging around to some degree or another. If conditions in the body become conducive to overgrowth once again, candida will take advantage of the opportunity and will proliferate. So we must never allow the body to become the type of environment that will encourage overgrowth. This takes hard work and commitment, and there is no magic bullet or miracle cure.

The same is basically true of any chronic health condition. Most of the health problems we see today are a result of eating the wrong diet, being exposed to environmental toxins, excess sympathetic nervous system activity, and making unhealthy lifestyle choices. The human body was simply not designed to be exposed to these types of conditions, and once the damage is done the damage is done. Regaining and maintaining any level of good health demands a long-term commitment to permanent changes in diet and lifestyle. However, I believe you will find that making this commitment is well worth your time and effort, because the changes in diet and lifestyle required to heal candida will not only help you manage yeast overgrowth but will also promote optimal physical, emotional, and spiritual health in general. You will be returning to the diet and way of living that nature intended for your body and mind.

The poor diet and lifestyle that foster overgrowth of candida and other microbes also lead to more serious health conditions and disorders, such as insulin resistance, type 2 diabetes, heart disease, cancer, obesity, Alzheimer's, depression, anxiety disorders, addiction, and poor physical and mental health overall. If you continue to eat and live in this manner, you will face far more serious diagnoses and deterioration in health at some point. You and your health are much better off in the long run by making these changes, which will protect you in the future.

For those who are just beginning the healing journey or who are resistant to giving up unhealthy foods and lifestyle choices, these concepts are often difficult to accept. However, they will get easier as you move through the process. Once your endocrine system and brain begin to heal, you won't be drawn to foods and actions that are destructive, and once you begin to feel better you'll become more motivated to be good to yourself.

During the healing journey, a person doesn't just employ a treatment plan; they change their values, beliefs, identity, choices, and way of interacting with the world. They redefine their life and who they are. Most aspects of modern society foster poor health; therefore, healing demands that you design a new life that supports health. It's about becoming someone new, and when you develop a new identity you will no longer want to eat and live in the same manner in which you used to. Yet, as you go through this book, you will discover that seeking health and designing the new identity is largely about returning to basic principles in diet and lifestyle that were followed by our ancient ancestors for millions of years. We are not reinventing the wheel.

Yes, there are a certain percentage of people who develop candida and get rid of it with a simple course of antifungals and who don't have to do ongoing maintenance. If you or someone you know is one of those people, then rejoice, because you are in the minority. This book is written for the person with chronic candida. *Chronic* refers to a condition that is persistent, long-lasting, constantly recurring, and difficult to eradicate. There is candida and there is chronic candida; they are two different beasts and must be treated as such.

Furthermore, there are many different levels of healing, and the level of healing that you can achieve is dependent on a variety of factors, such as how well you comply with the diet, your dedication to the healing journey, how long you have had candida overgrowth, the level of overgrowth, the extent of biofilms that are present, the species and strains of candida that you carry, the extent of damage to the gut, whether parasites and bacterial overgrowth are present, how many organs and systems have been affected, genetics, whether your candida is systemic or localized, severity of die-off, your age, the ability of your detoxification system to do its job, the level of stress in your life, other health issues that may have developed because of or in addition to candida, how much money you have to spend on healing, how many setbacks or roadblocks you come up against during your journey, whether you have a history of childhood abuse or neglect, and whether you have access to a physician with enough expertise on the condition and its many possible complications. Each of these topics is addressed in this book.

Although most people can make significant improvements at a minimum, improvements may range anywhere between mild and miraculous. Naturally, one who has a complicated case may be unable to achieve the same level of healing as someone who has a more clear-cut case. The experience of healing varies from individual to individual, depending on which of the aforementioned factors applies to each one. One may also move back and forth between different levels of healing at different points in his or her life in response to changes that may occur. For example, a person who has experienced a high level of healing may suffer a setback in response to stress, a virus, menopause, etc. Similarly, a person who has not achieved a high level of healing may be able to do so once they eliminate one of the complicating factors. Healing is dynamic and does not always occur in a linear fashion.

The healing journey requires that you become a diligent participant in the treatment plan and a passionate advocate for yourself and your health. Responsibility for your healing lies in your hands, not your doctor's. It's not as simple as taking an antifungal prescription and eating a yeast-free diet. Healing calls for a much more holistic, natural, and comprehensive approach that addresses each of the interconnected facets of the condition.

We must also detach ourselves from the unrealistic mind-set that everything should be quick, easy, convenient, and comfortable. Healing just doesn't happen that way. It takes time and a great deal of effort. It is vital that you develop tolerance for discomfort. Do not judge it or label it; just let it exist. We are conditioned by society to have zero tolerance for discomfort; we are encouraged to medicate it or run away in the opposite direction. Anything that you fight against seems to grow bigger and stronger. When you embrace your discomfort, it loses its power over you. You must learn to become comfortable with the uncomfortable. Seeking out quick fixes never works and only perpetuates the problem.

Healing also demands that we find a new definition for optimal health. Being healthy does not necessarily mean that a person has overcome all health limitations. It may also mean they are living life as fully as possible in the moment, despite the circumstances. It's about finding harmony, peace, and balance in the midst of the storm, while continuing to strive for a higher level of health. One does not have to be in "good" health to enjoy a peaceful, meaningful, and joyful life. Sometimes the most powerful transformation takes place internally on an emotional and spiritual level, prompting a change in one's perspective.

You will also need a high degree of patience, determination, commitment, diligence, and acceptance. In order to change the current circumstance, you must first accept where you are. The more you resist a circumstance (be it pain, loss, suffering, or any unpleasant situation), the more persistent and stronger it becomes. Acceptance reduces its impact on your life and allows you to move forward. You must fully embrace your pain, symptoms, losses, sorrow, grief, and suffering in order to move past them. My goal is not to hold you back by defining limits on what can or cannot be achieved, but neither do I want to set you up with false hope or unrealistic expectations. I'm not saying that you should approach healing with a mind-set that you won't get well. You should operate on the assumption that a full recovery is completely possible, but with an awareness of the challenges involved, and facing the reality of the situation head-on with courage. You want to continue to pursue options that may improve your health, but also have acceptance for wherever you are in the process at any given time. We don't want to dwell on the negatives, but we must have the facts if we are to make any improvements and to cope adequately.

I encourage you to approach your healing and all it entails with a sense of humor and an optimistic and hopeful attitude. As long as you have hope, you can get through anything. Hope reduces the stress and negative impact of a situation, changes our perception and outlook on life, motivates, inspires, comforts, supports, improves coping abilities, reduces feelings of powerlessness, and helps us to live more fully and to carry on regardless of the circumstance. Having hope is not about looking at the world through rose-colored glasses. It is simply believing that the current situation can change or get better. The key word here is *can*. Having hope does not require a guarantee that we will get the desired result. It is seeing the possibility for such an outcome. As long as there is a possibility that things can change or get better, all is not lost and we can go on. Find the humor in your situation. Instead of directing your attention on how awful a symptom or limitation might be, turn it around, and look at how ridiculous it is, and laugh in its face.

Travel the healing path with the mind-set of a curious and adventurous explorer, without judgment or expectations. Just observe, evaluate, and adjust accordingly. Try to appreciate the journey rather than being in a hurry to reach the destination. For example, instead of being horrified by the candida organism and biofilms that are taking up residence in your body or by the symptoms it produces, try to be awed by its remarkable ability to adapt and marvel at its will to survive. Objectively research and experiment with new healing modalities as though you are on a life-saving scientific expedition. Keep your attention on the fact that you are doing something good for your body and your life rather than on your symptoms or what you have had to give up. Direct all your thoughts and energy toward a passionate pursuit of healthy eating and living.

I also urge you to view your health condition not as a curse but as a learning opportunity. Look for its hidden gifts. Perhaps it helped you realize what was most important in life, taught you how to relax more often or how to appreciate yourself to a greater extent, or offered you important insights. Examine unconscious expectations and truths you live by that may no longer serve you well. There are always gifts amidst life's struggles and challenges. Instead of focusing on how difficult it is to make the changes required, keep the focus on what you can do to achieve the goal.

Sometimes it is hard to see that you are making any improvements on a day-to-day basis. However, if you look back to six months or a year ago, you are likely to see that progress has been made. Celebrate how far you've come, even if it is minimal. Be grateful for what you have. Learn to appreciate and enjoy the simple things in life.

Be your own best friend and give yourself love, support, and acceptance no matter what. Take it easy on yourself and really be there for yourself. Treat yourself the way you would treat a good friend. Say reassuring things to yourself out loud like, "It's okay," "You'll be all right," "You're so strong," "You're amazing," or "There's nothing to be concerned about." Be present with yourself.

Acknowledging that everything I have just suggested in this chapter is very difficult and that you will not always be able to rise to the challenge is also part of the healing process. There will be hours or days when you hang out in the dark pits, and that is okay, as long as you don't stay there. There must be acceptance for the inability to have acceptance as well. Crawl out, let it go, and get back on track.

You should also note that a holistic approach to healing does not completely exclude the use of pharmaceuticals. However, they are chosen only as a last resort and used in addition to the natural methods, never instead of. Adhering to a proper diet, lifestyle changes, nutritional supplements, herbs, and other natural strategies will be the first course of action. The decision about whether to use a pharmaceutical is influenced by a variety of factors, including the urgency of the problem at hand, the responsiveness of the condition to natural healing methods, the level of risk associated with the drug, severity of the drug's side effects, and the overall health of the individual. Most health conditions can be addressed quite adequately without the use of pharmaceuticals, and in many cases they only create new problems. However, when microbes like candida are involved, there may be times when a certain pharmaceutical is required and is the best course of action.

CANDIDA AND ME

Like many of you, I have been dealing with candida for the larger part of my life. I grew up in a violent and abusive home (emotional, physical, and sexual) and experienced loss of my primary caregiver at the age of seven, which, as you will learn later in the book, presents an extreme form of stress that poses severe consequences for the immune system, endocrine system, brain, and autonomic nervous system, leaving one vulnerable to a wide variety of health conditions like candida. Additionally, I believe my birth mother had candida when I was born because she exhibited all the symptoms; therefore, I think it is possible I picked up candida at birth.

When I look back on my life as a child, there were many signs that could have been candida-related. By my teens I was experiencing crippling anxiety attacks, suicidal depression, daily headaches, and chronic widespread pain. I turned to drugs and alcohol in an attempt to self-medicate these symptoms that impaired my ability to live a productive and fulfilling life. By the age of eighteen I was a full-blown alcoholic and drug addict (including being addicted to some pharmaceuticals like benzodiazepines), a state that continued until the summer of 1988 when I was twenty-seven, at which time my life completely fell apart and I entered a treatment program for addiction.

For the next year, I attended twelve-step meetings faithfully and worked the steps obsessively, engaged in heavy-duty psychotherapy, attended support groups of many different kinds, and managed to stay clean and sober. However, I was intensely miserable. My depression was slightly less severe than it had been in previous years, but my anxiety attacks had returned with a vengeance and were so acute I could barely function. I was hanging on by a fine thread. Additionally, my son, a child at the time, had such severe attention-deficit hyperactivity disorder that he was practically uncontrollable and had to be held back in the first grade. Life was challenging, to say the least.

Then I stumbled upon a book about candida, *The Missing Diagnosis,* by Dr. Orian C. Truss, given to me by a woman who ran one of my support groups. It completely changed the course of my life. I found myself on every page. It was as if the book had been written specifically for me. I knew instantly that the condition he described was not only my problem, but also my son's. I saw a doctor who specialized in candida, and he confirmed that both my son and I had the illness. We began the standard treatment protocol. As you likely know, the first step in the process when dealing with candida is to eliminate sugar from the diet. It was then that I discovered that I was as severely addicted to sugar as I had been to drugs and alcohol. I struggled for several months to give it up. Eventually I succeeded, and it was removed from our diets.

To my pleasant surprise, my disabling anxiety attacks completely disappeared, just like magic. Not only that, my son's ADHD improved by about 90 percent. I was astonished. To be certain that it was the sugar, we tested it on several occasions. It never failed: if either one of us ate sugar, the anxiety attacks and ADHD returned. I became passionate about healthy eating, and we remained committed to a candida diet and lifestyle. Not only was my anxiety relieved by these changes but so was my depression. Furthermore, I never experienced cravings for drugs and alcohol again. Attending a twelve-step program became counterproductive because of most members' heavy use of sugar, caffeine, carbs, and nicotine. And once I made the changes in diet and lifestyle required to address candida, I simply no longer needed the program's assistance. Staying clean and sober was no longer a struggle. It wasn't even an issue anymore.

Life improved significantly for my son and me, which compelled me to go to college and become a mental health counselor so that I could educate other people about how diet impacts mental and physical health. However, during this time, even though I had given up sugar, I struggled with bouts of intense carbohydrate bingeing, which continued for many years. Eventually I managed to regulate that behavior with portion control, but for decades I longed for carbohydrates. It was a constant battle to stay away from them—until I discovered the diet that I will present to you in this book.

Additionally, as I went through my healing journey, I began to notice that a lot of the guidance I received from health-care practitioners was not accurate. They said complex carbohydrates would not feed candida, but that wasn't true in my case. They said if you take probiotics and antifungals you will be cured, but that did not happen for me. They claimed it was easy to overcome candida and that pretty much everybody they treated recovered, but that was not my experience. When I tried to discuss these things with them, I was dismissed, brushed off, shunned, or labeled a difficult patient. I was basically forced to become my own doctor and driven to research the topic endlessly on my own.

At first I thought I was just an oddball with an unusual case. However, over the years, in both my personal life and as a holistic health counselor working with candida patients, I observed that practically every person I met who had candida had the same experience I had. It became undeniably clear that a very small percentage of people respond to traditional treatment for candida in the manner in which most of the experts claim they will. The majority of patients do not.

I came to understand that we were being misinformed or uninformed on a wide variety of issues related to candida—such as die-off, the appropriate diet, different strains and species of candida, sugar and carb addiction, testing procedures, biofilms, mutation, resistance, the extent of candida's ability to adapt and survive, limits of antifungals, length of treatment, nutritional supplements that feed candida, the role of parasites, bacteria, and autonomic nervous system dysfunction in relation to candida—all of which can significantly impede one's recovery process if not addressed in the appropriate way.

You have most likely read that if you eat a yeast-free, sugar-free diet and take some antifungals and probiotics, you will be cured quickly and easily. If you work with a health practitioner who really knows what they're doing, they may lead you to believe that you will be cured if you engage in the so-called 4R protocol: remove, repair, restore, and replace. But as someone who has battled candida for more than twenty-five years, that has not been my experience. Nor has it been the experience of hundreds of other people with candida whom I have worked with professionally for the past eleven years, many of whom have been treated by some of the greatest experts in the field. Although the traditional treatment regimen constitutes sound advice and is a necessary part of the healing journey, healing from chronic candida isn't that simple. A more holistic and permanent approach is required.

This is not a criticism of the pioneers in the field. Their work was groundbreaking and life-changing, but it was in its infancy. The full magnitude of the problem was not yet fully understood. We are still learning. Facts surrounding these additional aspects of recovery that need addressed are not well known or easily accessible; it has taken me decades to learn what I know, and I had to go out of my way to do so. My passion has been fueled by my own struggles and need for solutions, and then it became my mission in life to educate others about what I have learned. So here we are today. This book is informed by my own personal battle with candida, the decades of research I've undertaken on the topic, and the hundreds of clients I have worked with who live with candida.

My goal with this book is to thoroughly inform you about all aspects of candida. Gaining such knowledge is the first and most powerful step in the healing journey—not only by presenting you with the best treatment options but also by reducing feelings of fear, helplessness, hopelessness, and loss of control that often go hand in hand with a chronic health condition. Knowledge and information help you understand what's happening, what to expect, and how to remain involved in the process of your healing. They enable you to cope more effectively, prepare yourself emotionally and physically, take control of your own destiny, and minimize candida's impact on your life as you navigate the rocky roads. As I see it, there are few things more empowering than being adequately informed.

My candida diagnosis changed the quality and course of my life forever—for the better. Although it has been a challenging path, it has also been one of my greatest gifts. I am humbled and honored that my experiences have brought me full circle and now provide me with the opportunity to write this book and to help other people transform their lives and to achieve the highest possible level of healing for their circumstances.

CHAPTER 1

Candida:
The Basics and More

Candida is a yeast microorganism from the fungus family that under normal circumstances naturally resides in the human body in small amounts. It thrives in environments that are moist, dark, and warm, so it is typically found on certain areas of the skin and in the mouth, throat, gastrointestinal tract, and vagina. It can serve us beneficially by helping our bodies identify and exterminate pathogenic bacteria. It is also utilized by some of our healthy bacteria that aid in digestion and absorption as a food source. When we die, it helps our bodies decompose. However, under certain conditions, it can grow out of control, becoming pathogenic and causing a wide variety of negative effects in the brain and body of the host. You have probably heard of the conditions oral thrush, vaginal yeast infection, diaper rash, jock itch, and athlete's foot. The yeast organism that causes these conditions is the same one we are discussing: candida. When one has an overgrowth of candida, regardless of where in the body it occurs, the illness is referred to as candidiasis.

It is estimated that as much as 80 percent of the American population may have chronic candida overgrowth; most of these people are undiagnosed or misdiagnosed. Since candida overgrowth is largely dismissed by much of the medical society as a legitimate health condition, unless they are dealing with a patient who is severely immunocompromised, people inflicted are often labeled hypochondriacs or mentally ill. Many visit doctor after doctor for decades before getting an accurate diagnosis. Candida is considered by most enlightened physicians to be a major contributing factor to many common diseases, conditions, and syndromes. Prior to 1960 candida was rare, but it's now one of the most common organisms to result in infection at hospitals.

This increase in prevalence seems to parallel the increase in antibiotic use. Dr. William Shaw writes, "Oral antibiotics first appeared in the early 1950s, and the pharmaceutical companies actually included antifungal drugs along with the antibiotics because they knew about this problem. The FDA disallowed the addition, declaring that there was no approval for the prophylactic use of antifungals, thereby washing their hands of the whole business. It is significant to note that if individuals are given the same amount of antibiotics intravenously, their oxalate values do not rise because there is no effect on the GI tract. In some ways, the old medical treatment—a shot of penicillin—was a lot safer."[1] Dr. Warren Levin, in his book *Beyond the Yeast Connection,* writes that antibiotics should never be prescribed without antifungals and probiotics.

ANATOMY OF A FUNGUS

Candida is the name of the genus to which this organism belongs. Throughout the book I primarily use the form candida (unitalicized and in lowercase), which is typical in scientific lingo when referring casually to a genus name. It is the overarching term for all the species of fungi that exist within the genus *Candida*. Although *Candida albicans* is the species we hear the most about and is the primary cause of most fungal infections, there are more than two hundred known species of candida. *Candida albicans* (also referred to as *C. albicans*) is considered to be the one most commonly encountered by humans. However, overgrowth of *C. glabrata, C. tropicalis, C. parapsilosis, C. krusei,* and *C. lusitaniae* is becoming fairly common as well. *C. glabrata* is currently the second most common. *C. guilliermondii, C. dubliniensis, C. inconspicua,* and *C. kefyr* are also emerging more often. *C. inconspicua* may be underreported as it is often confused with *C. krusei*. Within each species, there is a vast array of different strains (genetic variations or subtypes). For example, there are *C. albicans* SC5314 and M61, *C. tropicalis* 1230, *C. parapsilosis* PA/71 and P92, and *C. glabrata* BG14, to name a few. Each species and each strain within a species may exhibit slightly different characteristics and behavior and may respond to treatment differently.

Over the years, we have seen an increase in the non-albicans species of candida, and it is expected that we will continue to see a rise in the incidence of infections from these other, less common species. It is not uncommon for an individual to have overgrowth of more than one species or strain, and species and strains may change over time. Additionally, there are many other types of fungi besides candida that can cause the same sorts of problems and require similar treatment. Aspergillus and geotrichum are two of the most common. Aspergillus is a very common airborne fungus that can enter through the lungs and lead to respiratory disorders.

Candida is a polymorphic or pleomorphic organism, meaning it has the ability to take on different morphologies or forms. It may exist as a single, oval, asexual yeast cell, which reproduces by budding (cell division that creates a new organism). The new organism remains attached to the parent until it is mature, at which time it separates, and then it is known as a blastospore or blastoconidium (plural: blastoconidia). Or it may elongate and form filaments, which are long, root-like, rod-shaped structures called hyphae or pseudohyphae (chains of cells), in which case they are multicellular and may reproduce with spores, through cell division, or by mating (two cells joining together to form a new one). The structure of pseudohyphae and hyphae and the manner in which they carry out cell division differ somewhat, but both the hyphae and pseudohyphae allow candida to travel and spread to other areas of the body and to penetrate deeper into the epithelial layer (innermost lining) of the gut and other tissues or organs. In order to morph into hyphal form, candida needs the right temperature, the presence of glucose, and an alkaline environment. Candida may also take on a cyst-like or chlamydospore form, described as "round refractile spores with a thick cell wall," which can invade tissue as well. Candida may even exist as a cell wall–deficient form. Cell wall–deficient forms are exceptionally small and difficult to identify except in the most advanced research laboratories. It is believed that cell wall–deficient candida may be able to hide inside the host's own bodily cells, which may be another reason why it is so difficult to eradicate.

Candida can change back and forth between forms (an ability known as morphogenesis), depending on its needs at any given time and the conditions it is under, and in response to changes in the environment. It can produce different types of colonies, which enables it to adapt and survive in a wide variety of conditions. Its morphogenetic quality is one of the primary factors contributing to its great virulence (severity of disease it is capable of producing). In yeast form, it appears to be a soft, flat, white colony, and in hyphal form it appears as a gray, rod-like colony. However, texture and color of the colonies may vary somewhat from species to species, ranging anywhere from white to gray to opaque, creamy or yellowish to waxy and smooth, or pale, dried, wrinkly, and muddy.

A mass of spreading hyphae is called mycelia. As the mycelia spread, they develop a biofilm, a sticky matrix that the cells use to conceal themselves from the host's immune system, from antifungal medication, or from anything else that may threaten its existence. Spores (units of asexual reproduction that can grow into a new organism) grow along the hyphae and may become active or lie dormant until a later date. The hyphae are also used to search for and obtain food, particularly glucose, and when they find it they excrete enzymes that digest the material they are attached to. Some species, like *Candida glabrata,* do not produce hyphae, only spores. Members of colonies engage in division of labor, share resistant genes with one another, and support each other for the good of the colony. As candida colonizes, it causes irritation and inflammation to that particular area.

Like all pathogens, candida forms a certain number of persister cells. Persister cells are a variant of a pathogen that are dormant and highly resistant to all antimicrobial agents. When an antimicrobial is administered, they are not affected. Once the concentration level of the antimicrobial begins to drop, the persister cells reestablish the colony. Only about 1 percent of the entire population consists of persister cells. However, that is all that is needed to repopulate if the rest of the population is eliminated.

Candida has an outer cell wall that exists to maintain integrity of the cell and ensure its survival. The cell wall is fundamental to just about all aspects of the pathogenicity and biology of candida. It serves as a permeability barrier, provides the structure for maintaining its shape, and provides it with a surface so it can interact with the environment. Although initially the cell wall was thought to be an inert and rigid structure, it is now understood to be a "complex and dynamic organelle" (a specialized subunit within a cell with a specific function). Since the cell wall dictates the shape of the cell, it is the "structure ultimately responsible for a given morphology."[2] The cell wall consists of polysaccharides (carbohydrates, including sugars) and protein matter, specifically mannans, mannoproteins, beta-glucans, and chitin. Eighty to 90 percent of the cell wall is carbohydrate. The outer cell wall may be comprised of several layers, and the number of layers that are present can vary from strain to strain. Inside the cell wall is a membrane that consists of fat and protein, as well as a mitochondria and a nucleus.

Candida has the ability to suppress or activate the immune response of the host, in this case the human body, and it appears that the constituents of the pathogen's cell wall play a vital role in this action. Mannans and mannoproteins have the most power because they have the ability to manipulate all structures and functions of the immune system, including phagocytes, natural killer cells, cell-mediated immunity, and humoral mechanisms. Mannoproteins have been shown to release histamine and prostaglandin E2 (PGE2), two substances involved in allergic reactions. With regard to the role of chitins in the cell wall: "Complex regulatory mechanisms enable chitin to be positioned at specific sites throughout the cell cycle to maintain the overall strength of the wall and enable rapid, life-saving modifications to be made under cell wall stress conditions."[3] However, like all microbes, candida will also settle into places in the body where the immune system can't reach it very well. Other research suggests that there are other ways that candida can evade the immune system that we have only just begun to understand. For example, candida and other pathogens "are able to develop high oxidative stress tolerance" which makes them "more resistant to killing by immune cells."[4]

Beta-glucan, a type of sugar in the cell wall of candida, can either suppress or stimulate an immune response, which can play a role in a variety of conditions related to inflammation and autoimmunity. For example, a study in Japan found that "fungal metabolites such as beta-glucans have the capacity to induce and exacerbate autoimmune diseases such as RA" (rheumatoid arthritis).[5] Researchers in the Netherlands found that even minute levels of candida can lead to more destructive arthritis.[6] Candida can also produce enzymes, such as phospholipase A, that affect joints and promote inflammation.[7]

In order to colonize, candida must be able to adhere to a host surface. It uses multiple types of mechanisms to adhere to human cells, enabling it to attach to many different sites within the body. Different mechanisms may be used depending on the form it is in and the surface it is adhering to, whether epithelial cells, an implant in the body, or another type of surface. The cell wall generates a large variety of substances, referred to as adhesins, that are used in this process.

Candida is a facultative organism, meaning it produces energy to survive through aerobic respiration if oxygen is present, but it's capable of switching to fermentation or anaerobic respiration if oxygen is not present. In other words, it is both aerobic and anaerobic, giving it the capacity to live in either an oxygen-rich or oxygen-depleted environment, but it prefers aerobic. The ideal temperature for its survival and the one that permits it to morph from a single-celled yeast organism into hyphal form is 98.6 degrees Fahrenheit, which, as you know, is the average temperature of the human body—making us the perfect environment for setting up house. However, it may sustain itself in any temperature between 68 and 100 degrees Fahrenheit.

In most cases, candidiasis develops endogenously (originating within the organism and arising from the normal gut flora), but it may also be transmitted from person to person through sexual contact, giving birth, or organ transplant, or acquired from an outside source such as a catheter or prosthetic device. Infection may be superficial or localized to a specific area such as the feet, scalp, vagina, throat, tongue, lungs, fingernails or toenails, skin, or gastrointestinal tract, or it may be widespread and systemic. When it is localized, it is much easier to treat.

Candida albicans may contain as many as 178 antigens[8] (substances that provoke an immune response primarily via the production of antibodies). It also generates numerous byproducts and toxins that can enter the bloodstream and cause widespread inflammation and many other consequences. Mycotoxins, toxins produced by fungi ("myco-" is from the Greek for fungus), are used by candida as a protective mechanism, to claim territory, support proliferation, and weaken the immune system of the host. Some of the toxins generated by candida include ammonia, acetaldehyde, ethanol, and carbon dioxide, all of which have a detrimental effect on the gastrointestinal tract, immune system, endocrine system, brain, and nervous system.

It is these toxins that are largely responsible for the wide array of symptoms that one experiences with candida overgrowth. When candida breaks through the intestinal lining and travels to other parts of the body it is considered to be systemic, and at this point its toxins, byproducts, and antigens may affect any tissue, organ, or system (e.g., digestive, nervous, cardiovascular, respiratory, reproductive, urinary, endocrine, lymphatic, musculoskeletal). Candida can grow very rapidly, with many species capable of doubling their population in under an hour in the right conditions (e.g., right temperature, pH, serum, food source, hormones). Generally speaking, the higher the degree of overgrowth, the higher the level of toxins, which means the higher the number and severity of symptoms experienced by the host. However, some people can have a high degree of sensitivity to a very small level of overgrowth, so quantity is not always the determining factor for severity.

Ammonia is of particular concern as it is a neurotoxin, which in excess can cause neuroinflammation and produce a wide array of symptoms, including fatigue, abdominal pain, muscle weakness, nausea, diarrhea, restlessness, headaches, irritability, inability to concentrate, confusion, and other brain impairments. High levels of ammonia can cause encephalitis and seizures, and elevated levels are often found in people with Alzheimer's and autism. Additionally, most other microbes—for example, bacteria and parasites—emit ammonia as well. Therefore, if an individual is harboring a variety of organisms, the ammonia level in his or her body can become significantly elevated. Some degree of ammonia is produced by the body in the digestion of protein, but the body is equipped to handle this amount. A healthy liver turns ammonia into urea, which gets excreted in the urine. However, if the liver is not functioning optimally, due to an overload of microbial toxins or for other reasons, it may be unable to convert ammonia to urea efficiently, causing ammonia levels to build up. Additionally, if there is a high rate of microbial overgrowth, the liver may have a difficult time keeping up with all of the ammonia emissions, again allowing for a buildup in ammonia levels.

After ammonia is converted to urea, it must be filtered by the kidneys before being excreted in the urine, so optimal kidney function is essential as well. Furthermore, the Krebs cycle (a metabolic pathway that produces energy) must function properly to rid the body of ammonia. The presence of higher than normal levels of microbes can impair the Krebs cycle, which in turn hinders the ability to detoxify the ammonia that is being released. Finally, high levels of ammonia deplete alpha-ketoglutaric acid, which is needed to detox ammonia out of the central nervous system, producing a detrimental cycle that allows ammonia to continue building up to toxic levels.

There is disagreement in the field over whether candida produces a mycotoxin known as gliotoxin; research has been inconsistent. Gliotoxin is a sulfur-containing mycotoxin produced by some fungi, including aspergillus. It is of particular concern because it suppresses the immune system, kills cells, produces free radicals, and squelches the sulfhydryl (thiol) group of proteins, which are needed to support a wide array of vital enzymes (e.g., alcohol dehydrogenase, creatinine kinase, and transcription factor NF-kB). One study found that gliotoxin inhibits platelet function.[9] Platelets are a component of blood used for blood clotting, wound repair, and other immune activities and has been found to contain a protein called platelet microbicidal protein (PMP) that has demonstrated the ability to kill some species of candida and other microbes.[10] Gliotoxin is believed to contribute significantly to virulence. In a 1991 study candida was found to produce gliotoxin in thirty-two of fifty isolates (isolated species of candida); a 1995 study by the same researchers yielded similar results.[11,12] However, in 2007 it was not found in any of the one hundred isolates studied, including *C. albicans, C. glabrata, C. tropicalis, C. krusei,* and *C. parapsilosis.*[13] I think the logical conclusion we can draw is that some strains of candida produce gliotoxin sometimes, but not always. It's interesting to note that one study found that production of gliotoxin by a yeast (aspergillus) was enhanced by biofilm formation.[14]

Several species of candida have the ability to produce substances known as proteases that can degrade SIgA, including the two subclasses IgA1 and IgA2, thus essentially inactivating SIgA's ability to do its job. SIgA (secretory immunoglobulin) is an antibody produced by B-lymphocytes that plays a critical role in protecting mucous membranes from toxins and pathogenic microbes. It is found in tear glands, salivary glands, mammary glands, the respiratory system, the genitourinary tract, and particularly the gastrointestinal tract. The protease activity can also trigger a polyclonal B-cell response (several different types of antibodies from several B cells launched at an antigen at one time) and inflammation. Candida antigens may also provoke mast cells to release histamine and prostaglandin (PGE2), each of which encourages inflammation. Some antigens, such as hyphal wall protein 1 (HWP1), which is expressed by hyphae and pseudohyphae, are critical to candida's ability to adhere to intestinal epithelial cells and thus colonize and cause disease. Some of the amino acids in HWP1 are very similar to wheat proteins and may contribute to celiac disease.

When the body's immune system launches an attack against candida, candida responds by releasing more toxins. The result is basically an internal war, which generates more inflammation. Furthermore, it appears that the combination of inflammation and the damage done to tissue and cells by candida fosters an environment that promotes more colonization and spreading of the organism, triggering a vicious cycle in which low-level inflammation encourages candida colonization, which promotes more inflammation, which stimulates more colonization, and so on.[15]

Inflammation is the body's normal response to many types of infection, illness, injury, or even stress. If the body is injured or if it senses that it is facing something potentially dangerous, it defends itself by releasing a variety of chemicals that produce pain, redness, heat, and swelling, the telltale signs of the inflammatory process. Inflammation is critical for our survival because it protects us from harm. It's what helps us heal when we cut ourselves or are bit by an insect; it protects us from pathogenic microbes by attacking fungus, viruses, or bacteria that manage to invade. It removes other harmful stimuli like toxins, irritants, or damaged cells. However, it is supposed to be short-lived, because the inflammatory chemicals are toxic to our cells. As David Perlmutter writes, long-term exposure to these substances "leads to reduction of cellular function followed by cellular destruction."[16]

If the inflammatory process gets out of control and we remain in a constant state of inflammation, inflammation spreads to parts of the body that weren't necessarily affected by the initial injury or illness. We are now coming to understand that inflammation plays a role in heart disease, cancer, arthritis, type 2 diabetes, obesity, autoimmune disorders, neurological disorders, and other conditions. Inflammation in the brain may manifest in conditions including depression, anxiety, attention deficit, hyperactivity, addiction, or even Alzheimer's. When candida is chronic, the body is continuously dealing with the inflammation cycle.

Research demonstrates that candida mutates (undergoes a change in genes to create a new form), rendering it resistant against not only antifungal medications but toward other methods of eradication as well, such as an increase in body temperature and oxidative stress. *Candida glabrata,* the second most common form of yeast to result in overgrowth, can mutate at a frightening speed by rearranging chromosomes and making copies of large chromosome pieces. It can also produce a mini-chromosome that enables it to remain alive even at a dose of antifungal that is ten times higher than normal.[17] Additionally, when candida is attacked, it releases spores that may lie dormant (unaffected by the antifungal) until the antifungal or other method of eradication is discontinued, at which time the spores repopulate. Candida will hide when it is under attack, burrowing deep into tissues, where it will wait until the coast is clear and then reemerge.

SYMPTOMS OF CANDIDA: AN OVERVIEW

Candida, its toxins and byproducts, its antigens, and the immune responses it generates may trigger or be an underlying factor in a wide variety of physiological and psychiatric symptoms, including, but not limited to, IBS (irritable bowel syndrome), allergies, skin rashes, asthma, acne, dermatitis, psoriasis, itchy skin, dry skin, hives, eczema, cold sores, overactive bladder and bladder infections (cystitis), bloating, abdominal pain, diarrhea, anal itching, constipation, gas, vaginitis, recurrent UTIs, celiac disease, inflammatory bowel disease (e.g., Crohn's), dehydration, fatigue, ulcerative colitis, infertility, heartburn, weakness, indigestion, acid reflux, bad breath, interstitial cystitis, urethritis, headaches, migraines, muscle and joint pain, dysuria (painful urination), changes in personality and mood, sinus congestion or sinusitis, dizziness, chronic earaches, muscle weakness, inflammation, endometriosis, decreased libido, impotence, prostatitis, insomnia, sleep disorders, recurrent vaginal yeast infections, diaper rash, athlete's foot, jock itch, fungal nail infections, gallbladder problems, hair loss, brain fog, white tongue or oral thrush, chronic pain syndromes, mood swings, sore throat and/or persistent cough that flares when carbs are eaten, addictions, vulvodynia, lethargy, impaired cognitive functions, and arthritis. If you feel sick all over, but doctors can't find anything wrong with you, candida may be to blame. It is almost always an underlying factor in fibromyalgia. Some practitioners believe that candida can injure DNA and provoke abnormal cell mutation in people who are genetically susceptible to cancers.[18]

Candida is a primary underlying cause of leaky gut and food sensitivities. The surface of the gut where candida colonizes becomes inflamed, and an inflamed gut is more porous. Additionally, when candida morphs into hyphal form, it can penetrate the gut wall, increasing inflammation and creating microscopic, Swiss cheese–like holes. This is leaky gut. Dr. William Shaw explains that when yeast is in the hyphal form it imbeds itself in the lining of the gastrointestinal tract like "ivy climbing a brick wall" and "this attachment is facilitated by the secretion of yeast digestive enzymes at the point of attachment."[19] Yeast enzymes—including phospholipase A2, catalase, acid and alkaline phosphatases, coagulase, keratinase, and secretory aspartate protease—literally digest the intestinal lining. Of most importance is the secretory aspartate protease, which can destroy the gut lining and may also digest IgA and IgM antibodies, which are used by the body to defend itself against yeast. Candida also increases levels of zonulin, a substance that controls the tight junctions (spaces that separate epithelial cells in the gut lining).

Zonulin regulates the opening and closing of these spaces so that nutrients and other molecules can get in or out of the intestine. It is zonulin that triggers diarrhea when you have ingested a harmful pathogen, in an attempt to flush it from your body. If too much zonulin is produced, it leads to weaker junctions, whereby the spaces open up too much, known as leaky gut.

The epithelial layer is all that separates the bloodstream from the contents of the small intestine. It allows nutrients into the bloodstream and keeps toxins, bacteria, antigens, and waste out. The tightness of the junctions between the cells takes on some of this responsibility as well. A leaking gut allows undigested food particles, toxins, candida, bacteria, and other pathogens to invade the bloodstream, where they are perceived as foreign invaders. The immune system is prompted to produce antibodies against these unwelcome substances, resulting in food sensitivities and inflammation. In a process called molecular mimicry, the immune system may become confused, producing antibodies that can cross-react with tissues in the thyroid gland, skin, joints, brain, or other areas, leading to more inflammation and the development of autoimmune disorders such as multiple sclerosis, rheumatoid arthritis, Sjogren's, Crohn's, or thyroiditis. Certain individuals who have a genetic vulnerability to autoimmune diseases are especially prone to such conditions.

Epithelial cells in the gut are referred to as enterocytes. In the colon they are called colonoyctes. Enterocytes in the colon absorb water and electrolytes. The surface of the small intestine is lined with small finger-like villi that protrude into the lumen (cavity) of the small intestine and house the enterocytes, which assist with nutrient absorption. In turn, these enterocytes are covered with microscopic, fuzzy, hair-like projections called microvilli, also referred to as brush border cells, which further aid in the absorption of nutrients. In the stomach, food is converted into a liquid substance called chyme. As it moves through the small intestine, chyme is sloshed around and mixed with digestive enzymes; nutrients are absorbed from this mixture with the assistance of the epithelial cells and brush border.

Embedded within the brush border cells are enzymes that are used in the digestion of fats, carbs, and protein, for example, amylase, cellulase, sucrase, peptidase, and maltase. Besides damaging the intestinal lining, candida or bacteria may release their own enzymes, which destroy the mucous coating of the small intestine and the brush border enzymes. A deficiency in both lactase and fructase (enzymes that break down the sugars lactose and fructose) may develop from damage to the brush border. Loss of the brush border also leads to more inflammation, perpetuating the cycle.

When enterocytes and the brush border are damaged, absorption of nutrients is impaired. When absorption is impaired, malnutrition may occur, possibly inhibiting the epithelial cells from healing (nutrients are needed for repair and regeneration of the epithelium) and leading to more damage to the epithelial cells and loss of brush border cells and enzymes.

The epithelial cells and brush border are also a critical part of the immune system as they help form a barrier that keeps pathogens from entering the body. Further, enterocytes manage transportation of antigens and present antigens to the T cells. Just under the mucous lining lies an abundance of T cells, B cells, and antibodies that the immune system uses to protect the body. As a matter of fact, approximately 70 percent of our immune system resides in and around the gut, so damage to the gut can significantly impair your immune function, which we will talk about in more detail in chapter 9. Under normal conditions, new epithelium is produced every three to six days, but if inflammation is present from candida, bacteria, or other sources, such as inflammatory foods, the process is inhibited. Damage to epithelial cells, regardless of whether caused by offending foods, bacteria, or candida overgrowth, results in inflammation that can encourage candida and other pathogenic microbes to overpopulate.

Zonulin also plays an important role in the blood-brain barrier in a manner similar to how it regulates the gut barrier. Typically, the blood-brain barrier allows necessary substances to enter the brain and blocks substances that are unnecessary or harmful. It consists of cells and tight junctions like the gut barrier. It is speculated that substances that affect zonulin also open the blood-brain barrier, allowing harmful substances to cross—for example, bacteria and other microbes, heavy metals, pesticides, and other environmental toxins. In other words, when there is leaky gut, there may be leaky brain. Leaky brain can lead to a wide array of neurological disorders and types of cognitive impairment, including Alzheimer's, dementia, depression, anxiety, bipolar disorder, panic attacks, Parkinson's, multiple sclerosis, schizophrenia, autism, seizures, ADHD, and others.[20]

The brain is one of the organs most affected by candida. Candida toxins can impair neurotransmitter production and function. Neurotransmitters (e.g., dopamine, serotonin, acetylcholine, GABA, glutamate, histamine, norepinephrine, endorphins/enkephalins) are chemicals produced by neurons that regulate processes such as thoughts, actions, behaviors, mood, appetite, and energy levels, as well as cognitive functions, metabolism, pain perception and management, circulation, gut functions, sexual arousal, vision, immune response, motor functions, and sleep. Problems with neurotransmitters may result in anxiety disorders, panic attacks, unexplained fear, depression, irritability, hyperactivity, attention-deficit and learning disorders, inability to cope, memory and concentration problems, obsessive-compulsive disorders, impaired cognitive functioning and problem-solving abilities, autism, Tourette syndrome, depersonalization, severe menopause, cravings for and addiction to sugar and carbs, cravings for and addiction to alcohol or drugs, compulsive overeating, conduct disorders, bipolar disorder, anger-management issues, rage, antisocial behavior, violence, low self-esteem, loss of self-confidence, mania, agoraphobia, schizophrenia, Alzheimer's, and other mental health conditions. Neurotransmitters are also responsible for peace of mind and feelings of overall well-being, serenity, and inner peace, and the ability to feel compassion and empathy, regulate impulsiveness and aggressiveness, and connect with self, others, and one's source of spirituality. When neurotransmitters are out of balance, one's spiritual health suffers greatly and so may their ability to fit into society. In one study, functional MRI testing "indicated that the serotonin system may serve as a biological basis for spiritual experiences . . . the several fold variability in 5-HT1A receptor density may explain why people vary greatly in spiritual zeal."[21]

One way candida overgrowth contributes to neurotransmitter imbalance is by inhibiting serotonin production through a variety of different means. Among other things, serotonin is our natural anti-depressant and appetite suppressant, and it plays a significant role in gut health. Insufficient serotonin levels are largely responsible for the high levels of depression experienced by people with candida and may contribute to cravings for sugar and carbs and compulsive overeating. Serotonin provides us with feelings of connectedness, self-esteem, self-confidence, and overall well-being. It is the precursor to melatonin, the primary sleep hormone. If serotonin is low, so is melatonin, which can lead to sleep disturbances and insomnia.

Most everyone with candida is familiar with brain fog, which results in a feeling of spaciness, inability to concentrate and focus, short attention span, mental fuzziness, and impaired memory. This phenomenon can be blamed on the disruption of neurotransmitters by toxins generated by candida and other microbes. A common complaint in the individual with candida is that when they read, they must read a passage several times, and they may still be unable to retain the material. Brain fog may occur for a variety of other reasons as well, such as low blood sugar due to the consumption of the body's glucose stores by the candida cells, weak adrenal glands, bacterial overgrowth, or food sensitivities.

As mentioned previously, two byproducts of candida are alcohol and acetaldehyde. Alcohol is a fermentation byproduct of candida's consumption of glucose. When an individual with candidiasis ingests an excess of sugar or other carbohydrates, alcohol levels can rise so high in the body that he or she may feel and appear drunk, fail a breathalyzer test, and experience a hangover after the sugar or carbs have left the system. This phenomenon is called auto-brewery syndrome, and it can lead to cravings for alcohol that advance to alcoholism or can perpetuate alcohol addiction in an alcoholic. When recovering alcoholics who unknowingly have candida eat sugar and carbs, their bodies produce alcohol, which commonly leads to relapse. Joan Mathews-Larson reports in her book *Seven Weeks to Sobriety* that at the Health Recovery Center, a treatment center for addiction in Minnesota that was founded by Mathews-Larson, histories indicating probable candida overgrowth are identified in approximately 55 percent of alcohol-addicted women and about 35 percent of alcohol-addicted men. However, since tests for diagnosing candida are poor at best, it is my opinion that the number is probably much higher. Most of the people I work with who have alcohol or drug addiction also have candida overgrowth. It can be difficult to know which came first, candida or alcoholism, but the two are often found together and perpetuate one another. As Joan states in *Seven Weeks to Sobriety,* "alcoholics are particularly susceptible to candida because their high intake of sugar (in the form of alcohol) provides a receptive environment for the growth of these intestinal fungi." Alcohol is a potent sugar that enters the bloodstream through the stomach wall (it doesn't have to be digested like a candy bar). Consumption of alcohol encourages candida overgrowth, which produces its own alcohol, leading to cravings for more alcohol.

Acetaldehyde, also produced abundantly by candida, has the uncanny ability to combine with two key neurotransmitters in the brain, serotonin and dopamine, to form substances called tetrahydroisoquinolines. These closely resemble opiates in structure, function, and potential for addiction, thereby producing an opiate-like high.[22] This process may generate cravings for addictive substances of all kinds, including sugar and carbs, alcohol, or even opiates. It may lead to opioid addiction or, in the case of an individual trying to recover from addiction to sugar/carbs, drugs, or alcohol, it may result in relapse. Since these substances interact with neurons that produce our natural opiates (called endorphins), the eventual result may be endorphin deficiency. Endorphins are critical for modifying emotional and physical pain, and for providing us with feelings of empowerment, self-esteem, self-confidence, joy, ability to relax, and well-being. When endorphins are low, cravings for sugar and carbs or drugs and alcohol often develop in an unconscious attempt to alleviate the symptoms.

Additionally, when acetaldehyde interacts with dopamine, one of the tetrahydroisoquinolines it is converted into is a neurotoxin called salsolinol, which kills off brain cells that contain dopamine, resulting in a deficiency in dopamine.[23] Insufficient levels of dopamine are associated with addictions of all kinds—including addiction to sugar and carbs, drugs, alcohol, gambling, and sex—as well as with attention-deficit disorder, depression, lack of motivation and ambition, an inability to feel pleasure, joy, and connectedness, and many other conditions. Recent research suggests that the killing off of dopamine by candida may be an underlying cause of Parkinson's.

Acetaldehyde also stimulates dopamine receptors (D2), inciting addictive behavior. When D2 receptors are overly stimulated it causes the brain to downregulate responsiveness, which then leads to a drive to find other substances to stimulate the receptors (drugs, alcohol, sugar, carbs, nicotine, caffeine, etc.).

Since serotonin and dopamine are highly involved in the process of addiction to any substance or activity, that means candida promotes addiction of all kinds and puts a person who is in recovery from addiction at high risk of relapse. Psychotropic substances can temporarily increase levels of neurotransmitters, providing relief of the symptoms, but then they lead to even lower levels of neurotransmitters, promoting more cravings for the substance. Candida's impact on dopamine and serotonin may also be one of the most common underlying causes of attention-deficit hyperactivity disorder in children.

Furthermore, acetaldehyde is a neurotoxin (destroys nerves and nerve tissue and impairs transmission between neurons), and it may accumulate in the brain, spinal cord, joints, muscles, liver, and kidneys, where it impairs their normal functions. It also obstructs normal function of the thyroid, pituitary, and adrenals, affecting the hormones produced by those glands. Acetaldehyde inhibits phase 1 detoxification, which can impair our ability to eliminate other toxins. It can change the structure of red blood cells, decreasing their ability to carry out their duties, which results in less oxygen getting to our brains.

It disrupts metabolism of prostaglandins, which are highly involved with immune function and inflammation. Acetaldehyde also decimates critical enzymes and produces deficiencies in various nutrients (e.g., vitamin B1, niacin, acetyl coenzyme A, and pyridoxal-5-phosphate [vitamin B6]) that are critical for neurotransmitter production and function, brain function, mental health, and immune function. Coenzyme A is a factor in numerous enzymatic pathways, such as production of adrenal hormones, sex hormones, cholesterol, hemoglobin, and bile; energy production and metabolism; and production of the neurotransmitter acetylcholine. Insufficient levels can lead to impairment in all these areas.[24]

Acetylcholine is the primary neurotransmitter used by the autonomic nervous system. It regulates functions associated with both the sympathetic nervous system and the parasympathetic nervous system, such as gut function, motility, and stress modulation. It is what makes the brain, nerves, and muscles work. Acetylcholine is also responsible for regulating attention, mood, arousal, memory, sleep, intelligence, movement, and stability. It is what supports the ability to think quickly and have a sharp and clear mind. Insufficient levels of acetylcholine produce brain cloudiness; difficulty assimilating new information, remembering details, staying focused, and falling asleep; fatigue; irritability; and problems with equilibrium. Low levels are associated with dementia, cognitive decline, and Alzheimer's. On the flip side, too much acetylcholine can overstimulate the sympathetic nervous system, producing depression, agitation, anxiety, insomnia, and nervousness.

Acetaldehyde and other candida toxins can also overburden the body's detoxification system, impairing the ability to clear toxins of all kinds (environmental, metabolic, microbial) and allowing them to accumulate in tissues and organs. Acetaldehyde is also present in cigarette smoke and car exhaust and is generated with alcohol consumption. The individual who is overloaded with acetaldehyde from candida often finds her- or himself highly sensitive to these other sources of acetaldehyde. Furthermore, when acetaldehyde accumulates in the liver it overtaxes the liver's ability to clear toxins, especially those that are similar to acetaldehyde, such as formaldehyde. Formaldehyde is found everywhere in our environment—department stores, clothing, cleaning supplies, construction of many products, building materials, carpeting, perfumes and colognes, and other personal-care products. People with candida often develop multiple chemical sensitivities, exhibiting a wide array of neurological and physiological symptoms when exposed to formaldehyde-containing products or other chemicals. These toxins may also impair the methylation cycle, an important chemical process in the body that is critical for detoxification, neurotransmitter production and function, hormone function, mental health, cognitive function, immune function, energy levels, reducing inflammation, and cardiovascular health. Finally, acetaldehyde is produced when we drink alcohol. It is believed to be largely responsible for the symptoms of a hangover (headache, widespread pain, fatigue, etc.).

As mentioned, antigens associated with candida incite the release of histamine. Additionally, in the presence of leaky gut, histamine is released each time a food or other substance breaks through the gut wall and into the bloodstream. That means an individual with candida may have elevated levels of histamine. Although most histamine is generated, stored, and released by mast cells or basophils as part of an immune response against foreign invaders, non-mast cell histamine is found in the brain, where it functions as a stimulatory neurotransmitter. As a neurotransmitter, it helps control or maintain the sleep/wake cycle, mood, learning, appetite, libido, body temperature, memory, pain sensitivity, release of other important neurotransmitters (e.g., dopamine, serotonin, and norepinephrine), and stability in the endocrine system, among other functions. In other parts of the body, histamine is an essential component of gastric acid production, cardiac stimulation, vasodilation, most smooth muscle contraction, and the immune response.

However, excessive levels of histamine create a vast array of negative effects, for example, brain racing, high levels of unexplained fear, excessive sex drive, obsessive-compulsive behaviors, anxiety, hyperactivity, aggressive behavior, sex and gambling addiction, depression, hives, sneezing, runny nose and eyes, itchiness, inflammation, motion sickness, migraine headaches, diarrhea, fatigue, constipation, and abdominal pain and swelling. Because the consumption of sugar, carbs, alcohol, or other mind-altering substances can temporarily offset the symptoms of histamine excess, cravings for these substances frequently develop in candida patients.[25]

The toxins released by candida can create surges in glutamate,[26] which may be responsible for a large number of symptoms associated with candida overgrowth. Glutamate is a neurotransmitter that is critical for stimulating brain cells, allowing us to think, talk, and pay attention, and to process, learn, and store new information. It is also associated with higher levels of intelligence. Glutamate is one of the most abundant neurotransmitters in the brain, but it typically exists in very small concentrations. Too much glutamate is toxic to the brain; it overstimulates brain cells, potentially causing neurological inflammation and cell death and resulting in a wide array of symptoms such as anxiety, agitation, restlessness, confusion, compulsive behaviors, insomnia, and seizures.

An excess of glutamate can be a primary contributing factor to a wide variety of neurological disorders, including autism, ALS, Parkinson's, schizophrenia, migraines, restless leg syndrome, Tourette's, PANDAS, fibromyalgia, multiple sclerosis, Huntington's chorea, and seizures. It is also implicated in atrial fibrillation, insomnia, bedwetting, hyperactivity, OCD, bipolar disorder, anxiety disorders, and panic disorders. It may play a role in stimming: repetitive self-stimulatory behaviors that are commonly seen in autistic children, such as rocking, pacing, body spinning, hand-flapping, lining up or spinning toys, or echolalia (unsolicited repetition of another person's vocalizations). It is associated with an increased risk of stroke, drug and alcohol addiction, and sugar and carb cravings/addiction.

Furthermore, high levels of glutamate increase eosinophils, white blood cells that contribute to inflammation. Many types of microbes thrive in an environment that is high in glutamate. Excess glutamate also depletes levels of glutathione, which is important for controlling inflammation and gut health, and for detoxification. High levels of glutamate increase the toxicity of mercury when it is present in the body, and also cause cancer cells to proliferate, increasing tumor growth and survival.

Elevated levels of glutamate trigger the brain to release high levels of natural opioids (endorphins/enkephalins) in order to protect the brain from damage, which can result in feelings of spaciness and eventually contribute to depletion of the body's natural opioids. It also causes an elevation of acetylcholine, which can lead to more overstimulation of the autonomic nervous system. As mentioned, acetylcholine in excess has a stimulating effect, resulting in high levels of fear, anxiety, restlessness, nervousness, insomnia, and depression.

Furthermore, when glutamate is high, the neurotransmitter GABA is low, because they balance one another. In the gut, GABA (gamma-aminobutyric acid) plays a critical role in bowel contractions; too little can result in abdominal pain, constipation, and slow transit time. A GABA deficiency may also contribute to excess stomach acid, heartburn, or GERD, as GABA is needed to regulate the lower part of the esophagus. GABA also assists with maintaining sufficient levels of IgA, the antibody that protects the gut and other mucous linings from pathogenic invaders like candida.

In the brain, GABA helps regulate mood, sleep, appetite, sexual arousal, and the autonomic nervous system. GABA is what enables us to relax, calm down, unwind, and deal with stress. It's like our natural Xanax. Low levels of GABA play a vital role in alcoholism, addiction to drugs such as benzodiazepines, and cravings for sugar and carbs. These substances temporarily and artificially increase GABA levels, so one is unconsciously drawn to them; however, GABA levels drop even lower after repeated consumption of these substances, so they actually further deplete GABA, perpetuating the problem.

GABA is critical for speech and language; without it, our conversations would consist of lots of run-on sentences, slurred speech, or loss of speech. We would have trouble comprehending language. It generates alpha brain waves and assists with sensory integration.

Insufficient levels of GABA result in nervousness, anxiety and panic disorders, aggressive behavior, decreased eye contact, antisocial behavior, attention deficit, problems with eye focusing (like that seen in autistic children, when both eyes are focused inward toward the nose or waver back and forth in a horizontal or vertical movement), and chronic pain syndromes.

GABA is found in almost every area of the brain, but the hypothalamus contains a great number of GABA receptors, making GABA vital for the gland's many functions: regulating sleep, body temperature, appetite, thirst, sexual arousal and desire, and controlling the action of the pituitary gland, HPA axis, and autonomic nervous system. The primary role of the hypothalamus is to maintain homeostasis throughout the body; without enough GABA production this will not happen.

Like all neurotransmitters, GABA and glutamate play a vital role in regulating the autonomic nervous system and maintaining balance between the sympathetic (stress response system) and parasympathetic nervous systems. The presence of too many excitatory neurotransmitters causes our sympathetic nervous system to take over, rendering us unable to return to the parasympathetic mode. Thus, depletion of GABA can be a major contributing factor to what is known as sympathetic dominance, resulting in disorders such as adrenal fatigue, insomnia, chemical sensitivities, chronic fatigue, and panic attacks. Maintaining sufficient levels of GABA is crucial to recovery from these conditions.[27]

THE STRESS CONNECTION

It's worth devoting a little more discussion to the phenomenon of sympathetic dominance. Candida overgrowth, through the many different mechanisms discussed in this chapter, sets off the body's stress response system, potentially leading to dysfunction in the autonomic nervous system, whereby the sympathetic nervous system becomes dominant.[28] The autonomic nervous system, also known as the involuntary nervous system, manages the bodily functions that occur automatically: breathing, digestion, circulation, heart rate, and blood pressure. It consists of the sympathetic nervous system and the parasympathetic nervous system. The sympathetic nervous system, also known as the stress response system or the "fight or flight" response, is triggered when a person is under stress. It provides the body with an immediate burst of energy to deal with the situation at hand. The parasympathetic nervous system takes over when the stressful event is over, returning the body and mind to a state of relaxation and rest.

When the body is in fight/flight, a cascade of physiological and psychological events takes place in the mind and body. Blood pressure and heart rate go up, digestion is shut down, metabolism and circulation are impaired, blood sugar rises (leading to high levels of insulin), other hormones are disrupted, neurotransmitters are drained, detoxification is impaired, sleep is interrupted, memory and cognition may be impaired, and immune function is weakened. Anxiety and fear increase. Our senses are heightened, particularly the sense of smell. (This may partially explain why individuals with candida have an intensified sensitivity to chemicals, fragrances, or sound.) This chain of events is designed to give us the laser-targeted focus and lightning-fast energy and stamina required to withstand an emergency. We are in a state of high alert—in other words, hypervigilance. Once we return to the parasympathetic state, breathing is slowed, blood pressure and heart rate drop, pupils constrict, circulation is increased, digestion runs smoothly, senses return to normal, the bladder contracts, and energy is conserved.

The stress response system is essential for our survival; however, it was only intended to be used for brief emergencies, not extended periods of time. When we remain in that state for too long it becomes degenerative. Physical and emotional health deteriorate, and we age quickly. All the organs and systems may be affected, and the body may begin to break down in many ways. Symptoms, conditions, diseases, and syndromes begin to develop—for example, multiple chemical sensitivities, chronic fatigue, adrenal fatigue, insomnia, high blood pressure, circulation disorders, gastrointestinal disorders, heart disease, headaches, addiction, panic attacks, ulcers, autoimmune disorders, anxiety disorders, depression, and more. The body prefers to be in the parasympathetic state, which is regenerative and healing.

When all is functioning as it should, the sympathetic nervous system turns on when we are under stress, the stress passes, and we return to the parasympathetic state. However, in the presence of some kind of constant stressor, the body remains in a perpetual state of sympathetic stress, referred to as dysautonomia or sympathetic dominance. In the case of candida overgrowth, the body is unable to return to the parasympathetic state, because the overgrowth is a constant source of stress. A vicious circle ensues, perpetuating the condition, because when the body is in sympathetic stress, the immune system cannot adequately fight candida, the gut is impaired, and glucose levels increase. Increased glucose levels feed candida and cause insulin to spike. Then glucose levels drop, leading to more cravings for sugar and carbs. The result is a negative feedback loop that keeps a person stuck in perpetual sympathetic overdrive. Additionally, the system can become hypersensitive and overreact to lower and lower levels of stressors.

Norepinephrine is responsible for setting off the stress response. It is released in an area of the brain stem called the locus ceruleus, which stimulates the amygdala, which in turn stimulates the hypothalamus. The hypothalamus triggers the pituitary to release the hormone

ACTH, which stimulates the adrenal glands to release cortisol and the adrenal medulla to release epinephrine. Epinephrine triggers the liver to release its stored sugar. Therefore, when stress is elevated due to candida overgrowth or for any other reason, norepinephrine is also elevated. Norepinephrine is another important neurotransmitter that provides us with energy and focus, but in excess it is toxic to the brain. When norepinephrine is elevated, it results in high levels of fear, anxiety, agitation, irritability, hyperactivity, an inability to relax or sleep, and other symptoms. Blood sugar (glucose) is also elevated, which feeds candida and fuels cravings for sugar and carbs.

Additionally, remaining consistently in the sympathetic state places excessive stress on the adrenal glands, two walnut-size glands that sit atop the kidneys. They produce cortisol and other stress hormones. Every time the stress response system is activated, the adrenals are called into action. At first this increases levels of cortisol, but if the state continues for long, eventually cortisol levels become depleted and can no longer meet the demands of stress. The adrenal glands produce more than fifty hormones, the most well known of which are cortisol, DHEA, aldosterone, and adrenalin. Each of these is critical for supporting the body during times of stress. If you lack sufficient levels of these hormones, then you won't cope well with stress, which creates more stress. Over time the adrenals begin to wear down, resulting in adrenal fatigue. Almost everyone with chronic candida develops adrenal fatigue.

Besides producing the main stress hormones, the adrenal glands are involved in many other functions and processes—for example, managing levels of blood sugar, converting protein, fat, and carbs into energy, regulating the immune system and inflammatory process, regulating blood pressure, electrolyte balance, the distribution of stored fat, cardiovascular function, producing sex hormones, and mental alertness. When they are not functioning up to par, a wide variety of symptoms may occur, including profound fatigue and lethargy, mild depression, low blood sugar, inability to lose weight, low blood pressure, inability to cope, nervousness, insomnia or sleep disturbances, impaired cognitive function, and cravings for sugar, carbs, caffeine, or other mind-altering substances. Cravings lead to the consumption of foods and substances that feed candida, perpetuating the cycle. At its worst, adrenal fatigue can lead to a nervous breakdown because the individual simply loses his or her ability to deal with the stress at hand.[29]

Furthermore, when the adrenal glands are weak, the body has a difficult time dealing with the stress that is associated with normal functioning, including energy production, so they downregulate production of energy and other metabolic functions, including thyroid activity, in order to conserve energy and rest.[30] This is one of the primary reasons why chronic fatigue is the predominant symptom when the adrenals are weak and why low thyroid function is so common in people with candida and adrenal problems.

The thyroid is a vital organ located in the front of the neck that is part of the endocrine system. It manufactures hormones that govern most functions in the human body, including metabolism (converting food we eat into energy), body weight, menstrual cycles, cholesterol levels, emotions, memory, skin conditions, heart rate, muscle strength, and more. Too much or too little of these critical hormones can lead to a vast array of psychiatric or medical problems, including weight gain, depression, fatigue, cravings for sugar and carbs, sleep disturbances, and irregular menstrual cycles.

When the thyroid slows down, all other organs and systems decelerate as well. Every cell in the body is dependent on thyroid hormone to activate its mitochondria and thereby produce energy. Thyroid hormone also enhances the ability of catecholamines (dopamine, norepinephrine, and epinephrine) to activate their receptors. If thyroid hormones are elevated, as is the case in hyperthyroidism, then catecholamines may be overactivated; if thyroid hormone levels are low, as is the case in hypothyroidism, catecholamine activity may be decreased.

The adrenal glands are part of the HPA (hypothalamic-pituitary-adrenal) axis. When adrenal function is not up to par, pituitary and hypothalamic action is depressed. Both the pituitary and hypothalamus are needed for thyroid hormone production. Stressed adrenals also inhibit conversion of the thyroid hormone T4 into its active form, T3, and decreases thyroid receptor sensitivity, meaning cells lose their sensitivity to thyroid hormone in a mechanism similar to that which occurs in insulin resistance.[31] Candida toxins can mimic thyroxin (a primary thyroid hormone), another way in which candida can inhibit proper function of the thyroid gland. Further, when liver function gets compromised because of the presence of candida toxins, then it can't convert T4 to T3, contributing to more thyroid dysfunction. Other functions of the pituitary and the hypothalamus may become impaired as well—for example, regulation of body temperature, appetite, thirst, sexual arousal, sleep, hormone production, fertility, and metabolism. When the adrenal glands become impaired for an extended period of time, cortisol and DHEA levels begin to drop. Both cortisol and DHEA are needed to modulate thyroid function.

Dr. Charles Gant explains that a phenomenon called cortisol steal occurs when the body remains in the sympathetic state. All the precursors that the body needs to produce cortisol are also needed to make other hormones (DHEA, aldosterone, progesterone, estrogen, testosterone). Cortisol is absolutely critical for life—we would die without it—so when the demands for cortisol are high, as they are when we are in sympathetic stress, the body will "steal" the precursors to make the necessary cortisol. This leaves nothing to make the other hormones, which leads to hormone imbalances.[32]

If cortisol levels are elevated for an extended period of time, as often occurs in early-stage adrenal fatigue, the liver's ability to eliminate excess estrogens from the blood decreases, which can lead to estrogen dominance. When estrogen is in surplus, it causes an elevation in TBG (thyroid-binding globulin), the group of proteins that attach to thyroid hormone when it is transported throughout the body. Elevation in TBG decreases the amount of free thyroid hormone available for use.[33] Estrogen dominance leads to a wide array of problems, which are discussed throughout the book.

OTHER WIDE-RANGING EFFECTS OF CANDIDA

Oxalates are formed in very high numbers by molds and fungi such as candida and aspergillus. Individuals with candida overgrowth or infection with aspergillus may develop higher levels of oxalates. Oxalates are a type of organic acid that occur naturally in plants, animals, and humans. Under certain circumstances, in the human body, high levels of oxalate can form sharp, razor-like crystals. These crystals can deposit in various places throughout the body, including the bones, kidneys, eyes, muscles, blood vessels, heart, lungs, sinuses, gastrointestinal tract, and brain, causing pain, inflammation, and other symptoms.[34,35]

Excessive oxalates can be a contributing factor in fibromyalgia, arthritis, vulvodynia (vulvar pain), kidney stones, chronic fatigue, depression, bladder pain and painful urination, interstitial cystitis, gastrointestinal distress, hives, Zellweger syndrome (a metabolic disorder that causes mental retardation and metabolic problems), autism and other developmental disorders, and thyroid disorders. In the gastrointestinal tract they can also inhibit absorption of certain nutrients, including calcium, magnesium, and zinc, leading to deficiencies. They may alter pH and antioxidant levels. In the skeleton, oxalate deposits "tend to increase bone resorption and decrease osteoblast" activity,[36] possibly contributing to osteoporosis. (Osteoblasts are cells that help to build bone.) Oxalate deposition may also "crowd out bone marrow cells,"[37] which can lead to anemia and immunosuppression. Deposits in the heart can tear tissue as the heart contracts.

If oxalate deposits form in the eyes, they can cause severe eye pain, which may result in eye-poking behavior, commonly seen in the autistic population. Oxalate crystals can combine with iron, decreasing iron levels that are needed for formation of red blood cells. They can increase oxidative stress, damage surrounding tissue, and interfere with transportation of glutathione. They may attach to heavy metals like mercury and lead, carry them into tissue, and keep them trapped. Once an oxalate attaches to a metal it becomes insoluble, which means it can't leave the body. In the mitochondria, oxalates can impair energy production, resulting in chronic fatigue. There has been a great deal of success in reversing vulvodynia by combining a low-oxalate diet with treatment for candida. (Vulvodynia can also be caused by yeast penetrating the vaginal tissue into the epithelial cells. Since it is embedded in the tissue, a vaginal swab for yeast will test negative.)[38]

Children with autism have a significantly higher level of oxalates in their urine than the general population. A low-oxalate diet has shown great improvement in many associated symptoms, including cognitive skills, motor skills, social interaction, speech, and more. Levels of oxalates in the autistic population are often as high as they are in someone who has hyperoxaluria (a genetic impairment to eliminating oxalates), even though they don't have the genetic disorder. It is believed this is due to candida overgrowth, because treatment with an antifungal will lower the oxalate levels in this population.[39]

Oxalates take on different shapes depending on which mineral they bind with. They most commonly bond with calcium, forming shapes that resemble a star, needles, a wedge, arrows, an envelope, or coral. They may also bind with iron, zinc, magnesium, or cobalt. Cobalt oxalates are shaped like a spear, while zinc oxalates are very thin and sharp discs.

Candida possesses an estrogen-binding protein (EBP) with a high affinity for estradiol and estrone, and a corticosteroid-binding protein with a high affinity for corticosterone and progesterone. When candida binds with any of these hormones, they are rendered unavailable for use by the body. In his book *The Yeast Syndrome,* Dr. Trowbridge states, candida albicans take the steroids (progesterone and corticosterone are its two favorites) into its "own cellular protoplasm" in the same manner in which a woman transports steroids into the cytoplasm of her body cells. "Bidirectional interaction is possible, meaning the yeast can potentially participate in and interfere with human hormone signal systems." Candida also produces a toxin that can mimic estrogen, possibly leading to estrogen dominance.

Corticosteroids are produced by the adrenal glands; therefore this ability of candida to bind with members of this class of hormones is another way in which it contributes to adrenal fatigue. The preferred corticosteroid, corticosterone, is the precursor to aldosterone, an important hormone for regulating sodium and potassium levels, blood pressure, and water retention. Common symptoms of adrenal fatigue are imbalances in sodium and potassium levels and low blood pressure.

Progesterone and estrogen counteract each other's effects; they must maintain a fine balance for optimal health. Each plays a critical role in the health of the brain and body; too much or too little of either leads to great problems. Thus, conditions related to hormones—for example, PCOS (polycystic ovary syndrome), PMS, endometriosis, and menstrual irregularities—occur in high numbers in women with candida. Sufficient levels of progesterone are critical for blood sugar regulation, for the prevention of endometriosis and endometrial cancer, for acting on GABA receptors to help prevent anxiety and increase relaxation, and for the prevention of osteoporosis by stimulating bone-building osteoblasts, among other functions. Too much progesterone is associated with urinary incontinence, depression, breast tenderness, and low sex drive.

Among its many other functions, estrogen plays an important role in managing blood sugar and cholesterol levels, preventing vaginal dryness and atrophy, preventing urinary tract infections, and managing neurotransmitter function to regulate mood and memory. It improves the receptivity of serotonin receptors. If estrogen levels are too low, symptoms of low serotonin result, including depression, increased appetite, and impaired gut function. Too much estrogen is associated with menstrual irregularities, mood swings, anxiety, headaches, digestive disturbances, weight gain, breast tenderness, depression, brain fog, insomnia, endometriosis, fibroids, endometrial cancer, uterine cancer, prostate cancer, inhibition of thyroid function, irritability and rage, breast cancer, and other conditions.

An imbalance in progesterone and estrogen may inhibit the friendly bacteria in the gut, encouraging candida to flourish even more and creating a vicious cycle of more imbalance in hormones. In turn, gut bacteria also influence whether estrogen is broken down and eliminated properly; with insufficient levels of friendly flora resulting from candida overgrowth, estrogen levels may be impacted. Candida toxins can block hormone receptors of all kinds, preventing them from being utilized. Studies have indicated that an excess of either estrogen or progesterone increases the virulence of candida overgrowth, which we will talk about in more detail further ahead.

Candida may lead to a wide array of nutritional deficiencies. For example, most species of candida need biotin (also known as vitamin B7 or vitamin H) for survival, so they steal it from the host's body.[40] Additionally, biotin is produced by the healthy bacteria in the gut, so when healthy bacteria are depleted, biotin levels may drop. A biotin deficiency is very common in people with candida, leading to hair loss, depression, lethargy, numbness and tingling in the extremities, hallucinations, birth defects, brittle fingernails, and a red scaly rash around the nose, eyes, mouth, or genitals. Biotin is also required for metabolism of fat and carbohydrates, supports the adrenal glands, helps manage blood glucose levels, and participates in energy metabolism.

Candida also uses iron, magnesium, and calcium for survival and development of the biofilm, so deficiencies may develop in these nutrients, which are critical for the immune system, brain health, nervous system, bones, oxygen transport, gut health, and much more. Magnesium alone is required for more than three hundred biochemical processes in the body. Thiamine is "stimulatory or essential for some strains." Some strains and species, particularly the C. *krusei* subgroup, need thiamine, B6, or nicotinic acid (B3) either singly or in combination in addition to biotin. Pantothenic acid "stimulates some strains of Candida pseudotropicalis."[41] Candida can also inhibit vitamin B6 from converting into its active form (pyridoxal-5-phosphate).[42] Some species of candida—for example, C. *glabrata*—require niacin and vitamin B6 for their survival, potentially depleting them from the body.[43] Furthermore, candida can bind to B6, making it inaccessible to the body. B6 is critical for neurotransmitter production, the nervous system, adrenal health, metabolism of fats, proteins, and carbohydrates, and methylation, and is required for the production of more than one hundred enzymes. Another byproduct of candida, arabinose, can block biotin, B6, and lipoic acid. This is all in addition to the deficiencies that can be caused by acetaldehyde, which we discussed on pages 26–29.

Because candida eats blood glucose, contributes to hormone imbalances, weakens the adrenals, triggers the stress response system, impairs gluconeogenesis (the conversion of protein or fat into glucose), and causes nutritional deficiencies, it is frequently accompanied by significantly low blood sugar and the vast array of symptoms that may be associated with this issue. These include trembling between meals, ravenous hunger, nervousness, light-headedness, headaches, weakness and fatigue, irritability, and mood swings. Low blood sugar also leads to cravings for sugar and carbs in an effort to quickly restore sugar levels; as discussed, foods that contain sugar and carbohydrate feed candida, perpetuating more issues with low blood sugar.

Candida may also play a pivotal role in obesity or the inability to lose weight, as it impairs metabolism and hormones that are needed to burn fat and inhibits your ability to break down fat tissue. Candida toxins can impair mitochondrial function, the Krebs cycle, and ATP production—all of which are involved in the production of cellular energy—another pathway through which it may contribute to chronic fatigue. Some candida toxins, such as tartaric acid, have an adverse effect on muscles, which may be exhibited as fibromyalgia. On the spiritual level, the symptoms of candida can significantly impede one's ability to experience serenity, inner peace, and well-being, live their life with the meaning, depth, and purpose they desire, and feel connected with self, others, and their spiritual beliefs.

Many people are under the impression that candida occurs in women more often than in men, but the reality is that it is under-reported in men. In my professional work, I see just as many men with candida as I do women. Men are much less likely to be diag-nosed because they ignore their symptoms and frequently don't seek help. Due to socialization they may feel it is unmanly to complain and instead just learn to live with them. The most common ways for candida to manifest in males are through irritability, being argumenta-tive, outbursts of anger, inability to concentrate, cognitive impairment, fatigue, low-grade depression, restlessness, anxiety, forgetfulness, diar-rhea, constipation, headaches, frequent stomachaches, indigestion, heartburn, excessive shyness or feelings of self-consciousness, rashes, jock itch, athlete's foot, and prostatitis. Even if they do go to the doc-tor, they end up with one of these diagnoses, instead of candida.

When they are children, males with candida are frequently diag-nosed with hyperactivity, attention deficit, learning and behavioral disorders, or chronic earaches. Earaches are treated with antibiotics, which perpetuate candida even more. Males with candida are often underachievers and have difficulty excelling in school due to impaired brain function. They may get into fights a lot as a child and as an adult. In *The Missing Diagnosis,* Dr. Orian Truss states, "In men it is expressed more as chronic fatigue and a bad disposition," or as low-grade depression, ill temper, a lack of ambition, acne, or intellectual impairment. Since males don't have the female hormones that promote candida overgrowth at different phases of the monthly cycle, resulting in intermittent changes in personality, males do not experience the extreme emotional fluctuations that women do. "As a result, this con-dition in men is less easily recognized; its constancy gives the impres-sion that this is normal character and personality."

Due to candida's ability to affect such a wide range of organs and systems, it has the potential to be an underlying contributor to just about any symptom or condition. By no means have I covered it all; there are numerous issues that I did not focus on because they have been extensively covered by other authors. My intention in this chapter is to highlight aspects of the condition that I feel do not get enough attention and that have had a significant impact on the people I have worked with over the years.

The level and severity of symptoms and how they manifest can vary widely from individual to individual and even within the same individual on a day-to-day basis, depending on the level of overgrowth that is present and how much damage has been done, whether it is localized or systemic, which organs and systems are being affected at any given time, other conditions that may exist, genetic vulnerabilities, status of the autonomic nervous system, and other unknown factors. Symptoms can range anywhere from mild and annoying to severe and completely incapacitating.

One person may develop an autoimmune condition and have no other symptoms, while another may endure a vast array of gastrointestinal and mental health symptoms. The condition may be expressed as endometriosis in one person, and other unlucky individuals may experience most of the symptoms listed. Symptoms may vacillate from system to system within the same individual, resulting in problems in the gastrointestinal tract any given day or hour, the musculoskeletal or reproductive system another day or hour, and the nervous system at another time—and then back again.

Generally speaking, the higher the level of overgrowth, the more toxins that are emitted, which means the more symptoms that will be experienced. However, one person can have a severe response to a very low level of overgrowth, while another individual may not experience that severity until there is an extremely high level of overgrowth, so biochemical susceptibility plays a role as well.

CHAPTER 2

Causes and Perpetuators
of Candida

Normally, candida lives in or on the human body in symbiosis with all the other microbes that inhabit the area. Overgrowth occurs when something allows candida to proliferate and become more dominant than other microbes. The human body is actually more microbe than it is human, with microbe cells outnumbering human cells ten to one.[1] "The ecological community of commensal, symbiotic, and pathogenic microorganisms that literally share our body space" is referred to as our microbiome.[2] Microbes live on all our mucous surfaces (mouth, nose, throat, lungs, and urogenital tract), on the skin, and in the gastrointestinal tract. The community of microbes that reside in the gut is referred to as the gut microbiome (or gut biome for short). It is estimated that the gut microbiome is made up of more than one thousand species of microbes with more than seven thousand strains; genetically speaking, the human gut biome collectively contains one hundred fifty times more genes than the human genome.[3] Some microbes are considered friendly or healthy, and others are considered bad, unfriendly, or pathogenic. The gut of the average healthy adult contains about one hundred trillion healthy bacteria, with a total weight of between three and five pounds. All these different microbes compete for space and nutrients within the body. Preferably, about 85 percent of the gut biome should consist of healthy bacteria, allowing less space and fewer nutrients for the pathogens so they will die off.[4,5] Some bacteria consume candida and other unfriendly microbes as a food source; they also release small amounts of lactic acid and acetic acid, which keep the gut acidic, preventing proliferation of pathogens and preventing candida from morphing into its hyphal form. All microbes can alter our genetic expression and thereby have significant influence on the human genome.

The friendly microbes live in colonies, form biofilms, and support one another in achieving their goals—just like pathogenic microbes. When all is functioning as it should, the healthy bacteria keep the bad microbes in check, so everything remains in balance and we all live in harmony together. If the healthy bacteria are present in insufficient numbers, they are unable to perform their proper function and candida can grow out of control and take over the domain. Two important friendly microbes are lactobacillus (acidophilus) and bifidobacterium (bifidus). Lactobacillus resides mostly in the small intestine and the vagina, and bifidobacterium dwells mostly in the large intestine. Acidophilus is also present in the lining of the cervix and urethra, where it inhibits the presence of pathogenic microbes.

Friendly microbes provide a variety of other valuable functions for our health. On the skin they break down dying skin cells and debris. In our eyes, mouth, sinuses, and gut they protect us from pathogens that can cause infection. In the gastrointestinal tract they help us digest food and absorb nutrients, metabolize lipids, break down cholesterol, improve peristalsis and bowel transit time, and eliminate toxins and waste. They also help produce digestive enzymes and nutrients like short chain fatty acids, B12, K, and biotin. According to Dr. David Perlmutter, the presence of microbes in your gut microbiome, or lack thereof, has also been shown to affect the integrity of the blood-brain barrier.[6] Approximately 50 percent of our stool consists of bacteria. Additionally, about 70 percent of our immune system resides in and around our gut, and our healthy bacteria play a critical role in immunity, which we will talk about in more detail in chapter 9. When the immune system fails to function optimally, it allows candida and other pathogens to gain the upper hand. So, essentially, the cause of candida overgrowth is an imbalance between the good and bad flora (a condition known as dysbiosis) and/or insufficient immune function. However, the factors that can lead to this state of affairs are many. This chapter outlines some of the main ones.

ANTIBIOTICS AND DIET

Dysbiosis is correlated with many other conditions and disorders besides candida—for example, IBS, anxiety disorders, hyperactivity, autism, depression, attention deficit, autoimmune disorders, colitis, and more. The primary contributing factor to dysbiosis, and thus candida overgrowth, is the widespread use of antibiotics. When you take an antibiotic, not only does it kill the bacterium that is causing the infection, but it also kills all your healthy bacteria, which are needed to keep candida in balance. Because candida is a fungus, antibiotics have no effect on it, so with the healthy bacteria wiped out, candida takes advantage of the situation and flourishes. Antibiotics also make the gut too alkaline, which encourages candida to spread (we will discuss this in more detail on page 51). Although there are certainly times when antibiotics can serve as a life-saving intervention, they are heavily overprescribed. Their overuse is resulting in more pathogenic bacteria becoming antibiotic resistant, which means the antibiotic may have no or little impact on the bad bacteria and instead will obliterate only the healthy ones, which then gives the bad guys the upper hand. The result is more pathogenic bacteria than healthy bacteria. Once healthy bacteria are eliminated and candida takes over, it is very difficult to restore the status quo. Additionally, it is standard practice in the conventional farming industry to administer antibiotics to farm animals either through injections or in their feed. Even if you're not taking antibiotics, if you're eating meat or other products (cheese, milk, yogurt, eggs, etc.) from animals that have been raised conventionally, you're consuming significant levels of antibiotics on a regular basis. In mice studies, infant mice are much more susceptible to candida than older mice. If the mice were exposed to antibiotics at an early age, the incidence of candida in their intestines increased by an average factor of 130.[7]

The second most instrumental factor leading to the development and perpetuation of yeast overgrowth is one's diet. Sugar, as well as any food that readily breaks down into sugar, are candida's primary food sources. Additionally, sugar is used in the formation of candida's cell wall, in the process of morphogenesis, and in the formation of biofilms—all of which enables its colonies to grow and expand and strengthens its ability to attach to the gastrointestinal wall. Therefore, a diet high in sugar and carbohydrates, including complex carbohydrates, feeds and supports candida, enabling it to morph into the more pathogenic hyphal form and develop biofilms. It also damages the gut, feeds other pathogens, promotes and perpetuates sugar and carb addiction, and weakens the immune system, all of which encourage candida to grow and multiply. Finally, a diet high in sugar and carbs is also lacking in many of the nutrients that are needed to support a healthy gastrointestinal tract, production of digestive enzymes, and healthy immune function, leaving the body more susceptible to candida and other microbes. As mentioned in chapter 1, alcoholic beverages are a potent source of sugar that is partially absorbed directly through the wall of the gut; it doesn't have to be digested, so it provides candida with an instant infusion of fuel for growth. Additionally, chlorinated water has a similar impact on the gastrointestinal tract as antibiotics. Chlorine is added to the water supply to kill bacteria, and it does the exact same thing in your gut— kills your friendly bacteria. Most water coming from the tap is chlorinated. We will discuss diet in great detail in chapters 10 and 11.

CHRONIC STRESS

Chronic stress can be a cause, a perpetuator, and a result of candida overgrowth for a variety of reasons. First, our primary stress-coping hormone, cortisol, is increased when we are under stress. When cortisol is high, immune function may be suppressed by as much as 50 percent, because all our bodily resources are redirected to managing the stressful event. Digestion is shut down, leading to insufficient gastric emptying, a decrease in secretion of stomach acid and digestive enzymes (and therefore in the absorption of nutrients), inhibited motility, and interference of vital communication between the gut and the brain via the vagus nerve (the commander of the parasympathetic nervous system). High levels of stress inhibit a transporter in the small intestine called GLUT2, which is needed for transporting glucose, leading to cravings for sugar and carbs when glucose levels decline. Furthermore, high levels of stress directly inhibit or kill the healthy gut flora that are needed for a healthy immune system and to keep candida and other unfriendly flora under control. Stress also increases gut permeability. Cortisol inhibits secretory IgA, the primary immunoglobulin in our mucous secretions (produced by the epithelium in the gut, mouth, etc.)

that protects our gut from pathogens like candida, bacteria, and parasites. Elevated cortisol levels activate tryptophan pyrrolase, a liver enzyme that breaks down the amino acid tryptophan, decreasing the level of tryptophan that is available to manufacture serotonin, which we learned in chapter 1 is vital for controlling appetite, modulating mood, maintaining gut health, and many more functions. If one is exposed to prolonged periods of stress, then gut health, brain health, and immune function decline, leaving the individual susceptible to overgrowth of candida and other pathogenic microbes. Infant mice that are exposed to the hormone cortisone have an eightfold increase of candida in the intestine; similar results have been found in humans.[8]

On the other hand, if chronic stress continues indefinitely, then eventually cortisol levels will decline because the adrenal glands will no longer be able to produce sufficient levels. Insufficient levels of cortisol are associated with chronic pain syndromes, chronic fatigue, asthma, allergies, and more, and result in an overactive immune system and autoimmunity. When our immune system attacks itself, as is the case in autoimmune conditions, high levels of inflammation follow. Cortisol is needed to counteract these effects, but if levels have declined then inflammation will be rampant. Additionally, cortisol plays a critical role in regulating our immune response; it both activates an immune response when necessary and prevents the response from becoming too aggressive. As discussed in chapter 1, the adrenal glands produce cortisol; in the presence of relentless stress, eventually the adrenal glands lose their ability to adequately produce cortisol and other stress hormones. Adrenal fatigue and sympathetic dominance develop, perpetuating the whole cycle.

A great deal of energy is needed to deal with stress, so when we are under stress epinephrine triggers the liver to release glycogen (stored glucose) into the bloodstream, increasing blood glucose levels. High levels of blood sugar encourage candida to proliferate and prompt an insulin response that results in a large decline in blood sugar. This cycle typically results in cravings for sugar and carbs to bring blood sugar levels back up again. At the same time, critical neurotransmitters in the brain that modulate mood, appetite, gut, and brain function will be in short supply, because they are being used to regulate the stress response system. Production of serotonin, which suppresses appetite, prevents depression, regulates gut function, and more, is curbed when cortisol levels are high. As mentioned previously, low levels of the neurotransmitters serotonin, GABA, dopamine, and endorphins often result in cravings for sugar, carbohydrates, caffeine, alcohol, and mind-altering drugs, and a wide variety of mental health symptoms. As you can see, high stress both feeds candida and makes it difficult to refrain from eating foods that will feed candida even more.

Our nutrient supply is used up faster when we are under stress, which can lead to deficiencies in critical nutrients that are needed for maintaining a healthy immune system and gut lining. Nutrient deficiencies also interfere with the creation of the neurotransmitters that are needed to control cravings for sugar and carbs and to reduce symptoms like depression, anxiety, hyperactivity, and attention deficit. Stress also produces higher levels of metabolic waste products, which can tax the detoxification system if it is dealing with a lot of other toxins like those created by candida. And our ability to think things through before acting, control our impulses, and utilize any stress-management skills that we may possess is impaired when we are under stress, which makes us more likely to make bad choices and turn to sugar and other carbs, caffeine, nicotine, drugs, or alcohol for a quick fix to get us through the stressful period.

A subcategory under the topic of stress is childhood abuse and neglect. When a child is trapped in an abusive or neglectful situation, he or she is subject to an extreme form of stress. This is also true for adults, but the developing brain of the child is exceptionally susceptible to the damaging effects of stress. Childhood abuse seriously wounds the limbic system (the area of the brain that controls the stress response system) and completely alters brain chemistry. The stress response system of an abused child becomes "sensitized" and remains on alert even when stress doesn't exist. Initially, the child's cortisol levels will be excessive, but over time they drop, even while the child's system remains in a hypersensitive state. Additionally, children of abuse have lower levels of the critical neurotransmitters dopamine and serotonin, and their GABA receptors are altered in a manner that reduces the function of this important neurotransmitter. All of these effects are carried with the child into adulthood.[9,10,11,12] This scenario makes one susceptible to a wide variety of mental health problems and medical conditions, including alcoholism, drug addiction, sugar and carb addiction, compulsive overeating, depression, anxiety, hyperactivity, attention deficit, adrenal fatigue, weak immune function, and autoimmunity. Childhood abuse is rampant in our society. Many children are unwillingly subjected to this prolonged source of stress, setting them up for a lifetime of health issues such as candida overgrowth. Any type of trauma, in either childhood or adulthood—for example, presence in a war zone, rape, domestic violence, living in poverty, a car accident, witnessing a murder, death of a loved one, or surviving a natural disaster—can have a similar impact.

In particular, studies have demonstrated that severe stress or trauma early in life (like childhood abuse, neglect, or loss of the primary caregiver) makes the individual highly susceptible to developing functional gut disorders like SIBO (small intestinal bacterial overgrowth) or candida overgrowth later in life. Acute, life-threatening events experienced in adulthood—such as those listed above—can also significantly increase vulnerability to functional gastrointestinal disorders. Both childhood and adulthood trauma have the ability to cause permanent and irreversible damage to the stress response system, triggering stress circuits to remain in a hypersensitive state and keeping one stuck in a perpetual state of stress. This state of affairs can lead to functional gut disorders (and mental health issues) later in life[13] and to sympathetic dominance, which we learned in chapter 1 can perpetuate overgrowth of candida. Similarly, even if one hasn't been subjected to trauma in childhood or adulthood, high levels of day-to-day stress or chronic stress can lead to or perpetuate the gut disorder and exacerbate symptoms.

On the other hand, as discussed earlier, when the body has to deal with an ongoing chronic health condition such as infection from candida or some other microbe, this is a form of stress that can lead to depletion of the adrenal glands, sympathetic dominance, and a vicious circle that encourages more overgrowth. That means candida itself contributes to the whole stress cycle: it causes stress, flourishes as a result of that stress, and then produces more stress.

Furthermore, we all live with an exceptional amount of stress each day just dealing with modern-day life. The stress response system is a survival mechanism designed to protect us from threats. In our earlier development as a species, it protected us from predators like wild animals or rival tribes. We would see the threat, and the stress response system would go into action to help us deal with the stress of escaping the situation. We would escape the threat, the sympathetic nervous system would turn off, and the body would return to its pre-stress state called the parasympathetic state. The problem in this day and age is that we are surrounded by "wild animals" (poor diet, pesticides, air pollution, EMFs, emotional stress, microbes, etc.) at every turn and we can't escape them, so we rarely return to the desired parasympathetic state, which leads to deterioration in health and complications as discussed previously.

Dr. Charles Gant teaches that there are at least twelve different types of stress that may contribute to the total stress load that the body must deal with on a daily basis: cognitive stress (e. g., thinking processes, living up to others' expectations, setting unrealistic life goals), sensory stress (e.g., artificial lighting, chronic pain, loud noise), toxic stress (e.g., pesticides, air pollution, perfume, cologne, air fresheners), emotional stress (e.g., financial problems, relationship issues, grief, internal conflict), immune stress (e.g., autoimmune disorders, food sensitivities), oxidative stress (e.g., circulation issues, sleep apnea, impaired detoxification), endocrine and neurotransmitter stress (e.g., neurotransmitter imbalances, adrenal fatigue, thyroid disorders), infectious stress (e.g., candida, bacteria, viruses), purposelessness (e.g., lack of meaning and depth in life, loss of connection with self, others, and spiritual source), energetic stress (e.g., EMFs, geopathic stress), structural stress (e.g., TMJ, cranio-sacral, posture, misalignment of spine), and metabolic stress (e.g., pH, blood sugar, improper exercise).[14]

GUT pH

The topic of pH is very confusing for many people, because a great number of health-care professionals are often focused on encouraging individuals to become more alkaline. Although it is true that our blood and body tissue pH should be alkaline and that acidosis can lead to a wide variety of health conditions such as muscle loss, osteoporosis, high blood pressure, kidney stones, and stroke, that is not the case for the gut and the vagina. Candida and other microbes flourish in an alkaline environment. The pH in most areas of the gastrointestinal tract needs to be acidic. The acid in your gut is your first line of defense against intrusion and proliferation of pathogens. This is one of the primary roles of the acidophilus microbe; it forms acids (e.g., lactic and acetic) that create an environment unfavorable for candida and other bad guys, killing them off.

Different parts of the body have different pH requirements. Body tissue and blood pH should be at about 7.3 or 7.4, which is slightly alkaline. The optimal range for blood and tissue pH is 7.365, but it will fluctuate somewhat throughout the day. (A pH of 7 is neutral.) The stomach, when empty, should range somewhere between 1 and 3, which is highly acidic, while the small intestine should be somewhere between 6 and 6.5, which is slightly acidic. The colon should be between 5.5 to 7, or slightly acidic, and the vagina should range between 3.8 and 4.5, or moderately acidic. However, conditions vary even within these areas. For example, the pH level may be slightly different in the duodenum than it is in the jejunum or ileum, although all these areas are parts of the small intestine.

All species of candida can exist and thrive in a broad span of pH levels, ranging anywhere from 2 to 10.[15] However, research has shown that *Candida albicans* needs an alkaline environment in order to morph into the pathogenic hyphal form that allows it to travel to other areas, invade deeper into tissues, and cause more damage. Hyphal growth is inhibited at a pH of 4 or below.[16] If the pH in the vagina goes above 4.5, then yeast and other pathogens (e.g., bacteria) will flourish. In fact, if candida finds itself in an environment that is too acidic, it will release toxins such as ammonia to alkalize the environment, allowing it to change into hyphal form. It has demonstrated the ability to increase pH from 4 to 7 in less than twelve hours,[17] once again demonstrating its remarkable ability to manipulate its environment in order to survive.

One of the primary factors that renders the gut too alkaline is antibiotics. When healthy bacteria levels are wiped out with antibiotics, they are present in insufficient quantity to keep the gastrointestinal tract acidic, which results in an environment that is too alkaline. So not only do antibiotics directly eliminate the rivals of candida and other unfriendly microbes; they also make the gut a habitat that is more amenable to candida and other pathogens. However, eating a diet that is too alkaline (e.g., that contains too many fruits and vegetables and not enough meat) can contribute as well, which we will talk about in more depth in chapter 10.

Additionally, as we age, our ability to secrete stomach acid (composed of hydrochloric acid, potassium chloride, and sodium chloride) significantly declines, making aging another factor that makes us more susceptible to candida overgrowth and other microbial problems. "In one study, researchers found that over 30 percent of men and women past the age of 60 suffer from atrophic gastritis, a condition marked by little to no acid secretion. Another study found that 40% of women over the age of 80 produce no stomach acid at all."[18] Obviously the use of over-the-counter antacids and other acid-suppressing medications, such as proton pump inhibitors and ulcer medications, plays a significant role in reducing acidity and contributing to candida. So does chlorinated drinking water.

Maintaining healthy levels of gastric hydrochloric acid (chemical symbol HCl) is critical for other reasons as well, because it affects numerous functions downstream. In the stomach, it works with other chemicals (potassium chloride and sodium chloride) to both digest food and to directly kill pathogens like candida, parasites, viruses, and bacteria, preventing them from traveling further into the gastrointestinal tract. The lack of sufficient levels can be a major contributor to candida overgrowth, parasite infection, or SIBO. HCl is important for the assimilation of certain nutrients such as vitamin B12 and protein, so a shortage of HCl may result in a deficiency of B12 or amino acids. Both of these nutrients are critical for the production of the neurotransmitters that regulate our mood, energy, appetite, cognitive functions, and gut health, and of the antibodies that protect us from pathogens. The release of HCl in the stomach also incites the pancreas to release enzymes that are needed for digestion, and the gallbladder to release bile to digest fats. If HCl is in short supply, then these actions will suffer and digestion may become significantly impaired.[19]

PESTICIDES, HEAVY METALS, AND OTHER ENVIRONMENTAL TOXINS

It is believed by many that glyphosate, the active ingredient in Roundup, the world's most popular broad-spectrum herbicide, may be the single most critical factor associated with the development of multiple chronic health conditions and diseases that are prevalent in our society today, including gastrointestinal disorders and diseases, inflammatory bowel disorders, autism, breast cancer and other forms of cancer, Parkinson's, Alzheimer's, depression, anxiety disorders, obesity, cardiovascular disease, infertility, ALS, multiple sclerosis, infertility, allergies,

ADHD, sleep disorders, developmental malformations, as well as violence and antisocial and aggressive behaviors.[20,21]

Approximately one billion pounds of glyphosate are used each year on both conventional and genetically engineered crops. Genetically engineered crops receive the most. If you're eating processed food or CAFO meat (meat from concentrated animal feeding operations, or factory farms), you are ingesting high levels of glyphosate. Roundup is also widely used by homeowners, in state and local parks, on golf courses, outside government buildings, in schoolyards, play grounds, along the shoulders and medians of highways, on athletic fields, and in many other places. You may not realize that you are being exposed to this toxin on a frequent basis. It is extremely persistent in the environment and has been found to last as long as three years.

Pathobiologist Stephen Frantz writes in regard to glyphosate (GLY), "And we now know that it bioaccumulates in lungs, lymph, blood, urine, bone and bone marrow and breast milk too. While Monsanto has consistently denied GLY bioaccumulation, their own studies found it in red cells, thyroid, uterus, colon, testes and ovaries, shoulder muscle, nasal mucosa, heart, lung, small intestine, abdominal muscle and the eyes. An insidious matter with GLY in mammals is that it manifests slowly over time as inflammation damages cellular systems throughout the body."[22]

Groundbreaking research by Drs. Stephanie Seneff and Anthony Samsel reveals that glyphosate disrupts the function and lifecycle of the healthy microbes in the gut, allowing pathogens like candida and other fungi, parasites, and bacteria to take over, creating dysbiosis, leaky gut, food sensitivities, inflammation, neurological disorders, and autoimmunity.[23] Glyphosate inhibits a large group of enzymes called cytochrome P450s that are crucial for the first phase of the body's detoxification system, and it interferes in the transport of serum sulfate, also needed for detoxification and many other vital functions. It may lead to nutritional deficiencies by chelating (binding with) the body's minerals, making them unavailable for use in important bodily processes, and by altering the nutrient content of the crop being treated.

Glyphosate depletes three very important neurotransmitters in the brain, serotonin, dopamine, and endorphins, which, as mentioned previously, help regulate the autonomic nervous system and help modulate mood, appetite, energy, pain, cognitive function, behavior, and thought.

Again, insufficient levels of these neurotransmitters are associated with a very long list of conditions and disorders, including cravings for carbs and sugar, compulsive overeating and other eating disorders, depression, panic and anxiety disorders, aggression and violence, suicide, obesity, Alzheimer's, alcoholism and drug addiction, Parkinson's, autism, ADHD, and insomnia. Stephen Frantz writes that glyphosate "Interferes with synthesis of aromatic amino acids and methionine leading to shortages in critical neurotransmitters and folate."[24] The aromatic amino acids include tyrosine, phenylalanine, and tryptophan. In a glyphosate webinar by Dr. Charles Gant, he explains that we need phenylalanine, tyrosine, and methionine to manufacture our endorphins and that tyrosine is the precursor to dopamine and tryptophan is required for serotonin production. Without sufficient levels of these amino acids, these neurotransmitters cannot be produced. Tyrosine is also needed for thyroid function. He also explains that among other things, methionine is the precursor to SAMe, which is needed for methylating away norepinephrine, which leads to sympathetic dominance when in excess and to synthesize melatonin. It is also the precursor to glutathione, a vital antioxidant and master detoxifier. "Phenylalanine and tyrosine are the precursors used in the phenylpropanoids biosynthesis. Phenylpropanoids are used to produce flavonoids, tannins and lignans, which are important antioxidants." Dr. Gant also warns that the effects of glyphosate affect our beloved pets in the same manner.[25]

It's alarming to note that the suicide rate among farmers in the United States is the highest of any occupation.[26] Farmers in India, who are forced to use glyphosate, commit suicide at a rate of about 1 every 30 minutes.[27] Although the cause of suicide is often blamed on other factors, I would say it is no coincidence that this is a population who is exposed to high levels of pesticides like glyphosate and we should strongly consider the impact this is having on neurotransmitter production and function.

Glyphosate contains an enzyme that breaks down the amino acid phenylalanine, releasing ammonia as a byproduct. As discussed, ammonia creates an alkaline environment that is conducive to microbial overgrowth. It is believed that glyphosate may also disrupt activation of vitamin D, synthesis of bile acid, and homeostasis of cholesterol. It encourages the overgrowth in the human gut of an organism called *Pseudomonas aeruginosa* that releases high levels of formaldehyde and other toxins. Formaldehyde is a neurotoxin and a class A carcinogen. Additionally, it encourages the growth of *C. diff (Clostridium difficile)*, a serious and aggressive bacterial infection that runs rampant in hospitals and is resistant to many antibiotics. Glyphosate kills off friendly bacteria but has no impact on pathogens.

Other studies reveal that glyphosate is lethal to human liver cells, increases oxidative stress, and is a known endocrine disruptor, which can result in a wide variety of diseases ranging from hormone imbalance to infertility to breast cancer and more. It causes cell mutations and DNA damage, both of which are precursors to birth defects and cancer, and has been linked to hairy cell leukemia and non-Hodgkin lymphoma.[28,29,30,31,32] There is a much higher incidence of Parkinson's found in farmers who use herbicides like glyphosate. It is also associated with a wide range of other reproductive effects in humans and other species. Researchers from Canada discovered that fathers in farm families who were exposed to glyphosate are linked to an increase in premature births and miscarriages.[33] Even in very small quantities (parts per trillion), glyphosate has been found to make breast cancer cells proliferate—meaning it stimulates tumor growth.

Dr. Gant's glyphosate webinar also cites Jeffrey Smith, director of the Institute for Responsible Technology and author of *Seeds of Deception*, as stating, "Monsanto's research on rats found that exposure did not cause medical issues, because they published short term exposure data (weeks)." "Because glyphosate accumulates slowly, Monsanto's research (not published) revealed that medical problems ensued later and eventually caused death."[34]

Studies demonstrate that Roundup and similar products are three times more toxic than glyphosate alone because it contains many other surfactants and chemicals to enhance its weed-killing ability, the combination of which increases toxicity. Glyphosate has been found in women's breast milk, in placentas and umbilical cords, in the urine of many Americans, and in the drinking water of many U.S. regions. Even more disturbing is that many of the people in these studies were actively trying to avoid GMOs, indicating that glyphosate is pervasive in our environment.[35] Many people believe they can remove herbicides such as glyphosate from their food by washing it, but that is not true. It is distributed systemically throughout the entire composition of the plant. It is impossible to wash off, because it becomes part of the plant.

Glyphosate is one of a class of compounds called organophos-phates. Be aware that most of the studies mentioned thus far in this section are focused specifically on the synthetic herbicide Roundup, but many other pesticides on the market contain organophosphates that are equally toxic and harmful to your health. For example, naled is an organophosphate that is currently being dispersed across some cities in the U.S. to eradicate Zika-carrying mosquitos. Among other things, naled is associated with birth defects in humans like microcephaly. Its breakdown product (dichlorvos) has been shown to cause degenera-tion of dopaminergic neurons (neurons that produce and transmit the critical neurotransmitter dopamine) and a decrease in dopamine levels. "The degenerative changes were accompanied by a loss of 60–80% of the nigral dopamine neurons and 60–70% reduction in striatal dopamine."[36] According to the *Journal of Pesticide Reform*, "like all organophosphates, naled [Dibrom] is toxic to the nervous system. Symptoms of exposure include headaches, nausea, and diarrhea. In laboratory tests, naled exposure caused increased aggressiveness and a deterioration of memory and learning. Naled's breakdown prod-uct dichlorvos (another organophosphate insecticide) interferes with prenatal brain development. In laboratory animals, exposure for just 3 days during pregnancy when the brain is growing quickly reduced brain size 15 percent. Dichlorvos also causes cancer, according to the International Agency for Research on Carcinogens. In laboratory tests, it caused leukemia and pancreatic cancer. Two independent studies have shown that children exposed to household 'no-pest' strips con-taining dichlorvos have a higher incidence of brain cancer than unex-posed children."[37,38] Naled is banned in Europe, and even Puerto Rico refuses to use it. Other examples of organophosphates include insecti-cides (malathion, parathion, diazinon, fenthion, dichlorvos, chlorpyri-fos, ethion), nerve gases (soman, sarin, tabun, VX), ophthalmic agents (echothiophate, isoflurophate), and antihelmintics (trichlorfon). Her-bicides (tribufos [DEF], merphos) are tricresyl phosphate-containing industrial chemicals.[39]

Organophosphates are transported directly into the nervous sys-tem (the brain, spinal cord, and long nerves), where they are con-verted into a metabolite called chlorpyrifos-oxon, which is three thousand times more potent than the original substance.[40] Organo-phosphates inhibit the conversion of tryptophan into serotonin, which as discussed, is critical for regulating mood, appetite, the autonomic nervous system, and gut function. Organophosphates also block the action of an enzyme called acetylcholinesterase, which is needed to break down the neurotransmitter acetylcholine, allowing acetylcholine to build up. This creates a "jam in the transmission system."[41] As mentioned in chapter 1, one of the primary roles of acetylcholine is to regulate the autonomic nervous system. When acetylcholine is in excess, it produces symptoms like high anxiety, panic attacks, fear, depression, restlessness, insomnia, and possibly seizures and loss of consciousness. It keeps one stuck in a hyper-aroused state that puts great stress on the adrenal glands and perpetuates sympathetic nervous system dominance.

A study from the University of California found that the children born from pregnant women who had organophosphates applied nearby their home during pregnancy had a 60 percent increased risk for autism spectrum disorder.[42] Organophosphates in general have been shown to affect the gut biome in a variety of ways. For example, "chlorpyrifos exposure during development affects the gut microbiota, impairs the intestinal lining, and stimulates the immune system of pup rats. Another study also shows that chlorpyrifos affects gut microbiota, resulting in intestinal inflammation and abnormal intestinal permeability." They also increase blood glucose levels and may contribute to insulin resistance and type 2 diabetes.[43]

Organophosphates are endocrine disruptors, which means they can attach to hormone-receptor sites and impair normal functioning of the endocrine system (hypothalamus, pituitary, thyroid, parathyroid, adrenals, pineal, pancreas, and reproductive organs). They may either mimic hormones like estrogen or disrupt the way they are produced or function in the body. This can contribute to a wide array of problems, including microbial overgrowth, cravings for sugar and carbs, blood sugar issues, thyroid disorders, inability to handle stress, infertility, unwanted weight gain and obesity, insomnia, low libido, erectile dysfunction, hyperactivity, endometriosis, addiction, low sperm count, depression, anxiety, hormone imbalances, and adrenal fatigue. Organophosphorous compounds are so toxic they have been used by governments throughout the word as chemical weapons. Some research suggests that approximately one third of the population may be deficient in paraoxonase, an enzyme that is needed to detoxify organophosphates. These people would be much more susceptible to herbicide poisoning and other negative effects from these types of chemicals.[44]

Pyrethroids, or permethrin, are another big problem. They are used widely in mosquito abatement and are also found in pesticides for fleas, lice, ticks, mites like scabies, ants, fleas, flies, and termites and are widely used in agriculture on cotton, wheat, corn, etc. Pyrethroids are one of the most common pesticides to be used in households. Studies on rats have found that low-dose exposure early in life to permethrin can "affect the fecal microbiota and could be a crucial factor contributing to the development of diseases."[45] In humans, permethrin has been shown to impair glucose homeostasis.[46] All of which creates an environment in the gut and body that would invite overgrowth of candida and other pathogens and contribute to cravings for sugar and carbs. Even the EPA, who is extremely reluctant to acknowledge toxicity of any chemical, says they are "likely" carcinogenic and high levels can affect the nervous system. In rats they cause hyperactivity, tremors, salivation, hyperexcitability, urination, defecation and incoordination, and liver damage. Baby rats are much more susceptible than adult rats and exhibit more severe symptoms. Other animals exposed may experience numbness of the lip and tongue, diarrhea, nausea, convulsions, aggression, seizures, paralysis, respiratory failure, and death. They also kill indiscriminately, meaning in addition to the bug you're trying to get rid of, it also kills a variety of beneficial insects, including bees, aquatic life, and small mammals like mice. It is highly toxic to cats, honey bees, and other beneficial insects and is considered mildly toxic to birds like mallards.

Common reactions in the human population include itching, burning and prickling sensations of the skin, headaches, convulsions, tremors, facial flushing, asthma, sneezing, nasal congestion, and nausea. Permethrin has been linked to a variety of serious health conditions like autism, Parkinson's, birth defects, depression, breast cancer, thyroid damage and disease, liver disease, kidney problems, learning disabilities, and damage to the immune, endocrine, and nervous systems.[47,48,49,50,51,52,53] A study in the *Archives of Neurology* found that "if you used the insecticide permethrin, you were three times more likely to develop" Parkinson's.[54] Permethrins kill their victim by modifying the normal biochemistry and physiology of the membrane sodium channels and altering the nerve function. In other words it paralyzes the nervous system.

Now, if all this isn't bad enough, here's the real kicker in regard to the usage of permethrin. Permethrins are only effective at knocking down and paralyzing its intended victim; it doesn't kill them. So another chemical is added with permethrins to give it more killing power called piperonyl butoxide. Piperonyl butoxide is a suspected carcinogen and believed to be highly toxic to the liver, kidneys, gastrointestinal, reproductive, and nervous systems. It is suspected of being connected to symptoms and conditions such as coma, convulsions, renal damage, hyperexcitability, prenatal damage, vomiting, weight loss, anorexia, and many more. It, too, is toxic to birds, fish, and other aquatic life.[55] Piperonyl butoxide works by inhibiting the detoxification pathways of its victim, which means the pesticide is then permitted to remain in its victim for a longer period of time, so that permethrins can kill it. In humans, this detox pathway is in the liver; this means this chemical targets the liver. So these two chemicals together knock down the intended victim by attacking its nervous system and then render it unable to detox the chemical out of its body by inhibiting its detox pathways.

Make no mistake, folks, this is exactly what these chemicals do to the human body as well—attacks the nervous system and inhibits detox pathways—but on a less noticeable scale for most. It's enough to kill the bugs, but only enough to result in a disrupted nervous system and impaired liver function in the human, which results in chronic health conditions. I can tell you this is true from personal experience. When I am exposed to pesticides, my body responds by having respiratory difficulty, severe tremors that border on convulsions, depression, numbness in lips and tongue, diarrhea, inability to think clearly, and thyroid dysfunction. I once had to move, throw away half of my belongings, and could hardly sleep at all for a year, because my neighbors sprayed herbicide to their fence post and it got in my house. I never fully recovered from the damage that was done. There are large numbers of people who respond the same way, but this information is not widely known, because the chemical companies don't want the public to know and government agencies and conventional medical doctors will deny it happens.

Even the botanical form of permethrins, which is often sold in health food stores as an alternative pesticide, called pyrethrum or pyrethrins is also a neurotoxin. In its natural organic form, it is a plant in the chrysanthemum family and the pesticide is made from the dried flower head. Although it is certainly a safer choice than most because it breaks down faster than the synthetic form, it too is harmful to birds, fish, and other mammals including humans. It too paralyzes the nervous system of the victim in the same way and is also linked to health conditions like autism, tremors, etc. Just because something is natural doesn't mean it won't hurt you. There are many things in nature that are intrinsically poisonous. I once sprinkled this stuff around my house and had similar symptoms to those I experienced from the synthetic type.

Many of the same problems occur with the use of any other type of pesticide under any other name. Pesticides of all kinds are neurotoxins that can disrupt the endocrine system, compromise neurotransmitter production and function, stimulate the stress response system, and impair gut function and immunity.

At the University of California at Berkeley, a study found that a pesticide called maneb increases your risk of developing Parkinson's by 75 percent. Additionally, when more than 90,000 licensed pesticide applicators and their spouses were followed closely, the risk of developing Parkinson's was found to be 2.5 times higher in people who used rotenone or paraquat, and a study in the *Archives of Neurology* found that you're twice as likely to develop Parkinson's if you use pesticides.[56] This should be of grave concern considering that Parkinson's is a disorder of the central nervous system, thus demonstrating the profound effect pesticides can have on the brain. "The World Health Organization estimates that at least three million people are poisoned by pesticides every year and 20–40,000 more are killed" and "over 1 million Americans will learn they have some form of cancer and 10,400 people in the U.S. die each year from cancer related to pesticides."[57]

It's important to remember that your public health and safety organizations and conventional medical practitioners are taking their information from the EPA, FDA, and the manufacturers of the chemicals. You are not getting the truth. The goal of chemical manufacturers is to keep their chemicals on the market so they make money, not to protect the consumer, and unfortunately the EPA and FDA are in their pocket. The government agencies hold out on listing the toxicity of a product until their hand is forced; they are often only concerned with whether a chemical causes cancer, when cancer is only one possible effect of toxicity. Many chemicals are not carcinogenic; however, they harm the brain, gut, nervous, endocrine, and immune systems and damage internal organs, which is just as serious. Additionally, they fail to take into account the issue of accumulation. When you consider the fact that the human body is exposed to an onslaught of chemicals every day, the combination of all them together creates even more toxicity. Pesticide sales generate trillions of dollars in our world and the truth about their toxicity would be detrimental to our economy, so it is covered up. It does not take a rocket scientist to put one and one together and see the dangers that exist. Pesticides are the new tobacco, but even worse. With tobacco, the government wasn't actively blowing smoke in your face, but our government participates widely in exposing us to pesticides. The repercussions of pesticide use are being downplayed, ignored, or intentionally concealed by the manufacturers and our own government agencies. We are only beginning to understand and reveal their full effects on human health and it may be too late by the time the masses become willing to recognize the extent of these ramifications.

The consequences of widespread pesticide use have a profound effect on not only each individual's health but on humanity as a whole. The areas of the brain affected by pesticides are the regions that allow us to feel compassion, patience, and empathy for one another, to control our impulses, to manage anger, irritability, and rage, which leads to acts of aggression, violence, and other antisocial behavior. Neuroscientist Dr. Bruce Perry tells us that "all" human behavior is mediated by the brain and the brain's ability to mediate impulse control is related to a ratio between the lower, more primitive areas of the brain, which are excitatory, and the higher sub-cortical and cortical areas of the brain, which are inhibitory. Any element that increases activity in the more primitive areas of the brain or decreases the higher, more modulating areas of the brain will "increase an individual's aggressivity, impulsivity, and capacity to display violence."[58] Combine pesticide exposure with the fact that most of the population is eating a nutrient deficient diet (which also impairs the brain in a similar way and can contribute to violence and anti-social behavior) and we have a recipe for social disaster looming overhead, which we can already see beginning to play out in our communities with a new act of violence being perpetrated nearly weekly and sometimes daily.

It is believed that toxic metals, especially mercury, promote candida overgrowth. Exposure to low-level mercury weakens the immune system, kills friendly flora in the gut, and directly inhibits the output of hormones produced by the adrenal glands. In addition, candida has demonstrated the ability to convert inorganic mercury into methyl mercury, which is much more toxic to humans. On the other hand, some studies have demonstrated that mercury can actually have an inhibitory effect on candida growth and morphogenesis.[59] Still, metal toxicity can inhibit and disrupt the production and function of the neurotransmitters that play a key role in appetite, mood, gut health, and managing stress. This can lead to a wide variety of psychological symptoms such as anxiety, depression, and insomnia, and can increase cravings for sugar, carbs, and alcohol, making it difficult to remain committed to your diet. Mercury and other toxic metals are commonly found in silver-metal fillings in the mouth, vaccines, seafood, broken thermometers, batteries, pesticides, acid rain, talc powder, CFL light bulbs, tattoo ink, cigarette smoke, refinery emissions, air pollution, the water supply, and other sources.

Besides pesticides and metals, toxins of all kinds are found in everyday products such as cosmetics, dish soap, laundry detergent, air fresheners, perfume, cologne, body soap, shampoo, household cleaning supplies, furniture, carpeting, treated drinking water, and plastic. These, too, can set off the stress response system and thus contribute to high blood sugar, insulin spikes, low blood sugar, and depletion of neurotransmitters. Additionally, they all have the potential to land on receptors for hormones or neurotransmitters, thereby disrupting normal production and/or function, and to weaken immunity or cause autoimmunity.[60] Many toxins in our environment today are estrogenic (e.g., certain pesticides, pthalates, BPA, and more), meaning they are causing abnormally high levels of estrogen in both men and women, which can then provide fuel for candida overgrowth. It is believed that estrogenic compounds are leading to a feminization of males in our society, resulting in testosterone deficiencies, erectile dysfunction, lower sperm counts, infertility, prostate problems, development of breasts, and other female characteristics.

We are all exposed to unprecedented levels of toxins on a daily basis, potentially overburdening our bodies' detoxification system and allowing toxins to accumulate in our tissues. Candida and other microbes can flourish in a body that is overloaded with toxins, and cravings for sugar, carbs, and alcohol can intensify, encouraging overgrowth. When toxins get embedded in the gastrointestinal tract, they can damage the gut lining and impair absorption of vital nutrients. At the same time, a high toxin load creates a much greater need for nutrients to remove the toxins from the system—another vicious cycle potentially leading to nutritional deficiencies. If the greatest share of nutrients is being utilized to remove toxins, there aren't many left over for other important functions (e.g., maintaining the immune system, regulating gut health, and making neurotransmitters). The higher a person's exposure to toxins, the more nutrients that are needed, and the greater the stress on the body.

Toxins can decrease the activity of important participants in the immune system such as macrophages, neutrophils, and natural killer cells. They may also poison bone marrow, where these cells (or their precursors) are produced, prompt an immune response and inhibit the communication system within the immune system.

Additionally, the elimination of toxins from the body generates high levels of oxidative stress. The higher the level of toxins in your body, the greater the oxidative stress. Increased oxidative stress boosts inflammation, and, as we learned previously, inflammation promotes overgrowth of candida and other microbes. Toxins also have the ability to alter gene expression, set off an autoimmune response, and inhibit BDNF (brain-derived neurotrophic factor), a substance used in the creation of new neurons and the protection of existing neurons. Low levels of BDNF are linked to an increase in appetite as well as a wide array of neurological conditions such as anxiety, depression, and Alzheimer's.

Exposure to environmental toxins of all kinds sets off the stress response system. Dr. Charles Gant explains that toxins of all kinds are able to cross the blood-brain barrier. In the brain stem we have sensors that identify foreign chemicals in the body. When a toxin is detected by a sensor it performs two functions. One, it sets off the fight/flight system, warning us that there is a threat to our existence; and two, it activates our detoxification system. So the fight or flight system warns us, "Hey, there's a threat to our being here and we need to take action," and the detoxification system is called in like the cavalry to eliminate the threat.[61]

As discussed, activation of the stress response system increases the amount of sugar in the bloodstream as a result of the liver's release of glycogen. Elevated blood sugar both feeds candida and triggers the release of insulin. Insulin causes blood sugar levels to drop, leading to cravings for carbs and sugar and activating the entire cascade of stress-related effects on the gut, immune system, neurotransmitters, etc. For this reason, frequent exposure to toxins encourages sympathetic dominance and perpetuates the whole cycle. Additionally, a high level of environmental toxins in the body may interfere in the ability of nutritional supplements to perform their job. Your body may be unable to absorb or utilize the nutrients they contain.

HORMONAL IMBALANCES

As discussed in the previous chapter, candida can bind to and mimic hormones, and interfere in their signals, leading to numerous hormonal problems. However, hormones can also be a cause of candida overgrowth. Candida can thrive in the presence of progesterone because of the hormone's vital role in regulating blood sugar (glucose). It helps move sugar into the bloodstream. When progesterone levels in a woman's body increase, so do glucose levels. The increase in progesterone levels that occurs during the week before menstruation and subsequent rise in glucose feeds the yeast, leading to cravings for sugar and carbs and to a wide variety of symptoms like irritability, anxiety, headaches, depression, and moods swings—often referred to as premenstrual syndrome, or PMS. Additionally, high levels of progesterone have been shown to decrease insulin sensitivity, which would also contribute to cravings for more of the sugar and carbs that feed candida.[62]

Other studies have demonstrated that estrogen appears to stimulate candida overgrowth, and "estradiol directly stimulates the dimorphic transition from yeast to the hyphal form and because the latter form is associated with tissue invasion, this hormonal action may increase fungal virulence."[63,64] Estrogen is another hormone that's important for managing blood glucose because it helps increase insulin sensitivity, thereby enabling cells to utilize glucose more efficiently. However, too much estrogen can increase glucose levels in the vagina, potentially feeding candida. It has been shown that excess estrogen decreases the ability of epithelial cells in the vagina to inhibit growth of *Candida albicans*.[65] Still, estrogen is vital for maintaining a vaginal pH level that is acidic, a necessity to prevent microbial overgrowth. As you can see, there is a delicate balance needed for both progesterone and estrogen. An excess of either one can contribute to yeast overgrowth.

Progesterone and estrogen levels increase at different times during pregnancy. Additionally, changes in vaginal pH that take place during pregnancy may contribute to vaginal yeast infections. The birth control pill and hormone replacement medications (including bioidentical hormones) are all substances that may increase estrogen or progesterone. Progesterone stimulates estrogen receptors in addition to progesterone, so when supplementing with bioidentical progesterone, if one is not taking a high enough dose of progesterone to offset this, it can contribute to estrogen dominance.[66] In summary, pregnancy, the birth control pill, and hormone replacement (including bioidentical) all make one more susceptible to hormonal imbalances that can lead to candida overgrowth.

Candida may also be passed from mother to child during childbirth and breast-feeding, and from one partner to another during sexual activity. When it is acquired through childbirth, the child often has chronic problems with ear infections, stomachaches and other gastrointestinal problems, headaches, sleep disturbances, attention deficit, hyperactivity and behavior disorders, or autism. The infant and mother can pass candida back and forth to one another through breast-feeding, as candida can colonize the tissue in nipples and breasts, resulting in cracked nipples and painful breast-feeding and pain in the breasts even when not feeding. The infant may begin to exhibit resistance or fussiness around feeding, which may result in abandonment of breast-feeding since the mother doesn't understand the cause.

OTHER CONTRIBUTING FACTORS

Other factors that may contribute to and/or perpetuate candida overgrowth include nicotine, steroids, NSAIDs, and immune-suppressing drugs. Immune-suppressing drugs temporarily inhibit immune function, possibly allowing candida to flourish. Steroid drugs suppress the immune system and also increase blood glucose levels, simultaneously allowing candida to have free rein and feeding it at the same time. Additionally, as we established earlier, candida has a high affinity for binding with steroids. Nonsteroidal anti-inflammatory drugs (NSAIDs) damage the lining of the stomach and the small intestine. Smoking (nicotine) increases proliferation, morphogenesis, and adherence of candida, causes nutritional deficiencies, introduces acetaldehyde and heavy metals into the body, and increases blood glucose, all of which impair brain function, weaken the immune system, and provide sugar for candida to feed on. Furthermore, nicotine is a mind-altering drug that disrupts neurotransmitters in the brain, again leading to cravings for sugar and carbs. We will talk about smoking and nicotine in more detail on pages 419–423.

The presence in the gut of some other type of microbe, like bacteria or parasites, can damage the epithelial cells and brush border, causing inflammation and creating an environment that is ripe for candida to multiply. Furthermore, both bacteria and parasites can harbor candida. We talk about parasites and bacteria in more detail in chapter 5. Additionally, the consumption of foods that cause inflammation and degrade the integrity of the gut, like grains, legumes, chocolate, and caffeine, can contribute to overgrowth as well, all of which are discussed in more detail in chapters 9 and 10. Damage to the gut lining from any source—be it candida, bacteria, grains, legumes, pharmaceuticals, etc.—can trigger inflammation and perpetuate candida overgrowth.

According to candida expert Dr. Michael Biamonte, current research suggests there are several genetic polymorphisms that may make one more prone to candida overgrowth, but especially the MMP-1 gene when it is inherited from both parents. Defects in the MMP-1 gene produce weak collagen in the gastrointestinal tract. The weaker collagen is less responsive to the intestinal immune system, thus making it more difficult for healthy bacteria that suppress candida to colonize. Mutations in the GPX1 and EPHX genes, which affect detoxification, can indirectly promote candida overgrowth by impeding elimination of the toxins that kill healthy gut bacteria.[67]

Additional risk factors for candida overgrowth that we will not discuss in detail include AIDS, cancer, diabetes, leukemia, neutropenia, hypoparathyroidism, Addison's, severe burns, surgery, prosthetic devices (including dental implants), chemotherapy, radiation, and IV drug use. When candida occurs in the severely immunocompromised, it can be quite serious and even life threatening. The immunocompromised are more vulnerable to Candidemia (candida infection in the blood), which has a very high mortality rate.

CHAPTER 3

The Biofilm: Candida's Secret Weapon

One of the most fascinating but alarming aspects of candida and other microbes is their ingenious survival mechanism known as the biofilm. A biofilm is a complex, dynamic, three-dimensional structure that microorganisms build on the surfaces they colonize; it provides them with a protective shield against the host's immune system, against antimicrobials (including antifungals), or against anything else that endangers them. With the help of a biofilm, instead of existing as single-celled yeast organisms, candida cells join together as a large population to form a highly sophisticated ecosystem that enables them to evade detection and eradication. We've come to understand in recent years that one of the primary reasons that it is so difficult to eradicate yeast overgrowth is due to their formation of biofilms.

BIOFILM BASICS

When free-floating plankton (e.g., yeast cells or bacteria) come in contact with a surface and attach to it, the cells divide and proliferate, eventually producing a sticky, slimy, glue-like substance that enables them to form a structure (referred to as the extracellular matrix) that promotes their continued growth and expansion. A biofilm community can develop within hours.

Biofilms can be found within industrial settings, which is where we have learned much of what we know about them, as they are easier to study there. Biofilms are a composite of liquid and solid, but in an industrial setting they can turn more solid and brittle as they gather sediment, rust, or calcium deposits. In the United States, billions of dollars are lost each year to damaged equipment, contamination of products, and medical infections caused by biofilm formation. Conversely, biofilms can be useful in certain situations, like hazardous waste sites, treating wastewater, and preventing the contamination of soil and groundwater. Water that is utilized for drinking is more stable biologically and has less need for disinfection if it has been exposed to microbes before treatment. In nature, biofilms are a food source for other organisms. So, as with all living things, biofilms fulfill a purpose in the ecosystem.

Biofilms may develop on any surface that provides the organism with the right combination of moisture and nutrients, including metal, plastic, natural materials, and bodily tissue. You may be unaware that you encounter biofilms on a daily basis. They may form in your sink, on your countertop, or in your toilet. The slimy gunk that clogs up your drain or that you see growing on rocks in a stream is an example of a biofilm. On the human body they may form externally or internally, in locations that include the gastrointestinal tract, mouth, genitals, feet, throat, teeth, blood, sinuses, adenoids, urinary tract, or medical implants. The plaque that forms in your mouth is a biofilm.

Most of the research on biofilms within the human body has been conducted on implanted medical devices such as prosthetic heart valves, artificial hip joints, intravenous catheters, and the like. Researchers extrapolate from those situations to draw conclusions about the behaviors of biofilms in other circumstances. If you have any medical implants, be aware that biofilm formation on and around these devices is rather common and can lead to serious complications. This applies to breast implants, hip replacements, teeth implants, pacemakers, IUDs, contact lenses, shunts, stents, endotracheal tubes, artificial joints, metal bars, or anything foreign that is placed in the body. Biofilm formation can become an ongoing source of infection and may cause the device to malfunction, necessitating its removal.[1]

A fully developed candida biofilm is a spaciously distributed and complex three-dimensional structure that is intentionally crafted to optimize the yeast organism's ability to acquire nutrients, eliminate waste products, and establish microniches throughout the matrix. The matrix, which may range in thickness from 25 to more than 450 micrometers, shelters a dense web of yeasts, hyphae, and pseudohyphae. In an industrial setting (e.g., a water-distribution plant) a biofilm can become so thick that it obstructs water flow. We can assume the same could happen in the gastrointestinal tract or other areas of the body.

Although it is possible that the population within a biofilm may be comprised of only one species, such as *Candida albicans,* a biofilm most frequently contains a variety of different species—not only of candida but of different types of microbes as well, including other fungi, protozoa, parasites, viruses, and bacteria. These opportunists will take refuge in the matrix. Literally hundreds of distinct and assorted microbes have been found to coexist together within a biofilm. A biofilm may house *Candida albicans, Candida parapsilosis, Candida tropicalis,* and many different strains of each of those species. It may contain *geotrichum* (another genus of fungi) as well as protozoa, nematodes, and bacteria such as klebsiella, clostridia, or others. Over five hundred species of bacteria have been identified as existing together within dental plaque biofilms.

The biofilm is constructed with gradients and niches that provide many diverse living conditions that are perfect for a wide array of microbes. For example, one gradient or niche may be lacking in oxygen, while another may be oxygen rich. Microbes that thrive on oxygen will inhabit the areas of the biofilm that have more oxygen, and those that can survive without oxygen will take up residence in the low-oxygen areas. Some microbes use the waste products of other microbes as a food source; these microbes will position themselves in an area of the biofilm where they can easily access the waste. It may be difficult to transport nutrients to some areas of the biofilm; the microbes in the less-accessible areas may grow slowly or stop growing altogether, making them less sensitive to agents that can eradicate them.

Since the candida biofilm may shelter a wide variety of organisms, and each organism may contribute to how the biofilm affects the body and its response to treatment, it is important that we understand the characteristics of all the organisms and their biofilms, and how their interactions with one another affect the biofilm.[2,3]

When candida (and other microbes) assemble together as a group, their behaviors and responses to treatment are greatly different from when they are individual units. Treatment methods that are generally effective against single cells may be ineffective against a bigger and well-organized society. As with any society, there is strength in numbers; the biofilm provides the organisms with many tools that enhance their survivability. The immune system typically recognizes foreign invaders by the proteins in their outer membrane, but the biofilm works as a cloaking device that prevents the immune system from identifying those proteins. As a result, the invading pathogens go undetected by the immune system, no antibodies are produced against them, no attempts to eliminate them are made, and they are free to multiply.

For example, if you were to inhale a single-celled organism, the cells in your lungs that are part of your immune system (phagocytes) would attack it, preventing infection from forming in your lungs. If, instead, you were to inhale a biofilm fragment, the pathogens it housed would go unnoticed by the phagocytes and you would develop an infection. Biofilms are often found in hospital settings and sick buildings, where they can lead to widespread infection. Outbreaks of Legionnaires' disease have been traced back to the distribution of biofilms in the air conditioning and ventilation systems of large buildings such as hotels.

The formation of biofilms is one of the primary reasons why many people do not test positive for candida, bacteria, or parasites in many of the common laboratory tests devised to identify them, despite the fact that the patients display all the symptoms of pathogenic overgrowth. Their concealment in the biofilm matrix enables these microbes to evade detection in the blood, stool, or other bodily fluids, preventing antibodies from being produced against them.

Research has found that candida and other microbes that dwell in a biofilm are substantially more resistant toward antifungals and other antimicrobials. As a matter of fact, organisms within the biofilm community can be as much as a thousand times more resistant than free-floating organisms.[4,5] The more fully developed the biofilm, the greater the resistance; and the longer candida has been present, the stronger and more well-established the biofilm. In one study, the MIC (minimum inhibitory concentration—the lowest concentration of a substance that prevents visible growth of a microbe) of amphotericin B, nystatin, fluconazole, and chlorhexidine was assessed for early, intermediate, or mature biofilms. In the early phase of biofilm development MICs were low, but "as the biofilms developed, the

MICs progressively increased." When the biofilm reached the mature phase of development they were "highly resistant." The researches concluded, "the progression of drug resistance was associated with the concomitant increase in metabolic activity of developing biofilms. This indicated that the observed increase in drug resistance was not simply a reflection of lower metabolic activity of cells in maturing biofilms but that drug resistance develops over time, coincident with biofilm maturation."[6] Other research has observed that candida housed within a biofilm can become 100 percent resistant to all antifungals.[7] However, "researchers have discovered that small molecules known as 2-amino-imidazoles disrupt biofilms, making antibiotic-resistant strains of bacteria more vulnerable to conventional drugs. Moreover, antibiotics enhance the ability of 2-amino-imidazoles to disrupt biofilms. Perhaps new antibiotics are not the only way to combat biofilm infections if we could make ineffective older antibiotics active again," says principal investigator Christian Melander, an associate professor of bio-organic chemistry at North Carolina State University.[8]

It seems as though resistance is achieved through many complex facets and processes that we do not yet fully understand. What we have learned has led us to surmise that resistance may result from the high density of cells within the biofilm, the effects of the biofilm matrix, decreased growth rate and nutrient limitation, the expression of resistance genes, and the presence of persister cells (cells that are dormant and highly resistant to all antimicrobial agents and that reestablish the colony after an antimicrobial is administered). All pathogens produce a small subpopulation of persister cells.

All life forms (including those within a biofilm) have DNA molecules constructed of genes that deliver instructions to dictate the characteristics and cellular activities of the particular life form, as well as what genetic material will be passed on to future generations through reproduction. For example, the genes of a microbe like candida dictate how it obtains nutrients, eliminates waste, responds to its environment, and what traits it will hand down to its offspring. This blueprint is what ensures survival of the organism and species. It has been found that microbes that dwell within a biofilm express a different set of gene instructions than planktonic (free-floating) organisms, leading them to participate in different activities and to respond to their environment differently.

Additionally, candida yeast cells, as well as other microbes, can engage in cell-to-cell communication with one another or with other species by using chemical signals that enable them to recognize the size of their population and to modify their gene expression accordingly. This process, known as quorum sensing, plays a critical role not only in the construction of a biofilm, but also in its attachment to a host surface, detachment from the surface, and other behaviors. Studies have found that when microbes are exposed to substances that can inhibit their cell-to-cell communication, the establishment of biofilms is inhibited as well.

Microbes' chemical signals, when transmitted in their planktonic state, are not strong enough to alter gene expression, but within the biofilm matrix their close proximity strengthens the signals, giving them the means to modify gene expression and, consequently, cellular behavior. Genes will be turned on or off as needed to benefit the population; some genes are not made active until they recognize through their chemical communications that the population is of a certain size.[9]

Research also implies that the cell-to-cell signaling system enables the microbes to generate subpopulations in which each one performs different activities that are essential to sustaining the population as a whole. For example, one subpopulation may focus on obtaining nutrients, while another produces offspring. Some cells may even be sacrificed for the good of the society. Some microbes are able to share information with one another—for example, by passing on a drug-resistant gene. Other behaviors within subpopulations that have been detected include wall-forming, swarming, and swimming. Wall formers are cells that line the wall of the matrix fortress; swarmers and swimmers produce daughter cells. As you can see, the methods utilized by single yeast cells (or cells of other microbes) to join together, coordinate behavior, and divide labor to advance their species and ensure their survival are similar to the ones we humans have adopted. Much as we do, they take the "I'll scratch your back if you scratch mine" approach.

The changes in gene expression that take place within the biofilm are what provides the microbes with the means to develop more resistance toward antimicrobials and to evade the immune system so effectively. Researchers speculate that these powers are obtained in the following ways: yeast and other microbes in the planktonic state carry a lot of genetic code that cannot really be expressed until they become a group; because they are so vulnerable to antifungal or anti-bacterial agents in the planktonic state, they die before the code can be activated. Additionally, they may be able to neutralize an antifungal or antimicrobial more efficiently as a group than they can as a single cell. Finally, persister cells that are spawned in the planktonic state are more vulnerable than persister cells spawned in the matrix.

A biofilm is responsive to its environment and can migrate across surfaces. Biofilms may disconnect as a cluster or release new cells to grow and spread into other areas. Organisms within the biofilm community can separate from the matrix and travel individually or as a mass. If they disengage as a group, they retain their increased resistance toward antifungals, antibacterials, and other antimicrobials.

Candida's morphogenetic abilities appear to be important in the formation of some biofilms, but not all. Some studies demonstrated that the hyphae were vital elements of the integrity and multilayered design of mature biofilms, but some biofilms consist of yeast cells only, and no hyphae. It is assumed that the hyphae are required in the more sophisticated designs. The ability to construct biofilms varies among the different species and strains of candida. In a hospital environment, biofilms are seen most commonly in *Candida albicans* and, next, in *Candida parapsilosis*. Biofilms created by *Candida parapsilosis* are less complex and comprise less matrix material than *Candida albicans* biofilms, but they possess just as much resistance, thus demonstrating there are other factors about how the biofilm contributes to resistance that we have yet to learn.

Adhesion of the biofilm to human tissue causes inflammation in the tissue, which perpetuates conditions that encourage more overgrowth. Additionally, the takeover of the tissue by pathogenic biofilms prevents our healthy flora from flourishing.

BREAKING DOWN THE BIOFILM

Research into biofilms in the human body is fairly new and much more difficult than studying microbes in their planktonic state, so our understanding of them at this time remains limited and is a work in progress. Like the yeast cells themselves, the biofilm matrix is exceptionally robust and hard to eradicate. Eradication may take years to achieve, if it is achieved at all. The longer a biofilm has been present in the body the stronger it is and the more difficult it is to penetrate. In the case of chronic candida, the biofilms have had a long time to establish a strong foothold. We do not yet have all the pieces of the puzzle. The treatment procedure is still experimental, and definitive guidelines for the standard of care have not yet been established.

Clinicians and researchers are still in the process of discovering which treatment methods are effective; what we have developed so far falls somewhat short of success. The methods being utilized at this time produce good results in some people, moderate results in others, and no results for some. Clearly, we have much yet to learn. Research in the field needs to be directed toward finding more effective methods for breaking down the biofilm. Due to the biofilm's complexity and the potential for complications, any protocol aimed at biofilm degradation is best embarked upon under the supervision of a knowledgeable physician.

As mentioned previously, it has been universally demonstrated that microbes within the biofilm community are much less vulnerable to the effects of an antimicrobial than the same microbes residing outside the biofilm. Research from the Center for Biofilm Engineering has demonstrated that treatment against microbial biofilms in an industrial setting is most effective when the antimicrobial is administered at a higher-concentrated dose. A brief exposure to a concentrated dosage has been shown to be more effective than a long exposure or a short exposure to a lower concentration. However, researchers point out that in a medical setting, the dosage of antimicrobial that may be required to wipe out the biofilm may also kill the patient.[10]

The material of which the biofilm matrix is constructed influences how it will respond to antifungals, with some being more resistant than others. This offers another explanation for why treatment with one antifungal can be successful against one species but not another. The biofilms of *Candida albicans* and *Candida tropicalis* are constructed from carbohydrate (polysaccharides, starch, cellulose, beta-glucans), protein, hexosamines, phosphorous, and uronic acid. The *Candida albicans* biofilm is composed primarily of glucose (32 percent), while that of *Candida tropicalis* is made primarily of hexosamine (27 percent).[11] However, biofilm materials can vary from biofilm to biofilm. And like everything else related to healing from candida, one's diet can play a significant role in the formation of biofilms, because sugar and carbs are used in the construction of biofilms, not just as a food source for the yeast cells themselves. The diet as described in chapters 10 and 11 is critical for restricting materials that can be used in biofilm development.

Biofilms of all microbes typically contain magnesium, calcium, iron, DNA, and fibrin (a protein created by the body for clotting the blood). Researchers speculate that the calcium, iron, and magnesium assist in holding the matrix together. Iron also serves as a critical tool for dodging the immune system, as the outer protein membrane of the pathogenic intruder is not expressed when iron is present, which prevents the immune system from seeing it. Under normal circumstances, the body manufactures two proteins, lactoferrin and transferrin, to soak up excess iron, which would prevent biofilm development. However, microbial invaders have the ability to emit iron chelators that compete with lactoferrin and transferrin and obtain the iron that is necessary for their existence. If you have the Lyme bacterium (*Borrelia burgdorferi*) in addition to candida, you want to be aware that it uses manganese for its survival instead of iron, which permits it to get around this whole process and avoid detection by the immune system.[12] Dietary supplementation with these minerals can unintentionally strengthen the biofilm matrix and may need to be avoided while working on this issue.

To break down the biofilm, several different agents are needed that can address each aspect of matrix development. Since multiple microbial species and strains may be involved, each of which adds something unique to the mix, agents that are effective may vary from species to species and even strain to strain. The matrix for each microbe may be composed of slightly different materials. Depending on the type of candida and other microbes you are dealing with, what works for one person may not work for another. That said, most biofilms share enough similar characteristics that we know what to target primarily.

Dr. Anju Usman, one of the leaders in biofilm education, has suggested that the protocol needs to contain an agent that detaches the matrix, an agent that restricts minerals, an agent that targets the microbe, and an agent that mops up the degrading biofilm and the toxins released in the process. Nutrients that provide support for the gut, for recovery from inflammation, and for the immune system are also needed.[13] We'll look at each of these features in a little more detail.

Most antifungals (or antimicrobials of any kind) are not capable of penetrating the biofilm to destroy the resident organisms, so the biofilm must be broken down beforehand. If this is accomplished, then the immune system can get back in the ball game and work in conjunction with the antimicrobial. An antifungal or other antimicrobial can't be effective without the immune system; it can simply tip the scales in the host's favor by wiping out some of the pathogenic population, which gives the immune system a fighting chance. If the biofilm is eliminated, that increases the body's chances of successfully reducing overgrowth of candida and other microbes.

To cite an example of this phenomenon from the world of bacteria, when *S. aureus* became resistant to penicillin, one of the antibiotics that we turned to was Vancomycin. However, it wasn't too long until some of the bacterium became resistant to vancomycin (VRSA). However, researchers discovered that if they first administered the chelating agent EDTA (ethylenediaminetetraacetic acid), the calcium, magnesium, and iron were removed, which eliminated the biofilm. Then the vancomycin was effective against VRSA once again, suggesting that we can take action against the candida biofilm in the same manner. Administer one agent to disintegrate the walls of the matrix, and then an antifungal agent to destroy the yeast cells as they are unleashed. The EDTA chelator is used to restrict the minerals in the matrix.

Two types of antifungals, amphotericin B in liposomal form and a class of drugs known as echinocandins, have been found to be effective against some candida biofilms, but not all. In some research, all the species and strains tested were resistant to everything but liposomal amphotericin B and echinocandins; this could be due to the fact that these drugs have not been around as long as the others. Both echinocandins and liposomal amphotericin have also demonstrated the ability to reduce the capacity of planktonic yeast cells to construct biofilms.[14] In regard to bacteria, an antibiotic called Tindamax (tinidazole) has demonstrated the ability to dissolve biofilms as well. Tindamax is often used in the treatment of protozoa, Lyme, vaginal infections caused by bacteria, and resistant forms of clostridia in SIBO—all of which may accompany candida.

Some natural substances that have demonstrated the ability to break down biofilms include bromelain, serrapeptase, nattokinase, lumbrokinase, and a variety of other enzymes, as well as lemongrass, clove, cis-2-decenoic acid (a fatty acid messenger), apple cider vinegar, lactoferrin, and NAC (N-acetylcysteine). Serrapeptase is an enzyme generated by serratia bacteria within the intestines of silkworms. Nattokinase is an enzyme derived from a Japanese food called natto (fermented soybeans). Lumbrokinase is an enzyme generated by earthworms. These three substances are some of the most common found in products on the market for breaking down biofilms.

In one study NAC decreased biofilm genesis by 62 percent for a number of different types of bacteria, including *Staphylococcus aureus, Staphylococcus epidermis, Escherichia coli, Klebsiella pneumoniae, Pseudomonas aeruginosa,* and *Proteus vulgaris.*[15] Candida was not part of this study, but it is presumed that NAC should have a similar effect on it since the biofilms are all similar in nature. It is unclear why NAC is effective. We know that it is an antioxidant that increases glutathione levels in the body and aids parts of the immune system that regulate mucosal surfaces, and we know that it can bind with acetaldehyde, but it is not understood how it has the ability to penetrate the biofilm. On the other hand, some practitioners feel NAC may feed candida, so monitor your responses carefully. Sometimes natural remedies may be combined with drugs. For example, a nasal spray that contains NAC may be used instead of EDTA in combination with a pharmaceutical based antifungal.

One of the most widely used products to dislodge the biofilm is called InterFase or InterFase Plus, by Klaire Labs. Both have been clinically proven to be effective against reducing biofilms. Each of them contains a specialized enzyme formula designed to degrade not only the biofilm but also the cell wall of the yeast and bacterial organisms themselves. The Plus version includes EDTA for binding the calcium, magnesium, and iron to make them unavailable for biofilm development.[16] Another similar, popular, and effective product is called Biofilm Defense, by Kirkman. It contains cellulase to break down cellulose in the biofilm, beta-gluconase to break down beta-glucans in the cell wall of candida, and chitinase to break down chitin in the cell wall.

There are a variety of other products on the market with a combination of enzymes designed for this purpose. However, do be careful, as some of them are combined with questionable bacteria that I warn you about (e.g., *B. subtilis* and *Enterococcus faecalis*) on pages

204–208. Sodium butyrate (a short-chain fatty acid) and *Saccharomyces boulardii,* both of which are discussed on page 181 (butyrate) and 205 (boulardii) in the antifungal section, have also shown the ability to inhibit biofilm formation.

Each of these substances achieves its effects by breaking down some of the substances (polysaccharides, fibrin, and others) that form the architecture of the biofilm, which brings the protective shield tumbling down. Once the yeast cells are no longer protected by the fortress, the immune system can recognize them and launch an attack, and antifungals can access them. Therefore, these biofilm breakers should be used in conjunction with antifungals or other antimicrobials, if you are dealing with a variety of microbes.

The chelating agent EDTA is also available in suppository form over the counter from a wide variety of manufacturers. Personally, I am hesitant to use chelators; removing minerals that are needed for the microbes' survival means that you are prohibiting your own body from acquiring these vital nutrients as well. If you are not careful, this could result in the development of new problems and more deterioration in health. If you use this option, I urge you to work with an experienced health-care provider and exercise the utmost caution—and be sure to replenish the minerals after your course of treatment. This is not something you want to engage in for the long term. As I see it, a better and safer alternative is to use lactoferrin and transferrin, which are discussed in more detail on pages 75 and 193–194. These substances bind with iron and carry it into the cell so that candida and other microbes cannot use it for their own purposes. Apple cider vinegar (2 teaspoons in 8 ounces of water) is also a mild chelator that may be effective for some. However, as mentioned elsewhere, vinegar often sets off allergic-like symptoms in people with candida and it is high histamine and high glutamate.

Not all practitioners agree that the all-in-one biofilm-buster approach is effective. In Dr. James Schaller's book *Combating Biofilms,* he states that not all biofilms are created equal, and treating them as if they were is as "flawed as saying every house key works in every house lock." He explains that biofilms are profoundly diverse in numerous ways. For example, there are vast differences between a new biofilm and a mature biofilm; in their responses to enzymes, essential oils, and antibiotics; in the type of infection involved (bacterial, parasitic, fungal, etc.); in the species inhabiting the biofilm; and in the materials available for building the biofilm based on such things as the species of host (materials available in a dog would be different from those available in a human) and the individual's diet. A person with a lung infection will have a different biofilm than someone with a sinus infection; a person with candida will have a different biofilm than a person with bacteria—and so on. Even individuals who have the same type of candida or bacteria may have a vastly different biofilm. You must have the right "key" for your biofilm "lock" in order for the treatment to be effective. A single master biofilm destroyer does not exist. If you have an overgrowth of a variety of different organisms, each one may have a different type of biofilm, which will likely increase failure rates for both of them.

Schaller discusses at length many different substances and their effectiveness, or lack thereof, against numerous organisms and their biofilms, including allicin, eugenol, carvacrol, linolool, farnesol, xylitol, lactoferrin, stevia, and others. He cites research that indicates that the allicin in garlic, the eugenol in cloves, and colloidal silver have each demonstrated a powerful ability to decrease biofilm formation. He also seems to disagree with many of the common agents being used for busting biofilms, stating they are not very effective—for example, lumbrokinase, nattokinase, and others. Schaller offers some novel approaches to breaking down biofilms—for example, the D form of amino acids, RNAII inhibiting enzyme, and vitamin D, which, as discussed on page 232, increases the production of cathelicidin LL-37, a peptide that has shown antibiofilm activity. Schaller states that combining several different biofilm breakers, which he calls stacking, enhances their effectiveness. This is a must-read book for everyone dealing with biofilms.

When the biofilm is broken, candida and other organisms that reside there, as well as their toxins, are released, which can result in an array of symptoms such as diarrhea, rashes, vomiting, and fever. The barrage of invaders that is suddenly released may surprise your immune system; it may take a while for the immune system to recognize them and go into action, or they may initially overwhelm the immune system's capacity to handle them. Further, once the immune system goes into robust action, medications such as antifungals and other antimicrobials will suddenly become effective, resulting in a high level of inflammation and microbial die-off.

Once the matrix is destroyed, an array of substances such as bentonite clay, alginate, activated charcoal, algae, zeolite, and pectin can be utilized to absorb the toxins and reduce die-off. Everything listed in chapter 8 as a treatment for reducing die-off can be beneficial here as well. To accompany the breakdown of the biofilm, you should consider supplementing with antioxidants and anti-inflammatories—for example, vitamin C, vitamin E, beta carotene, CoQ10, omega 3s, curcumin—to deal with the increase in oxidative stress and inflammation. Additionally, probiotics, which are discussed in more detail on pages 199–208, are believed to help dislodge the biofilm from the mucous membrane, but exercise caution if SIBO is involved.

As mentioned in other sections, research indicates that all resistant microbes flourish in a toxic environment; this is another reason why it is important to reduce your exposure to environmental toxins by living a "green" lifestyle as presented in chapter 13 and optimizing your detoxification system.

Additionally, it is thought that the biofilm matrix may harbor heavy metals; if that's the case, they will be released into the gastrointestinal tract during biofilm breakdown, potentially causing an array of symptoms that are associated with heavy-metal toxicity. Taking something to absorb the heavy metals, like activated charcoal or IMD (Intestinal Metals Detox), is typically recommended for this purpose. IMD is best consumed with food, but charcoal is best on an empty stomach as discussed on page 214. Using a far-infrared sauna may also be beneficial for excreting toxins.

You should note that some concern exists that breaking the biofilm can be counterproductive, because once it is open all the pathogens and toxins that were contained in one place can now be distributed throughout the body. As mentioned previously, our understanding of biofilms within the human body is in its infancy. Failure to mop them up effectively could perpetuate one's health problems. For this reason, it is critical to be aware of all the risks involved and to work with a knowledgeable practitioner who can help you troubleshoot. In *Combating Biofilms*, James Schaller suggests the following protocol to help address these potential problems: use many different agents for killing the organism, which should have a variety of mechanisms by which they work; start at a low dose and slowly work up to a larger one; and "pulse" (vary the treatment schedule)(e.g., use the remedies every other day, or stop treatment for a few days, or do one week on and one week off) when die-off is too intense.

Be aware, too, that the healthy flora in your gastrointestinal tract also form a biofilm, which you need to be careful to preserve in the process of treating the pathogenic biofilm. The biofilm of the resistant and pathogenic microbes takes over the healthy biofilm and prevents its resident microbes from thriving. In contrast to a pathogenic biofilm, a healthy biofilm is composed of a thin, moist, lubricated, and noninflamed mucus that allows nutrients to be transported through the gut wall.

Fry Labs offers a test for identifying biofilms in the blood. However, it does not provide any information about what is happening in the other bodily tissues. It is presumed that if biofilm formation is present in the blood, then it is in the other tissues as well, but better testing is needed in this area. I see no value in spending a lot of time, energy, or money trying to prove the existence of biofilms in your body. Biofilms are the rule in the microbial kingdom, not the exception. If candida, harmful bacteria, or other unfriendly microbes are present, we can safely deduce that biofilms are involved and we should take appropriate action.

It is believed that biofilms are involved in a considerable number of all human microbial infections (fungal, bacterial, viral, parasitic) and that the incidence of candida biofilms is escalating in frequency and severity. The National Institutes of Health estimates that biofilm colonies are involved in nearly 80 percent of chronic microbial infections.[17] They are believed to be the primary cause of chronic and recurring ear infections, strep and other throat infections, urinary tract infections, *H. pylori* infections, sinusitis, lung infections, Lyme, chronic low-grade infections of many kinds, peptic ulcers, tonsillitis, osteomyelitis (infection of the bone), gingivitis, periodontal disease, biliary tract infections, cystitis, prostatitis, bacterial endocarditis (infection of the inner surface of the heart and valves), cystic fibrosis, and Legionnaire's disease. They may also be a major contributor to a wide variety of conditions and disorders such as autism, depression, anxiety, chronic fatigue, OCD, ADHD, IBS, cognitive decline or impairment, colitis, Tourette syndrome, PANDAS, self-injury, or any persistent dysbiosis condition. Dr. Anju Usman has found that all her patients who do not respond to traditional treatment for microbes test positive for biofilm in their blood.[18]

Although the issues surrounding biofilms are frightening, they are also quite exciting. Research in this area may at some point lead to more effective treatment for chronic and resistant cases not only of candida but also of infection by bacteria and other microbes. New discoveries are on the horizon all the time, and individuals with candida should keep their eye on this topic. Research in this area could be a game changer.

CHAPTER 4

Diagnosing Candida

Absence of evidence is not evidence of absence.

—Carl Sagan

Although a wide array of lab tests may be used in the diagnosis of candida, and it can be highly beneficial to know what species of candida you are dealing with in order to use the right antifungals, it is critical to be aware that most testing for candida is not very reliable, and a high number of false negatives is the norm. Because candida can hide in the biofilm matrix, impair the immune system, exist in a hard-to-find cell wall–deficient form, mutate, run and hide, and lie dormant, it is a master at evading detection. Due to microbes' genius ability to survive, the lab tests available at this time are greatly limited in their ability to identify many of them. Although lab tests can be a valuable tool, they should be only one of several different considerations when making a diagnosis.

The most reliable way to diagnose candida is to look at current and past symptoms, your case history, and the response you have to treatment for candida. A positive lab test is just more confirmation, but a negative lab test should not be accepted as proof that candida does not exist. Additionally, since each test has strengths and weaknesses, you can get better results by using a combination of several different tests. If candida doesn't show up in one, it may show up in another, and the additional information that is gathered can help create a clearer picture of what is occurring in the body.

Another important point to be aware of is that even if someone doesn't have what are considered to be high levels of candida overgrowth, that doesn't mean their health can't be affected negatively. Some people can develop a great number of symptoms in response to a low level of candida, while others may have relatively few problems with a very high level of overgrowth. It depends on how tolerant one's body is of candida's byproducts and toxins and what other factors may be present.

COMMON DIAGNOSTIC TOOLS: PROS AND CONS

Stool Test

One of the most commonly used tests for identifying candida is a stool test, and it is also one of the least reliable. Candida rarely shows up in a stool test. Candida does not float around the colon freely; it attaches to the colon wall and may lie deep in the tissue. Therefore, it may not be present in the stool that is eliminated and collected for testing. Additionally, candida may be taking cover in the biofilm, or it may have left the colon and reside elsewhere. That said, if you are one of the few people who test positive for candida in a stool test, the result can be used to assess the pathogen's current susceptibility to antifungals (discussed in more detail on page 166).

A comprehensive stool test can also provide an abundance of other valuable information about your health—for example, the presence of inflammation, the state of digestion, bacteria levels, the presence of *H. pylori,* the existence of parasites, and the efficacy of nutrient absorption. Even if candida doesn't show up, other markers may indicate its presence and the existence of other microbes. A stool test may also indicate fat malabsorption, which is highly indicative of SIBO. For these reasons, even though a stool test may not provide an accurate diagnosis of candida, I believe it is one of the most valuable health tests available. If you can afford it, I recommend getting it done. I prefer the GI Effects Comprehensive Stool Profile, by Genova Diagnostics; it combines standard culture testing with DNA testing, which has proven to be a more reliable and accurate tool for assessment. It can be done with one sample or three samples. Always do three samples, which give you a better chance of finding parasites.

Another stool test, GI Pathogens Screen, by BioHealth Laboratory, is considered by many to be a good choice. (I haven't used it personally or professionally.) This test collects three stool samples and utilizes advanced staining and antigen techniques. Comprehensive Stool Analysis with Parasitology, by Doctor's Data, and the GI-Map Stool Test by Diagnostic Solutions are two other popular options. A very specialized stool test called CHROMagar can identify the species of candida. Dr. Warren Levin, in his book *Beyond the Yeast Connection,* states that swabbing the lining of the rectum (a test called anoscopy) is much more reliable for both candida and parasites. I have never used this test either, so I can't attest to its efficacy, but I trust Dr. Levin's opinion on this issue. An anoscopy will most likely require a visit with a specialist in infectious disease. Undergoing more than one stool test from different labs can improve your chances of obtaining an accurate diagnosis. The stool test is collected at home and sent to the lab, so it doesn't require a visit to the lab.

Spit Test

A popular test falsely believed to be reliable is the spit test. The instructions for doing the spit test are as follows:

- As soon as you wake up in the morning, before you put anything in your mouth or brush your teeth, pour a glass of water in a clear glass that you can see through. Don't use tap water.

- Collect saliva in your mouth with your tongue, and spit it into the glass.

- Keep an eye on your saliva in the glass for the next fifteen minutes, and observe what it does.

According to advocates of this method, any of the following indicates the presence of yeast colonies:

- Your saliva stays at the top and you see thin strands that look like strings or spider legs extending downward.

- Your saliva floats to the bottom and looks cloudy.

- Your saliva takes on the shape of little flecks that are suspended in the middle of the glass.

The spit test was created as a marketing tool in the mid 1990s by a large nutraceutical company that sells candida products, so there is a conflict of interest to consider. Additionally, there is no published medical research to support its validity. Many practitioners do not feel it is a reliable method of assessment. They report a high rate of both false negatives and false positives. Results are inconsistent, as responses can vary from day to day within the same person. The only factor the spit test actually assesses is the viscosity of the individual's mucus.

As candida expert Dr. Jeffery McCombs points out in one of his educational videos, many things can cause mucus to thicken, possibly resulting in any of the responses listed—for example, dehydration from not drinking water overnight, the consumption of dairy products, airborne allergies, food allergies, viruses, bacteria, mold, parasites, high levels of toxins in the body, cold weather, or other weather changes.[1] Whatever responses occur when you spit in the glass of water could be caused by numerous other factors and may have nothing to do with candida.

Antibodies Test

A lab test that looks in the saliva or blood for antibodies against candida (IgA, IgG, and IgM) can sometimes be a valid method. But, again, candida may be hiding in the biofilm, and/or the immune system may be impaired by candida itself, so antibodies may not be produced. Looking for candida in the blood or doing a live blood-cell analysis is not reliable either, as candida rarely appears in the blood of the average person with yeast overgrowth. Additionally, there are serious validity concerns with live blood-cell analysis for any purpose.

Organic Acids Test

The most reliable lab test for diagnosing candida is an organic acids test (OAT), by Great Plains Laboratory. A variety of different labs have their version of an organic acids test, but for the purpose of diagnosing candida and bacteria, in my experience, the one from Great Plains is superior and has a wider range of markers for identification. This test examines the urine for byproducts of candida and other fungi such as aspergillus. Although it is not foolproof, and a negative result should not lead you to disregard the possibility of candida over-growth, this test greatly increases your chances of an accurate diagnosis. It is also good for identifying bacterial overgrowth and SIBO, and it will provide you with a vast amount of other extremely useful information about your health, such as information about nutritional deficiencies or imbalances, absorption, mitochondrial function, energy production, methylation, the detoxification system, oxidative stress, metabolism, D-lactate, ammonia and oxalate levels, and neurotransmitter production and function (only serotonin, dopamine, and norepinephrine).

Additionally, the results of an OAT can indicate whether other tests are called for that could help identify deeper issues. Having this test done is well worth your time and effort. It is one test that I believe everybody should have, if possible. When combined with a good stool test, the organic acids test can give you a well-rounded picture of your gut health. It can also be used to track your progress during treatment. As overgrowth is reduced, levels of byproducts should begin to decrease. If overgrowth increases, byproduct levels will rise. However, an elevation in byproducts can also be the result of die-off, because yeast releases a lot of byproducts when it is killed, so that should be taken into consideration when reviewing results. Another benefit to this test is that it doesn't require a trip to the lab. You collect your own urine at home and mail it to the lab. Note that the organic acids test by Genova often finds things that are not found on the Great Plains test, so, again, undergoing more than one type of organic acids test can be highly beneficial.

Dr. Crook's Questionnaire

The most valid method for determining the presence of candida is not a lab test at all; it is the long version of the written questionnaire that was published by Dr. William Crook in his book *The Yeast Connection*. The questions relate to factors such as symptoms and lifestyle. When used in conjunction with a person's case history and response to treatment, it can be a highly accurate tool. Dr. Crook's questionnaire has been used for decades by alternative health practitioners to acquire an accurate diagnosis. Another benefit is that lab tests can get very expensive, and the questionnaire is highly affordable.

Numerous other tests are available that we will not discuss, and their use varies from practitioner to practitioner. Be aware that all lab tests have limits, and do not rely on them solely for a diagnosis.

I always tell people that if it quacks like a duck, it's a duck and should be treated accordingly. I also encourage them to try to let go of the need to have a lab test for validation. Lab tests should be used as guides, not gods. Many people get really hung up if they aren't able to get a definitive confirmation with a lab test, which only wastes a vast amount of time, energy, and money, and delays progress. Learn to listen to your body; your symptoms and your response to treatment can provide you with everything you need to know. This is true of testing for all pathogens, not only candida. Health-care providers who work heavily with pathogens like candida and its co-conspirators will tell you that we just do not have good and reliable tests available for the full range of microbes. A knowledgeable practitioner will make a diagnosis based largely on one's symptoms, case history, and response to treatment, not just a lab test.[2,3]

OTHER BENEFICIAL TESTS

Besides tests for candida, other tests can provide individuals with helpful information. Here are four of the most important.

Adrenal-Cortisol Saliva Test

As discussed, the adrenal glands are commonly burdened when one is dealing with candida overgrowth and other microbes. It is important to support the adrenal glands when addressing candida to prevent a vicious circle wherein weak adrenal glands perpetuate candida overgrowth, which in turn further weakens the adrenals.

Adrenal fatigue occurs on a spectrum. Individuals may fall at either end of the spectrum or anywhere in between. Knowing where you are on the spectrum is very important for determining your recovery plan. You can't know which direction to go if you haven't been tested. You don't want to take supplements or pharmaceuticals that increase cortisol if it's high, and you don't want to take supplements that lower cortisol if it's low.

The adrenal-cortisol saliva test measures levels of cortisol and

DHEA throughout the day. The data indicate how a person is being impacted by stress, the health of the adrenal glands, and where the person is on the adrenal-fatigue spectrum. This information can be used as a guide throughout the healing process, and you can retest periodically to monitor your progress.

The adrenal-cortisol saliva test is a very simple, do-it-yourself, home test kit. You collect your saliva and mail your sample to the lab, and the results will be sent directly to you. It is considered to be one of the most accurate and reliable indicators for how your adrenals are functioning. It is recognized by the World Health Organization, and it is covered by Medicare Plan B and many other insurance companies. It can usually be purchased online from one of a variety of labs without a doctor's order.

You should be aware that even if your cortisol levels are elevated, you may still not be producing enough of the hormone to meet the demands of the stressors in your life, especially if you are dealing with a lot of stress—such as that triggered by candida overgrowth. Adrenal reserve (the ability of the adrenal glands to produce cortisol in response to stress) can be inhibited, even if your test results indicate that your cortisol levels are normal. If you have all the symptoms of adrenal fatigue, but the test is normal, then this description may apply to you.

Here's a simple way to test your adrenals without a lab kit. Sit down in a chair and take your blood pressure. Record the numbers. While the cuff is still on your arm, stand up and immediately take your blood pressure again. In a healthy person blood pressure will rise upon standing, but in a person who has adrenal fatigue it will drop. Another sign of adrenal fatigue is lightheadedness when rising from a sitting or lying-down position.

Betaine HCl Challenge Test

As we learned in chapters 2 and 5, insufficient levels of stomach hydrochloric acid (HCl) can be a significant contributor to overgrowth of candida, SIBO, or parasites. Therefore, ensuring that you have adequate levels is an important part of the assessment process.

On the other hand, too much hydrochloric acid will produce serious discomfort, damage the stomach lining, and can lead to the development of ulcers. So we don't want to go too far in that direction either. One should know whether they *need* to supplement with HCl before doing so.

The betaine HCl challenge test is the easiest and most affordable way to assess hydrochloric acid levels and how much, if any, supplementation is needed. It should be repeated a couple of times on different days to confirm the results. Here's how you do it:

1. Purchase a bottle of betaine hydrochloride tablets with pepsin.

2. Take one tablet with a meal. If this results in burning in the abdomen area and/or indigestion, then you are producing enough hydrochloric acid and no supplementation is needed. If it does not generate burning or indigestion, then proceed to the next step.

3. Take two tablets of HCl with a meal. If burning or indigestion develop, this indicates that one tablet is sufficient to replenish your HCl levels. If no burning or indigestion develops, proceed to the next step.

4. Take three tablets of HCl with a meal. If burning or indigestion develop, this indicates that two tablets are sufficient to replenish your HCl levels. If no burning or indigestion develops, proceed to the next step.

5. Continue to increase tablets of HCl until you find the dose that works for you.

Please note that HCl should never be taken on an empty stomach.

According to Dr. Jonathan Wright, in his book *Why Stomach Acid Is Good for You,* HCl supplementation should not be combined with certain anti-inflammatory medications (e.g., corticosteroids, aspirin, Indocin, ibuprofen, other NSAIDs). Furthermore, these medications can damage the stomach lining to an extent that prevents your stomach from being able to handle HCl supplementation even when it is needed. Be sure to consult with your doctor prior to supplementation.

If you want to get more scientific than testing at home, there is a lab test for HCl called the Heidelberg test, but it is a lot more expensive.

As we have discussed in previous chapters, a variety of factors can contribute to low levels of hydrochloric acid, including over-the-counter antacids, other acid-suppressing medications (e.g., proton pump inhib-itors), ulcer medication, chlorinated drinking water, aging, and infec-tion with *H. pylori* if it inhabits the middle of the stomach, where it impairs the cells that produce HCl. (If *H. pylori* inhabits the duode-num, it can lead to excess production of HCl.)

Other conditions can lead to insufficient HCl. Peptides, found pri-marily in protein, stimulate the secretion of the hormone gastrin from G cells. In turn, gastrin stimulates the release of histamine, and his-tamine stimulates the parietal cells to secrete HCl. Thus, insufficient levels of histamine prevent the secretion of HCl. Additionally, the para-sympathetic nervous system, via the vagus nerve, works with gastrin to stimulate parietal cells. Too much sympathetic nervous system activity, a lack of parasympathetic nervous system activity, or problems with the vagus nerve may inhibit production of HCl.

As you can see, identifying and addressing the underlying cause of HCl insufficiency is important and can possibly reduce the need for betaine supplementation.

Food Sensitivity Testing

As discussed previously, food sensitivities frequently develop as a result of leaky gut caused by candida or other microbes. Food sensitivities perpetuate inflammation, leaky gut, autoimmune responses, and crav-ings for sugar and carbs, all of which can fuel overgrowth of candida and other microbes. Furthermore, the symptoms of food sensitivity can be very similar to the symptoms of candida overgrowth; it is often difficult to distinguish between the two. When you identify your food sensitivities and remove those foods from the diet, you help the gut heal, downregulate the immune response, and eliminate many of the disruptive symptoms that may drive you to consume sugar and carbs. A variety of tests are available for identifying food sensitivities, and each one has its strengths and weaknesses. I prefer the ALCAT test as it is more sophisticated than standard IgG testing.

Cholesterol Test

As you will learn throughout this book, having sufficient levels of cho-lesterol is critical for a healthy brain and neurotransmitter function, which in turn helps control cravings for sugar and carbs, modulate mood, decrease sympathetic dominance, and regulate gut function. Cholesterol is also needed for the adrenal glands to manufacture cortisol, DHEA, and other stress hormones—and it is involved in the production of vitamin D, which helps to fight off candida and other microbes and regulates blood sugar. Ensuring that your cholesterol levels are not too low is a vital step in the recovery process. Cholesterol is tested through blood and can be checked at any lab. It's a test that is commonly run by physicians as part of a checkup. Optimal levels for cholesterol are discussed on pages 307–309.

Other tests that are commonly performed on people with candida include, among others, immune-function tests to determine if the immune system is compromised, thyroid tests, blood sugar tests, autoimmune panels, and electrodermal testing. The tests you will be prescribed depend on the practitioner you are working with and other conditions you may be dealing with. In addition to the tests described in this chapter, be sure to read about tests for SIBO and parasites in chapters 5 and 6.

If you don't have a doctor to write prescriptions for the tests you desire, many online labs provide services directly to the consumer. However, some states (e.g., New York, New Jersey, and Rhode Island) restrict "over-the-counter" testing.

CHAPTER 5

Candida's Partners in Crime: Parasites, Bacteria, and Viruses

andida overgrowth rarely occurs alone. It is usually present in conjunction with parasites, viruses, and/or pathogenic bacteria. They all join forces and support one another to take over the domain. Each of the different types of microbes offers something unique that supports the community, resulting in a mutually beneficial arrangement for all involved. Additionally, it appears that many pathogens such as parasites and candida do not have the ability to significantly colonize the gastrointestinal tract unless there is a high level of gut dysbiosis (imbalance between good and bad flora).

As with candida, parasites and bacteria expel a variety of toxic byproducts such as ammonia and sulfur, which destroy healthy gut flora, inhibit absorption of nutrients, weaken or heighten immune response, change the bodily pH, inhibit digestive enzymes, cause significant damage to the gastrointestinal tract, disrupt brain chemistry, and perpetuate sympathetic dominance. The result is an internal environment that encourages overgrowth of candida and triggers an array of physiological and psychiatric symptoms, including issues with low blood sugar and nutritional deficiencies.

Addressing candida requires that the likelihood of infection by these other microorganisms be confronted as well. It is possible in some cases that parasites or bacteria may be the primary problem and candida the secondary problem. In that circumstance, an antifungal may do little good because it doesn't have any effect on parasites or bacteria. Furthermore, as is the case with candida, many of these other microbes have the ability to disarm the immune system. And each one can have a profound influence over a person's appetite, cravings, and mood—which can sabotage efforts to remain on the candida diet.

This chapter presents an overview of parasites, bacteria, and viruses that may coexist with candida. The next chapter is devoted to small intestinal bacterial overgrowth (SIBO). This serious health condition, although caused by bacteria and sometimes coexisting with candida, is complex and important enough to merit a chapter of its own.

PARASITES

Although intestinal parasites are believed to be restricted to third-world countries, this is an inaccurate perception. Undiagnosed parasite infection is very common in the United States and other industrialized countries within all social classes. Many practitioners believe they are one of the primary underlying causes of several chronic mental and physical health conditions that plague our society. As a matter of fact, it is quite easy to acquire a parasitic infection. Parasites are commonly found in water, food, day-care centers, preschools, lakes, streams, and rivers. Animals, even pets, are some of the biggest carriers—including dogs, cats, pigs, horses, goats, and rodents. If you have a pet in the house, you most likely have parasites. Parasite expert Dr. Klinghardt reports that a survey of salad bars in New York City found every one of them tested positive for ova and parasites, which may have been acquired from those who prepared the food, from patrons, or from the area where the food was grown.[1] If you eat in salad bars frequently, you have an increased risk of contracting an infection.

When these unwelcome visitors take up residence in your body, they consume your nutrients for survival and emit a variety of toxins such as ammonia that can impair not only your gastrointestinal tract but also your detoxification system, brain, autonomic nervous system, and immune system, leading to a wide variety of psychiatric and physical health conditions. Parasites not only feed on the food and nutritional supplements that you consume; they also feed on your cells, blood, and glucose. If you have a chronic health condition or psychiatric disorder, you should always explore the possibility that you've been infected by a parasite, especially if you have not responded to other treatments and interventions. Practitioners with expertise in this area feel that undiagnosed parasitic infection is one of the primary reasons that an individual does not recover from other chronic health conditions such as candida.

Cats can carry and excrete in their feces a parasite known as *Toxoplasma gondii* (*T. gondii*), which can cause toxoplasmosis, a condition that may lead to schizophrenia, bipolar disorder, addiction, sudden rage, poor school performance, and even suicide. The risk of toxoplasmosis is the reason pregnant women are told to avoid the cat litter box. The parasite can be transferred to the fetus and cause severe brain damage or death. It is also a big threat to people with a weak immune system. Until recently, it was thought to be harmless to most other people, but research now suggests it may be implicated in many mental health issues in the general population.[2,3,4]

T. gondii can sexually reproduce only in the intestines of cats, but it can hitch a ride with other animals including rodents, dogs, and humans, where it will infect the muscle and brain to avoid the host's immune system. Once in the brain, the organism appears to be able to manipulate the host's behavior to engage in activities that are beneficial to its survival, but may be harmful or even lethal to the host. In rats and mice, *T. gondii* has been shown to intentionally eliminate their innate fear of cats, and encourage them to engage in behaviors that will ensure they are eaten by the cat, so it can get into the cat's intestines to reproduce.[5] Neuroendocrinologist Robert Sapolsky states that *T. gondii* "rewires circuits in parts of the brain that deal with such primal emotions as fear, anxiety, and sexual arousal."[6]

Toxoplasma gondii may also be acquired by drinking water or eating undercooked meat, poultry, seafood, and unwashed vegetables and fruits, or exposure to soil that may be contaminated by cat feces.

The tapeworm (acquired from undercooked pork) can get in the brain as well where they can cause seizures, blindness, lack of balance, inability to speak, paralysis, and even coma. It is believed this may be a hidden epidemic that is affecting millions.[7]

Types of Intestinal Parasites

There are two primary types of parasites, worms and protozoa, and many different species within those types.

Worms include pinworms, tapeworms, hookworms, roundworms, whipworms, threadworms (e.g., strongyloides), schistosoma (blood flukes), liver flukes, and others. They attach themselves to the lining of the intestine, where they may cause internal bleeding, nutrient depletion, and anemia.

Protozoa are one-celled organisms. Examples include *Cryptosporidium parvum*, giardia, various entamoebas, babesia, *Dientamoeba fragilis*, *Blastocystis hominis*, *Chilomastix mesnili*, *Endolimax nana*, and others that are invisible to the naked eye, and they initially cause diarrhea that may become acute or chronic. The diarrhea may disappear completely, leading the individual to think the infection is gone, but then new symptoms may develop later.

Common Symptoms of Intestinal Parasites

abdominal pain

diarrhea

constipation

bloating

itching around anus or perineum

burning, stabbing, poking, cutting, or cramping in abdominal area and/or rectum

stinging (similar to a bee sting) in rectum

pain in lower right quadrant of abdomen (near appendix)

sudden urge to eliminate

sensation that something is moving around in the intestines

blood in stool

anal leakage

loose stools

rashes

itching

hives

joint pain

weight loss

weight gain

loss of appetite

increased and insatiable appetite

muscle pain and/or weakness

flu-like symptoms

unexplained sweating

enlarged lymph nodes

dizziness

anemia

seizures

vitamin B12 deficiency

shortness of breath or difficulty breathing

pain or congestion in lungs

crawling sensation under skin

bone loss

dermatitis

chronic fatigue

rosacea

hair loss

gas

foul-smelling gas

nausea

insomnia

hyperactivity

anxiety, depression, OCD, panic disorders, or any other mental health issues

arthritis

irritability

anorexia

muscle cramps

headaches

impaired concentration, attention, and memory

rheumatoid arthritis

extreme hunger (as distinct from cravings), even after eating

MS and other autoimmune conditions

IBS

Crohn's

colitis

appendicitis

irritable bladder or chronic bladder problems that don't respond to treatment

cravings for sugar and/or fat

hypersensitivity to chemicals, foods, electromagnetic fields, sounds, etc.

As you can see, there's a wide range of possible symptoms that one may experience with parasites, and many of them overlap with the symptoms of candida or bacterial overgrowth. Generally, one won't experience all these symptoms; it depends on the type of parasite, how severe the infection is, other health factors that may be present, how much inflammation the parasites cause, and how long they've been present. That said, if you have some type of GI or bowel disorder, chances are very good that parasites are present.

Symptoms may range from acute to chronic and may change from day to day. There may be periods when symptoms settle down and almost disappear, and there may be periods when they flare with a vengeance. Some people experience no gastrointestinal symptoms, while others are incapacitated by them. A single individual may alternate between constipation and diarrhea. It is also possible that an individual is asymptomatic at all times.

One of the systems affected most often by parasitic infection is the nervous system, particularly the autonomic nervous system. When that happens, the sympathetic nervous system becomes dominant, resulting in symptoms such as insomnia; sleep disturbances; hyperactivity; restlessness; nervousness; anxiety; hypersensitivity to chemicals, foods, and sounds; and feeling stressed out. If you have an autonomic nervous system disorder (e.g., dysautonomia, sympathetic dominance), parasites may likely be one of the primary underlying factors. This means parasites can be a major contributor to adrenal fatigue and all the associated consequences discussed throughout the book.

The toxins emitted by parasites can affect the brain and impair neurotransmitter function, resulting in depression, anxiety, mania, paranoia, fear, memory problems, learning disabilities, lack of focus and concentration, schizophrenia, and just about any other mental health, behavioral, or cognitive symptom. They can trigger cravings for sugar, carbs, caffeine, alcohol, and/or mind-altering drugs. They can also impair the detoxification system, making the individual more sensitive to the effects of toxins (e.g., chemical sensitivities) and making it difficult for them to eliminate toxins. When parasitic toxins combine with candida toxins, the result can be an overburdened detoxification system.

A parasite infection can be a primary contributor to or perpetuator of candida overgrowth, because the ammonia and other toxins emitted by the parasite kill the body's friendly flora, alter the pH, damage the gut lining, and create leaky gut, producing an environment that allows candida to take over. Additionally, it is believed that parasites can house candida inside themselves. For these reasons, candida infection may be secondary to parasitic infection, and most people with yeast overgrowth are also dealing with a parasitic infection. Parasites can make you crave certain foods, just like candida does. Some parasites like sugar and some like fat, so you may crave either, but they also eat protein. They also frequently occur in conjunction with pathogenic bacteria, and may house them as well. One parasite may carry another parasite inside it; therefore, having more than one type of parasite is very common.

Like all pathogenic microbes, parasites are very hardy and have crafted a variety of ingenious ways to evade elimination. They may mutate, develop resistance against medications and herbs, invade a cell so that the immune system cannot access them, and hide out in biofilms (discussed in chapter 3)—all of which make them very difficult to eradicate.

Parasites frequently migrate from the intestinal tract; they may be found in the blood, liver, gallbladder, lungs, bile ducts, kidneys, brain, or even the eyes. They may move around within the gastrointestinal tract; one of their favorite spots to congregate is in the cecum, the first section of the large intestine, which resides near the appendix. One's symptoms may vary depending on where the parasites are located at any given time. Since parasites consume the host's nutrients and glucose, nutritional deficiencies and low blood sugar are very common. If you are anemic and/or have a vitamin B12 deficiency, you should always explore the possibility of parasites. According to Dr. Leo Galland, iron supplements and probiotics are food sources for protozoa, so if you have protozoa you need to be careful with probiotic and iron supplementation.[8] On the spiritual level, as with all chronic health conditions, a parasite infection can wreak havoc on one's ability to experience inner peace, tranquility, and feelings of connectedness, creativity, and self-awareness, lowering quality of life.

We are all exposed to intestinal parasites, but they cause problems only in some people. It is believed by most practitioners with expertise in parasites that individuals who have intestinal permeability (leaky gut, insufficient friendly flora, and impaired immunity) are the ones who are vulnerable to infection. When the gut is healthy, the immune system takes care of the problem. Insufficient hydrochloric acid may also be a primary contributing factor in some cases. HCl in the stomach should prevent parasites from making their way into the gastrointestinal tract.

Diagnosing Intestinal Parasites

According to Dr. Dietrich Klinghardt and Dr. Charles Gant, two leading specialists in the field of microbes, you rarely see evidence of a parasite.[9,10] Their intention is not to deliberately harm the host but simply to have a comfortable place to live, so they lurk quietly in the background a lot of the time. Since most mainstream practitioners don't acknowledge that a condition exists without a lab test to prove it, most people with parasite infections go undiagnosed because all the lab tests for diagnosing them are unreliable. Parasites are masters at evading detection; therefore, most tests come back negative, even for people who are infected. Like candida, they may hide in the biofilm or other places in the body.

Ideally, stool should be examined within fifteen minutes of elimination, which almost never happens, because some parasites secrete an enzyme that digests themselves when exposed to air, and some parasites don't reside in the bowel. In a webinar by Dr. Charles Gant, he relates that a patient of his clearly passed a roundworm after taking an antiparasitic medication. His office sent the worm to one of the conventional labs to be tested, and still it came back negative.[11]

One of the most reliable lab tests available is the GI Effects Stool Profile, by Genova. It combines two different types of technology for identifying microbes, including looking for their DNA. However, it still produces a high number of false negatives. The GI Effects test often comes back with a result of "taxonomy unavailable," which means a parasite was found but its species is unknown. Many practitioners and the lab itself believe this is probably not a serious issue and don't strongly encourage patients to address the issue. That has not been my experience. Many people who've received this result have serious parasite infestation. Do not disregard treatment if you see this in your results. A well-trained practitioner will know that it should be treated in the same manner as any other positive result. The GI Effects test offers options for both a one-day stool collection and a three-day stool collection; the three-day collection should be used as it increases your chances of locating an organism.

Using older methods of diagnosis, Dr. Gant states that he observed an incidence of parasites in about 17.9 percent of samples submitted. With the GI Effects test, he observes an incidence of about 50 percent. This is a significant increase; it demonstrates that the prevalence of parasitic infection is very high. The other stool tests that we discussed in chapter 4—namely, the anoscopy, the GI Pathogens Screen, and the Comprehensive Stool Analysis with Parasitology—are also good tools for assessing the presence of parasites.

Ideally, a patient would undergo all of these tests because each has its own strengths and weaknesses. If one test does not identify the parasite or bacteria, another may. Additionally, if symptoms strongly suggest the probability of parasites but nothing is found on any of the tests, then one should retest several times. Evidence may not have been available the first time, but it may show up the second or third time.

For the most part, a diagnosis must be made based on symptoms and on the likelihood of incidence. On the authority of Dr. Charles Gant, other telltale signs that are indicative of a parasite infection include the following:

- Indistinct feelings of itching, skin irritations, or something crawling, particularly at night

- An imbalance between lactobacillus and bifidus, with the former being low and the latter being high

- Bloody stool, caused by parasites chewing through the lining of the gastrointestinal tract (yeast and bacteria are incapable of this activity; however, bloody stool can also occur from hemorrhoids and anal fissures)

- Anemia, or low iron, TIBC, and/or ferritin (if there's no other known cause)

- Pain or discomfort in the lower right quadrant of the abdomen (e.g., near the cecum, where parasites like to accumulate)

- Deficiencies in amino acids as indicated by an amino acid (plasma) test, despite adequate consumption of protein (parasites can consume the body's protein stores)

- Deficiencies in other nutrients, such as zinc and selenium, with no plausible explanation

- A positive response or worsening of symptoms when administered an antiparasitic medication

- A history of travel to foreign countries, especially if followed immediately by an acute episode of gastrointestinal distress that seems to clear up later (international travel significantly increases risk, but many people who have never traveled in a foreign country acquire parasites as well)

- Itching of anus or rectum

- Unsuccessful treatment of yeast or bacterial overgrowth even when the patient was completely compliant with the protocol

Please also be aware that many of these symptoms can result from small intestinal bacterial overgrowth (SIBO), which is discussed in the next chapter.

If you have one type of parasite, then you can assume you most likely have a variety of others, because if the gut and immune system are vulnerable to one microbe, they are vulnerable to many. Additionally, once a microbe takes up residence it impairs immune function and gut integrity even more, leaving the door open for others. For the same reasons, parasites rarely occur alone; they are nearly always accompanied by yeasts, fungi, viruses, and/or bacteria. Each of the other microbes must be addressed as well.

Treatment Options

Some of the most common natural remedies used for parasite infection include wormwood, black walnut hulls, clove, garlic, goldenseal, pumpkin seeds, gentian root, thyme, castor oil, neem oil, grapefruit seed extract, quassia, male fern root, coconut, pomegranate, diatomaceous earth, papain (from papaya), bromelain (from pineapple), fig, and mimosa pudica. A variety of homeopathic formulas are also used, and a device known as a zapper is advocated by some.

The most frequently used prescription pharmaceuticals for parasites include Alinia, Flagyl, albendazole, ivermectin, Biltricide, and iodoquinol. According to Dr. Klinghardt, the herb mimosa pudica is thirty times stronger than pharmaceuticals.[12] However, as is the case with antifungals, what works best for one person may not work best for another. It depends on many different factors, for example, the species you are dealing with, whether it has developed resistance to the substance, and what other pathogens you are carrying. A lot of trial and error will be required.

The pharmaceuticals for parasites are hard core and have the potential for a number of side effects. One must research the products and weigh the positives against the negatives when deciding whether to take them or not. Most of the pharmaceuticals used for parasite treatment are very expensive in the U.S. So expensive that it can prohibit treatment. I'd like to make you aware that you can order them from Canada at a fraction of the cost at one of their online pharmacies.

One must also be aware that herbs are like natural drugs and can generate a variety of unexpected side effects, some of which can be quite serious. For example, neem oil significantly lowers blood sugar. This could be a positive effect for someone with type 2 diabetes, but not so good for someone with low blood sugar issues, which is the case for most people with candida. I discovered this by accident when I almost passed out on several occasions because the neem I was taking caused my blood sugar to plummet. Please read page 138 for more information on neem. Additionally, I experienced severe inflammation and rectal bleeding in response to taking diatomaceous earth. Both prescription pharmaceuticals and natural remedies should be used only under the care of a knowledgeable physician.

My opinion about using herbs and other natural remedies to treat parasites is that they aren't strong enough to kill them off completely. Their use seems to increase the parasites' resistance to extermination, which results in a great deal of inflammation. Generally speaking, I am in favor of using pharmaceutical drugs only as a last resort, but I believe this is one of those situations when they are absolutely necessary. Other practitioners with expertise in parasite treatment agree. Dr. Gant, who practices integrative medicine and is also in favor of pharmaceutical drug use only as a last resort, believes that parasites cannot really be eliminated without prescription-based medications and in combination with other treatment protocols, for example, herbs, homeopathics, oxidative stress (e.g., hydrogen peroxide and oxygen based products), colonics, and the zapper.

Since people infected often do not know which parasites they are dealing with, a broad range of antiparasitic medications must be used to cover all the bases. The goal is to hit them with an arsenal. However, the medications must be taken in a specific order. If you attempt to kill the small parasites before killing the big ones, the large ones begin to migrate, often while carrying the smaller ones inside them. Treatment usually has to be repeated numerous times, as parasites lay eggs when they are threatened, and maintenance treatment should be done periodically. Furthermore, treatment requires a comprehensive approach that supports the liver and kidneys, keeps the bowels moving, and reduces exposure to electromagnetic fields. A strong liver and kidneys are needed to help eliminate toxins. Constipation may occur with treatment as a result of the parasites' last-ditch attempt to hold on by inhibiting peristalsis. Electromagnetic radiation may cause parasites to proliferate and release more toxins (discussed in more detail on page 382).

It is critical to keep the bowels moving so they can eliminate all the toxins that will be released as the parasites are killed. Please refer to chapter 8, where I discuss several ways this can be achieved and other ways to assist in die-off. Sometimes it is necessary to treat with some type of antibacterial (natural or pharmaceutical) in addition to an antiparasitical, since many parasites depend in part on pathogenic bacteria for their survival.

BACTERIA

Bacteria in the gastrointestinal tract can cause problems in a variety of ways. Pathogenic bacteria may be present anywhere in the gastrointestinal tract. In addition, as you will learn further ahead, even healthy bacteria can become pathogenic under certain circumstances. High numbers of good or bad bacteria may reside in the small intestine, where they don't belong. As with candida and parasites, bacteria can invade bodily tissues and release a wide array of byproducts such as ammonia and sulfur, which can impair health in numerous ways, for example by overloading the detoxification system, impairing brain function, causing mental health disorders, degrading the integrity of the gut, encouraging sympathetic dominance, and causing numerous gastrointestinal issues—all of which potentially perpetuate candida overgrowth. Bacteria can have a profound impact on mental health, and this issue is discussed in detail in the next chapter. Additionally, bacteria hide in places where the immune system can't reach them very well. They may go intracellular, even getting inside neurons or white blood cells.

An array of different types of pathogenic bacteria may inhabit the gastrointestinal tract; some of the most common include *H. pylori, Escherichia coli,* campylobacter, *Klebsiella pneumoniae, Staphylococcus aureus, C. difficile,* and other clostridium species. As candida does, pathogenic bacteria compete with the healthy bacteria for space and nutrients, thus preventing them from doing their work to keep the gut and immune system strong and to discourage yeast overgrowth. Additionally, candida can attach to bacteria and use them to take cover. Certain types of anaerobic organisms in the colon are a primary cause of constipation as they inhibit peristalsis. They can also inhibit the process of glucuronidation, one of the body's primary detoxification pathways. Among other things, glucuronidation is important for getting rid of estrogens. When the process does not work properly, estrogen dominance may result, which, as we learned in chapter 2 , provides fuel for candida growth.

Again like candida and parasites, bacteria have devised a variety of brilliant adaptive mechanisms to enhance their survival. They can alter gene expression in the host. They can share their DNA with future generations or among different strains and even with other species. If a bacterium alters its genes to become resistant to a particular treatment, it can share this modified DNA with other bacteria, allowing them to become resistant as well. They may change their structure so the antibiotic is no longer effective, or they may inactivate or neutralize an antibiotic. Resistance is a big problem in bacterial overgrowth. Taking an antibiotic that has no efficacy against a particular microbe increases resistance, and the more often an antibiotic is used, the more likely resistance is to develop. For example, the bacterium MRSA (methicillin-resistant *Staphylococcus aureus*) arose as a direct result of bacterial resistance. Shortly after penicillin was developed, some of the *S. aureus* bacteria acquired genes that made them resistant toward penicillin. After a while, the strains that weren't resistant were killed off, and the strains that were resistant became dominant. The penicillin molecule was modified into a substance to target the resistant bacteria, methicillin, but soon the bacteria developed strains that were resistant to this antibiotic as well.

Whether the bacterium in question is gram-positive or gram-negative may have some effect on treatment. Gram-positive and gram-negative bacteria are distinguished by structural differences in their cell walls. Gram-negative bacteria have a double membrane in their outer cell wall, whereas gram-positive have a single layer. The double membrane is impenetrable by many antibiotics, which makes these bacteria more resistant to drugs and antibodies than gram-positive bacteria. They also have a greater capacity to share DNA with other bacteria.[13]

I would like to focus on a few types of bacterial infection that occur most frequently in conjunction with candida—*H. pylori,* Lyme disease, and SIBO (small intestinal bacterial overgrowth)—because they can significantly impede the healing journey if they are present and not addressed. Infection with *H. pylori* and Lyme disease are discussed below; SIBO is addressed in detail in the next chapter.

H. Pylori

Helicobacter pylori is a gram-negative bacterium that inhabits the stomach and/or the first part of the small intestine (the duodenum). It is believed that 50 percent of the world's population carries *H. pylori,* but not everyone develops symptoms. *H. pylori* can produce a broad range of upper GI symptoms, including GERD, heartburn, acid reflux, a deep gnawing or burning feeling in the stomach or upper small intestine, bloating, nausea, and frequent and intense belching. It is the primary cause of ulcers and gastritis. It can also cause other symptoms, for example, coughing, sore throat, loss of appetite, vomiting, weight gain, anxiety, chronic fatigue, joint and muscle pain, depression, and brain fog with impaired cognitive functioning and ability to focus and concentrate. *H. pylori* can cause a great deal of inflammation in the stomach and the small intestine, contributing to leaky gut, which in turn encourages candida overgrowth, nutritional deficiencies, impaired immunity, autoimmune disorders, and anything else associated with leaky gut. The World Health Organization lists *H. pylori* as a class-one (definite) carcinogen, which means it significantly increases one's risk for gastric cancer.[14] However, I would like to point out that there is a study that found an increase in consumption of cruciferous vegetables is associated with an "11% and 22% (comparing the highest with the lowest category) decreased risks of gastric cancer in prospective studies and case control studies, respectively."[15] Be sure to eat lots of cruciferous vegetables if you have *H. pylori.*

H. pylori consumes hydrogen as an energy source. The body mixes hydrogen with chloride to make HCl (hydrochloric acid, the primary stomach acid), so if *H. pylori* is consuming your body's stores of hydrogen, then you may not have enough HCl. Conversely, *H. pylori* can also cause overproduction of HCl. If *H. pylori* colonizes the area where the stomach joins the small intestine (duodenum), it can affect the cells that control HCl production, resulting in too much HCl and leading to ulceration. But if it colonizes in the middle of the stomach, it can impair the cells that produce HCl, inhibiting production and resulting in hypochlorhydria, a state that can increase one's risk for gastric cancer.[16] Additionally, inadequate HCl can lead to a deficiency in vitamin B12, which can't be assimilated without HCl. Finally, HCl is what kills candida and other microbes and keeps them from spreading through the gastrointestinal tract. (HCl has been discussed in more detail on pages 52; 89–91.) Since hydrogen is *H. pylori*'s favorite source of energy, anything that increases hydrogen levels—including excess consumption of foods that result in hydrogen production (sugar, starches, grains, fiber, fruit, and other carbohydrates) and the presence of SIBO discussed in the next chapter—can exacerbate *H. pylori.*

Toxins from *H. pylori* may lead to lower levels of vitamin C and inhibit absorption of iron. In pregnant women, *H. pylori* can cause severe morning sickness. It is also able to evade the immune system by adhering below the mucosal lining. Like candida, *H. pylori* forms biofilms and can morph into a different form. Typically, *H. pylori* exists in a spiral rod shape, but when exposed to adverse environmental circumstances that threaten its survival, it can change into a coccoid (spherical) form as a protective mechanism.[17]

Gastric acid secretion influences *H. pylori,* but *H. pylori* also influences gastric acid secretion. Like candida, its ability to colonize is dependent on the pH of its surroundings; in order for *H. pylori* to survive in the naturally highly acidic stomach, it releases an enzyme called urease, which converts urea (a substance in the stomach) into carbon dioxide and ammonia.[18] The ammonia reduces the acidity, making the stomach a more hospitable place for *H. pylori.* The alkaline environment then encourages overgrowth of candida and other pathogens. (And, of course, as discussed earlier, ammonia is toxic to human cells and can produce a wide array of symptoms.) Furthermore, as also discussed, low stomach acid caused by other factors encourages microbes such as candida and *H. pylori* to multiply. *H. pylori* is the only bacterium known to have adopted a way to exist in the highly acidic environment of the stomach.

Tests used to diagnose *H. pylori* include a blood test, a breath test, a stool antigen test, and an endoscopy with stomach biopsy. As is the case with all testing for microbes, the typical tests result in a fair

number of false negatives. If symptoms suggest infection, then I suggest retesting if you get a negative result. The stool antigen test may be
more reliable than the other methods.

The primary treatment for *H. pylori* includes taking two different
types of antibiotics simultaneously with proton pump inhibitors, a
combination that is very toxic and in my opinion does more harm
than good. Proton pump inhibitors make the gut more alkaline, which
encourages overgrowth of microbes and is associated with numerous
problems, including impaired absorption of nutrients (magnesium,
calcium, and vitamin B12), potentially leading to deficiencies, an
increase in bone fractures, weight gain, pneumonia, and overgrowth of
Clostridium difficile, a very serious problem. This treatment protocol
rarely eradicates *H. pylori* completely and has a failure rate of more
than 20 percent.[19]

Some of the most effective natural remedies for *H. pylori* include
colostrum, bismuth citrate, mastica, zinc, lactoferrin, turmeric, cinnamon, garlic, citrus seed extract, cranberry extract, broccoli sprouts
or supplements containing their active ingredient (sulforaphane),
extra-virgin olive oil, berberine, vitamin C, and lactic acid probiotics (e.g., *L. acidophilus* and *Bifidobacterium bifidum*). Many of these
substances are discussed in more detail in chapter 7 because they also
demonstrate antifungal activity. Colostrum is also very effective for
reducing the inflammation and pain associated with *H. pylori* (discussed in more detail on pages 237–239).

Be aware that *H. pylori* frequently develops resistance to these substances before treatment has been completely effective. This bacterium
is exceptionally difficult to eliminate fully. To increase the chances of
preventing resistance, a combination of substances typically needs to
be used simultaneously and alternated in the same manner as described
for antifungals in chapter 7.

The reason that mainstream medical practitioners use two different antibiotics simultaneously is because they recognize that *H. pylori*
becomes resistant very quickly to a substance that is used solo, but
success is increased if two are combined. The same principle should be
applied when using natural remedies.

As with candida, different strains of *H. pylori* may respond to treatment differently, so what works for one person may be ineffective for
another. A bit of trial and error is required, and treatment typically

must be repeated whenever flares occur. In my own life, I had little success with the natural treatments for *H. pylori,* except sulforaphane. However, the sulforaphane would only keep it under control. As soon I discontinued use, it would return in full force. Mastica worked great for a few weeks, but then I got resistant. Eventually, I had to take several rounds of antibiotics for SIBO, and at some point I realized my *H. pylori* was gone. No proton pump inhibitor was needed. The antibiotics did the trick.

Of course, all foods that feed microbes such as *H. pylori* and that impair gut integrity should be avoided when dealing with *H. pylori.* These foods include sugar, grains, legumes, alcohol, caffeine, chocolate, processed foods, and even complex carbs that are high-carb and fruit. Like most microbes, *H. pylori* loves sugar, which allows it to reproduce rapidly. Gluten also causes surges in overgrowth. Following the diet in chapters 10 and 11 will support your efforts at eradicating *H. pylori.* Avoid overeating. Nutrients and herbs that help reduce inflammation—for example, vitamins A, C, and E, CoQ10, curcumin, and zinc—may be helpful as well (see page 465).

The symptoms of *H. pylori* can overlap significantly with those caused by candida and even more so with those of SIBO. *H. pylori* can also shelter candida inside itself. Please read pages 157–161 for information about how to differentiate between the three.

Lyme Disease

Lyme disease, which is caused by *Borrelia burgdorferi,* is another bacterial infection that commonly occurs in conjunction with candida. This is largely due to the fact that the standard treatment protocol for Lyme is long-term antibiotic therapy, which can result in a secondary candida problem. Individuals with Lyme usually also need to treat for candida at some point. On the other hand, it could be that a candida patient's weakened immune system allows *B. burgdorferi* to take hold in the body.

Many of the symptoms of Lyme overlap with those of candida—for example, brain fog, headaches, fatigue, joint pain, insomnia, rashes, impaired concentration—so it can be hard to differentiate between the two conditions. An individual with candida may be misdiagnosed with Lyme, and vice versa. Additionally, one may overcome Lyme without knowing it because they have contracted candida, which can feel just like Lyme. As is the case with all microbial testing, the tests for Lyme are not reliable. Of course, treating for candida when the problem is Lyme will be counterproductive, and vice versa. Lyme bacteria produce a toxin that inhibits the body's ability to use acetylcholine, which may contribute to the development of SIBO since acetylcholine is so critical for gut motility and the migrating motor complex (see chapter 6).

There is not space or time in this book to go into detail about Lyme disease as it is very complex and requires the care of a physician with expertise in the condition. Lyme is acquired through the bite of the blacklegged tick (or deer tick). It can be transmitted through a woman's placenta to her developing fetus if treatment isn't commenced in a timely fashion. In addition, some practitioners believe that infection can be spread through semen or breast milk, demonstrating that microbes have the ability to change their mode of transmission.[20] There is disagreement among experts on these modes of infection. Some of the natural antifungals for candida discussed in chapter 7 (e.g., cat's claw or samento) are highly effective against Lyme. Other herbs used specifically for Lyme include otoba bark and Japanese knotweed. According to Dr. Warren Levin, studies in Germany have demonstrated that the antifungal Diflucan suppresses growth of Lyme.[21]

Like candida and parasites, all bacteria form biofilms and use them as hiding places. Steps to break down the biofilm must be taken (described in chapter 3). Bacteria can become resistant to both natural and pharmaceutical antibacterials, so remedies must be diverse, must be used in various combinations, and must be modified regularly. The best treatment option for bacterial infection varies from person to person, depending on factors such as where in the body the infection is located, the species and strain of bacterium involved, how advanced the biofilms are, and whether the bacterium is resistant to a particular substance.

Not only does bacterial infection contribute to candida, but the toxins emitted by bacteria can overburden the detoxification system and the adrenal glands. They can impair the autonomic nervous system, and the production and function of neurotransmitters. Again, these complications can have a significant impact on mental health by contributing to depression, anxiety disorders, ADHD, cognitive impairment, behavioral disorders, OCD, psychoses, autism, and cravings for sugar, caffeine, carbohydrates or other mind-altering substances. Iron-deficiency anemia may result from bacterial overgrowth since all microbes use iron for their survival. Other nutritional deficiencies are common as well. Bacterial infection may also impair cells' mitochondria and the production of ATP, leading to chronic fatigue.

In his book *The Yeast Syndrome,* Dr. Trowbridge presented the work of Dr. Eunice Carlson, who demonstrated a profound relationship between bacteria and candida. Infection by both simultaneously resulted in a heightened level of virulence that was not exhibited when either pathogen existed alone. Dr. Trowbridge states, "If bacterial colonies are remaining in tissues after antibiotics are discontinued, safely shielded inside a colony of surrounding yeast, then only by killing the *C. albicans* at the same time can a physician effectively eradicate all of the patient's bacterial organisms. It's the only way to rid his patient of the bacteria that would remain to seed the next infection in the following weeks or months."

VIRUSES

People with candida commonly carry a variety of viruses, such as cytomegalovirus, Epstein-Barr, and herpes. These may contribute to symptoms including fatigue, aching, headaches, anxiety, fever, sore throat, swollen glands, and others. It is unclear whether they are a cause or a result of candida. It may be that the immune system is so weak from fighting candida that it leaves the door open for viruses as well, or it may be that a high viral load may make one vulnerable to candida. Many of these viruses lie dormant for long periods of time and then flare intermittently. The flare-ups seem to correspond to an increase in candida levels or to periods of high stress. Many of the natural remedies used for candida, parasites, and bacteria also work against viruses—for example, lactoferrin, colostrum, grapefruit seed extract, oregano oil, olive leaf, and colloidal silver. Viruses may live in a biofilm, so whatever steps are taken for reducing biofilms associated with candida, parasites, and bacteria are beneficial for reducing viruses.

A fascinating study by Johns Hopkins Medical School and the University of Nebraska stumbled upon a virus (chlorovirus ATCV) that can infect the human brain and significantly affect one's level of intelligence by altering gene expression within the brain. Individuals with the virus exhibit impairment in cognitive functions and spatial awareness, while apparently suffering no negative impact on other aspects of their health. "Many physiological differences between person A and person B are encoded in the set of genes each inherits from parents, yet some of these differences are fueled by the various microorganisms we harbor and the way they interact with our genes."[22,23] This finding demonstrates that viruses have the capability to manipulate the brain in ways similar to that of bacteria and candida.

All microbes (yeast, parasites, bacteria, and viruses) thrive on sugar and on foods that break down into sugar, so naturally the diet should be sugar-free and low in carbohydrates when dealing with any of these pathogens. The candida diet outlined in chapters 10 and 11 will fill the bill.

As you can see, many of the symptoms of candida, bacteria, parasites, and viruses overlap, and sometimes it can be difficult to know where your symptoms are coming from. I once had a chronic itch in the perineum area that I assumed was candida- or parasite-related. My efforts to address it from that angle met with no success. I was forced to take an antibiotic because of a persistent respiratory infection I had picked up, and to my surprise the itch cleared up as well. (Antibiotics are not always a bad thing.)

Be sure to read chapter 14 on nutritional supplements, chapter 9 on the immune system, and chapter 7 on herbal remedies. Each of them provides more information on steps that may be helpful for dealing with microbes other than candida. These issues can be very complicated and are best addressed with the help of a skilled practitioner who has expertise in microbes.

CHAPTER 6

Small Intestinal Bacterial Overgrowth (SIBO)

The small intestine typically contains relatively few bacteria. It houses less than ten thousand organisms per milliliter of fluid, compared to one billion per milliliter in the large intestine. Furthermore, the types of bacteria that reside in the small bowel are different from those in the large intestine. Most bacteria in the small intestine are *L. acidophilus*. Bacteria live throughout the entire digestive tract, from mouth to anus, but most of them reside in the colon.[1] When excessive numbers of bacteria end up in the small intestine, the resulting condition is called small intestinal bacterial overgrowth (SIBO). This disorder can have negative effects on both the structure and function of the small intestine that can result in an array of disruptive physiological and psychological symptoms.

SIBO may occur as an overgrowth of the bacteria that normally inhabit the small intestine (*L. acidophilus*), but most often it is caused when bacteria that reside in the large intestine migrate into the small intestine. Put more simply, there is an increase in the number of bacteria and/or a change in the type of bacteria that are typically present. Overgrowth usually involves a variety of different types of bacteria, not just one. According to Dr. Allison Siebecker, one of the leading experts on SIBO, the species most commonly found in overgrowth include both commensal anaerobes—*Bacteroides* 39%, *Lactobacillus* 25%, *Clostridium* 20%—and commensal aerobes—*Streptococcus* 60%, *Escherichia coli* 36%, *Staphylococcus* 13%, *Klebsiella* 11%.

A more recent study found the aerobes to be *Escherichia coli* 37%, *Enterococcus spp* 32%, *Klebsiella pneumonia* 24%, and *Proteus mirabilis* 6.5%.[2] In contrast to many other bacterial infections, SIBO is not contagious.

The small intestine is where food is digested and nutrients are absorbed. The presence of too many bacteria in this area interferes in these processes and gives the microbes premature access to the body's nutrients. Typically we get first dibs on our nutrients, and they get what's left over once it travels to the colon. If they are present in the small intestine, the arrangement is reversed. The consumption of vital nutrients by bacteria before our own cells have a chance to obtain them can lead to an assortment of nutritional deficiencies and negative consequences.

Bacteria need vitamin B12 and iron for their survival, so deficiencies of these nutrients are the two most common ones found in people with SIBO, but the bacteria also take calcium, magnesium, amino acids, and other nutrients. Diarrhea that results from the presence of bacteria can contribute further to malabsorption and malnutrition. Overgrowth of bacteria in the small bowel is the leading cause of fat malabsorption because it reduces the conjugated bile salts that are needed to absorb dietary fat. Fat malabsorption can lead to deficiencies in the fat-soluble vitamins (A, D, E, and K). Bacteria in the small intestine also consume the body's disaccharide enzymes, which are needed to break down carbohydrates, leading to carbohydrate malabsorption.

Colonization of bacteria in the small intestine can result in damage to the epithelial cells (cells lining the small intestine), otherwise known as leaky gut. (As discussed on page 22, this also occurs with candida overgrowth.) Leaky gut impairs digestion and the absorption of nutrients, contributing even further to nutritional deficiencies, and it allows toxins, pathogens, and undigested protein molecules to enter the bloodstream, causing food sensitivities, immune reactions, inflammation, and autoimmune disorders. SIBO causes an increase in zonulin, which as described earlier regulates the tight junctions between the intestine's epithelial cells. High levels of zonulin weaken the junctions, causing or exacerbating leaky gut. Recall that zonulin is also part of the blood-brain barrier; again, high levels weaken the barrier and lead to a condition known as leaky brain.[3]

Furthermore, since 70 percent of the immune system resides in or around the gut, bacterial overgrowth can significantly impede immune function. As you'll learn in chapter 9, the epithelium helps form a barrier that keeps pathogens from entering the body. SIBO is also commonly associated with elevated levels of endotoxin and other bacterial compounds that stimulate the output of proinflammatory cytokines (see chapter 9). Endotoxin is a toxic substance in the outer cell wall of gram-negative bacteria that is released when they are ruptured or disintegrate, prompting a strong immune response.

Like most microbes, the microbes responsible for SIBO prefer to feed on the sugar, starches, and other carbohydrates that are present in our diet by fermenting them, in the process releasing a variety of toxins and gases such as hydrogen and methane. When a high number of bacteria meet an abundance of dietary carbohydrate, the result can be excessive amounts of gases and toxins, leading to a wide variety of symptoms that include flatulence, diarrhea, bloating, abdominal pain, foul-smelling gas and/or stool, and increased or decreased motility (depending on whether hydrogen or methane is produced). The toxic bacterial byproducts may also overload the detoxification system, making it difficult for the body to eliminate both its naturally occurring toxins and the incoming environmental toxins, another scenario that can result in a buildup of toxins and lead to further degradation of mental and physical health. The combination of toxins from SIBO and toxins from candida form a double whammy. Because the bacteria in the small intestine have continuous access to a food supply, they proliferate, creating a vicious cycle: they consume the nutrients meant for us, which provide them with the energy to multiply, giving the colony even greater access to our nutrient supply.

As mentioned in the last chapter, chronic candida often occurs in conjunction with SIBO, and they perpetuate one another. The damage done by each creates an environment in the gut that encourages the other. If SIBO is not addressed, then reducing overgrowth of candida will be difficult to achieve, and vice versa. SIBO can certainly occur without candida overgrowth, but having candida overgrowth for a significant amount of time increases one's risk of developing SIBO at some point. On the other hand, the havoc inflicted by SIBO could make a person more vulnerable to candida overgrowth. SIBO damages the gut lining, can increase ammonia levels, alters pH, irritates the ileocecal valve (located between the small and large intestines), and weakens the immune system—any of which would create an environment that encourages the proliferation of candida. If both are present, an antifungal may do little if an antimicrobial is not also used, and vice versa. *H. pylori* can potentially precipitate SIBO as well. As described in the last chapter, if *H. pylori* colonizes the stomach it reduces hydrochloric acid levels, allowing other bacteria to overgrow; if it colonizes the small intestine it can create inflammation that encourages overgrowth of bacteria. Conversely, the hydrogen produced by SIBO can cause *H. pylori* to proliferate because it uses hydrogen as a food source.

Once I became aware of SIBO, which wasn't until recent years, I discovered that a very large percentage of my clients with candida also had SIBO. As I became more educated on this issue, I reflected on some of my clients over the years and realized that many of them, too, probably had SIBO. Symptoms and experiences that I was unable to explain or address effectively suddenly made sense. As I'll demonstrate below, the likelihood that you have SIBO in addition to candida is very high. When that is the case, treatment is much more complicated and needs to be tweaked a bit to enhance your healing journey.

COMMON SYMPTOMS OF SIBO

The symptoms and their severity may vary widely from person to person depending on what species of bacteria is overgrown, the extent of the overgrowth, where the bacteria are located, and other coexisting conditions. Different bacterial species have different behaviors, and different parts of the small intestine have different functions, so the types harbored and where they are located affect which functions will be impaired. Overgrowth may be mild, moderate, or severe, and symptoms will correspond accordingly. Some people may experience only a few symptoms that are mildly disruptive, while other people may become completely incapacitated—or anything in between. Additionally, symptoms and their severity can change within the same individual on a daily basis in response to the level of overgrowth or other factors. SIBO usually occurs in a gradual process; symptoms develop so slowly that one doesn't connect all the dots until it is full blown and they look back in retrospect. But, it may come on suddenly. The following are some of the most common symptoms reported:

- abdominal pain and cramping
- bloating and abdominal distension
- diarrhea and/or constipation
- excessive gas (may smell like sulfur)
- excessive belching (may smell like sulfur)
- feeling full after just a few bites

- nausea
- heartburn
- acid reflux
- headaches or migraines
- joint and muscle pain
- fatigue and/or weakness
- histamine intolerance
- steatorrhea (excess fat in stool)
- muscle spasms

Other symptoms I have witnessed in my clients and in myself include pain in the rectum, burning on the inside near the small intestine area that may radiate to skin on the outside, itching on the inside of the abdomen that radiates to the outside and may even make the skin in that area turn red, gallbladder pain and problems, lots of exceptionally loud intestinal noise after eating, dry cough, dizziness, bladder pain, chest pain, insomnia or disrupted sleep, persistent dental-plaque buildup, gingivitis or periodontal disease, ringing in the ears or head, back pain, spine pain, and shoulder pain.

Besides physical symptoms, numerous psychological disturbances are experienced by people with SIBO, and they are often not discussed in the literature. These symptoms can be much more frightening and disruptive than the gastrointestinal symptoms. Your gut bacteria can have a profound impact on your brain in a variety of ways that manifest as cognitive or psychiatric symptoms.

As explained earlier, when the gut lining is compromised, toxins from bacteria or other microbes that reside there (e.g., candida) can get into the bloodstream. Once in the bloodstream, they can travel to the brain, where they may impair the production and function of the neurotransmitters that regulate moods, thoughts, and behavior. If a person has leaky gut, they probably also have leaky brain, which means many substances can enter the brain that should not be there.

Our alimentary canal, from esophagus to anus, is lined with an extensive network of neurons (about one hundred million). The neurons contain neurotransmitters (more than thirty different ones). This network, known as the enteric nervous system, is often referred to as our "second brain." It not only regulates gut function and digestion; in conjunction with the brain in our head, it also influences our mental state and may affect other disease states like osteoporosis. The second brain may have a significant impact on our overall emotional well-being.[4]

Intestinal bacteria may use the vagus nerve to transmit signals to the brain that impair neurotransmitters. The vagus nerve consists of a variety of branches that travel from the brain to the gut. It is used by the brain to send messages to the gut (and vice versa), and it comes in contact with the heart and other organs along the way. Signals from the vagus nerve help modulate mood, including fear and anxiety. The vagus nerve is also believed to be associated with neurogenesis (the formation of new neurons) and with increases in brain-derived neurotrophic factor (BDNF), a substance involved in neurogenesis and in protecting existing neurons and encouraging synapse formation.

Bacteria can produce false neurotransmitters that interact with neurons, and they may interfere with enzymes that are needed to break down neurotransmitters. For example, bacteria from the genus clostridium are associated with conduct disorders, autism, depression, schizophrenia, and even psychoses by altering neurotransmitters in the brain. Certain species of clostridium can inhibit an enzyme called dopamine beta-hydroxylase that is needed to convert dopamine into norepinephrine. Dr. William Shaw explains that this "leads to overproduction of brain dopamine and reduced concentrations of brain norepinephrine, and can cause obsessive, compulsive, stereotypical behaviors associated with brain dopamine excess and reduced exploratory behavior and learning in novel environments that are associated with brain norepinephrine deficiency,"[5] a set of symptoms commonly seen in autistic children. Excess dopamine is also associated with schizophrenia and other psychoses. These disorders often respond favorably to treatment with the antibiotic vancomycin, which targets clostridia.

Like candida, bacteria can prevent tryptophan from being converted into 5-HTP in the gut. 5-HTP is needed to manufacture serotonin. As discussed previously, serotonin is critical for mood, appetite, gut function, and reducing sympathetic dominance, and is the precursor to melatonin, our primary sleep hormone.

Bacterial overgrowth may lead to a phenomenon called molecular mimicry. Rheumatic fever is a condition that can develop after an infection with a group-A streptococcus bacterium. Proteins in the cell wall of the bacteria are similar to proteins that exist in various places throughout the body—for example, in the heart, brain, and joints—and the immune system may mistake human tissue for the bacterial protein and attack it. Inflammation and damage to these tissues can lead to heart disease, arthritis, and/or a disorder involving abnormal movements called Sydenham's chorea or St. Vitus Dance. Another disorder known as PANDAS, which can develop in children after an infection with streptococcus, manifests as obsessive-compulsive disorder (OCD) or tic disorders. It is believed that PANDAS develops in a manner similar to how rheumatic fever develops: with the immune system attacking tissue in the brain, triggering inflammation and affecting the brain's functioning.[6]

One of the byproducts produced by some species of bacteria (predominantly gram-negative species like enterobacteriaceae, proteus, and clostridium) when they utilize protein is ammonia. As described in chapter 1, ammonia is a neurotoxin when present in excess and can lead to neuroinflammation, impairment of neurons, brain fog, mental confusion, impaired cognitive functioning, hepatic encephalopathy, and more. High levels of ammonia may produce numerous other symptoms, including headaches, irritability, fatigue, diarrhea, and nausea. It can overburden the liver and kidneys, further compromising the immune system. Bacteria's utilization of protein may also lead to protein deficiencies.

Some bacteria produce histamine out of the amino acid histidine (commonly found in the diet), which can cause an elevation of histamine. As discussed, high histamine levels can lead to a wide variety of psychological disturbances, including OCD, addiction, abnormal fears, brain racing, and schizophrenia, as well as physical symptoms such as hives, itching, weepy eyes, runny nose, and gastrointestinal symptoms. Some bacteria produce D-lactate, which at high levels is neurotoxic and may lead to symptoms including brain fog, disorientation, anxiety, obsessive-compulsive disorders, depression, and confusion. Please read more about D-lactate on pages 201–203.

Dr. Emeran Mayer, a professor of medicine and psychiatry at the University of California, Los Angeles, found that connections between regions of the brain differ depending on what species of bacteria is dominant in a person's gastrointestinal tract. According to Mayer, this suggests that "what kinds of brains we have—how our brain circuits develop and how they're wired" may be partly determined by the particular microbes that are present in our gut.[7]

Researchers at McMaster University in Hamilton, Ontario, discovered that if they transferred the gut bacteria from mice that were fearless into mice that were anxious, the anxious mice become less anxious and more gregarious. Likewise, if they replaced the gut bacteria of the fearless mice with those from the anxious mice, the fearless mice became more timid. Additionally, aggressive mice would become calm when their gut bacteria were altered with diet, probiotics, and antibiotics. Researchers in Ireland found that if they cut the vagus nerve in mice, the brain would no longer respond to changes in the gut biome.[8]

Dr. Mark Lyte, of the Texas Tech University Health Sciences Center, in Abilene, studies how microbes affect the endocrine system. He says, "I'm actually seeing new neurochemicals that have not been described before being produced by certain bacteria. These bacteria are, in effect, mind-altering microorganisms."[9]

Athena Aktipis, PhD, an evolutionary biologist and psychologist with the Arizona State University Department of Psychology, explains, "Microbes have the capacity to manipulate behavior and mood through altering the neural signals in the vagus nerve, changing taste receptors, producing toxins to make us feel bad, and releasing chemical rewards to make us feel good."[10]

Since we know that bacteria can have this impact on the brain, it is logical to assume that bacteria involved with SIBO would have the same capabilities. Furthermore, if SIBO leads to deficiencies of nutrients such as vitamin B12, iron, calcium, and magnesium, the result may be psychiatric symptoms as well, since these nutrients are vital for proper brain function and for producing the neurotransmitters that moderate our thoughts, mood, and behavior. People with IBS, which is frequently a SIBO-related condition, have been found to have excessive levels of short-chain fatty acids, likely due to the fact that these are byproducts of bacteria. Although short-chain fatty acids are beneficial to our health by providing us with energy, improving insulin sensitivity, and reducing inflammation, elevated levels can produce depression, anxiety, and migraines, and an increase in gastrointestinal symptoms.[11,12]

In a fascinating article out of Japan, it is hypothesized that when fermenting microbes are found in the gut, they are also located in the brain, where they may metabolize neurotransmitters, leading to depletion of the neurotransmitters. Or the neurotransmitters norepinephrine and epinephrine may be converted into amphetamine or methamphetamine and serotonin may be converted into LSD. All of which could lead to a wide array of psychiatric symptoms.[13]

Some of the most common brain symptoms experienced by people with small intestinal bacterial overgrowth include, but are not limited to:

- brain fog (possibly severe)
- obsessive-compulsive disorder
- attention deficit
- hyperactivity
- depression
- anxiety
- impaired memory and problem-solving abilities
- unexplained fear or paranoia
- choppy thought processes
- Tourette syndrome or tic disorder
- dyslexia
- loss of overall feelings of well-being
- songs or phrases getting stuck in the head but not in a normal or pleasant way

Severe SIBO may produce the following:

- weight loss (possibly severe)
- malabsorption malnutrition/ nutritional deficiencies (most commonly of iron and vitamin B12)
- anemia (from B12 or iron deficiency)
- failure to thrive
- hepatic encephalopathy
- possibly severe mental health issues (e.g., schizophrenia, psychoses)

CONDITIONS ASSOCIATED WITH SIBO

IBS, Fibromyalgia, and Chronic Fatigue

One of the conditions most commonly associated with SIBO is irritable bowel syndrome (IBS). Studies have found that SIBO is involved in more than half of all cases of IBS; in one study it was 84 percent.[14] Successful elimination of bacterial overgrowth in the small intestine leads to a 75 percent reduction in IBS symptoms. In another study, an even higher percentage of people with fibromyalgia tested positive for SIBO.[15]

High levels of hydrogen sulfide, a bacterial byproduct, may inhibit an enzyme needed for ATP production and thus impair functioning of the mitochondria (the cell's energy-producing "furnaces"). Some researchers believe that SIBO contributes to chronic fatigue in this way. Additionally, adrenal fatigue, which creates profound bodily fatigue, commonly occurs in conjunction with SIBO, triggered by the constant stress of the condition in a similar manner as candida does, described on pages 34–36.

GERD, Acid Reflux, and Heartburn

SIBO can be a major underlying cause of acid reflux, heartburn, and full-blown GERD. In his book *Fast Tract Digestion: Heartburn,* Dr. Norm Robillard has presented a strong case demonstrating how gas produced by SIBO puts pressure on the lower esophageal sphincter (LES), a muscular one-way valve at the bottom of the esophagus that allows food to pass into the stomach but typically keeps contents in the stomach from entering the esophagus. The pressure forces open the LES, allowing stomach acid into the esophagus. The more bacteria present in the small intestine, the more gas that is produced. The more gas produced, the more pressure will be exerted. Less bacteria equals less gas, and the LES can hold firm. Other practitioners, including Dr. Michael Eades, agree with this hypothesis. Dr. Eades explains that the LES weakens somewhat as we age, making it more vulnerable to gas pressure.[16] *H. pylori* is implicated in GERD, but, interestingly, *H. pylori* can proliferate by feeding on the hydrogen produced by SIBO, so it could be involved from this angle as well.

Autoimmune Disorders

Intestinal permeability (leaky gut), when combined with a genetic predisposition and an antigen or environmental trigger, is believed to be one of the primary underlying contributors to autoimmune disorders of all kinds. When the gut lining is damaged, permitting food, bacteria, and toxins into the bloodstream, the immune system launches an attack against these substances. Wherever the substances land (e.g., on an organ or tissue) becomes a target for the immune system. Molecular mimicry, described above, may play a role. Since SIBO does significant damage to the gut lining, it can play a major role in the development of autoimmune disorders.

Other coexisting conditions include, but are not limited to:

- rosacea
- hypothyroidism
- lactose intolerance
- chronic pancreatitis
- chronic pain syndromes
- hepatic encephalopathy
- interstitial cystitis
- restless leg syndrome
- acne
- nonalcoholic steatohepatitis (fatty liver)
- Crohn's
- celiac

- systemic sclerosis
- diabetes with autonomic neuropathy
- vitamin B12 deficiency
- gallbladder problems
- spastic colon
- fructose malabsorption
- hypoglycemia or low blood sugar issues
- chronic fatigue syndrome
- fibromyalgia
- osteoporosis
- appendicitis

Over time, SIBO compromises the immune system. It becomes stressed from dealing with the multiple invaders, toxins, and partially digested food being absorbed through the leaky gut. The antibody SIgA (secretory IgA) tags the toxins and invaders, notifying macrophages and other white blood cells to eliminate them. If too many toxins and undigested food particles enter the bloodstream, the system becomes overwhelmed. Many of the offending particles get missed, the immune system weakens, and the adrenal glands become stressed. As discussed, overworked adrenal glands lead to adrenal fatigue.

Recall that when candida or any other microbe colonizes the small intestine, it damages the epithelial cells and brush border that line the intestine. A damaged epithelium can encourage pathogenic bacteria to overpopulate, causing more damage to the epithelium, and so on. This is one way in which SIBO and candida perpetuate one another.

CAUSES OF SIBO

The causes of SIBO are not completely understood. It is believed to arise from a complex interplay of factors. Several protective mechanisms in the body are in place to prevent SIBO. They are summarized below.

1. *Adequate small-intestine motility by virtue of the migrating motor complex (MMC).* Lack of motility promotes bacterial overgrowth. The migrating motor complex triggers a wave-like action (peristalsis) in the GI tract that moves undigestible substances such as fiber, other foreign bodies, and bacteria out of the stomach and small intestine and into the large intestine. When functioning adequately, this cleansing process occurs every 90 to 120 minutes during fasting (between meals and overnight).[17] When food enters the digestive system, the process is inactivated, and digestive motility takes over. MMC is thought to be regulated in part by serotonin and a polypeptide hormone called motilin, which itself is initiated by vagal nerve stimulation.[18] Problems with MMC could be related to serotonin insufficiency or underactivity of the vagus nerve.

   Dr. Mark Pimentel, one of the leading experts on SIBO, believes that SIBO and, consequently, IBS are caused by an autoimmune response to a toxin (cytolethal distending toxin, or CDT) released by bacteria that cause food poisoning. The small intestine houses a particular type of nerve cell (ICC cell) that is in charge of regulating the migrating motor complex. These cells are very similar in structure to CDT, so the immune system confuses them for the toxin and develops antibodies against both the toxin and the ICC cells. This causes damage to the cells, resulting in impairment of the migrating motor complex and leading to overgrowth of bacteria.[19]

2. *Proper functioning of the ileocecal valve.* The ileocecal valve is

positioned between the ileum, the end of the small intestine, and the cecum, a pouch at the beginning of the large intestine. It prevents bacteria in the colon from entering the small intestine. Put more simply, it connects the small intestine to the large intestine and prevents backflow. If the valve fails to shut properly, it can allow bacteria, parasites, or candida to cross into the small intestine.

3. *Sufficient production of gastric secretions (HCl), pancreatic secretions (enzymes), and gallbladder secretions (bile).* Each of these substances helps to kill bacteria. As we age, our ability to produce stomach acid decreases, so aging makes all of us vulnerable to microbes of all kinds. Reduction in levels of any of theses secretions for other reasons already discussed leaves us at risk for SIBO.

4. *Immunoglobulins (antibodies) in the intestinal fluid.* They are part of the immune response to fight bacteria. People with SIBO frequently don't have sufficient levels to provide adequate protection.

Now let's look at some of the primary risk factors for SIBO.

1. *Heavy or moderate alcohol use.* "Moderate" alcohol consumption is defined as one drink per day for women and two drinks per day for men.[20,21] Alcohol may feed some species of bacteria, contributing to overgrowth.[22] It also damages the gut lining, which can contribute to leaky gut, and decreases muscular contractions. As mentioned previously, alcohol also feeds candida, which confounds the problem.

2. *The use of proton pump inhibitors.* They reduce the acidity of the gastrointestinal tract, which allows bacteria to multiply.

3. *Candida overgrowth.* Candida produces a toxin called acetaldehyde, which interacts with serotonin and dopamine and creates a very powerful opiate called tetrahydroisoquinoline. Opiates inhibit the migrating motor complex and gut motility overall. Candida creates inflammation in the gut lining, which encourages proliferation of pathogenic bacteria. Acetaldehyde can also deplete acetyl coenzyme A, which is needed to combine with choline to make the neurotransmitter acetylcholine, which may result in acetylcholine deficiency. Acetylcholine is used by the vagus nerve to regulate the parasympathetic nervous system, needed for gut motility and

to initiate the migrating motor complex. Serotonin is also needed to modulate the migrating motor complex, and, as noted, candida causes serotonin depletion. Candida increases histamine and norepinephrine levels, thereby keeping the body in sympathetic stress, another factor that inhibits the migrating motor complex. Candida disrupts proper functioning of the thyroid gland, which can inhibit gut motility. Candida releases ammonia, which lowers the pH of the gut, another factor that can inhibit the migrating motor complex and encourage overgrowth of bacteria. Candida weakens the immune system, decreasing the immunoglobulins that fight off bacteria. It may cause irritation to the ileocecal valve, affecting the way it functions. Some yeasts can create somatostatin, which inhibits the motilin that is needed to activate the migrating motor complex.

4. *Chronic or acute stress.* As discussed, when we are under stress, gastric emptying does not occur, digestive motility is impaired, stomach acid and digestive enzymes are inhibited, healthy bacteria are killed off, immune function is impaired, communication between the brain and the gut via the vagus nerve is disrupted, nutrient absorption is impeded, the bloodstream is infused with glucose, our nutrient supply is drained to deal with the situation at hand, and inhibitory neurotransmitters like serotonin are suppressed—all situations that will encourage the overgrowth of bacteria and other microbes such as candida and *H. pylori*. Stress may also cause pathogenic bacteria to cling to the gut wall. If one remains in a state of stress on a continuous basis, they are susceptible to sympathetic dominance.

Recall that the vagus nerve is how the gut and brain communicate with one another. It is deactivated when we are under stress. It uses afferent neurons to send messages to the brain about the state of affairs in the gut and other areas of the body, and it uses efferent neurons to send information from the brain to the gut and the rest of the body. The vagus nerve is also the commander-in-chief of the parasympathetic nervous system, which controls digestion and the relaxation response. The parasympathetic nervous system is part of the autonomic nervous system, which regulates all aspects of the body that occur automatically: digestion, breathing, heart rate, blood pressure, body temperature, sexual response, and other processes. The sympathetic nervous system is also part of the autonomic nervous system. It is activated when we are under stress.

After a stressful event, the vagus nerve activates the parasympathetic nervous system to return the body back to its normal mode of rest, digestion, and relaxation. The two systems work together to assure that the body responds to different situations in the appropriate manner; they have different effects on the same organ. For example, the sympathetic nervous system increases heart rate and blood pressure, while the parasympathetic decreases them. The sympathetic nervous system slows digestion, while the parasympathetic stimulates it. The parasympathetic nervous system controls the contractions that move food through the gastrointestinal tract. Stress hormones prevent the vagus nerve from turning on the relaxation response. If stress is ongoing, then the sympathetic nervous system will remain in overdrive, and communication between the gut and brain will be disrupted. The migrating motor complex is partly regulated by motilin, which is initiated by the vagus nerve. Therefore, stress inhibits the migrating motor complex as well.

As discussed, severe stress or trauma early in life, such as childhood abuse, neglect, or loss of the primary caregiver, makes an individual highly susceptible to developing functional gut disorders like SIBO or candida overgrowth later in life. Acute, life-threatening events in adulthood such as rape, a car accident, a natural disaster, or being present in a war zone can also significantly increase vulnerability to functional gastrointestinal disorders. Both acute, life-threatening episodes and early-life stress or trauma have the ability to cause permanent and irreversible damage to the stress response system. Stress circuits remain in a hypersensitive state, leading to functional gut disorders (and mental health issues) later in life. High levels of day-to-day stress or chronic stress can also lead to or perpetuate the gut disorder and exacerbate symptoms. Furthermore, overgrowth of bacteria or any other microbe such as candida is a form of stress and thus can create a vicious circle: overgrowth causes stress, which creates conditions that encourage more overgrowth, which causes more stress, and so on.

Autonomic nervous system dysfunction that leads to sympathetic dominance can also be caused by a variety of other factors, including depletion of inhibitory neurotransmitters, hormone imbalance, environmental toxins, too much exercise, electromagnetic fields, physical trauma, high levels of histamine and/or glutamate, and more. For these reasons, managing one's stress, as described in chapters 12 and 13, is critical for treating any gut disorder such as SIBO.

Some of the other possible risk factors for SIBO include damage to nerves in the gut, opiate addiction, bowel surgery, diabetes, hypothyroidism or any other condition that affects gut motility, anatomical abnormalities like diverticula, and pancreatitis.

HYDROGEN- OR METHANE-PRODUCING SIBO

According to health practitioner Chris Kresser, bacteria are not the only organisms involved in SIBO.[23] As you may know, one of the most commonly used tests for diagnosing overgrowth of bacteria in the small bowel is a breath test, which measures one's level of hydrogen and methane, two byproducts of microbe metabolism that indicate bacterial overgrowth. Hydrogen is produced by bacteria, but methane is produced by a group of ancient single-celled organisms called archaea. Archaea were once classified as bacteria, but now they are understood to be a different type of organism called prokaryotes. Archaea live in extreme environments, like salt lakes and hot springs, or any other habitat where biodegradation of organic compounds takes place, for example, the gut of the human being or an animal. Bacteria produce hydrogen gas when they ferment dietary carbs, and archaea produce methane by consuming the hydrogen produced by the bacteria. This is one of the ways that the body deals with excess hydrogen in the gut. Some bacteria may also convert excess hydrogen into sulfites,[24] which is one of the reasons why the breath, gas, or stool may smell like sulfur in a person with SIBO. Both archaea and bacteria may convert dietary sulfur into hydrogen sulfide. Hydrogen sulfide is believed to be eliminated with two enzymes called thiol methyltransferase and rhodenase, but some people may have insufficient numbers of these enzymes, which allows the hydrogen sulfide to accumulate and cause damage to the gastrointestinal tract (e.g., inflammation, ulcerative colitis). If you have a high level of methane at baseline or after consumption of the sugar solution in the SIBO breath test (discussed further ahead), this indicates an overgrowth of archaea. If you have a high level of hydrogen with no elevation in methane, this indicates an overgrowth of bacteria only.

Methane is an odorless, colorless, inert gas. At high levels in the body it creates bloating and distention and is associated with a variety of disease states. The research suggests that approximately 45 percent of individuals with SIBO have methane-producing archaea, and the level of methane produced is significantly higher in people with bacterial overgrowth than it is in people with fructose- or lactose-malabsorption issues.[25] According to Dr. Pimentel, SIBO expert, methane levels of over three parts per million indicate a methane producer, even if it is at baseline. Another indicator that one is carrying methane-producing archaea is constipation, as these organisms are associated with chronic constipation.[26] The higher the level of methane, the slower the colonic transit time. One study found that if the breath test was positive for methane, there was a 100 percent association with constipation-predominant IBS.[27] However, it's important to note that constipation can be caused by other factors besides methane-producing archaea, like hypothyroidism or magnesium deficiency. If methane production is not elevated and constipation is present, then there may be another underlying contributor. People who have an inflammatory bowel disease like Crohn's or ulcerative colitis, which typically present with diarrhea, have low levels of methane. On the other hand, it may be that constipation produces methane because slow transit time encourages methane-producing archaea organisms.

The neurotransmitter serotonin may be involved in this process. Serotonin, as you recall, is produced in the brain and the gut. One of the roles it is believed to play in the gut is intestinal motility. Studies reveal that people with high levels of methane have lower postmeal serotonin levels than people with high levels of hydrogen. Hydrogen production is associated with diarrhea. If one is producing both hydrogen and methane, both constipation and diarrhea may present, depending on the dominant gas at any given time. This explains why many people vacillate between diarrhea and constipation. IBS-C tends to indicate the presence of archaea methane producers, and IBS-D indicates the presence of hydrogen-producing bacteria only.

Studies have demonstrated that reducing methane levels improves symptoms. If SIBO doesn't improve when addressed from the hydrogen angle, this indicates that methane-producing archaea are present. Chris Kresser states that people with methane-producing archaea may also have a higher level of rectal hypersensitivity, which manifests as pain in the rectal area, the feeling of urgency, and a lower pH in a stool test. This condition occurs more often in women than men. You should also note that methane is produced by archaea in the colon in people without SIBO, but at lower and nonpathogenic levels. Note that methane production does not begin until after age three, methane is found in lower levels in people under age ten, and not everyone produces methane—indicating that not everyone is colonized with archaea.[28]

Why does it matter if you are a methane producer or a hydrogen producer? Because the answer to some degree affects how you'll approach treatment. Antibiotics or herbs that are effective against hydrogen producers are not always effective against methane producers. We will discuss this topic in more detail a little further ahead, in the SIBO treatment section.

SIBO TESTS AND DIAGNOSIS

SIBO is underdiagnosed for a variety of reasons. First, many doctors are not trained to recognize the disorder, so people are diagnosed with GERD, IBS, autoimmune disorders, OCD, or other conditions instead. Furthermore, since many of the symptoms overlap with other microbial infections, it is frequently misdiagnosed as candida or *H. pylori*. Or, because it often exists simultaneously with *H. pylori* and candida, all symptoms are assumed to arise from one of those disorders. On the other hand, many people don't seek help for their symptoms; instead, they medicate them with over-the-counter products like antacids, laxatives, etc. It is also underdiagnosed because the lab tests we have available are not always reliable.

As mentioned above, the most commonly used test for diagnosing SIBO is the hydrogen/methane breath test. It measures the levels of methane and hydrogen present in the breath after a twenty-four-hour prep diet (void of fermentable carbs) and an overnight fast. A fasting baseline level of the two gases is collected first. Then the patient consumes a nonabsorbable sugar solution, and breath samples are collected every twenty minutes for the next three hours. Breath is collected by inhaling into a specially designed vial and then analyzed with a machine called the BreathTracker. If hydrogen or methane is elevated, small intestinal bacterial overgrowth is indicated. If methane or hydrogen is elevated at baseline (prior to consuming sugar solution) overgrowth is indicated as well. As explained previously, elevation in hydrogen alone indicates that bacteria are involved; if methane is elevated, archaea are involved. The hydrogen test can also be used to diagnose *H. pylori* and carbohydrate malabsorption.

Testing may be done at a center that has the proper equipment to do so, or samples may be collected with a do-it-yourself home kit and then sent to the lab for analysis. Not all labs have the proper equipment to test for methane, so be sure the lab you use does. If methane is present, a slightly different treatment strategy will be required. It's important that one has abstained from using antibiotics, both natural and pharmaceutical, prior to testing.

The hydrogen/methane breath test results in a substantial level of false negatives, meaning that the test results are negative even when SIBO exists. This may occur for a variety of reasons. "Hydrogen breath tests are based on the fact that there is no source for hydrogen gas in humans other than bacterial metabolism of carbohydrates." But not all bacteria produce hydrogen, and if overgrowth consists of one of the species that doesn't produce it, then testing will yield a false negative.[29]

Additionally, the small intestine is approximately twenty feet long, and overgrowth may occur in one spot and not another, potentially affecting test results. The breath test may use lactulose or glucose as the substrate. Lactulose cannot be digested or absorbed by humans, only by bacteria. When bacteria consume lactulose, they produce gas. If an excess level of gas is produced, it indicates overgrowth. According to Dr. Allison Siebecker, lactulose is better at diagnosing bacteria located in the distal (lower) end of the small intestine, where most overgrowth is thought to occur. However, it is less effective overall than glucose. Glucose, on the other hand, is absorbed by both humans and bacteria. We absorb glucose within the first three to five feet of the small intestine; therefore, if high levels of gas are produced in response to glucose, it means the bacteria are present in the proximal (upper) end of the small intestine. But it also means the glucose substrate cannot diagnose bacterial overgrowth located in the remaining seventeen feet of the small intestine, where it is most likely to occur.[30] If a patient gets a negative test result with one or the other, but symptoms indicate SIBO, then it seems logical to me that the patient should have the test done with both glucose and lactulose. However, many practitioners feel that lactulose is the better substrate.

Delayed gastric emptying (time required for food to move from stomach to small intestine) and slow motility are other causes of false negatives. Smoking increases hydrogen levels, and exercise decreases hydrogen levels, so both of these can influence results as well. To complicate things further, not all practitioners interpret the test in the same way. One practitioner may interpret a result as negative, while another may interpret the same result as positive. As with candida, looking closely at your case history, current symptoms, and response to treatment is the best way to diagnose SIBO.

A false positive on the hydrogen/methane breath test is also possible if a patient has chronic pancreatitis, celiac disease, rapid transit through the small intestine, or high levels of oral bacteria, or if he or she failed to adhere to a low-fiber diet the day before the test. That said, most problems with the test are with false negatives.[31] If test results are negative, but the symptoms of SIBO seem apparent and other causes have been ruled out, most physicians will treat accordingly. If one has a positive result in response to treatment, they know they are on the right track.

The GI Effects Stool Profile, described earlier, can be used to see what's in the colon, but not in the small intestine. However, since SIBO often involves bacteria that have migrated from the colon into the small intestine, the test can give you a general idea of what's migrating. This test can also diagnose fat malabsorption, which indicates a high likelihood of SIBO. Still, it cannot provide a diagnosis by itself.

Another test that may be used in diagnosing SIBO is the organic acids test (OAT), particularly the one from Great Plains Laboratory. As I mentioned previously, although all organic acids tests can be highly beneficial for assessing underlying factors contributing to one's health condition, it is my opinion that the Great Plains Laboratory test is superior to those marketed by other labs in its ability to identify both bacteria and candida. The OAT looks for high levels of byproducts in the urine that indicate the presence of bacteria or yeast. However, like any lab test, it is not foolproof. As I see it, the OAT should be done in conjunction with the breath test. Also, as mentioned in chapter 4, the organic acids test provides an abundance of information on other problems that may exist—for example, nutritional deficiencies, mitochondria function, detoxification, and serotonin, norepinephrine, and dopamine levels—allowing you to achieve many different goals at one time.

Dr. Allison Siebecker lists the following additional signs that indicate the presence of SIBO:[32]

1. Dramatic improvement in symptoms when you take an antibiotic

2. Worsening of symptoms when you take a probiotic (especially if it contains a prebiotic, which feeds bacteria)

3. Worsening of constipation or other symptoms with the consumption of fiber (soluble fiber feeds bacteria)

4. For a person with celiac, little improvement with a gluten-free diet (they replaced gluten with other starches)

5. Developing gastrointestinal problems after taking an opiate drug (opiates slow motility and migrating motor complex)

6. Persistent low ferritin levels with no apparent cause (note that parasites can also cause low ferritin levels)

7. Pancreatitis is concealed by a gas bubble on a CT scan (bacteria makes so much gas that it obscures the pancreas)

PHARMACEUTICALS AND HERBALS FOR SIBO

If you take the pharmaceutical route, the most common treatment for SIBO is the antibiotic rifaximin. However, by itself, it is not very effective for the methane-producing archaea organisms. Recall that SIBO may involve both hydrogen-producing bacteria and methane-producing archaea. According to Chris Kresser, research indicates that individuals with only methane-producing SIBO have clinical improvement about half the time with rifaximin; it clears methane from a breath test only about 28 percent of the time. The antibiotic neomycin produced a clinical response about 63 percent of the time and cleared methane from a breath test about 33 percent of the time. If rifaximin and neomycin are combined, then improvement rates go up to about 85 percent, and methane is cleared from the breath test about 87 percent of the time. Therefore, if a person tests positive for hydrogen only, then rifaximin is used alone, but if she or he tests positive for both methane and hydrogen, it is critical to use both rifaximin and neomycin in order to target the archaea. It's also important to be aware that archaea are resistant to most other antibiotics that are typically used on either gram-positive or gram-negative bacteria, which makes them much more difficult to treat.[33]

Fortunately, rifaximin and neomycin both are broad-spectrum drugs, but they are poorly absorbed (they remain mostly in the gut). They do not wipe out all the healthy bacteria the way a broad-spectrum antibiotic that is systemically absorbed would, which means they are less likely to contribute to serious side effects. According to Dr. Allison Siebecker, rifaximin doesn't contribute to yeast overgrowth and it actually decreases antibiotic resistance rather than increasing it; therefore, resistance is less likely to develop against it. Since treatment commonly has to be repeated, rifaximin may continue to be effective.[34] However, in Dr. Pimentel's book *IBS: A New Solution,* he states that resistance to rifaximin and neomycin does sometimes occur. In my practice, it is not uncommon for me to work with people who have no response at all to rifaximin or neomycin. And some people report that rifaximin is very effective the first time they take it, but less so on the second time around, indicating that resistance is developing. Additionally, rifaximin caused a significant flare in yeast overgrowth (more than most) when I took it myself. It also caused a lot more side effects than I experience with most other antibiotics that are systemically absorbed, like severe acid reflux, muscle spasms, and an increase in chemical sensitivities. Not only that, it made my SIBO worse than ever and caused horrific abdominal pain throughout the whole GI tract and all my internal organs. It was one of the worse things I've ever taken. I had to discontinue usage a little before the treatment course was over and the symptoms did not abate. Two weeks after discontinuing rifaximin, I developed a severe respiratory infection and had to take some systemically absorbed antibiotics, and they cleared up most of the symptoms that were caused by the rifaximin, but pain throughout the colon persisted and this was pain that was not present until the use of rifaximin. Other people have reported development of yeast overgrowth and a worsening of health after treatment with rifaximin as well. So, I don't agree with the stance that rifaximin doesn't promote yeast overgrowth or prevent resistance. And I question whether it is a good choice for treatment. Rifaximin supposedly has an anti-inflammatory effect by decreasing intestinal proinflammatory cytokines and inhibiting NF-kB via the PXR gene, making it less harmful than most antibiotics. However, it caused horrific inflammation for me, so I question whether this is true. Neomycin is slightly more absorbable than rifaximin and can be associated with some rather serious side effects. For these reasons, some practitioners use allicin from garlic in conjunction with rifaximin, to target the methane-producing organisms. Another antibiotic, Tindamax, may be used if a resistant clostridia species is involved.[35] In my own life, I've had good results with full-dose erythromycin, cefdinir, and doxycycline. Another good option might be minocycline or vancomycin. Prior to the emergence of rifaximin, the tetracyclines were the drug of choice for SIBO and in my experience seemed to work better in some cases. Rifaximin is outrageously priced in the U.S., making it hard for many people to afford. Be aware that you can purchase rifaximin from one of the online Canadian pharmacies and have it shipped to you at a significantly lower price.

Although I am not typically in favor of antibiotic use unless absolutely necessary, considering the serious deterioration in health that can result from SIBO, this may indeed be one of those times that meets the criteria of necessity. In some cases, it is the only way to keep it under control.

Nevertheless, be aware that research indicates that one out of every two SIBO sufferers treated successfully with antibiotics relapses within a year and requires retreatment, typically numerous times or even ongoing. In the real world, I think this number may be even higher. If you visit any Internet forum on SIBO, you will discover that almost everyone has relapsed and must be treated repeatedly. On the other hand, forum participation is probably skewed toward those whose treatment hasn't been successful. Even still, it is clear that the success rate is very low. I haven't worked with anyone who didn't have SIBO return after treatment and most people coming to me have already been to a handful of practitioners including some of the most well-known SIBO experts. The manufacturers of rifaximin state on their website that people using it for IBS-D (typically caused by SIBO) get relief from symptoms for an average of ten weeks.

One study found that herbal antibiotics can be just as effective as pharmaceutical-based antibiotics against SIBO. This study used one of the following protocols: either Dysbiocide with FC-Cidal (by Biotics Research Corporation) or Candibactin-AR with Candibactin-BR (by Metagenics).[36] Although at this time no other true studies have been done on herbals for this condition, other herbs that are commonly reported to be effective by practitioners include cat's claw, uva ursi, Tanalbit, allicin from garlic, olive leaf, grapefruit seed extract, berberine, Oregon grape root, goldenseal, lactoferrin, colostrum, monolaurin, pau d'arco, artemisia, yerba mansa, coptis, thyme, neem, oregano oil, cinnamon, and peppermint. Many of these herbs are discussed in more detail in chapter 7, if they contain antifungal capabilities.

As is the case with antibiotics, not all herbs that are effective against hydrogen producers are effective against the archaea methane producers. Most practitioners use high-potency allicin, which is obtained from garlic, to address the methane producers. However, if lactobacillus is involved in your overgrowth, know that garlic is ineffective against these species of bacteria. A case study involving only one person found peppermint oil to be effective against both hydrogen and methane.[37] Despite the lack of large-scale studies, many practitioners recommend the use of peppermint oil in the treatment plan. Peppermint has also been found to be effective for reducing methane in rumen microbiome production. (The rumen is the first chamber in a cow's alimentary canal.) Clove, eucalyptus, and oregano oil have also been effective at reducing methane production in cattle rumen.[38] There's a fairly new product on the market called Atrantil that is supposed to be effective against methane producers. Atrantil is an herbal combination that contains a couple of unique herbs along with peppermint leaf. I have not used this product personally as of yet, but some of my clients have reported mixed results. It's effective for some, but not others.

The herbs that work for one individual may not necessarily work for another. Results may depend on what species of bacteria the person is carrying, whether the bacteria are resistant to the particular agent used, potency of the herb, level of overgrowth, where the offending bacteria are located, or other biochemical factors—so some trial and error will be required. Herbs may have to be exchanged for other herbs if resistance develops, which it frequently does. Ideally, the herbs used against bacteria should be rotated in the same manner as described for antifungals in chapter 7, to help prevent mutation and resistance. In contrast to pharmaceutical-based antibiotics, since herbs contain many different compounds rather than just one, the upside is that they have a wider spectrum of activity that may enhance their efficacy against SIBO and other microbes. Many of the herbs that have antibacterial qualities are also powerful antifungals (e.g., cinnamon, berberine, cat's claw, oregano oil, Tanalbit, pau d'arco, grapefruit seed extract), making them effective against candida. Some may contain antiparasitical and antiviral qualities as well. Many of these remedies are discussed in chapter 7. Since candida frequently accompanies bacterial overgrowth, using the right herbs may permit you to kill two or three birds with one stone. Additionally, several different kinds of herbs can be combined to create a synergistic effect, which may also help prevent resistance and target more microbes at once.

The downside to some herbals is that die-off or side effects like inflammation or disruption to neurotransmitters in the brain can be so severe that they inhibit the individual's ability to work or fulfill daily obligations and responsibilities. Since they have to be taken for a minimum of four weeks, the disruption may go on for an extended period of time. This means herbs may not be an option for some people. In some cases, the pharmaceutical route can address the problem quicker and with less disruption to one's life. Additionally, many people with candida and SIBO just don't do well on herbs for one reason or another. It is important to give the body a break from herbs rather than taking them nonstop for months, as some of them do have the potential to kill friendly bacteria as well as pathogens, or to affect neurotransmitters in the brain.

Herbs, like pharmaceuticals, are seen as foreign substances by the body and can trigger numerous adverse effects. Before taking any natural-health remedy it is very important that you do your homework and have a thorough understanding of the whole scope of the particular remedy you are exploring, as well as of your condition. Be aware of all possible complications, side effects, and outcomes. Preferably you should work with a skilled professional to help you find the most beneficial mixture of herbs and supplements for your symptoms. Be sure to disclose to all health-care practitioners you work with all the medications or natural-health remedies you are taking and all the health conditions you have. You should practice the same precautions with herbal and natural remedies that you would with prescription drugs. Please read pages 174–178 for more information on precautions with herbal remedies before use.

Some herbs should not be taken for long periods of time. Uva ursi is an excellent antimicrobial and commonly prescribed for urinary tract infections, SIBO, and other bacterial infections. It has demonstrated strong antibacterial activity against a variety of bacteria, especially against *E. coli*.[39] Before the discovery of sulfa drugs, uva ursi was a common treatment for bladder infections. It also helps reduce inflammation and pain, heal tissue, and may contain some antifungal and antiviral characteristics. However, uva ursi is toxic in high doses and can cause liver damage if taken for too long. It should never be taken for more than two weeks tops. Some medical sources, like the University of Maryland Medical Center, recommend taking it for no longer than five days.[40] Uva ursi can have a diuretic effect, which causes one to lose too much potassium, and can affect how quickly the body gets rid of lithium, which can cause an elevation in lithium levels. If one is taking lithium, lithium dosage may need to be modified while taking uva ursi. I call this specific herb to your attention because I have encountered many people on Internet forums—as well as some of my own clients—who mention that they have been using it long term.

I also offer an extra word of caution in regard to neem. Neem is a favorite among many health-care practitioners because it affords antiviral, antibacterial, antiparasitical, antifungal, and anti-inflammatory characteristics, which means it can be used for candida, parasites, bacteria, and viruses, targeting all of them at once.[41] However, it can also significantly lower blood sugar levels. It is so effective at lowering blood sugar that it may be used for managing diabetes. When I took neem, my gastrointestinal tract felt absolutely wonderful, which indicates it is very effective against microbes. However, it lowered my blood sugar so dramatically that I nearly passed out on several occasions and therefore had to discontinue use. One of these occasions occurred while I was taking a bath, which could have resulted in drowning had I lost complete consciousness. People with low blood sugar issues, which are very common in candida overgrowth, SIBO, and adrenal fatigue, may have to avoid neem. Please read pages 174–178 for cautions in regard to other herbal remedies.

As mentioned in chapter 7, oregano oil was found to be as effective as streptomycin, penicillin, and vancomycin for killing bacteria. This same test found that oregano oil was more powerful than carvacrol (a chemical extracted from oregano oil) alone, and that it had antibacterial activity against twenty-five different bacteria.

Considering the fact that at least 50 percent of the people treated successfully for SIBO will experience a relapse within one year, and a large percentage of people don't achieve complete eradication and may need to undergo treatment numerous times, it can make more sense to try herbals before pharmaceuticals. Depending on how quickly overgrowth repopulates, one may need treatment several times a year or more. Most of us in the natural-health field would not be comfortable using an antibiotic so frequently. Another option would be to alternate pharmaceuticals and herbals with each treatment round. The option I like most is to hit them hard with a pharmaceutical and then maintain those improvements with herbals. People who have problems with the herbals may tolerate them better at this point, as there will be fewer organisms to kill, resulting in less inflammation and die-off. Then use pharmaceuticals again periodically as needed to keep overgrowth under control.

The decision about whether to use herbals or pharmaceuticals should be determined by weighing the positives against the negatives, how severe the level of overgrowth is, to what extent health has been compromised, the urgency for relief, other health conditions that may be present, and what allows the individual to function most optimally during treatment. Someone who has mild overgrowth and mild impairment to their health may be better off going the herbal route, while someone who is experiencing severe malnutrition and a failure to thrive may need to address the problem immediately with pharmaceuticals.

I'd like to share an observation that can affect treatment. When a severe flare in my SIBO levels occurred, I experienced most of my pain, inflammation, and gas in the duodenum area (center of my stomach), pancreas, and gallbladder. After I began using herbal antibiotics, most of the pain in that area went away, but it moved down to the cecum and ileocecal valve area (lower right quadrant). It appeared that the bacteria relocated to that area to try and escape the herbs, and it seemed that the herbs I was using were less effective at killing them when they get that far down in the gastrointestinal tract. Furthermore, I had a lot of brain symptoms and felt very ill when the bacteria were located in the duodenum, but not nearly as many problems when they moved to the cecum. Location definitely affects the type of symptoms one may experience. Additionally, in my experience, none of the herbs provide the same level of relief as a pharmaceutical-based antibiotic.

Bacteria also form biofilms within the body. Recall that a biofilm is a sticky matrix that allows microbes to hide from the immune system and from antimicrobials. Bacteria in the biofilm are much more resistant to treatment—as much as a thousand times more. Agents that can help break down the biofilm should accompany any antimicrobials used. Please read chapter 3 for more about how to address biofilms.

Taking an antimicrobial for the right length of time is very important. Dr. Allison Siebecker recommends fourteen days with an antibiotic and four to six weeks with herbals (length of treatment will vary with practitioners). She also states that treatment will be much less effective if the proper diet is not in place, the topic of the next section.[42] According to Dr. Pimentel's book, *A New IBS Solution,* he uses only a ten-day course of antibiotics, and he recommends consuming carbohydrates while taking an antibiotic to entice the microbes out of dormancy and make treatment more effective. However, I have found eating a lot of carbs during treatment creates unbearable symptoms, so I am not convinced that this is the right course of action. Especially with the herbals, as they do not kill it off as quickly as a pharmaceutical and overgrowth is continually becoming elevated with consumption of carbs. Additionally, if you have candida in addition to SIBO, the consumption of carbohydrates is going to exacerbate this situation. Furthermore, I have experienced good results with antibiotics even though I eat very low carb. So, I encourage you to experiment with your carb consumption while treating with antibiotics to see what is most effective and tolerable for you.

SIBO AND DIET

The diet for treating SIBO is very similar to the one for candida, except it is even lower in carbohydrates and fiber. The optimal diet for dealing with candida is addressed in chapters 10 and 11. Everything in those chapters applies to SIBO as well, just tweaked a little bit as described below.

Most bacteria prefer carbohydrates and soluble fiber as their primary sources of fuel. They produce gas when they ferment these substances. If one's diet contains a lot of carbs and fiber, the bacteria will multiply quickly, producing an abundance of inflammation, gas, and all the associated symptoms. The higher the level of carbohydrates and fiber in the diet, the more the bacteria will proliferate. The higher the number of bacteria, the more toxins and gases created, and the more symptoms one will experience.

If protein and fat are the predominant macronutrients in the diet, then fewer bacteria will grow, and those that do exist won't produce as much gas. Therefore, a low-carbohydrate diet can be used to reduce bacteria's food sources (polysaccharides, oligosaccharides, and disaccharides), ultimately leading to a reduction in symptoms. Many people can achieve dramatic improvements in a short amount of time by following the right SIBO diet.

This is true regardless of whether you have hydrogen- or methane-producing microbes. When you limit foods for the hydrogen-producing bacteria, you starve them out, which reduces the hydrogen that the archaea would convert into methane. In turn, this reduces archaea and methane levels as well, since archaea won't have as much hydrogen for fuel to survive and to convert into methane.[43] However, archaea are very robust and can survive a significant amount of time without hydrogen and may also metabolize other substances like sulfur and ammonia.

The primary foods these bacteria use as nutrient sources are called fermentable carbohydrates. They include the following:[44]

- starch (grains, beans, legumes, starchy vegetables)

- resistant starch (whole grains, seeds, legumes, potatoes, potato flour, green bananas, plantains, other starchy veggies)

- soluble fiber (grains, legumes, beans, nuts, seeds, vegetables, fruit, pectin, psyllium)

- sugar (in all forms, including fruit, lactose, fructose, sucrose)

- prebiotics (inulin, FOS, MOS, GOS, arabinogalactan) also found in beans, agave, vegetables, roots/herbs, bone broth, and some nuts

- alcohol (feeds bacteria, damages the gut, and inhibits DAO enzyme)

- sugar alcohols (also known as polyols; found in some fruits and vegetables, as well as maltitol, sorbitol, isomalt, mannitol, erythritol, xylitol, and inositol

Many of the above foods are eliminated not only because they feed bacteria and candida, but also because they promote inflammation, which encourages proliferation of pathogens. Grains and legumes contain high amounts of antinutrients that are damaging to the gut. Nuts and seeds also contain some degree of antinutrients that can cause inflammation and inhibit absorption of minerals. In people with healthy guts, nuts are not much of a problem as long as they are consumed in moderation. However, in the individual who has inflammation from SIBO or candida, they may contribute to the problem. Nuts and seeds are also exceptionally high in omega-6 fatty acids, which also promote inflammation when they're not in balance with omega-3 fatty acids. Other foods not listed above can be inflammatory if the gut is damaged—for example, nightshades, casein, and egg whites. Some people with SIBO report problems with ghee. Perhaps it is because some short-chain fatty acids (propionate and acetate) are converted into glucose or because their overgrowth involves a microbe that favors fat.

Raw foods (vegetables and fruit) should be avoided or limited because they are higher in fiber and resistant starch than cooked foods. Cooking vegetables and fruit until soft will lower the content of fiber and resistant starch. Additionally, fruit that isn't ripe is higher in resistant starch than ripe fruit, so be sure any fruit eaten is ripe.

Caffeine (including that contained in chocolate, raw cacao, and green tea) should also be avoided as it stimulates the liver to release sugar into the bloodstream. Caffeine depletes vital neurotransmitters in the brain (acetylcholine, GABA, dopamine, and serotonin) that are critical for regulating appetite, brain function, gut motility, and the migrating motor complex. Caffeine also triggers the stress response system, which can weaken immunity, inhibit motility and the migrating motor complex, kill friendly gut bacteria, and cause other issues. Please read more about caffeine on pages 290–294.

As discussed in chapter 10, artificial sweeteners should also be eliminated because they are chemicals, not real food substances, and they contribute to leaky gut, kill friendly flora, feed pathogenic bacteria, disrupt the endocrine system, and inhibit those vital neurotransmitters in the brain and gut. Their use is often associated with an increase in cravings for sugar and carbohydrates, a larger appetite, bingeing, weight gain, panic attacks, hyperactivity, depression, nervousness, attention deficit, headaches, irritability, seizures, dizziness, joint pain, and more. They can also cause numerous digestive disturbances, including abdominal pain and cramping, diarrhea, and nausea. Please refer to page 280–281 for more information.

Many practitioners recommend the Specific Carbohydrate Diet, a low-FODMAPs diet, or the GAPS diet for the treatment of SIBO. Each of these diets has produced a significant amount of success and is certainly a step in the right direction. But based on my experience and that of many of my clients, I don't believe that any of these diets are ideal because they permit an array of foods that are harmful to the gut and produce symptoms in some people. I feel that the best diet for SIBO, candida, or any other gut disorder is a low-carb paleo diet that also moderates the high-FODMAPs group of foods, high-histamine foods, high oxalate foods, and high-glutamate foods. The diet plan should be tailored specifically to each person according to their unique biochemical needs in what I call the Individualized Paleo Plan, all of which is discussed in great detail in chapters 10 and 11.

In most cases, total carbohydrate intake will need to be under 50 grams per day if SIBO is present. If overgrowth is severe, then it may need to be at 25 or 30 grams per day, until some improvements have been made. Some people with SIBO may need to go even lower or eliminate carbs all together to get relief. This includes complex and paleo-friendly carbs like sweet potatoes, yams, winter squash, taro, fruit, and nuts. As a matter of fact, as discussed in Dr. Norm Robillard's work, complex carbohydrates can be even more problematic for the individual with SIBO than simple carbs. Simple carbs are metabolized quickly, while complex carbs sit in the GI tract for a while, which means bacteria have access to them for a longer period of time.[45] I'm not saying that one should eat simple carbs, because they are bad for us for other reasons (e.g., they cause spikes in glucose and insulin, and they contribute to type 2 diabetes, obesity, heart disease, etc. and disrupt neurotransmitters). I just want to call to your attention the fact that complex carbs are problematic in other ways.

One's intolerance to the foods that feed bacteria can vary widely. Each person may have a different threshold depending on the severity of overgrowth, what types of bacteria are involved, where they are located, stress levels, other health conditions that may exist, damage to the gut, and whether candida is present as well. One person may be completely intolerant to all the foods on the list, while someone else may have to limit only a few of them. It may not always be necessary to eliminate a food completely; in some cases the food may simply need to be reduced to a smaller serving size or eaten less frequently. An individual's threshold can change from time to time in response to changes in their body and life. Carbohydrate tolerance may increase after overgrowth is reduced, or it may decrease if overgrowth increases.

For example, when my SIBO level was low, I could eat small servings of fruit and nuts ($^1/_2$ cup fruit and 2 tablespoons nut butter) three times a week with minimal discomfort. But when my SIBO was at its highest, I couldn't touch fruit and nuts. After an experiment with resistant starch, my SIBO level went through the roof. I completely lost my ability to consume fruit or nuts and had to stay under 30 grams of carbs per day. Additionally, if I experience a high-stress event, my abdominal pain increases significantly, and I can barely eat anything. When the stressful event passes, I return to baseline.

You, too, will need to experiment to learn how your body responds and adjust accordingly. Since many of the foods that feed bacteria can be beneficial to our health when eaten in moderation (like vegetables, fruit, and nuts), we don't want to remove foods unnecessarily. Additionally, be sure to challenge yourself periodically to see if your threshold has changed. However, do be careful when reintroducing carbs. It may take a while for the bacteria to recolonize, so you may get away with increasing your carb intake for a while—until the bacteria levels reach a certain point and symptoms return. Dr. Siebecker and Dr. Pimentel state that a low-carb diet must generally be continued even after successful treatment for SIBO to prevent overgrowth from returning.[46] Additionally, in regard to food sensitivities, memory B cells can cause inflammation and leaky gut to persist when the particular food reenters the diet.

Although thousands of different species of bacteria inhabit our gastrointestinal tract, most of them fall into two primary classes: the bacteroidetes and the firmicutes. Some may be friendly and beneficial, and others may cause disease. Whereas in a healthy gut, a vast array of different bacterial species compete for space and nutrients, in an unhealthy gut, the microbes are less diverse, and one individual type may become dominant. Your gut is an ecosystem, and like all ecosystems it is healthiest when there is greater diversity. Bacteroidetes eat a more diversified diet of protein, fat, and carbs, while firmicutes eat primarily carbs, including starches and fiber. Therefore, if firmicutes are present in abnormally high numbers, and the diet is heavy in carbs, overgrowth of firmicutes is encouraged. If these bacteria have wandered into the small intestine, as is the case in SIBO, they will make SIBO proliferate.

Research has found that people with IBS (which can be caused by SIBO) tend to have a higher number of firmicutes and less microbial diversity overall. It is theorized that most bacteria involved in SIBO are the ones that thrive on carbs. A diet that is high in the foods that firmicutes feed on may be what causes the overgrowth in the first place. In *Fast Tract Digestion: IBS,* Dr. Norm Robillard cites a variety of studies indicating that a diet high in complex polysaccharides encourages an increase in firmicutes, actinobacteria, and some strains of clostridia, but a decrease in bacteroidetes and other strains of clostridia. This scenario can lead to production of excess gas and toxins—and all the associated symptoms and conditions—as well as an increase in "microbe-mediated formation of carcinogenic compounds." Robillard explains that by eating a diet low in carbs, starches, and fiber, and richer in animal protein and fat, we create an environment that encourages healthy competition between our gut microbes, thereby favoring "survival of the well-adapted organisms best suited to be our partners in digestion and health." He writes that limiting food sources for the "polysaccharide loving microbes" puts them on a diet. Eating a diet rich in animal-based foods combined with a limited amount of fermentable carbs promotes an environment wherein species of bacteria that metabolize amino acids and other animal-based macronutrients can compete with the firmicutes and clostridia that prefer carbs, without allowing one or the other to become dominant.

By contrast, if overgrowth involves bacteroidetes, which feed on protein and fat as well as carbohydrates, restricting carbs may fail to provide complete relief of symptoms. Furthermore, just like candida, bacteria are exceptionally adaptable, and although they would rather have carbs as their food source, they will make do with whatever is present. They may also feed on blood glucose, which is always around to some degree even when dietary carbs are low, due to gluconeogenesis. Keep in mind that bacteria in soil and groundwater will even break down industrial solvents for energy. They are so effective at consuming industrial byproducts that they are often used to clean up toxic waste sites. This demonstrates how bacteria can adapt to and thrive in just about any environment or situation. Some will even survive in radioactive waste sites.[47,48] Again, how much relief is experienced with a change in diet will be influenced by how severe the overgrowth is, what species of bacteria are involved, and their adaptability.

To cite another example from my own life, when my SIBO level was mild, I could pretty much control my symptoms with a low-carb, low-FODMAPs, paleo diet. However, when my SIBO level was at its highest, and I was down to consuming no more than 25 to 30 grams of carbs per day, the same diet no longer provided complete relief. It was simply impossible to eat more carbs without triggering unbearable suffering. Then the bacteria began eating my protein and fat stores. If my carb consumption went over 30 grams per day, I had horrific abdominal pain and excess gas that smelled like sulfur. When I ate nothing but protein and fat, I had a milder level of pain and less production of gas. Still, I produced some gas, and it smelled like ammonia, which is an indication that bacteria are eating protein. For a while it was extremely painful to eat anything at all until I began using herbal antibiotics and eventually a pharmaceutical—which brings me to the next point. In most cases, diet alone will be insufficient for managing SIBO. It should be combined with one or more of the herbal or pharmaceutical antimicrobials discussed previously. According to Siebecker, diet alone has been successful in infants and children, but not adults.[49]

It is also recommended that one should not eat between meals. Allowing four to five hours between meals enables the migrating motor complex to move bacteria from the small intestine to the colon. Snacking between meals interrupts this process. Drinking water is permitted.

Bone Broth and Fermented Foods in Regard to SIBO

You may have noticed that many natural-health practitioners recommend the use of bone broth to remineralize and heal the gut from a variety of gastrointestinal disorders. Although bone broth can be highly beneficial in some conditions, that is not the case with SIBO. According to Dr. Siebecker, the joint and cartilage tissue that remains attached to the bones contains mucopolysaccharides (MOS), substances that feed bacteria, potentially exacerbating SIBO. She recommends that people with SIBO make broth from meat, not bone.

Bone broth is also exceptionally high in glutamate, which as discussed in chapter 10 can contribute to an imbalance in GABA and glutamate in people who lean toward glutamate excess. Excess gluta-mate is toxic to the brain, causing overstimulation and neurological inflammation, killing brain cells, and leading to the slew of mental health symptoms described earlier. It also impedes regulation of the lower part of the esophagus, interferes with bowel contractions and transit time in the gastrointestinal tract, inhibits IgA in the mucous linings, increases eosinophils, encourages overgrowth of microbes, fuels sympathetic dominance, and drives cravings for sugar and carbs. Please read about the importance of preventing excess glutamate on pages 30–31 and 435–444.

Bone broth is also high in histamine, which can be problematic for people who have high brain histamine (histadelia) or histamine intoler-ance. As mentioned previously, high brain histamine is associated with obsessive-compulsive disorders, sex and gambling addiction, brain racing, abnormal fears, attention deficit, hyperactivity, aggressiveness, disrupted sleep or insomnia, and even schizophrenia. Histamine intol-erance may be exhibited as hives, itching, flushing, wheezing, watery eyes, runny nose, nasal congestion, gastrointestinal distress, or motion sickness, to name just a few indications. Furthermore, some of the symptoms associated with histamine intolerance include constipation, diarrhea, abdominal swelling and pain, and fatigue—which pretty much mimic the symptoms of SIBO. High levels of histamine also pro-mote sympathetic dominance. Please refer to pages 29; 444–449 for more information on histamine.

Fermented foods, including cultured vegetables and kefir, are also high in histamine and glutamate. They contain a significant amount of alcohol, which, as you will learn in chapter 10, can make a person feel drunk and can lead to relapse in the alcohol addicted. Additionally, alcohol feeds bacteria and candida. Fermented foods also contain high levels of the bacteria that can exacerbate SIBO in some people, depend-ing on which types of bacteria are involved in the overgrowth. We will discuss this topic in more detail below, in the probiotics section.

To summarize, for people with high histamine and/or high gluta-mate, the consumption of bone broth or fermented foods can result in numerous symptoms associated with excess levels. Many people with gut disorders such as candida and SIBO may already have high hista-mine and glutamate levels, since both conditions can cause an increase in either one, so this is something to watch out for and moderate.

High levels of histamine and/or glutamate activate the stress response system and may keep one stuck in sympathetic dominance, which, as discussed, can inhibit gut motility and the migrating motor complex, kill friendly bacteria, and weaken the immune system.

While it is true that histamine intolerance can be caused by small intestinal bacterial overgrowth or candida, and that intolerance may improve if overgrowth is reduced, that is not always the case. Some species of bacteria have the ability to convert histidine in the diet into histamine. If these bacteria are present in high numbers, histamine levels may be elevated, which makes one more vulnerable to high-histamine foods. Additionally, the enzymes DAO (diamine oxidase) and HMT (histamine N-methyltransferase), which break down histamine, are created by enterocytes (cells) in the gut. Damage done to the gut from bacterial overgrowth or candida can impair adequate production of these enzymes, leading to buildup of histamine. In each of these situations, histamine intolerance may improve when overgrowth is addressed. However, until one is successful in eliminating SIBO, reduction in high-histamine foods will most likely be necessary.

Certain genetic polymorphisms can impair one's ability to produce both DAO and HMT. Additionally, DAO production can be inhibited by a deficiency in vitamin C or copper, both of which are needed for synthesis of the enzyme, and in vitamin B6, which is required as a cofactor to DAO to break down histamine. HMT requires the methylation process to inactivate histamine, so deficiencies in the nutrients required for methylation (e.g., folate, vitamins B12 and B6, magnesium, and SAMe), as well as genetic polymorphisms that affect methylation, like the MTHFR gene, may lead to undermethylation, impairing one's ability to break down histamine. Deactivation of histamine in the central nervous system is always achieved through HMT, because DAO does not exist in the central nervous system. Therefore, in some of these situations it becomes necessary to permanently avoid high-histamine foods, even if candida or bacterial overgrowth isn't present. Even when everything is working right, if one eats a diet high in histamines, the enzymes may be unable to keep up. Avoiding or limiting other high-histamine foods is usually required as well. You can find a list of high-histamine foods on page 347–348.

As mentioned in chapter 1, histamine is released from mast cells every time an antibody attacks a protein that escapes from the gut into the bloodstream, so histamine levels are elevated in patients with leaky gut, which commonly occurs in people with candida and SIBO. Toxins from candida can also trigger histamine release, so if one has candida and SIBO, the histamine load may be even higher. Please read chapter 13 for more information on keeping histamine in balance.

Elemental Diet

A diet called the elemental diet has been quite successful in addressing small intestinal bacterial overgrowth without any type of antibiotic. The elemental diet removes all solid food for two to three weeks, during which time the patient consumes only powdered, predigested nutrients mixed with water. It is commonly used in hospitals to treat a variety of gastro-intestinal disorders by giving the digestive tract a break. It completely starves out the bacteria because the nutrients are absorbed so quickly that the bacteria do not have a chance to access them. It has a success rate of 80 to 85 percent. Although elemental diets are available over the counter, I would not recommend attempting this diet without being under the care of a physician who has expertise in SIBO. Additionally, I believe that this option is best utilized only in extreme cases in which the individual is severely malnourished, is experiencing a failure to thrive, has symptoms that are disabling, or is on a diet that is too restricted.

The elemental diet formulas on the general market are loaded with ingredients we don't really want to put in our bodies. To avoid these ingredients, a homemade formula can be designed with amino acid formulas and a good source of fat like medium-chain triglycerides. I think it's best to leave out any sweetener, especially if you have candida in addition to SIBO.

However, like treatment with antimicrobials, overgrowth typically returns when one returns to eating normal. So, treatment with other methods must be ongoing.

OTHER FACTORS TO CONSIDER WHEN TREATING SIBO

Probiotics and SIBO

If you have SIBO, or suspect you have SIBO, be sure to read pages 199–204 before supplementing with probiotics or consuming probiotic foods. Probiotics and foods that are high in probiotics (cultured foods, fermented foods, etc.) can make SIBO proliferate and cause a significant decline in health. It may be best to avoid probiotics until the gut achieves a certain level of healing at the very least, and possibly long-term. Be sure to note that you may have SIBO and be unaware of it since many of the symptoms overlap with candida. Other conditions commonly associated with SIBO include GERD, IBS, autism, OCD, and autoimmune disorders, so if you have one of these conditions, chances are good that SIBO is present. As Dr. Pimentel points out in his book *A New IBS Solution,* if the migrating motor complex is not working properly, as is the case in SIBO, taking a probiotic may cause more bacteria to accumulate in the small intestine, making the problem worse. Considering all this, it is unclear whether probiotic use is advisable for the person with SIBO. Additionally, some bacteria in probiotics can increase D-lactate and histamine, both of which can create a wide array of neurological and gastrointestinal problems. Please also read on pages 475–484 about the potential dangers of supplementing with resistant starch as it can significantly increase SIBO levels and make the condition very difficult to turn around.

Supplementing with HCl, Enzymes, and Other Nutrients

Hydrochloric acid is frequently used to help modulate incoming bacteria levels. However, this is only called for if you have low stomach acid levels. Not everyone with SIBO does. You may have high levels of HCl, in which case supplementation would be counterproductive. HCl levels can be determined with an HCl challenge test; instructions are found on pages 89–91.

Supplementing with digestive enzymes like pancreatin may be beneficial. In *A New IBS Solution,* Dr. Pimentel states that pancreatic enzymes taken with meals can help digest food before bacteria have a chance to get them. This will not eradicate bacterial overgrowth, but it may improve the condition by 30 to 50 percent. It is critical to avoid anything that inhibits stomach acid production, for example, antacids, H2 inhibitors, and proton pump inhibitors.

Once overgrowth is eradicated, a variety of nutritional supplements may be used to help heal the gut lining (enterocytes and the brush border). High doses of vitamin C powder (buffered with calcium, magnesium, and potassium) can be used to promote gut motility until it begins to work better on its own. Many practitioners recommend a variety of mucilaginous herbs, including licorice, slippery elm, marshmallow, and aloe vera, which have proven beneficial for soothing the gut. That said, if SIBO has not been treated successfully, these herbs may encourage overgrowth of bacteria due to their high content of mucopolysaccharides, which feed bacteria.

If a patient has developed nutritional deficiencies due to candida or SIBO, nutritional support for the deficiencies should be implemented. But be aware that certain nutrients (e.g., iron, calcium, and magnesium) can be a food source for bacteria and candida and their biofilms; supplementing with them should be held off until bacteria and candida levels are decreased. Sometimes lactoferrin or an oral chelator are used to restrict the microbe's access to these minerals. There are a variety of other supplements that can be counterproductive for SIBO, please be sure to read chapter 14.

Sources of Inflammation

Anything that can contribute to inflammation and leaky gut needs to be addressed when treating SIBO, including candida overgrowth, parasites, and *H. pylori,* as well as the intake of substances including sugar, grains, legumes, caffeine, chocolate, food additives and preservatives, pesticides, herbicides, artificial sweeteners, heavy metals, birth control pills, and too many omega-6 fatty acids. Other potentially inflammatory factors include zinc deficiency, lack of sleep, casein, stress, chlorinated water, alcohol, food sensitivities, steroids, proton pump inhibitors, and NSAIDs. Although each of these factors may cause damage in a different way, the bottom line is that they all cause inflammation in the gut, and inflammation, regardless of where it comes from, may encourage overgrowth of bacteria, candida, or parasites.

Stress Management

As discussed, stress can play a major role in SIBO, candida, and other functional gut disorders because it weakens the immune system, impairs digestion, decreases gut motility, reduces secretion of stomach acid and digestive enzymes, kills friendly flora, inhibits nutrient absorption, floods the bloodstream with glucose, drains neurotransmitter levels, and deactivates the vagus nerve—all of which can encourage overgrowth of bacteria or other microbes. Chronic stress can cause dysfunction in the autonomic nervous system, triggering sympathetic dominance. It is critical that one manage stress on a daily basis.

Anything that stimulates the vagus nerve can be beneficial. One of the most effective methods for activating the vagus nerve and consequently the parasympathetic nervous system and the relaxation response is performing deep-breathing exercises. Please read chapters 12 and 13 for more information on proper breathing technique and other ways to manage stress and reduce sympathetic dominance.

Since optimal functioning of the vagus nerve is vital for stimulating the migrating motor complex, other factors that damage or inhibit its performance, like heavy metals and pesticides, would be critical to address as well.

Pesticides and SIBO

As discussed on page 53, pesticides like Roundup (glyphosate) and others impair the life cycle and function of healthy gut bacteria but don't affect clostridia or *E. coli,* potentially allowing these guys to become dominant. Glyphosate also impairs cytochrome P450 enzymes (which are critical for detoxification), contributes to nutritional deficiencies, and depletes serotonin and dopamine levels. It fosters overgrowth of an organism called *Pseudomonas aeruginosa,* which releases high levels of formaldehyde (a neurotoxin and a carcinogen) and other toxins.[50] Any of these reactions may create an environment that encourages overgrowth of bacteria and cravings for sugar and carbs. Other pesticides may have a similar effect. Many different types of pesticides increase blood glucose levels.

Other Environmental Toxins

Environmental toxins of all kinds—including those found in everyday products like dish soap, personal care products, perfumes and colognes, air fresheners, laundry soap, household cleaning products, and industrial solvents—can trigger the stress response system and deplete or inhibit the neurotransmitters serotonin, dopamine, and GABA, keeping one stuck in sympathetic dominance if they are exposed on a daily basis. Toxins can also get lodged in the small intestine and cause more damage to the already vulnerable gut, allowing pathogens to thrive. Living an environmentally friendly lifestyle, as described in chapter 13, is a critical component of healing SIBO.

Sleep

Getting adequate sleep is absolutely essential for proper functioning of the neurotransmitters that help regulate the stress response system, the immune function, and the hormones that moderate appetite and blood sugar levels. Lack of sleep causes neurons to become less sensitive to neurotransmitters, which impairs cellular communication. Sleep also plays a role in modulating gut motility and the migrating motor complex.[51] Sleep is discussed in more detail on page 399–402.

Electrosmog

As discussed in chapter 13, electrosmog (electromagnetic radiation fields discharged from wireless devices and other electronic equipment) has been found to cause pathogens like bacteria, mold, candida, and viruses to multiply in numbers and release higher levels of toxins. It may also alter cells within the brain, other parts of the nervous system, and the immune system, and disrupt cell-to-cell communication. Furthermore, electrosmog triggers the stress response system. Any of these reactions would hinder the treatment of SIBO.

Thyroid Function

One of the primary symptoms of an underactive thyroid is slow gut motility. The thyroid may be underactive because of weak adrenals, and weak adrenals often go hand in hand with candida or SIBO. Support for the adrenal glands is critical for thyroid function. Adrenal function is also vital for reducing sympathetic dominance. Please read chapters 12 and 13 to find how to support the adrenal glands and consequently improve thyroid function.

Other factors that may inhibit thyroid function include candida toxins, pesticides and herbicides, tyrosine insufficiency, selenium insufficiency, iodine deficiency, heavy metals, halides, problems in the pituitary or hypothalamus, neurotransmitter disruption, and insulin resistance.

Ileocecal Valve

Problems with the ileocecal valve, including those associated with SIBO, may respond positively to direct massage of that area. Gas created by SIBO can put pressure on the ileocecal valve and cause it to open. Any other issues that may be impairing function of the ileocecal valve should be addressed.

Gut pH

The pH level of the gut is important; a gut environment that is too alkaline will encourage overgrowth of many types of bacteria. As discussed in chapter 2, an alkaline gut environment is also a potential cause of candida. It can occur due to antibiotic use, a diet that is too alkaline, failure to produce enough stomach acid due to age or impaired production, chlorinated drinking water, a lack of acid-producing bacteria, and the use of certain drugs such as antacids, proton pump inhibitors, and ulcer medication. However, candida and other microbes release ammonia to lower the pH and create an environment that allows them to thrive, so try as you might they will try and undo all your efforts.

Enemas or Colonics

Studies have found that colonics or enemas can lower or even eliminate methane levels, thereby reducing symptoms of SIBO.[52] Either can be highly beneficial for eliminating toxins caused by candida or other microbes, and can even physically remove the organism itself. Be sure to use colonics or enemas sensibly. Using them every day could potentially do more harm than good. Additionally, an enema or colonic removes toxins and organisms from the colon only, not the small intestine. This means they will not fix the problem of small intestinal overgrowth, but they can be used to assist with symptom relief. Enemas are discussed in more detail on page 415–419.

Physical Activity

Getting regular physical activity is vital for gut motility. Mild to moderate exercise has been shown to stimulate the vagal nerve activity that stimulates gastric motility and to enhance the stomach's processing of food.[53] However, it is critical that exercise be mild to moderate—not too excessive or undertaken for extended periods of time. Too much exercise depletes neurotransmitter levels, releases histamine, weakens immune function, increases blood sugar levels, and triggers the stress response system. Please read page 407–413 to learn how to exercise properly.

Migrating Motor Complex

To review, the migrating motor complex (MMC) can be impaired by surgery, nerve damage, opiate use, stress, intestinal scarring, gastrointestinal infection, proton pump inhibitors, antacids, anatomical abnormalities, and some disease processes. Anything affecting the migrating motor complex should be addressed.

MAINTENANCE FOLLOWING TREATMENT FOR SIBO

As mentioned previously, at least 50 percent of the people treated successfully for SIBO will relapse within a year. Further, between 15 and 50 percent of SIBO sufferers fail to achieve successful eradication. One study found that treatment with antibiotics eliminated symptoms for an average of only twenty-two days.[54] Bacteria can repopulate in as little as two weeks, but it may happen gradually or be set off by something like a major life stressor or a change in diet or supplementation.

For example, I had significant improvement in my SIBO symptoms with an antibiotic I had taken for a respiratory infection, and the improvements remained steady as long as I stayed with a diet low in carbs and FODMAPs, in addition to my standard paleo regimen. Then I experimented with resistant starch, and things got worse than they had ever been.

The possible reasons for a setback are many, but they are most likely due to the fact that the underlying cause of SIBO was not corrected. Underlying problems may have to do with the ileocecal valve, the migrating motor complex, chronic stress, or inflammation and per-petuation from some other microbe like candida. They could also be due to the fact that some bacteria are spore formers, and spores are resistant to antimicrobials; when treatment subsides they repopulate. Additionally, some bacteria have the ability to make the body excrete zinc in the urine, weakening the immune system. Gram-negative bac-teria are more resistant to antibodies and antibiotics, so their presence could influence success rates. Furthermore, many of the bacteria may take refuge in the biofilm, which can be very difficult to penetrate. As we learned in chapter 3, the substances currently available for break-ing the biofilm are not always effective. Some bacteria may be resistant to any ingredient used. According to Siebecker, other factors that have been found to contribute to unsuccessful eradication include chronic narcotic use, anatomical abnormalities, Addison's disease, sclero-derma, inflammatory bowel disease, NSAID-induced ulceration, and colonic inertia (inability to properly move waste from the cecum into the rectosigmoid area).[55]

I haven't seen the experts mention this, but I think it is entirely possible that the bacteria send out some kind of signal via the vagus nerve that inhibits the migrating motor complex so they can remain where they want to be. Since we know they have the ability to send out signals that alter thoughts, mood, and behavior, change our internal environment to suit their needs, and disarm the immune system, this seems a logical conclusion.

Regardless of the reasons why, ongoing maintenance using all the methods presented in this chapter (adhering to a low-carb diet, man-aging stress and sympathetic dominance, supporting gut health, main-taining pH, avoiding acid blockers, etc.) will be required to prevent overgrowth from returning or to keep symptoms at a minimum in people who do not achieve complete eradication. If treatment failed to achieve complete eradication, or if overgrowth returns, treatment needs to be repeated periodically.

Both Dr. Pimentel and Dr. Siebecker, the two leading experts on the topic, state that following the low-carb SIBO diet must be continued after treatment to prevent relapse, even if one is 100 percent success-ful at eradication. Restriction of fermentable carbs at this point may or may not need to be as strict as it was pretreatment, because the threshold may change and can vary from person to person. One should experiment to find what works for them, and they should continue to keep meals spaced four to five hours apart (with water allowed) to encourage the migrating motor complex to function optimally.

Since it is believed that dysfunction of the migrating motor complex is a primary underlying cause of SIBO, Drs. Siebecker and Pimentel encourage the use of substances that stimulate the MMC, called prokinetics. Prokinetics are taken for a minimum of three months— or potentially very long term—after antimicrobial treatment. They include low-dose naltrexone, low-dose erythromycin, and low-dose tegaserod.[56] However, each of these comes with a substantial risk of creating new problems. I cannot say I support the use of any of these options. Naltrexone targets endorphin receptors; any time an artificial substance is used to manipulate neurotransmitters it results in more disruption of the neurotransmitter, possibly leading to addiction and to a wide array of physiological and psychological symptoms. Erythromycin is a broad-spectrum antibiotic, so naturally it would be counterproductive to take it on an ongoing basis. Additionally, low-dose erythromycin has been found to increase biofilm formation in some organisms.[57] Tegaserod was removed from the market by the FDA because it was associated with an increased risk for heart attack and stroke, but it may still be obtained for emergency situations with permission from the FDA.[58] It is my opinion that each of these methods are too risky; research needs to focus on searching for more natural forms of prokinetics. It appears that the herb ginger-root has some natural prokinetic properties; it may work for some.[59]

CANDIDA, SIBO, OR *H. PYLORI?*

Candida, SIBO, or *H. pylori* may occur alone, but they frequently exist in conjunction with one another, or one leads to another at some point. Since many of their symptoms overlap, testing for each is unreliable, and complete eradication is very difficult to achieve for each, differentiating between them or getting an accurate diagnosis can be a challenge.

Gut dysbiosis makes a person vulnerable to any microbe, so the presence of any of the conditions may open the door for one or both of the others. Sometimes it can be hard to know which came first; however, one thing is certain: they can all perpetuate one another. Each can cause inflammation and degradation of the gut lining, compromise the immune system, and incite sympathetic dominance, creating an environment that encourages proliferation of the others.

To review, overgrowth of bacteria in the small intestine may cause elevated levels of ammonia, which increases gut pH, weakens the immune system, impairs function of the ileocecal valve, and creates leaky gut—any of which would create an ideal environment for candida. Hydrogen, which is produced by bacteria, is *H. pylori*'s primary source of energy, so SIBO provides a constant source of food for *H. pylori*. Candida can attach itself to bacteria, protecting it from antifungals. Candida can also create opiates, deplete acetylcholine and serotonin, increase histamine and intestinal permeability, impair thyroid function, disrupt immunity, damage the ileocecal valve, and cause sympathetic dominance, encouraging small-intestinal bacterial overgrowth. *H. pylori* can hide inside candida yeast cells. If *H. pylori* colonizes the small intestine, it will contribute to inflammation and leaky gut, which can encourage both SIBO and candida. If it colonizes the stomach, it will reduce hydrochloric acid levels, which fosters the overgrowth of other bacteria and candida. Intestinal parasites may perpetuate SIBO or candida. It has been found that bacteria can attach to parasites, and parasites may harbor candida.

If SIBO or *H. pylori* is present and not addressed in a person who has candida, they may fail to make much progress in eradicating yeast overgrowth—and vice versa. It is important to know which microbe(s) you are dealing with and to address each of them accordingly. Taking a pharmaceutical-based antibiotic may be necessary to address bacterial infection before undergoing antifungal treatment—even though doing so may seem counterintuitive due to antibiotics' impact on candida. Recall that many of the herbal antibiotics (e.g., oregano oil, cat's claw, berberine, cinnamon, turmeric) are effective against bacteria *and* candida; they may allow an individual to address both conditions simultaneously.

The symptoms of these three conditions are so similar that SIBO is often mistaken for candida or *H. pylori*. I've listed below a few characteristics of SIBO that I've experienced and witnessed in the people I work with and that set it apart from either candida or *H. pylori*.

- SIBO is more painful, and the symptoms (particularly in the upper

GI if located in the duodenum area, and center of the abdomen or lower right quadrant if located in the distal) can be much more severe.

- The psychological symptoms of small intestinal bacterial over-growth are much broader and more disruptive.

- With SIBO, the diet needs to be lower in carbs and more restrictive with fruit and nuts. Bacteria are much less forgiving than candida when you stray even a little bit from those limitations, and the complications can be harsher.

- The overall health of the individual with SIBO tends to be significantly more compromised than it is in candida or *H. pylori*.

- SIBO gastrointestinal symptoms are more concentrated around the center of the stomach (near the navel).

- Acid reflux, GERD, heartburn, indigestion, and belching tend to be related more to SIBO or *H. pylori* than to candida.

- SIBO is noisy (causes lots of gurgling, rumbling, moaning, and squirting in the midsection). Candida isn't.

- With candida, you may indeed have excess gas after eating carbs, but the gas that is produced by SIBO is much greater in quantity and much fouler. It may smell like ammonia or sulfur.

As someone who has dealt with candida for decades and SIBO for only a few years, I can tell you that candida is a walk in the park compared to SIBO.

H. pylori and SIBO can be hard to differentiate as well because they both can produce upper-GI symptoms such as acid reflux, burning sensation in the abdomen, heartburn, and belching. However, *H. pylori* symptoms are typically experienced higher up in the abdomen. That said, SIBO symptoms can radiate outward and upward.

SIBO and *H. pylori* both produce a great deal more belching than candida. SIBO belching originates from lower in the stomach, near the belly button or cecum, while *H. pylori* belching originates higher up. If you pay close attention when belching, you can feel where it originates from.

If you get really in tune with your body, you can also identify where your gas is originating from. When you expel gas, if you feel it in your upper abdomen, then it is likely caused by SIBO. If you feel it in your lower abdomen, it is likely caused by bacteria or candida in the colon.

Symptoms that develop as soon as food hits the stomach are more likely to be caused by *H. pylori* because it is the only microbe that can survive in that acidic environment. However, candida and bacteria do reside in the mouth and esophagus, and they become active as soon as food enters the mouth. If gas begins within about thirty minutes of eating, it indicates that fermentation (due to the presence of candida or bacteria) is taking place in the small intestine. It typically takes about five or six hours after eating for food to make it to the colon. Yet *H. pylori* may also inhabit the first section of the small intestine (duodenum), so it could be the source of belching and pain that begin within thirty minutes.

You can get a general idea of where the bacteria or candida are colonized by the timing of your symptoms. Symptoms occurring earlier in the digestive process indicate that the microorganisms are located higher up in the small intestine; their occurrence later in the process indicates they are farther down in the small intestine; occurrence after five or six hours indicates they are in the colon. Transit time varies from person to person, so these estimates may be inexact for any given individual. Additionally, once overgrowth becomes elevated in the small intestine, then symptoms may be constant, making it difficult to differentiate.

Candida responds very well to a low-carb diet; many symptoms will resolve with changes in diet alone. SIBO requires significantly more restriction of carbs and fiber, including vegetables, fruit, and nuts. If SIBO is severe, it may fail to improve much with diet alone, or the complete elimination of nuts and fruit may be required. In some cases, even the low-carb vegetables may need to be strictly limited as well. Not following the diet makes SIBO symptoms unbearable. Additionally, some bacteria feed on protein and fat, so even those macronutrients can become problematic to some degree in SIBO.

H. pylori symptoms will also persist to some degree even in the face of a low-carb eating plan. If you are following the paleo for candida diet faithfully, as I suggest, but still have a lot of upper and middle GI symptoms and/or psychological symptoms (depression, anxiety, unexplained fear or paranoia, OCD, brain fog), then you need to focus more on addressing SIBO and *H. pylori,* and you should explore the possibility of other bacteria and parasites.

MY SIBO STORY

I've been managing my candida for more than twenty-five years pretty successfully. But, around the age of fifty, I developed new GI problems that didn't respond very well to my usual regime. The new symptoms were much more severe and were located more in my upper GI and small intestine, where I had never really experienced symptoms before. The low-carb paleo diet I had been following for years wasn't working to alleviate these new symptoms. I had to reduce my carb intake even further, down to 25 or 30 grams on most days, with an allowance of around 60 or 70 grams three times a week. This helped a lot for a while, but gradually things got worse, despite the very low carb diet and the removal of FODMAPs. Weird brain symptoms began to develop intermittently, including intense brain fog, a choppy thought process, the unwanted repetition of songs or phrases, and high levels of fear. At one point, I feared I might be getting Alzheimer's and even began to have conversations with my adult son about what should be done if he began to notice more deterioration. I knew I wasn't dealing with candida, because candida had never been so painful, produced gas with that particularly foul smell, or triggered those types of brain symptoms.

Initially, my health-care team and I attributed the setback to *H. pylori* and parasites. Parasite treatment helped some, but not completely, and I managed to keep *H. pylori* to a minimum, but was unable to eradicate it completely until I treated for SIBO. I came to realize that I had developed SIBO when I was forced to take an antibiotic for a persistent respiratory infection. It coincidentally cleared up my gastrointestinal and brain symptoms and made me feel better than I had in a long time. In the past, antibiotics had caused a flare in my candida symptoms. I did some research and discovered that improvement of one's symptoms on antibiotics is an indication for SIBO.

At first I thought I felt better because the antibiotic had cleared up my *H. pylori,* but several months later I experimented with resistant starch, and all those gastrointestinal and brain symptoms returned with a vengeance. I wondered what the heck was going on. The symptoms were excruciating, and I couldn't touch fruit or nuts at all without severe brain symptoms and unbearable gastrointestinal pain. Even protein and fat became problematic because the bacteria began to eat them as well.

More research led me to discover that a negative reaction to resistant starch is an indication of SIBO. Bacteria feed on it as they do any other starch. I realized that resistant starch fed SIBO, causing them to produce hydrogen, which in turn fed *H. pylori*. My main focus now needed to turn to SIBO, without ignoring candida or *H. pylori*. I started herbal antibiotics, and my symptoms once more began to dissipate, which confirmed that the major problem was bacterial. However, the herbals weren't strong enough, and I was forced to take a pharmaceutical-based antibiotic. By accident, I had discovered that supplementing with resistant starch can be downright dangerous in the presence of small intestinal bacterial overgrowth. Please read page 475–484 to educate yourself further on resistant starch. Currently, I still must retreat my SIBO a couple times a year with a broad spectrum, systemically absorbed pharmaceutical based antibiotic, remain under 25 grams of carbs per day, and use herbal antibiotics periodically throughout the year, to keep it manageable.

I share my experience with you to demonstrate how confusing it can be to identify the right condition you may be experiencing. SIBO can develop so gradually that you don't realize you have it until months or years after its onset, when you can look back and see how it unfolded. I hope my story helps you know what signs to look for and identify the problem more quickly.

Fortunately, most of the steps that are required to improve candida overgrowth will also be beneficial for *H. pylori* and SIBO, if you have them. That said, if SIBO and/or *H. pylori* are present, treating candida alone will be insufficient. The healing plan must address each of the disorders.

CHAPTER 7

Antifungals and Probiotics

Now we'll turn our attention from the numerous *problems* presented by overgrowth of candida and other pathogens to the various options for treating them. This chapter discusses two methods for targeting the microbes directly: antifungal medications and probiotics.

ANTIFUNGALS

As you may know, an antifungal is a substance that is taken to kill the candida organism directly. In combination with the diet, it is the next critical element of the healing plan. There are many different types of antifungals, both prescription-based and natural. Some of the natural antifungals can be as powerful as the pharmaceuticals. Some are applied topically, while others are ingested. A topical antifungal is used to target a specific area of the body externally—for example, the toenails or vagina—while an oral antifungal is directed at the gut and/ or other areas internally or systemically. Prescription antifungals that are designed for topical use should never be ingested, as they contain a variety of ingredients that would not be suitable for consumption.

Strategies for Antifungal Use

The first vital point to be aware of in regard to antifungals is that different species of fungi and even different strains within a species respond differently to various antifungals. An antifungal that is effective against one species may be ineffective against another species or even against a different strain within the same species. An antifungal that is effective for you may not produce the same result in someone else with candida. Additionally, since candida has the ability to mutate, an antifungal may be effective for you for, say, one week, but not for the next week. Some species and strains of candida can be highly resistant to all treatment. Furthermore, remember that an individual may harbor more than one species or strain of candida, and even those can change over time. For all these reasons, I cannot recommend a particular antifungal, because the ideal one for you depends on the species and strains of candida you are carrying. Generally, each person has to experiment with various types and combinations of antifungals to find what works best for them, and they must remain aware that their needs may change over time.

The second vital point to know about antifungals is that they should be alternated in order to reduce adaptation, mutation, and resistance of the targeted microbes. If you pick just one or two antifungals and take them indefinitely, it is only a period of time before candida will mutate and develop resistance or find another way to adapt. The longer candida is exposed to one particular antifungal (or other type of treatment), the greater the chance it will adapt, mutate, and develop resistance. I've seen candida mutate against an antifungal in as little as two weeks. My recommendation is that a specific antifungal should be taken for no longer than a week, but definitely no longer than two weeks.

I propose that an individual select four different antifungals that appear to be effective against their candida. We will call them antifungal 1, antifungal 2, antifungal 3, and antifungal 4. In week one, antifungal 1 is taken; in week two, antifungal 2 is taken; in week three, antifungal 3 is taken; and in week four, antifungal 4 is taken. In week five, you restart with antifungal 1. Periodically, to maintain diversity, you may want to choose another set of four antifungals and rotate them along with your first set.

However, research suggests that we can decrease resistance and increase effectiveness by combining two or more different types of antifungals. Candida finds it more difficult to mutate when confronted with several different compounds at once, and the combination of compounds produces a synergistic effect. Therefore, you may get even better results if you use a couple of different antifungals in combination per week so you have one set that is taken in week one and a different set in week two and another set in week three and a whole new set in week four. Then in week five, go back to set one. Each of the different types of antifungals has a distinct way of killing and contains unique compounds. If a variety of antifungals is used simultaneously, candida is exposed to a number of different attacks, which will increase your chances of success. When you keep candida guessing, throw many different things at it at once, and change your plan of attack periodically, it doesn't know what to expect or have time to adapt and mutate. This is true of all treatment strategies, not just antifungals; the name of the game is change and diversity.

The labels of many herbal antifungal formulas state that the product needs to be taken for two to four weeks to be effective. If you choose to use one of these products, you can try taking it for the prescribed amount of time to see what kind of response you get. Resistance may not develop during the recommended time period. However, the next round of antifungals should consist of herbs that were not present in the last combination. Some formulas contain ten or twenty different kinds of antifungals. Although confronting candida with such a wide array of compounds at once can provide a variety of benefits, it is also extremely dangerous. You are at great risk of becoming resistant to every antifungal in the formula simultaneously. Combining different types of antifungals decreases resistance, but it does not eliminate the occurrence. I have grown resistant to formulas containing several different antifungals when I've taken them for long periods of time. The same is true for many of my clients. If you use one of the formulas that combine a large number of antifungals, be sure that you have a list of other antifungals that are not present in the combination to use at another time in case resistance develops. I think it is best to limit the number of antifungals in the combination to two or three. That way, if you become resistant to the formula, you still have many other choices at your disposal.

It is also critical to be sure that your species and strains of candida are susceptible to each of the antifungals used in your rotation. Using one or more antifungal that your candida isn't sensitive to could be counterproductive and contribute to resistance and adaptation, besides the fact that you'd be throwing money away. How do you know if your candida is susceptible to an antifungal? You should feel it. There may be an increase or a decrease in symptoms, you may feel worse or better, but it should be clear that something is happening. If you don't get any kind of effect, then most likely your candida is not susceptible to that particular antifungal and it should be eliminated from your rotation. Don't just jump in and start rotating any antifungal combinations you've read about. Take some time, experiment, test different formulas, and monitor how you respond—then design your protocol based specifically on your observations. You will consistently need to stay alert and watch for signs of resistance as you proceed with your rotation because things can change at any time. If you grow resistant to one of the antifungals in your rotation, it should be replaced with something else that has demonstrated effectiveness.

A variety of stool tests are available to assess one's susceptibility to different antifungals. However, the drawback to this method is that before testing for susceptibility, the stool test must first identify the presence of candida, which, as we established in chapter 4, doesn't happen very reliably. If you're fortunate enough to be one of the rare few whose candida shows up in a stool test, then testing for antifungal susceptibility can be a valuable tool. Since the stool test most frequently demonstrates false negatives for candida overgrowth, most people won't have this option. Additionally, keep in mind that just because your candida shows up as susceptible on the test to a particular antifungal today doesn't mean it will be susceptible next week. It could mutate and become resistant shortly after being exposed to the antifungal. Susceptibility testing can be a good guide for getting started, but anyone who relies on this method would have to test repeatedly to make sure sensitivity hasn't been lost.

I would like to make you aware that there are different schools of thought on this topic. Rather than rotation, some practitioners may recommend increasing the dosage of the antifungal or taking it for a longer period of time to help overcome resistance, but I have not found either of these methods to be effective in the long run. Increasing the dosage may demonstrate some effectiveness initially, but it is only a matter of time before the dosage needs to be increased again and the antifungal eventually stops producing results. Other professionals may suggest that you stick with a formula if you find that it works, but my experience has proven that if one particular antifungal or combination is used continuously, it is only a matter of time before resistance develops and it is no longer effective. That said, this method could work as long as you make sure to have a very long list of antifungals that you have tested and that can replace the current one. So, in other words, one could take an antifungal that is effective until resistance develops, then switch to another product until resistance develops, and so on. The risk here is that you could potentially become resistant to every antifungal used. Rotating helps decrease this risk. It is my opinion that the combining and rotating of antifungals achieves the highest level of effectiveness. Still, different things work for different people, so you're certainly free to experiment with different approaches, but do so with awareness of the risks, and protect yourself from inadvertently eliminating all the effective antifungals from your arsenal. You should note that taking a dosage that is too low can also contribute to resistance.

The patient's failure to be aware of or to address these three factors (susceptibility, combining, and rotating) is a primary reason why so many antifungal treatment regimens are ineffective. Dealing with each of them is crucial to achieving success in one's healing protocol. I learned this fact early in my candida journey through personal experience. When I first began treatment more than 25 years ago, I would take a particular drug or natural remedy for candida, and it worked great for a while. I would think I was about to be cured. Then the remedy would suddenly become completely ineffective, and my symptoms returned. None of the doctors I saw had an explanation for what was happening. It occurred with every antifungal I used, both natural and prescription. Then, I came upon an article about candida in *Discover* magazine that discussed mutation, and I understood why I'd had this problem. I had grown resistant to all the antifungals that were known to be effective in the 1990s because I had used them all and my candida had mutated. Later, as new antifungals were discovered, I learned that if I alternated them I could prevent mutation and resistance. I have heard this same story more times than I can count from my clients over the years. The following statement encapsulates one of the most common reasons people come to me for a consultation: "I was taking X, Y, or Z antifungal, and it worked absolutely great for a period of time, but all of a sudden it stopped working. Why is this happening to me?"

There is a slight catch-22 in regard to the need for alternating antifungals when it comes to pharmaceutical-based options. Generally, the pharmaceuticals need to be taken on a consistent basis to achieve optimal results. For example, nystatin is typically prescribed for three to six months or longer, and Diflucan is prescribed for anywhere from ten days to a month or longer. Many people grow resistant within this time frame. I believe the best course of action with the pharmaceuticals is to take them as prescribed and make as much progress as you can before mutation and resistance happen. A pharmaceutical can be a good way to make a lot of progress quickly, but once the treatment is over you should switch to a combination of natural antifungals on a rotating basis for maintenance. Hit the microbes hard with pharmaceuticals, and maintain any improvement with natural options. Alternatively, as you'll learn further ahead, some studies have found that the combination of certain pharmaceuticals with certain natural-based options can enhance the effectiveness of both. Adopting this protocol is another option. And, some practitioners may have you rotate the pharmaceuticals as well.

As anyone with chronic candida knows, or as the astute practitioner who works with candida patients has witnessed repeatedly, when one discontinues their antifungals and/or their diet for candida, symptoms generally return in full force. The reasons for this are many: The substances available at this time for breaking down the biofilm are not very effective for everyone, so the antifungal is unable to reach all the colonies of candida (recall that those inside the biofilm are much more resistant to treatment than free-floating organisms). A certain degree of improvement will be made while the antifungal is in the system, but once it is gone the remaining colonies multiply. Candida and other microbes are able to disarm the immune system. When attacked, candida releases a lot of spores, which are not affected by the antifungal. They lie dormant until the antifungal is out of the system and then return when the coast is clear. Candida hides or hibernates by burrowing deep into tissue where the antifungal cannot reach it and then repopulates when the antifungal is discontinued. Alternatively, it may convert into a cell wall–deficient form, which enhances its ability to hide. Dr. William Shaw, founder of the Great Plains Laboratory, who has done extensive and superb work with candida and autism, has the following mind-boggling theory for another possible explanation: "The yeast have genetically transformed some of the human cells that line the intestinal tract so that some of the human cells now contain yeast DNA. These genetically transformed human cells produce both yeast and human products and are somewhat sensitive to antifungal drugs but are not killed by them and produce yeast products whenever antifungal drugs are absent."[1] The bottom line is that it doesn't matter how long one takes an antifungal; most people with chronic candida see it return to some degree once they discontinue the antifungal. Future treatment needs to focus on preventing morphogenesis and resistance in addition to tackling biofilms.

For these reasons, in most cases, antifungals must be used on an ongoing or intermittent basis. How often they must be used varies from person to person—depending on how severe the overgrowth is, how quickly and to what extent they repopulate, the biofilms that are present, whether improvement in dysbiosis is achieved, how strong the gut lining and immune system are, other microbes that may be present, and possibly other unknown factors. One person may be unable to stop the use of any antifungals without a significant decline in health, and another may only need to do maintenance several times a year—or anything in between. Each person can gauge how often they need to use antifungals by how quickly their candida repopulates, which is determined by noting when their symptoms return after the antifungal is discontinued.

If the individual has strong biofilms, as described in chapter 3, then no antifungals may be very effective. Remember that candida in a biofilm may be one thousand times more resistant than candida outside the biofilm. It is critical that antifungals be taken in conjunction with products that break down the biofilm, all of which are presented in Chapter 3. Additionally, if a patient has issues with bacteria, viruses, or parasites, then the agents that are effective at killing them need to be taken as well, and they, too, should be alternated and combined to minimize mutation and resistance.

Let's take a closer look at some of the specific antifungals that are available to treat candida.

Pharmaceutical Antifungals

There are a wide variety of pharmaceutical-based antifungals to choose from. This section outlines some of the most common. They include the following (brand names are capitalized; generic names are lowercased):

- nystatin
- Nizoral (generic name: ketoconazole)
- Diflucan (generic name: fluconazole)

- amphotericin B
- Sporanox
- voriconazole
- posaconazole
- echinocandins (capsofungin, micafungin, and anidulafungin, which is marketed under the brand name Eraxis and is given intravenously)
- Lamisil (generic name: terbinafine, which is for topical use only, typically on the toenails, fingernails, and scalp)

Pharmaceuticals can be very effective if your particular species and strain of candida are susceptible to the particular drug. However, many of them also come with an array of side effects, some of which can be very serious. The biggest concern is that they can harm the liver. This is especially true of the azole class of drugs. If you're taking any of these drugs, your doctor should order blood tests on a regular basis to monitor your liver enzymes. If your doctor isn't doing this, you should request that she or he do so. I am shocked by the number of my clients who report that their doctors hand out antifungals and do absolutely no monitoring of the liver. My liver enzymes became elevated on all the pharmaceuticals I tried except nystatin.

Pharmaceutical-based antifungals can be obtained only with a prescription, so it will be necessary to have a doctor who has at least some knowledge of candida if you want to take this route. I talk more about finding the right physician in chapter 15. Again, keep in mind that not all species and strains of candida are susceptible to all drugs, even coming out of the gate. Some are highly resistant to any type of treatment, even initially. For example, all strains of *Candida glabrata* are resistant to the azole drugs (both Diflucan and Nizoral), but not to amphotericin or nystatin. Taking azole drugs can make you susceptible to developing one of the azole-resistant strains of candida. *Candida krusei* is intrinsically resistant to fluconazole and has a decreasing sensitivity toward amphotericin.[2,3]

Polyene antifungals, which include nystatin and amphotericin and others not mentioned here, bind with sterols (particularly with the ergosterol in fungi) contained within the cell wall of the organism, causing the internal contents to leak out and consequently death to the cell. Human cells contain cholesterol instead of ergosterol, so they are less susceptible to the effects of polyenes. However, at some dosages, amphotericin B may have the ability to bind with cholesterol, which increases its risk for toxicity. Amphotericin B also has antiprotozoal capabilities and is effective against geotrichum (another type of fungi), so it could address those issues as well.[4]

Nystatin is probably the most widely used prescription-based anti-fungal and can produce good results if one is not resistant to it. It is also the safest antifungal drug because it does not enter the blood-stream. Dr. William Shaw believes that nystatin is just as safe as the natural antifungals.[5] It remains in the gut and doesn't elevate liver enzymes; therefore, it can be taken for long periods of time with little risk. Remember, if you are not seeing some type of effect, it means resistance has developed. So if you're taking nystatin and symptoms return, then it should be discontinued. Nystatin is available in a variety of different forms, including tablet, lozenge, and powder. Avoid the tablet form and take the powder form instead, because Nystatin needs to coat the entire alimentary canal (mouth, throat, esophagus, intestines) as candida can reside in all those places. The tablet form doesn't come in contact with all those areas, which would permit the yeast to repopulate. The lozenge form doesn't allow the patient to start with small doses and work up to larger ones, and it may contain a variety of undesirable additives.

On the negative side, nystatin can cause die-off symptoms that are brutal and sometimes unbearable. In order to minimize a big die-off event, I was taught by my first candida doctor many years ago that one should begin treatment with nystatin by dipping the end of a toothpick into the nystatin powder and stirring it into a small glass of water three or four times per day. Each day you can slowly increase how much powder you put on the toothpick, gradually working your way up to a teaspoon three or four times a day. Be sure to swish the solution around your mouth. There is a powder that is designed for topical use and one for oral use. Be sure your doctor knows the difference (many do not); you don't want to consume the one that is designed for topical use as it contains unhealthy additives. Unfortunately, it is becoming increasingly difficult to find a pharmacy who carries the oral powder form. A compounding pharmacy is your best bet.

Nystatin powder is great for vaginal yeast infections. You can purchase empty cellulose capsules, fill them with the powder, and insert a capsule into your vagina like a suppository. It is also very effective in an enema as it will kill candida in the colon on contact, lowering one's candida level very quickly and providing dramatic and immediate improvements in symptoms. Nystatin powder can also be used nasally, by sniffing the powder, to help with fungus in the sinus cavity. The powder can also be mixed with water to form a paste and applied to any area desired.

Since nystatin stays in the gut and doesn't enter the bloodstream, it is not effective for systemic candida. If candida is systemic, nystatin must be used in conjunction with something that gets into the bloodstream, like Diflucan or Nizoral. Amphotericin B is also restricted to the gut, so the same would be true for it as well. According to Dr. William Levin, if one is taking amphotericin B, renal function must be monitored by measuring serum creatinine, blood urea nitrogen (BUN), and serum potassium levels.[6]

The azole class of drugs—which includes Nizoral, Diflucan, voriconazole, posaconazole, Sporanox, and many others—inhibits cytochrome P450-dependent enzymes within the organism that are required for biosynthesis of ergosterol. As mentioned, ergosterol is essential for structure and function of the fungal cell membrane. Since humans also have cytochrome P450 enzymes that play a critical role in their health, these types of drugs have the potential for toxicity.

Diflucan can initially produce dramatic improvements. However, candida grows resistant to Diflucan very quickly. In my experience, and that of nearly every person I have worked with, Diflucan makes you feel absolutely wonderful at first, but within a month or so it is no longer effective and symptoms return. Then what, you may wonder, is the point in taking it? You can significantly lower your candida level before resistance sets in, then follow up with some of the natural-based antifungals to maintain your level of healing. As noted in chapter 5, Diflucan may be effective for suppressing Lyme bacteria as well, so if you have Lyme in addition to candida, it may benefit you.

Note that Nizoral and Diflucan do not kill very much candida that resides in the gastrointestinal tract. These drugs enter the bloodstream and travel to various parts of the body, so they are beneficial for systemic candida, but they must be accompanied by another antifungal that targets the gut, like nystatin.

Systemic candida is much more difficult to treat than candida restricted to the gut. A patient with systemic candida may be unable to achieve the same level of improvement as an individual who has overgrowth in the gut only. Antifungals that target both the gut and the bloodstream must be used simultaneously. This is true of the natural antifungals as well; some of them are poorly absorbed, so they may work great for the gut, but not for systemic candida. Some antifungals do not make it to the bloodstream, and some may lose their potency by the time they get there. That said, aggressively reducing the level of overgrowth located in the gut is still beneficial for systemic candida, because it will prevent more candida and candida-related toxins from making their way to other parts of the body. The same is true for mycelial candida: it is much more serious and difficult to treat than planktonic yeast organisms.

Allylamine antifungals, which include Lamisil as well as others not mentioned here, also inhibit biosynthesis of ergosterol, so they could hold the same risk for toxicity that the azole antifungals do. However, these drugs are used topically, not orally.

Echinocandins, which include capsofungin, micafungin, and anidulafungin, inhibit synthesis of the polysaccharide glucan. We learned that glucan is a fundamental component of the cell wall of yeast and other fungi, as well as of bacteria, lichens, and some plants. It is also a primary constituent of the biofilm. Therefore, echinocandins can be effective against a wide variety of species and their biofilms when other drugs don't work. They are also less toxic. However, they are administered through an IV, which makes them inconvenient. Pathogenic resistance to echinocandins at this time is much less frequent than with other antifungals, but it does occur. I believe this is because they have been in existence for a shorter period of time, so candida hasn't yet been exposed to them very much. I suspect resistance will increase over the years.

Gentian violet is a dye that has antifungal, antibacterial, and antihelminthic properties. It is applied topically. It can be effective for breast-feeding mothers when applied to the nipple area. However, it can cause drying, so it is a good idea to combine it with an oil of some kind. Gentian violet may also put the health of the infant at risk, so it may not be a good choice. Other ways to address candida on the breast include applying baking soda to the nipples, which changes the pH, and washing nursing bras frequently.

Although I am in favor of natural treatments as the first course of action for most conditions, there is a time and a place for some types of pharmaceuticals, particularly when dealing with microbes. I am not opposed to the use of pharmaceuticals in addition to the natural options as long as you are educated about the potential problems and take the necessary precautions. I don't advocate taking most of the pharmaceuticals for extended periods of time. Instead, they work well as a short course at the beginning of treatment to help move things along a little faster and gain some ground in reducing overgrowth, or periodically when there is a significant flare of overgrowth, or if symptoms are severe and require immediate action. However, since antifungals typically have to be taken on an ongoing and sometimes lifelong basis, natural antifungals should be the primary choice and pharmaceuticals should be used adjunctively. Taking prescription drugs for an extended period is not conducive to healing.

Natural Antifungals

Before we discuss the natural-based options, I would first like to make you aware that "natural" does not always equal safe or side-effect free. You may find a lot of information on the Internet about herbal remedies that fails to present the possible side effects or complications. Even many alternative medicine practitioners may be ill informed about this aspect of natural remedies. It is your responsibility to be educated about everything you put into your body. I list some of the most common side effects further below, but this information is not necessarily inclusive.

Although herbs can be safer and less destructive than pharmaceuticals in many cases, they are still powerful substances that are foreign to the body. Herbs are not the same as nutritional supplements. Nutritional supplements contain nutrients that are familiar to and needed by the body. Herbs are not needed by the body; they are basically natural drugs. Plants, from which herbal remedies are derived, contain compounds called phytochemicals. Many of them evolved to ward off insects, pathogens, and consumption by animals, including humans. They have pharmacologic actions similar to those of synthetic drugs and sometimes can have profound side effects and negative consequences. Many pharmaceuticals are derived from natural herbs, thus demonstrating their potency. Although less likely, it is possible to have an allergic and life-threatening reaction to an herb, just as you can to a pharmaceutical. Some herbs can elevate liver enzymes or damage the liver and kidneys, just like pharmaceuticals. Some herbs should be taken for only short periods of time. Taking herbs in supplemental form is different from using them to season your food, because in supplemental form the most potent phytochemicals have been extracted and concentrated, which significantly increases their potency. Many people with candida (or other microbial issues) are often highly intolerant of certain herbs for one reason or another.

The body has a built-in detoxification system that gets rid of toxins and foreign invaders when they are detected. Detoxification occurs in phases. Phase one involves the cytochrome P450 enzymes, and phase two involves a process known as conjugation. Phytochemicals from herbs activate both phases, in the same manner as any other foreign chemical does, and the body attempts to get rid of them. Phase one oxidizes the toxin, and phase two adds molecules to the oxidized toxin so that it can be eliminated via urine or feces. Even many foods contain phytochemicals that have to be eliminated.

In some cases, herbs can speed up (induce) or slow down (inhibit) the detoxification system, which can affect how the body handles other drugs or toxins that are present in the system. This means the body may either get rid of the herb or other pharmaceutical before it has a chance to work, or keep it around for too long. Alternatively, the herb may speed up phase one and inhibit phase two at the same time, which increases toxicity because an oxidized toxin is much more toxic than it was in its original form.

Additionally, the liver and other parts of the detoxification system in people with candida may already be overwhelmed with toxins produced by candida or other microbes. Adding an herb or a pharmaceutical may overload the system even more, exacerbating symptoms and further degrading health. Die-off caused by herbs can be just as strong as that caused by pharmaceuticals, which also adds to the load of toxins that must be eliminated. Furthermore, any kind of genetic polymorphism that affects a person's detoxification system can also influence their response to an herb and their ability to eliminate phytochemicals.

Response to and benefits from herbs can vary widely from individual to individual. Even when you share the same health condition with someone, you each have a unique biochemistry that causes variations in the disease process and influences the results that can be achieved. How well your liver, lymphatic system, endocrine system, and autonomic nervous system function can have a powerful impact on your response to herbs and other treatments. A lot of trial and error may be required to find what works best for your biochemistry and unique set of circumstances.

Many herbs can stimulate neurotransmitters in the brain in a manner similar to the effects of pharmaceuticals. Artificial stimulation or overstimulation of neurotransmitters, regardless of the source (pharmaceuticals, recreational drugs, herbs, sugar, other carbs, etc.), can produce many adverse reactions and result in an excess or a depletion of the neurotransmitter. Herb-herb interactions can also occur, so be careful when combining. You could end up combining two or three herbs that overstimulate neurotransmitters or increase blood pressure or lower blood sugar and be in real trouble. On the other hand, one herb can counteract the actions of the other. For example, uva ursi and cranberry should not be taken together as they may negate one another.

Many potential herb-drug interactions can also occur; an herb can cause a drug to be more potent or to be less effective or to create new problems. If you are taking any type of pharmaceutical drug, then you should talk with your doctor before supplementing with herbs. This is especially true if you have kidney, liver, or heart disease, diabetes, Parkinson's, or another serious health disorder. For example, herbs can increase blood pressure, set off the stress response system, lower blood sugar, disrupt neurotransmitters in the brain, thin the blood, and much more. Additionally, herbs contain many different compounds, each of which has different actions. When you have several different health conditions present at once, as is often the case in the individual with chronic candida, one of those compounds may be helpful for one of the conditions, but one of the other compounds can exacerbate another condition. Herbs can even interact with foods you have eaten or other nonsupplemental treatment strategies you may be using, like acupuncture or massage.

Herbs may be less likely to result in tolerance than drugs because

Antifungals and Probiotics   177

they afford a variety of positive effects that are powered by many different compounds rather than just one. Their vitamin, mineral, and antioxidant content may provide a buffer that helps them be assimilated by the body. They possess many different active chemicals, whereas a pharmaceutical has just one toxin (active compound) that is typically combined with a variety of additives that are toxic as well, which triggers the immune and detoxification systems to get rid of them. Even nutritional supplements have additives that must be eliminated. That said, in the long term herb tolerance can develop, because over time the liver enzymes that target and break down the herbs will become more efficient at doing so. Or the body's cells may become resistant to an herb as the receptors that originally responded to it are downregulated. Either case may lead to ineffectiveness of the herb. Finally, there's a lot about herbs that we don't know; most of them have not been rigorously researched, so they may produce unexpected effects.

Be sure to purchase your herbs and other natural remedies only from reputable sources. Herbs and other natural remedies are not regulated like foods or drugs, and there is inconsistency in the industry in regard to safety, effectiveness, and potency. There are many low-quality products on the market that may contain fake herbs or be diluted, and some brands are loaded with heavy metals like lead, arsenic, and mercury. Your herbs should state on the bottle that they are standardized for maximum potency.

Having said all that, herbs are still preferable to drugs when it's possible to use them. The greatest benefit of herbs over drugs is that by combining several different types of herbs we can create a potent, broad-spectrum antimicrobial that can simultaneously target many different species and strains of candida, bacteria, and other microbes. This allows us to achieve many different goals at once. Research also suggests that the effectiveness of some pharmaceuticals can be enhanced by combining them with certain herbals.[7] However, one should approach the use of herbs in the same manner as one does pharmaceuticals: with caution and armed with information. Be sure to do your homework on potential adverse effects and contraindications, learn about the manufacturer, weigh risks against benefits, and communicate with your health-care professional before and during the use of herbs. Don't take a bunch of different herbs at once. Go slow, and introduce one product at a time to monitor how your body responds. The sicker you are the more important this is and the slower one should proceed with any remedy.

The huge array of natural antifungals available prevents me from discussing them all. I will highlight some of those that have been found to be most effective and are backed by research. As mentioned in chapter 5, many of the herbs that are effective against candida are also effective against bacteria, parasites, and viruses, so if one is dealing with these microbes as well, then many of the herbs can be chosen to target all of them at once.

At the same time, keep in mind that just because an herb offers antifungal or antibacterial activity does not mean it will automatically be right or effective for you. Again, it will depend on your strain, species, level of overgrowth, biofilms, resistance, and other unknown factors. Many antifungals in the following list (e.g., undecylenic acid and monolaurin) produced absolutely no antifungal activity in my body. Others produced mild results, and still others were excellent. I have worked with clients who had the exact opposite experience. There is no one-size-fits-all antifungal or antimicrobial; you must experiment to find what works best for you while being aware that your needs may change over time as circumstances change.

Oregano Oil

Oregano oil contains two substances, thymol and carvacrol, that are believed to react with water in the bloodstream to dehydrate and consequently kill candida yeast cells. One study found that origanum oil completely inhibited the growth of *Candida albicans,* both germination and mycelial. In this study, researchers tested mice with carvacrol alone and with oregano oil; the mice treated with oregano oil faired better than those treated with carvacrol alone, suggesting that other components besides carvacrol and thymol are involved in the antifungal effect.[8]

A study from Georgetown University Medical Center demonstrated that oregano oil is as effective against bacteria as prescription-based antibiotics like streptomycin, penicillin, and vancomycin. Additionally, mice that received 50 percent oregano oil survived, while mice that received carvacrol in an olive oil base died, again suggesting that other substances within oregano contribute to its antimicrobial capabilities besides carvacrol.[9] In another study, oregano oil demonstrated anti-bacterial activity against twenty-five different types of bacteria.[10]

Oregano oil also possesses antiviral, antiparisitical, antitumor, anti-inflammatory, antihistamine, and antioxidant abilities. One study found it to be more effective than tinidazole against the parasitic amoeba giardia.[11] It is even effective for breaking down the cell wall of norovirus and against MRSA.[12,13]

On the downside, oregano oil can impede the body's ability to absorb iron; therefore, iron supplements should be taken two hours before or after taking oregano oil. It can also increase blood flow to the uterus, potentially weakening the lining surrounding the fetus and leading to miscarriage. It may cause rashes, induce menstruation, increase risk of bleeding, lower blood sugar, and potentiate or amplify the action of some medications. It has anticoagulant properties. It should be avoided if you have an allergy to the Lamiaceae family of plants (e.g., mint, lavender, sage, and basil), and it is not advisable for infants and children. Because oregano oil is so potent, many practitioners believe it should not be taken long term as it has the potential to kill friendly bacteria.

Caprylic Acid and Undecylenic Acid

Caprylic acid, a fatty acid derived from coconut oil, has been shown to demonstrate potent antifungal characteristics against many species and strains of candida by disrupting the cell wall. In one study, researchers concluded that it was superior to Diflucan.[14] Another study found that it inhibited both the yeast form and mycelial form of candida, and it required very low concentrations to inhibit the mycelial growth.[15] Researchers concluded that it may also have potential against cancer, aging, infection, autism, and Alzheimer's, and that it improves circulation. It produces activity against other types of fungi and yeast, including geotrichum and rhodotorula, as well as having antiviral and antibacterial properties.

One caveat about caprylic acid: in its liquid form it is very quickly absorbed by the small intestine and metabolized by the liver, meaning it moves so quickly that it does not have time to exert its powerful antifungal activity against candida. Steps must be taken to slow absorption. Some people achieve this goal by combining it with psyllium husks or another type of fiber. I am not really in favor of psyllium because it is so abrasive and it feeds SIBO. Taking caprylic acid in a gel cap is another way to slow down its absorption. And there are several sustained-release forms of caprylic acid on the market that would distribute it slowly throughout the gastrointestinal tract as well.

Since caprylic acid is derived from coconut oil, coconut oil is often used as an antifungal. Coconut oil also contains capric acid and lauric acid, which also afford strong antimicrobial capabilities. On the down side, it can cause nausea and be very hard on the gallbladder, which is commonly affected in people with candida or bacterial overgrowth.

Monolaurin, a substance made from lauric acid, has demonstrated some antimicrobial activity, including against candida, bacteria, and viruses.[16] Some studies suggest that monolaurin is most effective against gram-positive bacteria, but it has also demonstrated significant activity against *H. pylori,* a gram-negative bacterium.[17,18] Many practitioners hail this product as one of the best, but I have just not witnessed this high level of effectiveness for candida or bacteria. Please read about possible contraindications with monolaurin in chapter 14.

In large doses, caprylic acid can cause irritation to the intestinal tract, nausea, and diarrhea. According to Dr. William Shaw it is safe for children in most cases, but a rare genetic disorder called medium-chain acyl dehydrogenase (MCAD) deficiency can impair children's ability to process caprylic acid.[19]

Undecylenic acid, another fatty acid similar to caprylic acid, which is derived from castor bean oil, has been found to be about six times more powerful than caprylic acid.[20] It inhibits morphogenesis of candida into mycelial form and disrupts the pH of the cell. It is the active ingredient in a wide variety of over-the-counter topical antifungals. The calcium, magnesium, and sodium salts of undecylenic acid have been shown to possess four times the fungicidal activity of undecylenic acid and thirty times more than caprylic acid. However, fatty acid salts are not very effective if the pH of the gut is above 6.0. Since candida often releases toxins to make the gut more alkaline, this can inhibit the effectiveness of undecylenic salts. The salts need to be delivered to the gastrointestinal system accompanied by an acid, which is typically done with a small amount of betaine HCl. This would be true for all fatty acid salts.

Be aware that one study looked at whether undecylenic acid was effective against candida biofilms in dentures. It found that *Candida albicans* biofilms were thinner and had less viable cells, but *Candida glabrata* biofilms actually exhibited higher cell counts, greater metabolic activity, and increased proteinase activity.[21]

Sodium Butyrate

Sodium butyrate, also a short-chain fatty acid, inhibits yeast growth, filamentation (formation of hyphae and pseudohyphae), and biofilm formation. It also enhances functioning of the macrophages, the white blood cells that gobble up pathogens like candida. Studies have demonstrated that it enhances the antifungal activity of azole-type drugs. Combining butyrate with amphotericin B completely eliminated biofilm populations of *C. albicans*.[22]

Garlic

Garlic contains a substance called allicin that is released when the root is crushed or chopped finely. The chopping or crushing process creates a chemical reaction that produces another substance called ajoene. Ajoene has been demonstrated in numerous studies to possess broad-spectrum antibacterial and antifungal characteristics. One study found that "garlic extract was more effective against pathogenic yeasts, especially *Candida albicans,* than nystatin, gentian violet or methylene blue."[23] Garlic also has antiprotozoal, antiviral, and antitumor properties, and it can boost the immune system. Allicin and other components in garlic have demonstrated a strong ability to inhibit biofilm formation.

Although allicin is the most extensively studied compound in garlic, the herb contains other substances that contribute to its health-promoting effects; therefore, it is most effective when ingested directly as raw garlic so you can acquire all the constituents rather than just isolating the allicin. Additionally, allicin is destroyed within an hour of chopping or crushing, so it is best obtained with fresh garlic that is consumed immediately. Dr. Joseph Mercola warns that you should not consume the clove of garlic whole, as it is the crushing or chopping that releases the beneficial compounds. If purchasing it as a nutritional supplement, be sure to use a reputable brand that ensures potency, as many versions may have lost their allicin content if not processed properly.[24]

Another great aspect of garlic is that it shows no activity against the friendly lactobacillus bacteria in the gut. However, this also means it won't be effective against SIBO if the organisms involved include lactobacillus. Allicin is considered by most SIBO experts to be the most effective herb against the methane-producing archaea.

It appears that garlic works in a manner similar to that of other antifungals by disrupting the cell membrane. However, ajoene has also been found to disrupt quorum sensing (the system microbes use to communicate with one another),[25] thereby disabling the organisms from performing many functions.

Garlic is safe for most people, but like anything else it is possible to have an allergic reaction to garlic, and it can potentially interact with drugs. Garlic contains blood-thinning properties,[26] making it potentially dangerous for those with bleeding disorders, those preparing to undergo surgery or dental work, or those about to give birth.

Kolorex (Horopito)

Horopito contains a substance called polygodial that has been proven in a variety of studies to have powerful antifungal activity (comparable to that of amphotericin B) against *Candida albicans, Candida krusei,* and some other species of candida and fungi.[27] Horopito is marketed in a product called Kolorex. A study conducted on Kolorex by ReGenera Research Group and the University of Milan, Italy, demonstrated it to be more effective than itraconazole against recurrent vulvovaginal candidiasis, with fewer side effects and a decrease in relapse rates.[28] It has also been found to be more effective than a blend of garlic and caprylic acid, and a blend of caprylic acid, pau d'arco, black walnut hulls, and oregano oil extract.[29] When combined with a substance called anethole that is found in anise seed, horopito becomes even more effective.[30,31] Horopito pokes holes in the organism's cell walls and then directly infiltrates the cells, while anethole prevents cells from recovering.

Thyme

Thyme oil has demonstrated strong antifungal and antibacterial properties. In one study that looked at thyme and clove oil, all twenty-five genera of bacteria tested were sensitive to both clove and thyme, but thyme exhibited more activity than clove.[32] In another study, thyme stopped the overgrowth of *Candida albicans* and clove inhibited it, but candida was more susceptible to both clove and thyme than any of the bacteria in the study.[33] Many other resistant species of candida are susceptible to thyme as well.[34] Thyme is a potent expectorant and cough suppressant, and is used commonly for upper respiratory infections.

On the "con" side, thyme can lower blood sugar and blood pressure and increase the risk of bleeding. It may also induce menstruation, promoting the risk of spontaneous abortion, so it should be avoided by pregnant women. It interferes with cytochrome P450, potentially affecting the body's response to a wide variety of pharmaceuticals. Large doses of thyme may result in nausea, headache, dizziness, heartburn, vomiting, upset stomach, and headaches. One particular species of thyme may have a stimulating effect on thyroid function, so it is not recommended for people with hyperthyroidism. Nor is it recommended for children or infants.

Berberine

Berberine is a substance found in Oregon grape root, goldenseal, barberry, coptis (huang lian), and other plants. It has been demonstrated to afford a wide range of activity against many different species of candida—including *krusei, kefyr, glabrata, tropicalis, parapsilosis,* and *albicans* (in that order of susceptibility)—and other fungi, as well as against bacteria, viruses, and parasites.[35] When used in conjunction with fluconazole it has a synergistic effect against resistant strains of candida and also inhibits biofilm formation.[36] Berberine stimulates the immune system, lowers cholesterol, triglycerides, and blood sugar, and suppresses proinflammatory cytokines. This means it may be beneficial in reducing inflammation and healing the gut and may suppress tumor growth. It has been found to be as effective as the drug metformin for lowering blood sugar levels in people with type 2 diabetes.[37,38]

However, berberine affects numerous neurotransmitters in the brain; therefore, it should not be used long term. It inhibits acetylcholinesterase, the enzyme needed to break down acetylcholine. This may lead to an excess of acetylcholine and all the associated problems we discussed in chapters 1 and 2. Berberine may also increase norepinephrine and serotonin, but suppress dopamine.[39,40,41] As I have mentioned, I am not in favor of herbs that manipulate neurotransmitters because this effect is no different from what a pharmaceutical might do, and artificial stimulation of neurotransmitters always has the potential to lead to depletion and create new problems. One should be extra cautious about using berberine if he or she suffers from depression, anxiety disorders, attention deficit, addiction, OCD, or other mental health issues—all of which are very common in the individual with candida.

Berberine can cause uterine contractions and may affect the development of an embryo or fetus, leading to birth defects, so it should not be taken during pregnancy. Additionally, its blood sugar-lowering effects can be problematic for people with low blood sugar issues. That said, in my observation, its impact on blood sugar is much less powerful than that of neem.

Cinnamon

Several studies have demonstrated that cinnamon has strong antifungal and antibacterial properties against a variety of different species of candida and bacteria.[42,43,44] It is one of the herbs of choice that Dr. Allison Siebecker uses in the treatment of small intestinal bacterial overgrowth.[45] Cinnamon can also lower blood sugar and increase insulin sensitivity, so it can be used in the diet to help regulate blood sugar spikes. It decreases the amount of glucose that enters the bloodstream after a meal. (Do be cautious in regard to low blood sugar.) It is high in antioxidants and offers anti-inflammatory properties.

A substance in cinnamon called coumarin can cause liver damage in a small percentage of people if too much is consumed, so it should be avoided by people who have a liver disease.[46] There are two types of cinnamon: Ceylon cinnamon, which is true cinnamon, and cassia cinnamon. True cinnamon contains very little coumarin, but cassia cinnamon may contain a significant amount. Cassia cinnamon is cheaper, and thus it is used most commonly in foods found on the supermarket shelf. Cinnamon sticks from cassia have a thick layer of bark with a hollow middle. Ceylon cinnamon consists of several thin layers and is solid in the middle. When supplementing with cinnamon, look for versions that clearly state on the package that it is derived from Ceylon cinnamon.

Coumarin is similar to the drug warfarin, which is used to keep blood from clotting, so cinnamon could interact with that drug.

Additionally, cinnamon stimulates the release of histamine, so using it could be problematic if you have histamine intolerance or histadelia.

Pau D'Arco

The South American tree pau d'arco has been well known for many decades for its antifungal properties and has been used by indigenous populations for centuries. It has been found to have activity similar to that of amphotericin B against *Candida albicans, Candida tropicalis,* and *Cryptococcus neoformans.*[47] It offers effective antimicrobial activity against a variety of both gram-positive and gram-negative bacteria, including *H. pylori,* staphylococcus, streptococcus, enterococcus, bacillus, and clostridium, as well as against some strains of the flu and herpes viruses. Additionally, it is believed to inhibit histamine-releasing cells, consequently reducing inflammation.

The active compound in pau d'arco is lapachol. According to the Phytochemical Database housed at the U.S. Department of Agriculture, lapachol has been documented as being "anti-abscess, anticarcinomic, anti-edemic, anti-inflammatory, antimalarial, antiseptic, antitumor, antiviral, bactericidal, fungicidal, insectifugal, pesticidal, protisticidal, respiradepressant, schistosomicidal, termiticidal, and viricidal." Many studies have demonstrated its benefits in the treatment of cancer.[48] Pau d'arco may loosen the bowels, which can help with motility issues.

The inner bark of the pau d'arco tree is where its most powerful properties reside, so be sure that the brand you purchase states that it is derived from the inner bark. There are many cheap and lower-quality sources of pau d'arco on the market. Furthermore, the tree is on the endangered species list, so some companies may market other bark as pau d'arco. Be sure to buy from a reputable source.

Although pau d'arco can be obtained in capsules, it is most effective when consumed as a tea. The tea can also be used as a vaginal douche or in an enema. Tinctures may be applied topically to toes, fingernails, skin, etc.

In high doses, pau d'arco may cause nausea, vomiting, abdominal discomfort, diarrhea, and weakening of the immune system. It should not be used during pregnancy or breast-feeding as it has been shown to cause birth defects in rats.[49] Pau d'arco can cause thinning of the blood, and long-term use may cause anemia.

Clove

Clove oil has been found to have powerful antifungal activity against a wide variety of fungi, including candida, aspergillus, and fluconazole-resistant strains.[50] In one study, clove demonstrated a significant ability to reduce ergosterol (a component of fungal cell membrane) and to completely or almost completely inhibit germ-tube formation (outgrowth produced by spores) in *Candida albicans*.[51]

It has also been found to have strong antibacterial qualities against a variety of species, including *H. pylori, Pseudomonas aeruginosa, Staphylococcus aureus, Salmonella choleraesuis, Klebsiella pneumoniae,* as well as the ability to disrupt bacteria's quorum sensing (their communication system). Impairing microbes' ability to communicate with one another reduces virulence and resistance.[52,53] Clove is commonly used for killing parasite eggs and to repel mosquitoes.[54]

Even in low doses, eugenol, one of the most potent components of clove, has shown a powerful ability to inhibit biofilm formation by disrupting the communication system of organisms, which impedes their ability to form communities.[55] Clove is often used to alleviate pain and inflammation, particularly in the mouth and throat.

Clove is a very potent herb and can produce a variety of side effects if consumed in large amounts, including abdominal pain, nausea, vomiting, diarrhea, sore throat, difficulty breathing, burns in the mouth and throat, rapid heartbeat, sleepiness, seizures, liver or kidney failure, and intestinal bleeding. Smaller doses have produced serious effects in young children, so clove oil, which is a more potent form, may be best avoided in children. In animals it can cause blindness, so keep it away from the eyes. It is not recommended during pregnancy. Eugenol can slow blood clotting, making clove potentially problematic for people with bleeding disorders or preparing to undergo surgery. Some people are allergic to clove; anyone who is allergic to balsam of Peru may also be allergic to clove.[56,57]

Cat's Claw

Cat's claw (botanical name *Uncaria tomentosa* and also known as samento) has powerful immune-boosting qualities that are considered to exceed those of many other herbs with the same ability. It enhances phagocytosis, the process whereby white blood cells engulf and destroy pathogens within the body. It is also an adaptogenic immune modulator, meaning it can either slow down immune response if it is too active or increase it if it is underactive, making the herb beneficial for autoimmune disorders.[58,59] It adapts to each situation depending on what is needed. It may directly help the body fight off candida and other microbes by enhancing the immune system's ability to do so.

Cat's claw also contains antifungal, anti-inflammatory, antibacterial, antiviral, and antioxidant characteristics, so it can both help kill microbes and reduce inflammation.[60] It may possibly shrink tumors and inhibit cancer, and it has a cleansing effect on the intestinal tract. It is commonly used for a wide variety of conditions, including candida, herpes, SIBO, and more. It is one of the herbs of choice for treating Lyme and is typically combined with otoba bark for this purpose.

There are two types of cat's claw: *Uncaria tomentosa* and *Uncaria guianensis*. Tomentosa is considered to be a better form and the one that should be chosen.

Cat's claw may induce miscarriage, so it should be avoided by pregnant women. It may also interact with drugs designed to suppress the immune system, cause thinning of the blood, and interfere with blood pressure regulation during or after surgery.[61] It may also cause an increase in dopamine, norepinephrine, serotonin, and acetylcholine, which can be problematic for those with elevations and/or lead to more imbalances with long-term use.

Turmeric

Turmeric, primarily due to its compound curcumin, has long been known for its powerful anti-inflammatory and antioxidant capabilities, which have been demonstrated to be about as effective as those of corticosteroids and even more effective than those of NSAIDs.[62,63] One of the ways it does this is by activating genes that control inflammation, rendering it able to alleviate the gut pain and inflammation associated with microbial overgrowth. Not only does it act as an antioxidant, but it can also increase the body's own antioxidant and detoxification enzymes.[64]

Curcumin has also been found to offer potent antifungal, antibacterial, and antiviral activity. In one study, it demonstrated anticandida activity (cell death and inhibition of hyphale formation) against thirty-eight different strains of candida, "including some fluconazole resistant strains and clinical isolates of *C. albicans, C. glabrata, C. krusei, C. tropicalis,* and *C. guilliermondii.*"[65] In another study, it was found to be more effective than fluconazole at inhibiting candida from adhering to human buccal epithelial cells (cheek cells).[66] Using curcumin as the agent in photodynamic therapy (combining a drug with a particular type of light to kill microbes) reduced "the biofilm biomass of *C. albicans, C. glabrata,* and *C. tropicalis,*" and also reduced planktonic activity.[67]

Combining curcumin with antifungal drugs like voriconazole, itraconazole, ketoconazole, miconazole, fluconazole, amphotericin B, and nystatin for a synergistic effect significantly increased their effectiveness against twenty-one clinical isolates of *C. albicans.*[68] Another study found that the effectiveness of curcumin against various strains of candida could be enhanced by five to ten times if it was accompanied by ascorbic acid (vitamin C). Vitamin C also enhances its antioxidant activity.[69]

A variety of studies have found that combining curcumin with an antibiotic produced a synergistic effect that enhanced the drugs' effectiveness against resistant strains of bacteria like *Staph. aureus* and MRSA. The combination was also shown to reduce biofilm formation, inhibit quorum sensing, and downregulate virulence factors in a variety of bacteria, and to exhibit pronounced eradication of *H. pylori* and associated inflammation.[70]

Curcumin may also stimulate dopamine and serotonin in a manner similar to that of antidepressants, which could be counterproductive and lead to depletion of those neurotransmitters.[71] As we learned earlier, artificial stimulation results in downregulation of production or responsiveness. Be cautious of this element. I developed depression and excessively high levels of fear after one dose of curcumin, demonstrating its powerful potential for a negative impact on neurotransmitters.

On a completely different note, curcumin can increase BDNF (brain-derived neurotrophic factor), a protein that plays a vital role in developing new neurons, protecting neurons, and encouraging synapse formation.[72] This substance is found to be low in people with depression, Alzheimer's, OCD, and other mental health issues. A higher level of BDNF is associated with controlling appetite. Curcumin may also help prevent or reverse heart disease, and may inhibit cancer cells.

Turmeric as a cooking spice does not contain very high levels of the potent compound curcumin. Most studies used curcumin extract, not turmeric as a spice. The curcumin content that is present in your table spice won't be high enough to produce these results if you sprinkle the spice on your food or put it in smoothies. Using it as a seasoning won't hurt, but to achieve the benefits outlined here you need to use curcumin extract, which will be in a base of turmeric.

Optimal benefits that can be achieved by curcumin are limited because it is poorly absorbed and quickly metabolized by the liver. One of the ways to overcome this obstacle is to combine curcumin with piperine, a substance found in pepper.[73] Other methods include combining curcumin with a nanoparticle like polylactic-co-glycolic acid (PLGA), used in time-released capsules, or extracting curcumin with heat.

Other potential side effects of turmeric may include allergy, nausea, dizziness, diarrhea, increased risk of bleeding, lowering of blood pressure, uterine contractions, increased menstrual flow, lowering of blood sugar, and gallbladder contractions. It may also interfere with certain medications like anticoagulants, and non-steroidal, anti-inflammatory drugs.

Black Walnut

Black walnut contains tannins and a substance called juglone that have been shown to generate activity against yeasts, fungi, and parasites. In one study, black walnut's efficacy was comparable to that of two common antifungals: zinc undecylenate and selenium sulfide.[74] It is also high in antioxidants and fatty acids, and has been shown to have potent activity against *H. pylori* and other bacteria.[75]

Black walnut can be irritating to the kidneys and liver, so it should be avoided by anyone with diseases involving those organs. It is unknown if black walnut is safe for pregnant women, but due to its ability to stimulate bowel contractions it should be avoided during pregnancy.

Grapefruit Seed Extract

Grapefruit seed extract has been shown to exhibit very powerful antimicrobial abilities. One study found that it performed as well as thirty different antibiotics and eighteen fungicides against gram-positive bacteria (*Streptococcus sp.*, staph, aureus, enterococci) and gram-negative bacteria (enterobacter and *E. coli*). The same concentration was reportedly highly effective against certain yeasts and molds (candida, geotrichum, aspergillus, and *Penicillium sp.*).[76]

Grapefruit seed extract is very popular in the natural health world and recommended by most practitioners for everything from acne to warts. That said, according to the Organic Consumers Association, grapefruit seed extract has been found to be contaminated with benzalkonium chloride (most commonly), parabens, and triclosan.[77] Benzalkonium, a synthetic chemical used for disinfection and for cleaning drains, is known to be toxic to the immune system and respiratory system and may be carcinogenic.[78] Some studies have demonstrated that grapefruit seed extract does not inherently contain any antibacterial qualities without the presence of these contaminants.

Grapefruit seed extract is derived through a very long process that uses ammonia chloride and hydrochloric acid. The end product contains 60 percent diphenol hydroxybenzene, "a chemical classified as a quaternary ammonium chloride—the same as benzethonium chloride. In fact it is nearly chemically identical to benzethonium chloride."[79]

Triclosan is a pesticide with neurotoxin capabilities. It has been linked to immune system and endocrine system damage and is believed to contribute to resistant strains of bacteria. Parabens are preservatives that are endocrine disruptors and have been linked to cancer.

In summary, it is seriously debatable whether grapefruit seed extract is natural and whether it should be used. On the other hand, it may still be less toxic than some pharmaceutical-based antimicrobials, and the benefits may outweigh the risks, so I leave it up to you to decide. As I see it, short-term use may be acceptable, but not long-term. The company who manufactures the brand Citricidal guarantees that its product is free of pesticides, triclosan, and parabens, so if you take the remedy be sure to stick with a more reputable brand like them. This doesn't eliminate the fact that the processed product is closely related to benzethonium chloride, but it eliminates two of the risks.

Other Plant Tannins

Many herbal remedies are effective because of their high tannin content. Tannins are natural substances found in a variety of plants that have demonstrated potent antifungal activity. A variety of products on the market consist of isolated and concentrated sources of tannins and are commonly used to treat yeast overgrowth. Tannins are also effective against other fungi (e.g., geotrichum) and against a variety of bacteria and parasites. One of the most popular tannin formulas for treating candida is Tanalbit, and one of the most popular for treating bacteria is Viracin.

Olive Leaf Extract

Olive leaf is another popular herb used widely by natural health-care providers for treating yeasts, other fungi, parasites, viruses, and bacteria. Several studies have demonstrated that olive leaf exhibits anti-fungal activity.[80,81] Oleuropein, one of its primary active ingredients, has been "shown to have strong antimicrobial activity against both gram-negative and gram-positive bacteria as well as mycoplasma."[82] When using olive leaf, be sure it is "extract" and not just leaf, and it should be at least 18 percent oleuropein (standardized) for maximum effectiveness. Oleuropein content should be listed on the bottle. It is also very high in antioxidants. However, olive leaf can significantly increase the neurotransmitters norepinephrine and phenylethylamine, so exercise caution. Phenylethylamine has an amphetamine effect and may increase dopamine. As mentioned previously, norepinephrine in excess is toxic to the brain. It incites the stress response system, wears down the adrenal glands, and incites anxiety, fear, and insomnia. On the other hand, it is possible for some people to take olive leaf for a period of time before the elevation gets too high. So, if you are using it in your rotation regimen, it may be possible that your switch to your other options occurs before the excess builds up. Olive leaf may increase blood flow and lower blood sugar, so it may need to be avoided in people who are diabetic or taking blood pressure medication, as well as pregnant and breastfeeding women.

Chitin Synthesis Inhibitors (Cell Wall Suppressors)

You may see a lot of hype around products that are marketed as candida cell wall suppressors, also known as chitin synthesis inhibitors. One of the newest on the scene is lufenuron, which is the active ingredient in some veterinarian flea-control products and parasite medications. It is a pesticide that inhibits the production of chitin. Chitin, a derivative of glucose, helps form the hard outer shell (exoskeleton) of insects and crustaceans and the cell wall of fungi like candida.

Chitin helps provide the candida cell with a protective shield.

Although it plays an important role in this function, it is a minor constituent of the cell wall (forming 0.6 percent–9 percent) in comparison with beta-glucans, which constitute 47 to 60 percent of the cell wall. Candida changes its cell wall composition depending on what form it is in, so the degree of chitin that is present may vary depending on the form candida is taking at any given time. For example, hyphal cells contain at least three times more chitin than yeast cells.[83] If candida is in an environment where chitin inhibitors are present, it will simply alter the amount of chitin in its cell walls to preserve itself.

As described earlier, one of the forms candida may take is a cell wall–deficient form, meaning it exists without a cell wall. It's critical to understand that any substance that targets the cell wall, like lufenuron, is going to be ineffective against these forms. Chitin synthesis inhibitors may get rid of some colonies of candida, but the ones without cell walls will survive and repopulate. Additionally, as discussed, the cell wall–deficient form is very small and has the ability to hide in human cells, and one must still get beyond the biofilm before the cell wall can be destroyed.

Although lufenuron has been proven to be effective against fungal infections in dogs, cats, and chimpanzees,[84,85] it has not been proven effective against candida specifically, and it is not approved for human consumption. A study on lufenuron at the University of California, San Francisco, found that it demonstrated no antifungal activity against aspergillus or *Coccidioides immitis* (two other types of fungi),[86] so it is unclear whether it would truly be effective against candida.

Proponents of lufenuron claim it is a nontoxic pesticide. However, it has been found to be harmful to epithelial cells and to the tight junctions that line the gut and ovary cells in animals, which means it may contribute to leaky gut and possibly affect reproduction.[87,88] It may also bioaccumulate in fat and interfere with absorption of N-acetylglucosamine, a substance that is needed for the formation of the cell wall in many healthy bacteria.[89]

Furthermore, once lufenuron is in the body, it takes weeks to clear from the system. That means if you have a negative reaction to it, simply discontinuing use may fail to provide immediate relief. For these reasons, it is my opinion that the safety of lufenuron is uncertain, and one should exercise caution when considering whether it should be used. I would not recommend its use until more information is acquired on how it affects humans.

The human body actually produces its own enzymes, called chitinases, that degrade chitin.[90] A variety of natural products on the market contain enzymes for this purpose as well. They may be referred to as cell wall suppressors or cell wall digesters. Many of these formulas combine enzymes that digest the cell wall with enzymes that break down the biofilm. These products are a better choice than lufenuron and can be beneficial when used in conjunction with some of the other antifungals presented above (along with the diet, of course). However, they are not a "cure" in and of themselves, for all the reasons we've discussed.

Food-Grade Hydrogen Peroxide

Food-grade hydrogen peroxide can be used to brush the tongue and as a mouthwash to kill candida and other microbes. As discussed elsewhere in this book it is also beneficial as a douche, in an enema, or for a soak in the bathtub. Brushing your tongue can sometimes provide significant relief from brain fog and other cognitive symptoms you may be experiencing from the presence of organisms in your mouth. Brushing your tongue, even without hydrogen peroxide, should be a regular practice if you have a white tongue, which indicates the presence of candida.

Some people take food-grade hydrogen peroxide internally to treat candida, but this is a controversial method. Although some evidence exists that consuming hydrogen peroxide can kill candida and other microbes, the substance is also a strong oxidizer that can harm cells and tissues and cause inflammation, and it kills friendly microbes as well. One must weigh the benefits against the risks if they choose to explore this option. Additionally, there is evidence that candida can adapt to and use hydrogen peroxide for its own benefit, and it can generate enzymes that break down hydrogen peroxide into its individual parts, rendering it ineffective.[91]

Lactoferrin

In previous chapters, we learned that the protein lactoferrin binds to iron and delivers it to cells, preventing candida and other microbes from acquiring it for their existence and the formation of biofilms. We also learned that lactoferrin activates the phagocytes, macrophages, neutrophils, and natural killer cells that engulf candida, bacteria, viruses, and parasites. It can enhance cell-to-cell communication in the immune system and reduce inflammation. All these actions can be helpful in reducing overgrowth and symptoms of candida and other microbes. It has even been found to effectively inhibit hepatitis C.

Lactoferrin also possesses peptides (short chains of amino acids) that are lethal not only to candida and other types of fungi but also to numerous types of bacteria—including *E. coli,* clostridia, *Staphylococcus aureus, H. pylori, Klebsiella pneumoniae*—and to some viruses, like HIV.[92] Peptides damage the cell membrane, enter the cell, and disable its ability to produce energy. They impede viral replication and block viruses from entering cells by occupying receptors. So not only can lactoferrin enhance immune function, reduce biofilm formation, and inhibit growth and travel, but it can also directly kill the microbes.

One study has demonstrated that lactoferrin can prevent *Candida albicans* and *Candida glabrata* from adhering to mucosal linings in the vagina, and can even help to break candida's hold if it has already attached.[93] We can conclude that if it has this ability in the vagina, the same is most likely true for other parts of the body.

Regardless of the other antifungals used, lactoferrin should probably be a fundamental component of all healing plans for candida and other microbial overgrowth due to the fact that it enhances all aspects of recovery: killing the microbes directly, boosting the immune system, and preventing biofilm formation. Some research found that combining lactoferrin with azole drugs inhibited hyphal growth, and combining it with other types of antifungals or antibiotics enhanced their effectiveness by 50 to 90 percent, depending on the concentration used.[94,95]

Lactoferrin is found in breast milk, where it occurs naturally with short-chain fatty acids like lauric acid and caprylic acid, which suggests they work well together. Combining lactoferrin with one of these fatty acids (discussed earlier) may produce a more potent antifungal effect.

Lactoferrin should be avoided by women who are pregnant as its potential immune-system stimulation could target the developing fetus.

A variety of other herbs and substances have been found to afford antifungal and antibacterial properties, including ginger, tea tree oil, peppermint, apple cider vinegar, iodine, colloidal silver, aloe vera, and others. We will not go into detail about them here.

Optimizing Antifungal Effectiveness

It is best to start antifungal treatment a week or two after beginning the paleo for candida diet (presented in chapters 10 and 11) to allow for some reduction in overgrowth prior to an aggressive attack. This sequence will prevent severe die-off and will avoid overwhelming the detoxification and sympathetic nervous systems. Lowering your carbohydrate intake will decrease the number of organisms present that will be killed by the antifungal, which means fewer toxins and less inflammation for the body to deal with at one time. For the same reason, it is well advised to start with small doses of whatever antifungals you choose and slowly work your way up to larger doses. We talk about die-off in more detail in chapter 8.

Be aware that antifungals are much less effective if they aren't used in conjunction with the paleo for candida diet. You cannot actively feed your candida while you are attempting to kill it; to do so will keep you spinning your wheels and getting nowhere. Each of these steps supports and enhances the effectiveness of the others.

Fascinating research has demonstrated that active bacteria "talk" with dormant spores to encourage them to join forces in the cause. Some experts believe that if a substance could be developed to keep a microbe in a state of dormancy, we could prevent it from repopulating. When a microbe is in a dormant state, it is resistant to antimicrobials. However, it is also inactive. Keeping it inactive would keep it in a state of "suspended animation." It wouldn't be dead, but nor would it be able to grow or spread.[96] Ongoing research in this area is something to look for in the future.

Treatment for Miscellaneous Fungal Infections

Let's take a brief look at natural treatment methods for various types of fungal infections localized to specific areas.

Athlete's Foot

The feet are a very common spot for candida to populate due to the moist, dark, warm environment provided by socks and shoes. Some antifungals that can be used specifically on the feet include garlic, tea tree oil, black walnut, and hydrogen peroxide. In order to prevent reinfection, take the following additional steps:

- Avoid tight-fitting shoes. A tight shoe does not allow air to circulate around the foot. Additionally, the feet and toes rub against the shoe, which can lead to small cuts and abrasions where yeast can dwell. This can also occur along the toenail and is a common cause of toenail fungus.

- Wear clean socks every day.

- Choose cotton socks, as they permit air to circulate around the foot more easily.

- Keep your feet clean and your shoes dry.

- Allow your feet to be uncovered and exposed to the air for at least some amount of time each day.

- Make sure your feet are dry before putting on socks.

- Don't share personal grooming tools like toenail clippers or towels.

- Keep toenails trimmed.

- Wash socks and towels with hydrogen peroxide.

- Lightly spray hydrogen peroxide in your shoes. Let them dry before wearing.

- Bake your shoes in the sunlight to dry them out and kill organisms.

- Protect your feet whenever you're in public areas by wearing at least thongs or sandals. Athlete's foot is highly contagious. It can be transmitted very easily from person to person in locker rooms, shower rooms, swimming pools, gyms, and spas, and via towels.

If you get athlete's foot frequently, it suggests that candida is in the gut or systemic. In that case, these remedies must be accompanied by the whole healing plan presented in this book for long-lasting results.

Genital Yeast

The genital area is another common trouble spot for people with candida due to the dark, moist, warm environment it provides. In women, genital yeast is referred to as a vaginal yeast infection; in men, it is commonly referred to as jock itch. Following the diet and taking the antifungals discussed in this book will benefit the condition, but genital yeast must typically also be addressed locally by applying an antifungal agent directly to the area.

As mentioned in other sections, nystatin, yogurt, acidophilus, and food-grade hydrogen peroxide can be used on the genitals as a douche, suppository, or paste. However, other steps need to be taken to prevent reinfection:

• Avoid tight-fitting clothes, which prevent circulation of air in this area.

• The birth control pill, steroids, certain personal-care products, or synthetic undergarments and a sensitivity to latex condoms or spermicides—all have the potential to encourage genital yeast. Eliminate use of such products as needed.

Women's and men's symptoms differ. Women typically experience intense and relentless itching, burning, redness, swelling, and inflammation of the vagina and surrounding tissue. If the culprit is hyphal yeast, these symptoms may be accompanied by a thick white discharge that looks like cottage cheese. Be aware that vaginal yeast infections don't produce much odor. If your vaginal infection has a strong odor, then it is most likely bacterial.

By contrast, men may exhibit no symptoms at all. When men do have symptoms, they are also experienced as itching, burning, and redness, or as a rash. Men's genital yeast infection may also be accompanied by a thick yellow discharge.

Men are often carriers of genital yeast and reinfect their female partners unintentionally. Both partners can pass it back and forth repeatedly. If you develop a vaginal yeast infection every time you have sex, chances are good that your partner is infected and also needs treatment. Friction from sexual activity can be a contributing factor as well. It can also be transmitted through kissing or oral sex.

Although a genital yeast infection may occur even if no candida exists in the gut, frequent genital yeast infections suggest a systemic yeast problem. If this is the case, treating genital yeast locally only will fail to produce long-lasting results.

Sinusitis

The sinuses are another common place for fungal infections to occur. In fact, the primary cause of persistent (non-seasonal) sinusitis is fungus. Fungus-caused sinusitis may respond to some degree to a treatment such as Diflucan, but it usually must be treated locally as well. The antifungal needs to be delivered directly to the sinuses in a spray. Common antifungals used for this purpose include amphotericin B or itraconazole (Sporanox) spray combined with NAC or EDTA for biofilms.

Beware of Miracle-Cure Scams

The Internet contains so much misinformation, so many lies, and so many scams about candida that it's enough to make your head spin. Websites often provide guidance that is ineffective and/or counterproductive. People are desperate and willing to try just about anything, so many of them fall prey to charlatans who take their money and compromise their health even further. There are also many well-meaning people on the Internet who simply do not have a thorough understanding of candida and who offer advice that is detrimental to people's recovery. Many books and websites on the topic of candida just regurgitate what the writer has been told by someone else or read elsewhere without having any real first-hand knowledge. This state of affairs results in a lot of tail chasing, wasted time and money, and further deterioration in health, leaving those who are inflicted feeling alone, confused, frustrated, and exhausted. Additionally, many people get into trouble when they try to follow too many different protocols at one time.

Beware of any products that claim miraculous and effortless cures for candida, especially those that don't require changes in diet or that claim candida can't grow resistant to their product. Anyone who makes this type of assertion clearly lacks a thorough understanding of candida. As I have stated previously, research demonstrates that candida can become resistant or adapt to just about anything, and its ability to do so should never be underestimated and treatment without changes in diet is futile.

PROBIOTICS

Probiotics are considered a key element in the treatment of candida by pretty much everyone in the field. They are used to help restore healthy bacteria levels to the gut, where they crowd out candida and other pathogens by competing for space and nutrients, keep the gut acidic, heal the gut, support the immune system, improve digestion and absorption of nutrients, enhance elimination, disrupt biofilms, and help produce digestive enzymes and nutrients like vitamin B12, vitamin K, biotin, and short-chain fatty acids. When more healthy bacteria are present to compete with candida, less space and fewer nutrients are available for candida, and candida will begin to die off. Some friendly bacteria actually eat candida.

As with antifungals, it is vital to be aware that there is no one-size-fits-all probiotic. The gut biome of each individual is as unique as his or her fingerprint. What promotes health and healing in one person could be disastrous for another. Additionally, our understanding of the gut biome at this time is a lot like our knowledge of a deep ocean floor: it's dark down there, and we still have much to learn. Recommendations are changing rapidly in response to new knowledge. The type of probiotic that is beneficial for any individual depends on what microbes exist in her or his gastrointestinal tract, and supplementing with the wrong type can bear serious negative consequences.

As described in chapters 5 and 6, our bodies house thousands of different species of bacteria, and even the good guys can become bad guys under certain circumstances. As in any community, some members may not play well with others and may become troublemakers, while others are good at keeping the peace. A comprehensive digestive stool analysis, like the GI Effects test (see chapter 4), can be helpful in identifying what types of bacteria and how many are present in your colon. Additionally, the Organic Acids Test, from Great Plains (also discussed in chapter 4), can help determine bacterial overgrowth. Performing the two tests together can provide you with a general idea of what is residing in your gut. That said, to some degree we're all swimming in the dark and hoping for the best when it comes to probiotic supplementation.

Strategies for Probiotic Use

Most health-care practitioners tell their patients that a good probiotic should have many different species of lactobacillus and bifidobacteria, with a minimum of five. However, when severe gut dysbiosis is present and a lot of damage has been done, many people do better with only one or two strains. They can experiment later with increasing the number of species or strains as improvements are made. Some people do well by staying with one or two species permanently. In some cases—for example, in the case of severe dysbiosis—it may be best to suspend use of a probiotic until some healing has occurred. Certain strains of bacteria may not be suitable for children. The dosage for children is typically less than an adult dosage and should be based on their age and weight. When children are involved, choose probiotics designed specifically for children. Be sure to consult with your physician before administering probiotics to your child.

It may be advantageous to rotate and alternate probiotics in the same manner as you do antifungals to foster more diversity. Probiotics that are being used for vaginal yeast should consist primarily of lactobacillus, because those are the bacteria that are needed in the vagina. Probiotics can be inserted directly into the vagina in capsule form like a suppository and are highly effective against vaginal infections. Yogurt can be used in this manner as well, but it's a little more messy. In either case, you want to wear a panty liner for protection. It's important to choose a reputable source for your probiotic to ensure potency and quality.

Health professionals don't agree about when is the optimal time to consume probiotics. Some practitioners and manufacturers recommend taking them with meals so the organisms will be sheltered from stomach acid and increase their chances of survival, but others recommend taking them on an empty stomach in order to avoid the digestive enzymes and bile that could exterminate the organisms. As of this date, there isn't any research to support either stance. Klaire Labs, one of the world leaders in the probiotic industry, encourages consumption with meals, because from an evolutionary perspective our probiotics were always consumed with food.[97] This is what makes the most sense to me, but I cannot say with certainty which stance is accurate. You will need to make a judgment call, or you could take them at both times, just to be sure your bases are covered. You should also note that when you're actively taking a formula to kill bacteria, it can impact your healthy bacteria, so probiotics should be taken at different times than antimicrobials. You may want to take probiotics by themselves for a period of time without any antibacterials to get them implanted, and then continue with the probiotics when you resume antibacterials.

Probiotics may be delivered to the colon through a retention enema. First, cleanse the colon with a plain-water enema. Next, mix the probiotics into a cup of water. Using an enema bag (available at any drugstore), slowly inject the water into the colon. Retain the solution in the rectum rather than expelling it right away. You can find further instructions for an enema in chapter 13. Because it bypasses the small intestine, this method may allow someone with SIBO who doesn't tolerate probiotics to recolonize the colon with healthy bacteria. However, it is also possible the implanted microbes will cross over into the small intestine. Many colon hydrotherapy clinics offer retention enemas if you don't feel confident doing it yourself.

Precautions for Probiotic Use

One has to be very careful in their choice of probiotics when a gut problem exists, and extra caution must be exhibited if they are dealing with SIBO in addition to chronic candida. As mentioned in chapter 6, small intestinal bacterial overgrowth can be caused by an overgrowth of D-lactate–producing bacteria like *Lactobacillus acidophilus.*

As mentioned above, the most commonly used probiotics consist of bacteria from the two genera *Bifidobacterium* and *Lactobacillus,* both of which ferment sugars to produce lactic acid. Within the lactobacillus genus, some strains produce mostly L-lactic acid (L-lactate) and others produce mostly D-lactic acid (D-lactate). L-lactate is most predominant in the body and is easily metabolized. D-lactate is not an issue for most people, but in high amounts it can be difficult for some individuals to break down, particularly those who already have impairment with carbohydrate malabsorption, which is the case in SIBO and a variety of other conditions like IBS, autism, immune disorders, fibromyalgia, and chronic fatigue. Unlike lactobacillus, bifidobacterium produces acetic acid and only L-lactate.

When present in excess, D-lactate is a neurotoxin that can cross the blood-brain barrier, disrupting brain cells and producing a wide variety of neurological problems such as confusion, brain fog, attention deficit, depression, slurred speech, disorientation, aggression, headaches, impaired coordination, anxiety, nausea, nervous shuddering, tics, OCD, and in extreme cases encephalopathy. It can also cause weak, aching, or painful muscles, create extremely painful muscle spasms and cramps, cause difficulty concentrating, and impair mitochondria function and the production of ATP (our primary source of fuel), leading to chronic fatigue. ATP is also needed in gluconeogenesis (conversion of protein and fat into glucose), so impaired production of ATP may contribute to low blood sugar issues. It may also be implicated in fibromyalgia, autism, and autoimmune disorders. Excess *L. acidophilus* has even been found in people with Crohn's.

Other species of bacteria, for example commensal bacteria in the genera streptococcus and enterococcus, both of which may be involved in SIBO, produce D-lactate as well. If an individual's SIBO involves any of the D-lactate–producing bacteria, supplementing with a D-lactate–producing probiotic will not only encourage more overgrowth, but it will increase D-lactate levels even further.

The same would be true of consuming probiotic foods that contain *L. acidophilus*—for example, yogurt, fermented or cultured vegetables, or kefir. These foods may or may not be helpful depending on the types of bacteria involved in one's overgrowth. In some cases, they could do more harm than good.

The two D-lactate producers commonly found in probiotic supplements include the very popular *L. acidophilus* and *L. plantarum*. If your SIBO involves D-lactate–producing bacteria, look for a probiotic that is labeled "D-lactate free." Some studies have found that *Bacillus clausii, Bifidobacterium brevis,* and *Lactobacillus casei* are beneficial for SIBO. If symptoms worsen when one supplements with *L. acidophilus,* it is a strong indication that overgrowth in the small intestine is caused by the D-lactate–producing bacteria.

An Organic Acids Test can tell you if you have an excess of D-lactate in your body, which would indicate that small intestinal bacterial overgrowth with a D-lactate–producing bacterium may be present. However, you should note that a diet high in carbohydrates can also cause a buildup of D-lactate. A variety of other factors can lead to high D-lactate, which we will not discuss at this time; they are mentioned in the notes accompanying the OAT test. Be aware, too, that some D-lactic acid–producing bacteria are resistant to antibiotics, potentially leading to dominance of these organisms after antibiotic use.

On the flip side, bifidobacteria can grow out of control and contribute to gastrointestinal and neurological symptoms if *L. acidophilus* is not present in sufficient numbers. In such a case, supplementing with bifidobacteria would be counterproductive and taking *L. acidophilus* would be beneficial. As you can see, there may be times when either bifidus or lactobacillus may be the right or wrong choice, depending on the gut biome of each individual. It's worth noting that *Lactobacillus acidophilus* GG is a particular strain that was formulated specifically for the control of clostridia.

Prebiotics, substances that accompany the probiotic to keep the bacteria alive (e.g., FOS, inulin, and maltodextrin), are food sources both for the bacteria involved in SIBO and for candida. Probiotics containing a substantial amount of prebiotics should be avoided. A small amount of prebiotic may be tolerated in some people, while none may be tolerated in others.

Strains of bacteria that generate histamine are commonly used in probiotic supplementation. The person with histadelia or histamine intolerance (see pages 444–451) would do best to avoid these species. They include *Lactobacillus casei, Lactobacillus reuteri, Lactobacillus delbrueckii,* and *Lactobacillus bulgaricus.*

Dosage

The optimal dosage of a probiotic can vary widely from person to person, depending on age, the bacteria involved, the extent of imbalances, how well the detoxification system is working, and other unknown factors. Generally speaking, most practitioners believe that the more severe the dysbiosis, the higher the dose needs to be to achieve positive and measurable results. They often prescribe a dose of fifty billion and more. Many of the organisms will not get past the stomach's acid, and a higher dose may help ensure that some will survive. That said, in some cases less is more. Many people don't need the recommended dose, at least in the beginning. When severe dysbiosis is present, starting at a low dose and slowly titrating up to higher doses may work best. If symptoms get worse, one should cut back on the dosage and increase slowly. If at any time throughout the process symptoms increase, go back to the dose that did not produce symptoms for a few days and try again. Some people may do best staying with a low dose indefinitely.

I am not convinced that taking high-dose probiotics is a good thing. I suspect that my supplementing with high-dose probiotics contributed to my development of SIBO, because that is when it first began to present. I had no problem taking low-dose probiotics for decades, but increasing my dosage incited new problems. I have also worked with several clients in whom it appears that taking high-dose probiotics for candida led to the development of SIBO. I recommend caution with high-dose probiotics and think it is best to stay in the range of 10 to 14 billion organisms.

Symptoms that are often attributed to die-off may actually be caused by taking either the wrong type of bacteria or a dosage that is too high. Such symptoms can be the same as those produced by the condition one is trying to treat, so it can be difficult to differentiate between the three scenarios. If you still experience symptoms of die-off after a week or so on a probiotic, chances are good that it is not die-off causing the symptoms. Of course, if symptoms grow significantly worse, even if they are caused by die-off, it is counterproductive.

As mentioned in chapter 6, Dr. Pimentel points out in his book *A New IBS Solution* that if the migrating motor complex is not working properly, as is the case with SIBO, taking a probiotic may cause bacteria to accumulate in the small intestine where we don't want them, making the problem worse. Considering everything discussed, it is unclear whether probiotic use is beneficial or advisable for the person with SIBO. As mentioned in chapter 5, according to Dr. Leo Galland, protozoa feed on probiotics, so if you have this particular parasite, this is another precaution to be aware of and consider.

And finally, according to Dr. Leonard Smith, who quotes pediatric gastroenterologist Timothy Buie, "about 15% of people with autism (and maybe the general population) can't tolerate any type of probiotic supplements."[98]

Other Types of Probiotics

For people who must avoid D-lactate–producing bacteria, or to enhance eradication of both candida and certain types of bacterial overgrowth in people who don't, some practitioners recommend probiotics based on microbes other than bifidobacterium and lactobacillus. Instead, they may suggest *Saccharomyces boulardii* (a type of yeast that eats candida and bacteria) and/or soil-based organisms that secrete antimicrobial peptides that kill candida, other yeasts and fungi, and bacteria. *Saccharomyces boulardii* also inhibits formation of filaments (hyphae and pseudohyphae), adherence, and biofilm formation.[99] Again, both these types of microbes can be helpful for some people, but they can become pathogenic. There is evidence in the literature of both *B. subtilis* (the most commonly used soil-based organism) and *S. boulardii* becoming pathogenic on occasion. When dysbiosis is present, the potential exists for any microbe to gain the upper hand.

Saccharomyces boulardii demonstrates several types of beneficial activity in a wide variety of gastrointestinal disorders, including "regulation of intestinal microbial homeostasis, interference with the ability of pathogens to colonize and infect the mucosa, modulation of local and systemic immune responses, stabilization of the gastrointestinal barrier function and induction of enzymatic activity favoring absorption and nutrition." However, efficacy varies greatly from product to product depending on the strains used and the number of organisms present. Many saccharomyces formulas on the market do not meet adequate standards. To ensure quality, one should choose a product that has been involved in clinical trials. Additionally, the temperature at which it is stored is critical, and so is the dosage.[100]

Since the 1990s, an increasing number of reports have emerged describing instances of saccharomyces infection. Most of these cases have involved individuals who were immunocompromised or who had an indwelling foreign object (e.g., medical device).[101,102] Furthermore, there are many undocumented reports of saccharomyces becoming pathogenic. Individuals with candida or SIBO are often immunocompromised to some degree or another, so, as I see it, this probiotic should be used with extra caution. If you do take saccharomyces, be aware that it is a yeast, which means antifungals will kill it. It must not be taken in conjunction with antifungals.

The bacterium B. *subtilis,* one of the most popular soil-based organisms, has been clinically proven to effectively kill candida and other yeasts and fungi, as well as bacteria. Like an antibiotic, however, it also kills friendly bacteria, which means it could contribute to dysbiosis and become the dominant organism in the gastrointestinal tract. A lot of controversy surrounds the question of whether soil-based microbes are beneficial.

As the term suggests, soil-based organisms live in the soil, where they execute a variety of beneficial activities like protecting plants from fungi, mold, yeast, and other pathogens. Some theorize that before the modernization of our food supply, humans ate soil-based organisms on a daily basis by ingesting small amounts of dirt that accompanied their food, and that the organisms contained therein helped keep our bad microbes under control. In an evolutionary context, these proponents claim, the lack of soil-based organisms in our diet may be a primary cause of many gut and colon disorders. In contrast to other gut bacteria, soil-based organisms are supposedly transient, meaning they do not take up permanent residence in the gastrointestinal tract. They organize short-term colonies until they die, and then they are cleared out of the system naturally through the digestive process and peristalsis.

As with saccharomyces infection, most documented reports of B. *subtilis* infection are associated with immunocompromised individuals or those who had an indwelling foreign object.[103,104] And again, many undocumented reports exist that describe a worsening of symptoms or the development of new symptoms from the consumption of B. *subtilis* and other soil-based organisms.

It is my opinion that there is not enough information on the use of soil-based organisms to draw a conclusion. Since I've experienced some negative effects first hand and have witnessed them in clients, I recommend that you exercise caution with these types of probiotics. When we are dealing with people who have damaged guts, impaired digestion and peristalsis, and compromised immunity, as is the case in individuals with chronic candida and SIBO, then many unexpected and out of the norm events may take place in our internal environment. For example, when I took B. *subtilis,* I experienced disturbed sleep, colorectal inflammation, significant psychological disturbances, and brain dysfunction—not to mention an array of new gut problems. In response to probiotics that were high in acidophilus and bifidus, I experienced increased levels of anxiety, insomnia, muscle pain, and plaque and biofilms in my mouth. I've heard reports of similar experiences with probiotics, saccharomyces, and *B. subtilis* from my clients over the years.

Another questionable organism that is frequently marketed to candida patients and that I would like to warn you about is *Enterococcus faecalis* (EF). Enterococcus has demonstrated the ability to inhibit hyphal morphogenesis and virulence in *Candida albicans*; therefore, it is marketed as an anticandida product.[105] However, it is a gram-positive, opportunistic bacterium that can also make you quite sick. According to researchers at the University of Texas, "*Enterococcus faecalis* accounts for approximately 5%–8% of hospital-associated bacteremia and approximately 5%–20% of all cases of endocarditis."[106] The *New England Journal of Medicine* tells us, "Although *Enterococcus faecalis* was once regarded as nonpathogenic, this opportunistic gram-positive coccus now ranks among the most troublesome hospital pathogens. It has intrinsic resistance to many antibiotics and a remarkable capacity for developing resistance to others."[107] The Canadian government lists enterococci as infectious agents and health hazards that are responsible for 10 percent of hospital-acquired infections in the United States.[108] Enterococci are consistently the second or third most common agent in urinary tract infections, wound infections, and bacteremia in hospitals. They are responsible for about 16 percent of nosocomial urinary tract infections. They can be transmitted on food products, person to person, and likely animal to human. Additionally, enterococci are lactic acid producers, so they may contribute to an excess of lactic acid and the associated problems discussed above. Although EF may reside in the colon of humans, it is a bad guy that is usually kept under control by our healthy guys. If dysbiosis is present, then this bad guy, like any of the others, can become pathogenic and cause disease.

I tried one of the popular products that contains EF. To prevent severe die-off, I always start an antifungal with a smaller dose than what is recommended, so I took only one-quarter of the recommended dose. Within a few days I developed a severe vaginal yeast infection. I also developed a high fever, sore throat, aches, pains, chills, hot breath, and chest congestion. I discontinued usage for a few days and then tried again to make sure I had not contracted an infection coincidentally with using the product. I went back to feeling normal. After a few days I resumed taking a quarter of the recommended dosage; I once again developed a vaginal yeast infection, sore throat, high fever, etc. I again discontinued and then resumed usage. I developed the same symptoms, after which I discontinued usage. My adult son tried the product. He also took only one-quarter of the recommended dosage and was flat in bed for three days after the first dose. He was much sicker than I had been, with a very high fever, severe migraine, chills, aches, pains, hot breath, etc. He wasn't willing to try it again.

Many of my clients and more than seventy-five people on my blog have shared horrific stories about their experiences with products that contain *Enterococcus faecalis* as the primary ingredient. Some of their reported symptoms include stabbing pain in the perineum, shakes and shivers, inability to sleep, burning throat, burning eyes, anxiety, appendicitis, strep throat, severe brain fog, diarrhea, headaches, urinary tract infections, vaginal infections, profuse sweating, fatigue, aggressiveness, OCD behaviors, weakness, and inability to function, to name only a few. Many of these people reported that their symptoms lingered for weeks after they discontinued use. You can find similar stories on other forums across the Internet.

Many of these controversial organisms are found in numerous probiotics on the market. Be sure you read labels and know what types of organisms are present in the probiotics you purchase. Please be aware that the large companies that make these products sometimes hire people to write convincing positive reviews and engage in other unscrupulous marketing tactics.

As you can see, probiotic supplementation is not a black-and-white issue. Each person needs to experiment with different types of probiotics to find the right species, strains, and dosages that work best for their body and current situation. The human gut flora is complex and dynamic, and it is influenced by a wide variety of factors such as age, sex, diet, nutritional status, genetics, and stress levels. Your probiotic needs may change over time in response to these factors. Do your homework, know the potential risks and benefits, and make an informed decision.

CHAPTER 8

Minimizing Candida Die-Off

D ie-off, otherwise known as the Jarisch-Herxheimer response (or just the Herxheimer response), is a phenomenon that occurs when an antifungal or other treatment causes candida to die in very large numbers, and consequently to release high levels of mycotoxins. These toxins can prompt an immune response, increase oxidative stress and inflammation, and make the individual quite ill. The Herxheimer response was first discovered in 1895 by two dermatologists, Adolf Jarisch and Karl Herxheimer, when they were treating syphilis patients. Treatment initially provoked an inflammatory response and a temporary worsening of symptoms, followed by an immediate improvement in health.

The term has been adopted to describe a similar experience in many different diseases, including candida. Symptoms may worsen and/or new symptoms may develop for a period of time before beginning to abate. Symptoms may mimic the flu. Die-off may occur to some degree when one begins following the diet or taking probiotics, but it is mostly associated with antifungals and other methods that directly kill the organisms. The more aggressive the treatment, the more severe the die-off is likely to be. In addition, some people have a genetic susceptibility that impairs their body's ability to recognize and eliminate mycotoxins effectively.[1] People with this genetic predisposition may also have an inhibited ability to deal with other types of toxins, including pesticides, solvents, petrochemicals, and formaldehyde. Essentially, the detoxification system may develop a traffic jam, so to speak, when dealing with candida toxins.

Experiencing a little bit of die-off is a good sign; it means your treatment strategy is effective. But die-off can be so severe and debilitating that it becomes unbearable to endure, significantly impeding the recovery process. Too much die-off can put you in bed flat on your back and significantly disrupt your ability to function. The "cure" can be worse than living with candida itself. If the individual is unaware of the steps that can be taken to reduce the severity of die-off and their practitioner does not inform them, they often abandon their treatment protocol. Additionally, severe die-off is counterproductive because it overwhelms the detoxification and sympathetic nervous systems. Overloading the detoxification system results in the recirculation of toxins throughout the body, which will further intensify die-off. Overstimulating the sympathetic nervous system, as previously discussed, perpetuates sympathetic dominance, which in turn promotes overgrowth of candida and other microbes. Further, the destruction of candida results in high levels of inflammation, which promotes more colonization.

SYMPTOMS OF DIE-OFF

The symptoms of candida die-off can vary widely, but most commonly they involve an exacerbation of the physical or psychological symptoms that an individual already experiences. Here are some of the most common:

brain fog

headaches

impaired concentration and focus

generalized anxiety or anxiety attacks

depression

irritability and crankiness

tightness in the chest

increased heart rate or palpitations

heightened fatigue and weakness

dizziness

fever, chills, and sweating

aching joints or muscles

sore throat or swollen glands

diarrhea and/or constipation

itching, hives, or rashes

nausea

breakouts on the skin

sinusitis

increase in gas or other gastrointestinal symptoms

overwhelming cravings for sugar and other carbs or caffeine

cravings for alcohol or other mind-altering substances

feeling intoxicated

flu-like symptoms

STEPS YOU CAN TAKE
TO REDUCE SEVERITY OF DIE-OFF

Stay on the Diet

The first and most important step for minimizing die-off is to remain on the diet described in chapters 10 and 11. As discussed in the chapter on antifungals, it is best not to begin taking any antifungals until after you have been on the diet for a couple of weeks. This will gently lower the level of yeast in the body before killing it directly. If while taking an antifungal you eat sugar in any form, honey, or even a lot of complex carbohydrates, then you're also feeding candida while you're killing it, which will make the symptoms of die-off more brutal. In addition, you need to provide your body with the nutrients it needs to support your detoxification system and the optimal functioning of organs.

Go Slowly

The more candida that is killed at one time, the greater the number of toxins produced and the worse the inflammation. Killing too many organisms at one time will worsen die-off. Treatment with antifungals should begin at a low dose and gradually work up to a higher dose. If at any point too much die-off occurs, reduce the dosage for a while and then move forward even more slowly.

Sometimes a particular antifungal may be too powerful for you, which creates intense die-off. If reducing the dosage doesn't work, it may be necessary to use a different, less potent antifungal until candida levels are reduced. As discussed in chapter 3, pulsing (taking the remedy every other day, or even every two days, rather than every day, or one week on and one week off) may be necessary as well.

Supplement with Molybdenum and Pantethine

Molybdenum is a trace mineral that helps the body produce two crucial enzymes: aldehyde dehydrogenase and aldehyde oxidase. Both enzymes are used to eliminate acetaldehyde, the primary toxic byproduct of candida. As we learned in Chapter 1, acetaldehyde is responsible for many of the symptoms experienced in candida overgrowth and is significantly increased during die-off, so eliminating it reduces symptoms. These two enzymes also help break down other toxins like alcohol and formaldehyde. Molybdenum is discussed in more detail on pages 459–460.

Pantethine, the active form of vitamin B5 (pantothenic acid), has been shown to boost levels of aldehyde dehydrogenase.[2] It also increases levels of coenzyme A (CoA), a cofactor in numerous enzymatic pathways. For the purpose of this discussion, however, we are focused on its role in the detoxification pathway known as acetylation. The acetylation pathway uses CoA to attach to toxins and carry them out of the body. Improving function of the acetylation pathway also helps reduce levels of candida byproducts, which in turn helps reduce die-off. In addition, pantethine is critical for the adrenal glands (see chapter 14).

One of the first practitioners to promote the use of molybdenum was Stephan Cooter. In his book *Beating Chronic Illness,* he suggests an optimal dose of 300 micrograms (mcg) per day divided into three doses. I have used 300 mcg in two divided doses daily for many years with great success. For the purpose of breaking down acetaldehyde, pantethine is typically used at a dosage of 600 mgs per day in divided doses.

Acetaldehyde in its original form cannot be eliminated from the body, so the body converts it into acetic acid, which the liver either eliminates or converts into CoA. In order to make this conversion to acetic acid the body needs sufficient levels of vitamins B6, B3, and B12, selenium, glutamine, folic acid, iron, and molybdenum. However, if acetaldehyde levels are high due to candida overgrowth, the body can have a hard time keeping up, even if the necessary nutrients are available.

Supplement with Vitamin C

High doses of buffered vitamin C powder can help significantly reduce die-off symptoms in a variety of ways. Vitamin C helps improve acetylation and other detoxification pathways, which, as described, can move candida byproducts out of the body. It is a powerful antioxidant with anti-inflammatory and antihistamine effects, which can buffer reactions, and it boosts the immune system. Vitamin C should be taken to bowel tolerance—meaning to the dosage your body can handle without producing diarrhea. Vitamin C is also critical for the adrenal glands (see page 455–457).

Support the Liver

Milk thistle, also known as silymarin, is an herb that has been proven in laboratory studies to repair and protect the liver, the primary organ involved in eliminating candida toxins. Silymarin can both optimize liver function and improve its detoxification abilities. It is so effective that it is commonly used for treating alcohol-induced liver disease and hepatitis. Silymarin exerts its effects in a variety of ways. It protects liver cells by binding to them directly and blocking toxins from entering, and it neutralizes toxins that are already present in the liver. It helps regenerate damaged liver cells and encourages the growth of new cells. It increases production of bile (used to transport toxins to the colon) and of glutathione and SOD, two powerful antioxidants that play a critical role in detoxification and in reducing inflammation.

When choosing a brand of milk thistle for optimum potency and effectiveness, look for one whose label states it is standardized to contain 80 percent silymarin extract. In most cases, milk thistle is considered very safe even for long-term use. It doesn't tend to produce many significant side effects; however, some reports of nausea, headache, rash, gastrointestinal upset, and other effects have emerged. If you're allergic to ragweed, you should avoid milk thistle, as it is in the same family. And since milk thistle targets the liver, it could affect other medications or natural remedies you may be taking. Milk thistle may lower blood sugar, so exercise caution if low blood sugar is pronounced for you or you're taking medication for diabetes.

Other supplements that can boost liver function and enhance detoxification include alpha-lipoic acid, glutathione, lecithin, N-acetylcysteine, vitamin B6, artichoke root, burdock root, and dandelion root. As noted elsewhere, N-acetylcysteine should be accompanied by vitamin C at two to three times the dosage of NAC. Some of these substances can have contraindications that are discussed in chapter 14.

The liver uses sulfur compounds to make the antioxidant glutathione, which enhances its ability to detoxify substances of all kinds, including mycotoxins like acetaldehyde and others. Vitamin C, alpha-lipoic acid, high-sulfur foods (broccoli, cabbage, kale, cauliflower, eggs, garlic, onions), milk thistle, NAC, glutamine, and whey protein can all help increase glutathione production. Glutathione also improves immune function and reduces inflammation. Mycotoxins can inhibit the body's ability to produce glutathione, so it may be low in individuals with fungal infections. On the flip side, as mentioned on page 470, glutathione can elevate glutamate levels in people with already high glutamate, and it can inhibit methylation in some individuals, so exercise caution. Additionally, it is believed by some practitioners that NAC, alpha lipoic acid, cysteine, and other sulfur-based supplements may actually make candida proliferate when taken orally. One may be able to get around this issue with transdermal supplementation.

The kidneys are also important in detoxification because they filter the blood and produce urine to remove toxins, waste products (including urea, a byproduct of protein metabolism), and excess water. They are best supported by avoiding sugar, alcohol, and high-carb foods, ensuring adequate amino acid intake, and drinking plenty of water.

Utilize an Enema or Colonic

Candida frequently resides in the colon. Furthermore, the detoxification system moves many toxins (e.g., those generated by candida) from other parts of the body into the colon to be eliminated through the stool. Physically removing candida and its toxins from the colon with an enema or colonic can provide immediate and significant reduction in die-off symptoms and enhance liver function. Enemas and colonics (including instructions) are discussed in more detail in chapter 13.

Bind Mycotoxins

Activated charcoal capsules taken orally are effective for absorbing toxins of many different kinds, including mycotoxins released by candida and the dead cells of candida itself. This prevents the toxins from being taken up in the bloodstream and carries them to the stool to be eliminated, which reduces die-off symptoms. Bentonite clay has a similar effect. Both charcoal and clay need to be taken without food, other supplements, or pharmaceutical drugs, as they can bind to nutrients and other substances. High-dose chlorella also binds to mycotoxins.

Calcium-D-glucarate can be used to improve the glucuronidation detoxification pathway, which may be inhibited due to bacterial overgrowth. This pathway, which helps eliminate pharmaceutical drugs, chemicals, estrogen, and corticosteroids, may become overloaded during die-off. Calcium-D-glucarate may also bind with some mycotoxins.

Stay Hydrated

Staying sufficiently hydrated is critical for moving toxins out of the body. The human body is about 75 percent water, and the human brain is about 70 percent water. Water is essential for every basic function in the body, including flushing away toxins. Without sufficient water, toxins will not move. This becomes even more critical when toxin levels are increased, as they are during die-off. Additionally, blood needs water to carry oxygen and nutrients to the brain and all the cells in our body.

Keep Physically Active

Being sedentary encourages toxins to accumulate, which increases symptoms of die-off. Remaining physically active throughout the day keeps toxins moving and boosts the immune system, helps the bowels function more effectively, enhances liver function, and improves the detoxification process. As noted, an improved detoxification pathway helps the body rid itself of candida and its byproducts (e.g., ammonia and acetaldehyde), consequently boosting mood and alleviating pain in the muscles, joints, and bones and other related symptoms. Regular exercise affords numerous other benefits as well. However, the way you exercise is critical. Be sure to read pages 407–413 to learn how to exercise properly.

Make Sure the Bowels Are Moving

Since many bodily toxins are transported to the colon and eliminated through the stool, it is essential to maintain regular bowel movements. If stool sits in the colon for too long, toxins get recirculated, placing more burden on the detoxification system and increasing symptoms.

Although constipation or slow transit time is a common occurrence in people with candida and other microbial overgrowth, the bowels can be kept regular with the daily use of high-dose buffered vitamin C powder.

High-dose vitamin C produces diarrhea in everyone because it pulls water into the colon, so it can be used as a natural laxative. You don't want to take a dose that produces diarrhea, but you want to take enough to make your bowels move. Dosage is determined in each individual by taking it to bowel tolerance, meaning consuming as much as the body can take in without producing diarrhea. If diarrhea is produced at a particular dosage, cut back on the dosage just a little until diarrhea stops but bowels continue to move smoothly. High-dose vitamin C provides an abundance of other benefits for the individual with candida—for example, supporting the immune system and the adrenal glands.

Another cause of constipation may be a deficiency in magnesium. Consider having your magnesium levels tested with a magnesium-loading test. Supplemental magnesium can be used occasionally to help the bowels move even if a deficiency does not exist, but it should not be used long term independently. Long-term magnesium use without calcium supplementation can lead to an imbalance in the levels of these two important minerals, which can result in a wide array of problems. Herbs like *Cascara sagrada* may be used on occasion to promote bowel movement, but they can produce dependency if used long term. Sufficient water and fat intake and regular physical activity are critical for motility as well. Constipation can also be the result of hypothyroidism, which is discussed in more detail in chapter 13, or from archaea organisms discussed in chapter 6.

Another major factor contributing to the large number of colon problems we see in our society is the shape of the modern toilet. Human beings are supposed to squat when having a bowel movement. Squatting allows the colon to completely empty itself, which is necessary to keep things flowing smoothly and to prevent buildup of waste materials along the colon wall. The toilet we use today is in complete contradiction to what is healthy. It does not allow for squatting; therefore, complete evacuation of the colon does not take place, and constipation and other colon problems develop. If you have ever gone to the bathroom in the woods, you will know this is true. When squatting in the woods, the bowel movement comes out with such ease and the bowel feels so complete and empty afterwards that it is actually renewing. You'll say, "Wow, that felt great."

There are a variety of steps you can take to address this problem. While sitting on the toilet, put something under your feet (e.g., a stool, a brick, etc.) that raises your legs to simulate a squatting position. There are products on the market designed specifically for this purpose, like the Squatty Potty. Another option is to install a new toilet with a shape that allows you to squat. If you happen to be in the process of remodeling or building a new home, it could be incorporated into your building plan. A less desirable option could be to place a bedpan on the floor, squat over it, and then empty it in the toilet.

Increase Parasympathetic Nervous System Activity

As discussed, candida overgrowth can be both a cause and a symptom of chronic stress and sympathetic dominance. If stress is high and the sympathetic nervous system is in overdrive, die-off symptoms can be significantly amplified. In turn, die-off further activates the sympathetic nervous system. In some cases, hyperactivity of the sympathetic nervous system can make it impossible to get through die-off and treatment is abandoned. Therefore, it is vital to decrease stress and sympathetic dominance and increase parasympathetic nervous system activity. Many techniques for doing so are discussed in great depth in chapters 12 and 13, including deep-breathing exercises, mindfulness-based meditation, communing with nature, smiling, and others.

Reduce Toxin Load

When the body is dealing with candida die-off, its total toxin load is increased. The presence of additional toxins adds even more to its burden. Minimize your exposure to other toxins, as suggested in chapter 13, by living a green and environmentally friendly lifestyle.

Take Enzymes

Some enzymes—for example, cellulase, protease, amylase, hemicellulase, and chitosanase—can help degrade the dying yeast cells, which may help decrease symptoms of die-off.

Use a Sauna

Far-infrared sauna has been shown to help mobilize toxins of many different kinds, including mycotoxins.

For most people, die-off is a temporary situation that diminishes slowly with time. It is usually at its worst during the first week of treatment and decreases in severity thereafter. However, duration and severity are influenced by the type of antifungal one is taking (depending on their method of eradication, some antifungals produce more die-off than others), the ability of the body's detoxification system, and the level of overgrowth that is present. Some people may experience die-off to some extent throughout the entire course of treatment, while others may get through it within a couple of days. Responses vary widely from person to person. Don't push yourself too hard, be compassionate, cut back and go slower when needed, don't give up, and remind yourself that it won't last forever. However, do not ever force yourself to endure die off-that is too severe. It will do more harm than good.

CHAPTER 9

Supporting the Troops:
Boosting Your Immune System

Your immune system is an astonishing, fascinating, and complex network of organs, tissues, and cells that exist to protect your body from foreign invaders and tumors. You might think of it as a superhero or a branch of the military. It forms natural barriers to keep invaders out of the body and launches direct attacks to get rid of any that manage to penetrate the barriers and infect the body. Immune cells travel around the body looking for bad guys (bacteria, viruses, yeast or other fungi, toxins, cancer cells, or anything foreign) that will harm you; when the immune cells find these unwelcome characters, they destroy and dispose of them quite efficiently.

The ability of the immune system to distinguish between "self" and "nonself" is crucial to prevent it from attacking bodily tissue. The body's cells (self) are distinguished or "marked" by particular types of proteins. This allows immune cells to identify and coexist peacefully with other bodily cells and also to recognize the invaders. A nonself substance that has the ability to incite an immune response is called an antigen. The immune system launches an attack anytime it encounters an antigen. An antigen may consist of a microbe—a virus, bacterium, yeast, or parasite—or it may consist of only a fragment of that microbe, such as a molecule. Antigens may also consist of chemicals, environmental toxins, pollens, undigested food particles, or toxins produced by a bacterium, yeast, or other microbe. Cells and tissues from another human being are also marked as nonself and are perceived as antigens (unless they are from your identical twin). This is why transplanted organs are sometimes rejected.

THE IMMUNE SYSTEM'S ARSENAL

When a foreign invader is found, the immune system has a variety of different weapons in its arsenal to get rid of it, depending on the situation. These weapons are white blood cells and antibodies. The big guns are the lymphocytes, neutrophils, eosinophils, macrophages, basophils, and natural killer cells (all types of white blood cells) and immunoglobulins (also called antibodies), which can travel through either the blood vessels or lymphatic vessels. Some cells display a wide variety of skills and can destroy many different kinds of invaders; others are highly specialized (like the Navy Seals) and go after only a particular type of pathogen. They rally together as a team and use an elaborate communication system to devour, puncture, blow up, inject, or spray the invaders with chemicals. One cell may flag an invader as an antigen and call in another type of cell to gobble it up or spray it with a chemical. Another cell hangs around and keeps watch to make sure the invader doesn't come back.

B Cells and T Cells

Some lymphocytes mature within the bone marrow (B cells); others are sent to the thymus to mature (T cells). Both identify and destroy invaders, but they do so in slightly different ways. B cells produce antibodies against the invader (called humoral immunity or antibody production), but they are not capable of penetrating a cell. Each B cell is hardwired to produce only one particular type of antibody and is activated whenever it encounters the antigen it is designed for, at which time it produces plasma cells that in turn produce the antibodies. T cells don't identify free-floating antigens; they may instruct and regulate the immune response or attack an infected or cancerous area directly. They destroy the invading organism by killing the bodily cell that is infected with the microbe, or by releasing chemicals called lymphokines that incite an immune response to attack the invader (cell-mediated immunity). They destroy cancer cells in the same ways. Some lymphocytes travel through lymphatic vessels and the blood vessels and patrol the body, while others are stored in the lymphoid organs. Most lymphocytes are T cells.

There are several types of T cells, and each one has a unique job:

Helper T cells, as the name implies, help to support the rest of the immune system. They use cytokines to call in macrophages, activate B cells that produce antibodies, and fuel production of cytotoxic T cells and suppressor T cells. Helper T cells are the cells that are affected in HIV.

Cytotoxic T cells excrete chemicals that fracture and destroy foreign invaders (e.g., viruses, bacteria, or fungi), cancer cells, or other cells that have been harmed in some way.

Natural killer cells (NK cells) are a type of cytotoxic T cell that bind with cancer cells or with other cells that have been infected with a microbe. NK cells then inject a deadly toxin to kill the affected cells. You can think of them as the Special Ops branch of your immune system: They move in very quickly and stealth-like and do not need prior information about the antigen to make a strike. They may slay on contact anything that is nonself. NK cells also assist in regulating the immune response by releasing cytokines that instruct other parts of the immune system to kill an invader. If natural killer cells are not functioning properly, the risk may be increased for certain autoimmune diseases such as type 1 diabetes or asthma, or for certain types of cancer.

Memory T cells stick around after an attack in case the invader returns to the scene. They are quite "intelligent" in that they keep a "record" of all the invaders that have affected your body. If the same pathogens try to invade the body again in the future, memory T cells can fight them off more easily.

Suppressor T cells keep the immune system from getting out of control and harming healthy cells.

Antibodies

Antibodies, also known as immunoglobulins, are Y-shaped molecules that ambush and bind to antigens, causing them to be neutralized or broken open and destroyed by other parts of the immune system. They may mark a particular pathogen so that it can be found by another immune cell for elimination, or they may take steps to neutralize the microbe by damaging its ability to survive or invade the host's bodily cells. There is a specific antibody for each individual antigen: one takes care of the flu virus; another targets a particular bacterium; another goes after candida. They are not interchangeable. Essentially, the antibody puts a little flag on the antigen that tells the white blood cells, "Hey guys, here's one, come and get him." Antibodies also activate the complement system (discussed below).

The five primary types of immunoglobulins are IgA, IgG, IgM, IgE, and IgD. They function as follows:

IgA is present in and guards all the mucosal surfaces throughout the body, including those inside the nose, ears, eyes, gastrointestinal tract, respiratory tract, and vagina. It is also present in fluids such as saliva, blood, and tears. Approximately 10 to 15 percent of the antibodies in the body are IgA.

IgG puts a coat on microbes to increase the speed at which other cells in the immune system can gather them up. IgG is found in all bodily fluids. It is vital for eliminating bacteria, viruses, and candida. IgG antibodies are the smallest and the most common in the human body, making up about 75 to 80 percent of all antibodies. They are the only antibody that can travel across the placenta to protect an unborn child.

IgM antibodies are potent against bacteria and can be found in the blood and lymph fluid. About 5 to 10 percent of all antibodies in the body are IgM. It has the largest molecular structure of the antibodies. IgM antibodies are the first to be made when a response is launched, and they assist other immune cells in destroying foreign invaders.

IgE is in charge of safeguarding against parasites. It is also what prompts the reaction to allergens such as animal dander, pollen, mold, food, medications, and poisons. IgE antibodies are found on the skin, lungs, and mucous membranes.

IgD remains connected to B cells, where it plays a primary role in promptly launching B cell responses. It is found in tissues that line the stomach and chest. At this time, all the roles of IgD are not completely understood.

If your body does not produce enough antibodies, you may be more vulnerable to infection and disease. Some people are born with a reduced capacity to produce antibodies, and production may also be stunted in response to some diseases like cancer.

Other White Blood Cells

Phagocytes—which include neutrophils, eosinophils, and monocytes (macrophages)—are white blood cells that gobble up, devour, engulf, or eat pathogens. They also absorb dead cells and help wounds to heal. Neutrophils and macrophages take care of bacteria and fungi; eosinophils primarily target parasites. Macrophages are monocytes that are present in tissue; when they are in the bloodstream they are called monocytes. A macrophage may present an antigen to other lymphocytes and produce a chemical signal called a monokine that is used in the immune response. Neutrophils contain chemicals that break down the invaders they consume. Eosinophils and basophils spray harmful microbes or cells with chemicals to damage them.

The white blood cells known as granulocytes contain granules that are filled with powerful chemicals to kill microorganisms. One of these chemicals is histamine, which contributes to allergy and inflammation. Basophils are a type of granulocyte that are connected with allergy-related antigens. Mast cells—which are not really blood cells but function similarly to basophils—are found in the nose, lungs, tongue, and skin; they also play a significant role in allergy symptoms. Mast cell granules are filled with histamine and heparin (an anticoagulant). Basophils are in the blood; mast cells are in the tissue. Platelets, which are used for blood clotting and repair of wounds, also activate some immune activity. Dendritic cells, which reside in lymphoid organs, help stimulate T cells and present antigens to the T cells.

ON THE DEFENSIVE

The body makes use of two kinds of immunity: natural immunity (also called innate immunity) and acquired immunity (also adaptive immunity). Natural immunity is conferred by barriers you are born with, such as skin, epithelial cells, and antibodies passed from mother to child. Acquired immunity results from exposure to a particular antigen, whereby the immune system learns and remembers how to eliminate it most effectively if it returns. Acquired immunity is utilized in vaccinations. If you give the body a diluted amount of a particular antigen, the body will learn how to get rid of it. If the same antigen presents itself in full force later, the body will already know what to do to keep you from getting sick. Some researchers believe that vaccines contain a variety of toxins that are harmful to the body, making their overall effectiveness questionable. There are numerous other risks that may be associated with vaccines as well.

Cytokines are small proteins that are used in cell-to-cell communication within the immune system. Types of cytokines include interleukins, interferons, growth factors, and others. A key element in the inflammatory response, cytokines help regulate the immune system by amplifying activity when there is an invasion, turning it down when the coast is clear, and quieting the immune system when it is overactive. One type of white blood cell will use cytokines to notify another type of white blood cell about an invader and instruct it to strike. Cytokines can turn on or off particular types of immune cells and stimulate the production of T cells. Some cytokines are proinflammatory and others are anti-inflammatory. The proinflammatory cytokines produce inflammation when fighting off an invader, and the anti-inflammatory ones are activated to reduce inflammation once the invader is eradicated.

Organs in the immune system, referred to as lymphoid organs, are located throughout the body. Lymphoid organs house and deploy the immune cells. They are attached to one another and to other organs in the body via the lymphatic vessels. The lymphoid organs include:

- tonsils (back of throat)

- adenoids (between nose and back of throat)

- thymus (in center of chest)

- spleen (left side of abdomen)

- bone marrow (soft center of all bones)

- lymph nodes (distributed widely throughout the body, e.g., armpits, neck, breasts, etc.)

- lymphatic vessels (distributed widely throughout the body)

- appendix (lower right of abdomen)

- Peyer's patches (organized lymphoid nodules in the lower part of the small intestine)

Microbes can enter the body through the mouth, nose, lungs, gastrointestinal tract, eyes, genitals, or skin. First, though, each of these organs has a variety of protective mechanisms in place that the microbe must penetrate. The skin is like a suit of armor and can only be penetrated by a cut or abrasion. The stomach secretes a variety of enzymes that destroy microbes, the nose produces mucus, and the lungs cough. If the microbe manages to get past these front-line barriers, then it must penetrate the second line of defense, which consists of a thick, protective layer of epithelial cells covered with mucus and lining all the passageways (respiratory, gastrointestinal, and urogenital). The mucous lining secretes IgA antibodies that capture approaching invaders. If the microbe manages to get past this epithelial layer, it will encounter B cells, T cells, and macrophages lying in hiding just below. There the invader will be attacked by phagocytes, natural killer cells, and the complement system. The innate immune system is always present; its initial response is immediate, short-lived, generic, and nonspecific. The complement system, which is part of the innate system, supports antibodies and assists other parts of the immune system such as neutrophils and macrophages.

Next the microbe faces the adaptive immune system, in which T cells and antibodies are armed with ammunition that is designed specifically for each type of microbe. The adaptive immune system is called on when invaders overcome the innate immune system. It provides highly specialized and long-lasting immunity that has been acquired from encountering pathogens and learning how to handle them better next time. As mentioned above, there are two types of responses within the adaptive immune system: humoral immunity (moderated by antibodies that are produced by B cells) and cell-mediated immunity (moderated by T lymphocytes).

This brief description is a really condensed and simplified explanation for immunity, but it should give you a general idea of the many parts involved in your immune system and how it works. Now, imagine that you have cut your finger. The amazing immune cells immediately gather around the source of injury, send an alarm to other cells, share information with one another, call other cells in to help them, generate powerful chemicals, kill the invaders, help the wound heal, and leave sentries behind to watch out for reinfection—all while patrolling the rest of the body for potential trouble spots. This happens automatically for you, without any effort on your part, a fact that is nothing short of astounding and should leave you with a sense of awe.

WHEN THINGS GO WRONG

Sometimes things can go awry in the immune system. It may become suppressed or overactive; it may confuse self for nonself or hit the wrong target. When this occurs, any of several disorders may develop (e.g., allergies, autoimmunity, certain types of arthritis, cancer), and one may be left vulnerable to invasion by a wide variety of microorganisms. For example, if the immune system confuses self for nonself, it may produce antibodies against the body's own tissue or cells and launch an attack against itself, resulting in an autoimmune disorder such as lupus, rheumatoid arthritis, or thyroiditis. If the immune system becomes hypervigilant and goes after substances that are not really harmful to us, like pollen or animal dander, then allergies develop. If immune cells become impaired for some reason or are not available in sufficient numbers, then a microbe may enter the body and get the upper hand, leading to infection, or cancer cells may not be kept under control.

As we learned in chapter 1, candida and other microbes can significantly impair the immune system and manipulate it to evade detection. They can directly suppress or activate the immune system. Some microbes can make the body excrete zinc in the urine to intentionally disarm the immune system. (Zinc is vital for the immune system to function properly.) In chapter 3, we learned that biofilms keep the immune system in a disabled state by shielding the harmful organisms from detection. The body may have insufficient numbers of natural killer cells, other lymphocytes, neutrophils, macrophages, or other phagocytes—all of which hunt down and annihilate pathogens like candida, other fungi, bacteria, parasites, and viruses, as well as cancer cells, toxins, or other foreign invaders. Compromised immunity encourages proliferation of candida and other microbes, which in turn further disrupts immunity.

About 70 percent of the immune system is located in and around the gut. As mentioned above, the gastrointestinal tract is lined with specialized cells (enterocytes) and mucus—together called the epithelium—that form a protective barrier to keep pathogens from entering the body. In the small intestine, enterocytes also generate enzymes that break down food and absorb nutrients. In the large intestine, enterocytes absorb water and electrolytes. Enterocytes also manage transportation of antigens and present antigens to the T cells. Since candida and other microbes reside primarily in the gastrointestinal tract, they can do exceptional harm to this barrier in a variety of ways.

First, the healthy gut flora help form the epithelial lining. When candida and pathogenic bacteria are taking up most of the space in the gut, there are fewer good guys around to help shape a sturdy and secure physical barrier. Friendly gut bacteria use the lymph nodes to share information with the immune system to help it differentiate between good microbes and bad ones. They also help regulate the growth and formation of organs like the thymus that play a critical role in immunity. Friendly flora also help activate phagocytosis (the eating of pathogens by immune cells) and the manufacturing of lymphocytes and antibodies. They generate hydrogen peroxide and other natural antimicrobial substances called bacteriocins, which retard pathogenic activity and generate organic acids that help sustain the right gastrointestinal pH to inhibit the growth of pathogens. When the friendly folk are taken over and replaced by candida and other harmful microbes, or when they are wiped out due to other factors such as poor diet or drug use, immune function declines. Additionally, if epithelial cells are damaged by other causes (examples listed below) inflammation is promoted that encourages overgrowth of candida and other pathogens.

Enterocytes die and are regenerated every few days. They develop within the villi (small, finger-like protrusions) then migrate to the tips of the villi, where they are sloughed off and replaced with new ones. This process is conducted by the gut flora. If the friendly flora have been wiped out by candida and pathogenic bacteria, fewer enterocytes will be regenerated and the barrier will weaken. This perpetuates the whole cycle, creating an environment that encourages more overgrowth and a weaker immune system. Your friendly flora also assist with digestion, nutrient absorption, construction of digestive enzymes, metabolization of lipids, and breakdown of cholesterol, and generate nutrients like B12, vitamin K, short-chain fatty acids, and biotin. Without sufficient levels of good guys, these actions will be impaired.

As discussed previously, both candida and bacteria increase levels of zonulin, the substance that controls the tight junctions between enterocytes, which leads to weaker junctions and the development of leaky gut. Candida can also penetrate directly through the wall of the gut lining, contributing to leaky gut. A leaking gut allows undigested food particles, toxins, candida, bacteria, and other pathogens to get into the bloodstream where they do not belong, prompting the immune system to create antibodies against these substances and potentially producing food sensitivities. In a process called molecular mimicry, the immune system may become confused, causing antibodies to cross-react with bodily tissue in the thyroid, skin, joints, brain, or other areas, leading to more inflammation and the development of autoimmune disorders.

When the body becomes chronically infected with a stubborn microbe like candida, the immune system remains in constant battle with the organism. This results in a high level of oxidative stress and inflammation, which can lead to a wide variety of other health problems and premature aging. Inflammation is considered to be a major contributing factor to just about every health condition, including heart disease, type 2 diabetes, obesity, cancer, depression, Alzheimer's, and more. As time goes on, the immune system may simply become overwhelmed by continually fighting candida and other pathogenic microbes, resulting in an inability to perform its job as effectively.

On the flip side, if one's immune system is weak or is challenged for other reasons, one is more vulnerable to overgrowth of candida or other microbes. The immune system is inhibited in its ability to fight a good fight. Impaired immunity can be both the cause and the result of overgrowth of candida or other microbes. Taking as many steps as possible to enhance immunity is an important component of the healing journey.

FEED YOUR TROOPS WELL

The first and most important way that you can support your troops is by eating the correct diet. A good general wouldn't send her troops into battle without proper nourishment. Nor would she feed them substances that would slow them down or impair their ability to do their job or weaken the integrity of their attack plan. Like all cells, enterocytes require nutrients (protein, fat, vitamins, minerals, etc.) for their survival. These nutrients are acquired from the food you eat. If you're not supplying enough of them for the gut, then cellular regeneration may be inhibited.

On the other hand, certain foods can be destructive to the epithelium and thus contribute to weakened immunity or autoimmunity.

At the top of this list are grains (wheat, corn, rye, sorghum, oat, rice), sugar, and legumes. Both grains (including whole grains) and legumes contain high levels of lectins, naturally occurring, sticky, but toxic substances comprised of part protein and part carbohydrate, produced by some plants to protect themselves from predators. The human body doesn't break down lectins very well. Lectins exert a wide variety of negative effects against the gastrointestinal tract to deter you from eating those plants again. They attach to the epithelium in the small intestine, particularly the villi, causing the same kind of damage as candida and other microbes and leading to the development of leaky gut and consequently impaired nutrient absorption, inhibition of friendly flora, food sensitivities, production of enzymes, inflammation, and autoimmunity.

When lectins cross into the bloodstream, the immune system perceives them as foreigners and goes after them. Once in the bloodstream, lectins can attach to the cells of organs; when the immune system attacks the lectin, it also attacks the bodily tissue that the lectin is binding to, which leads to more inflammation and possibly the development of autoimmune disorders. For example, if lectins attach to thyroid cells, thyroiditis or Grave's disease may develop. If it binds to cells in the joint tissue, arthritis may appear. Lectins are connected to a wide array of autoimmune disorders, including, but not limited to, lupus, colitis, multiple sclerosis, Crohn's, and rheumatoid arthritis.

All this havoc demands that a tremendous amount of resources be aimed at the affected region, which means there are fewer resources available for fundamental tasks like tissue growth and repair. This scenario creates an environment that encourages the overgrowth of candida and other pathogenic microbes. Lectins also have the ability to cause abnormal cell division, which may lead to cancer. Lectins have a variety of other negative effects, which you can read about on page 252.

In addition to lectins, both grains and legumes contain proteins that are similar to those contained in some bacteria and other microbes.

For example, candida contains HWP (hyphal wall protein), as discussed on pages 19–20. The immune system may get confused, mistake the food for an invader, and launch an attack against it and consequently against your own body. Grains and legumes also contain other destructive substances called phytates (phytic acid). Phytates can bind to minerals that are critical for immune function and gut health—for instance magnesium, iron, zinc, and calcium—inhibiting the body's ability to access them and leading to deficiencies in these nutrients. High levels of phytic acid may also reduce the activity of some digestive enzymes, aggravate the gut, and become a factor in leaky gut.

Grains and legumes contain high levels of protease inhibitors, substances that inhibit the capability of digestive enzymes to break down protein, which in turn impairs the body's ability to absorb amino acids. Amino acids are vital for the production of antibodies. Protein also plays a vital role in the healing process at the cellular level if a pathogen successfully invades the body. When protease inhibitors interfere with the activity of one enzyme, other enzymes like trypsin may accumulate in excess, which can lead to the release of antibodies and proinflammatory cytokines, culminating in more inflammation. Animal protein is the best source for all the essential amino acids. Protein from nonanimal sources is either incomplete or does not contain sufficient levels of the essential amino acids. A diet that is lacking in animal protein will leave you susceptible to invasion and infection by microbes of all kinds and impair your ability to heal.

Besides protein, another vital macronutrient is fat. White blood cells' ability to recognize and destroy pathogens like candida, bacteria, viruses, and cancer is compromised if there is not enough saturated fat in the diet. Fifty percent of every cell's membrane is made of saturated fat; it is what supplies the cell with integrity and stiffness.[1] Fat also transports the fat-soluble vitamins (A, D, E, and K), converts dietary beta-carotene into vitamin A, and aids in the absorption of minerals—all of which are needed for a strong immune system. Medium-chain and short-chain fatty acids hold some antimicrobial characteristics, which can help safeguard you from microbes. They also possess other attributes that support immunity.

Too much dietary fiber can make pathogens multiply, and a byproduct of fiber fermentation can destroy healthy flora. Fiber intake should not be too high.

As mentioned in other areas of this book, many other substances besides legumes and grains are destructive to your healthy flora and your gut lining and can therefore impair immunity. These include chlorinated drinking water, chocolate, caffeine, alcohol, food additives and preservatives, artificial sweeteners, sugar, high-carb foods, excessive amounts of omega-6 fatty acids, NSAIDs, proton pump inhibitors, acid reducers, prednisone or other corticosteroids, birth control pills, antibiotics, pesticides and herbicides, genetically modified foods, and heavy metals. Sleep deprivation, enzyme deficiencies, insufficient nutrient intake, and chronic stress can also have negative effects.

High blood glucose (caused from the consumption of sugar and carbs) decreases blood circulation,[2] which consequently reduces the ability of the white blood cells to expediently travel to the areas where they are needed and in adequate quantities to protect the body from pathogens. It also curtails phagocytosis activity (the process by which white blood cells consume pathogens), inhibits neutrophils from being able to stick to the endothelium or the inner lining of blood cells, and disrupts chemotaxis, a chemical-signaling system that directs neutrophils to the areas where invasion or injury exist. Neutrophils are some of the most powerful weapons we have against candida. Thus, the consumption of sugar and carbs directly impedes our ability to protect ourselves from candida and invasion by other microbes. Studies have demonstrated that immune function can be inhibited for at least five hours after the consumption of sugar.[3] The body can get all the vitamins, minerals, and antioxidants it needs for a strong immune system with the consumption of low-carb vegetables; no other carbohydrates are really necessary.

Furthermore, the immune system needs a wide variety of nutrients in order to function optimally, including zinc, selenium, vitamins A, C, E, B12, and B6, chromium, copper, iodine, and manganese. If your diet does not provide these nutrients in adequate amounts, immune function may be inhibited. Vitamin A is required for the production of white blood cells as well as regeneration of the mucosal lining in the gut. Zinc is essential for the production and activation of lymphocytes, strengthening the gut lining, and preventing intestinal permeability. Studies have shown that zinc tightens up leaky gut.[4] A recent study at Cornell University has found a correlation between zinc levels and the number and diversity of microbes in the guts of chickens.[5] Vitamin E stimulates B cells. Vitamin B6 is required for manufacturing red blood cells, protein metabolism, and cell growth. B12 is needed for cell growth and maturity. Manganese reinforces the cell wall and provides support for natural killer cells and macrophages. Vitamin C is required for both the production and activation of immune cells. Vitamin C also helps boost interferon, antibodies, and white blood cells and most other cells involved in the immune system. High-dose vitamin C has been very effective as an adjunctive treatment for serious health conditions like hepatitis C, HIV, and cancer.[6]

Vitamin D manufactures antimicrobial peptides that protect the body from yeasts and other microbes. About 70 percent of the population may be lacking in sufficient vitamin D levels.[7] Dr. Robert Atkins states that the immune system's vitality rises and falls directly with vitamin D's concentration in the body.[8] (A vitamin D measurement is one of the factors doctors use to predict the length of survival in AIDS patients.) Vitamin D (more specifically, the active form, 1a,25 dihydroxyvitamin D3) increases the production of cathelicidin LL-37. In *Combating Biofilms,* Dr. Schaller explains that cathelicidin is a collection of peptides that can inhibit or kill the "growth of microorganisms and activate the two main systems of immunity (innate and adaptive) to attack more aggressively." We have one cathelicidin gene, which can be processed into "different forms of anti-infection chemicals," but LL-37, the most commonly studied form of cathelicidins, specifically kills bacteria, increases the body's attack against infections, increases movement of cells, increases blood vessels, assists in wound repair and "handling cancer metastasis," and "activation of chemicals to focus the body systems on killing infections." It has been shown to have antibacterial, antibiofilm, and antiviral activities. It is believed to be essential for disrupting superbugs like MRSA, bacterial biofilms, and viruses like HIV. Please read pages 403–406; 461–462 for more information on acquiring adequate levels of vitamin D.

In summary: the diet should be void of grains, legumes, sugar, and other high-carbohydrate foods (including complex carbs); be rich in animal protein; contain moderate levels of fat; and be nutrient dense. Details for an eating plan that will fight candida and boost your immune system are found in the next two chapters.

AVOID YOUR IMMUNE SYSTEM ADVERSARIES

The rest of this chapter summarizes other important factors that can contribute to a compromised immune system.

Chronic Stress, Sympathetic Dominance, and Adrenal Fatigue

Cortisol plays a critical role in regulating the immune response; it both activates the response when needed and prevents it from becoming too aggressive. As we learned in chapter 2, high levels of cortisol are released when we are under stress. One of the roles of cortisol is to downregulate the immune system because all resources need to be aimed at coping with the stressful situation. It inhibits secretory IgA, the chief antibody in our mucous secretions (found in the epithelium in the gut, mouth, respiratory tract, and urinary tract). IgA defends us from invaders like candida and other microbes. Immune function may be decreased as much as 50 percent during periods of high stress. Additionally, stress hormones can directly kill the friendly microbes in the gut lining that play a critical role in immunity. They also reduce secretion of digestive enzymes and absorption of nutrients, and impair communication between the gut and brain. If stress and sympathetic dominance are ongoing, immune function will be consistently challenged.

If stress continues for an extended period of time, the adrenal glands may lose their ability to produce cortisol and other hormones efficiently. Although high cortisol can be detrimental, so can low cortisol. Low levels of cortisol incite overactivity of the immune system and autoimmunity. Cortisol is the most powerful anti-inflammatory substance in the human body; if it is present in insufficient amounts when the immune system is attacking pathogenic invaders, it will be unable to reduce the immune-triggered effects of inflammation such as redness and swelling. Additionally, cortisol is critical in reducing inflammation during autoimmune attacks. Insufficient cortisol is also associated with chronic pain syndromes, chronic fatigue, asthma, allergies, and more. Supporting the adrenal glands, managing stress, and reducing sympathetic dominance (as discussed in detail in chapters 12 and 13) are critical for immune health.

Environmental Toxins

Environmental toxins can depress immune function or overexcite the immune system and cause autoimmunity. Besides air pollution, insecticides, and herbicides, toxins are contained in everyday chemicals such as those in cosmetics, dish soap, laundry soap, shampoo, air fresheners, colognes, carpeting, plastic, paint, and perfumes. As described earlier, candida, bacteria, and other microbes release toxins as well, so toxins can come from both external and internal sources. Your own body produces a variety of toxic metabolic byproducts. Although the body has a built-in detoxification system designed to remove these waste products, it can become overloaded by man-made toxins or by those released from invasive microbes.

Toxins of all kinds generate free radicals that can bind with cytokines (proteins involved in communication within the immune system), preventing the immune system from instructing cells to go after pathogens. They may reduce activity of natural killer cells, inhibit macrophages and neutrophils, and poison bone marrow. Toxins can spur an immune response similar to that produced by lectins and undigested food particles. The presence of all toxins is a form of stress. High levels of toxins will culminate in high stress, which suppresses immunity.

Even electrosmog (electromagnetic radiation fields from electronic and wireless devices), discussed on pages 382–384, can interfere with cell-to-cell communication, impair immunity, and make candida and other microbes multiply in numbers and spew out more toxins. Electrosmog also triggers the stress response system and increases cortisol.

Minimizing your exposure to environmental toxins by living an environmentally friendly lifestyle as discussed in chapter 13 is critical to supporting optimal immune function.

Marijuana, Nicotine, and Caffeine

On pages 420–428, we will discuss many issues related to nicotine and marijuana and how they may promote overgrowth of candida and other microbes. With regard to the immune system, marijuana inhibits neutrophil activity, and nicotine suppresses the immune system in a variety of ways. Smoking cigarettes also impairs the body's ability to absorb many nutrients that are critical for a strong immune system, such as vitamin A, vitamin E, selenium, zinc, and calcium.

Avoiding marijuana and nicotine is critical for the health of your immune system.

Also as mentioned previously, caffeine sets off the stress response system and damages the adrenal glands. Caffeine consumption interferes with absorption of a variety of nutrients, including iron, calcium, vitamin D, zinc, potassium, and many of the B vitamins (e.g., B1, inositol, and biotin), many of which are needed for a strong immune system. Avoid caffeine to support the immune system.

Too Much Exercise

Mild to moderate exercise enhances circulation of immune cells throughout the body, boosts their ability to protect the body from foreign invaders, and creates more macrophages. Individuals who exercise on a consistent basis are less vulnerable to a wide range of health complaints, conditions, and illnesses. However, immune function is considerably lower in people who exercise too much. Done in excess, exercise generates free radicals, and it is a form of stress, both of which inhibit immune function. We should move frequently, but most of the time at a slow pace with occasional bursts of intensity. This topic is discussed in more detail on pages 407–413.

Lack of Sleep

We will discuss the importance of sleep for remaining committed to your diet and other factors related to healing in chapter 13. In addition, when we are sleep deprived we produce fewer antibodies and fewer granulocytes (phagocytes that consume microbes). Lack of sleep can both reduce the number of natural killer cells and decrease their activity. The immune system appears to fight a better fight while we are sleeping, and the body does all its healing and regeneration during sleep (including cellular repair and regeneration).[9,10] Sleep deprivation also triggers the stress response system and can perpetuate sympathetic dominance, and promotes inflammation. Laura Schoenfeld, staff nutritionist with Chris Kresser, explains, "When circadian rhythms get misaligned from weeks or months of inadequate sleep, inflammatory immune cells are produced excessively, leading to an increase in 'friendly fire' against the body's own tissues."[11] Ensuring that you get adequate sleep each night, as discussed on pages 399–402, is critical for your immune health.

CONSIDER REINFORCEMENTS

There's a wide range of choices in supplements that can enhance immune function. Here are a few worth noting that may be particularly helpful in tackling candida, bacteria, parasites, and their biofilms.

Beta Glucan

Beta-glucan is a polysaccharide that is found in the cell wall of a variety of fungi. Taken as a supplement, it can significantly enhance immune function. It is extracted from the cell wall of baker's yeast, but all the yeast is removed through the purification process. Beta-glucan stimulates neutrophils, macrophages, and cytokines, improving cell-to-cell communication and enhancing cells' ability to kill yeast and other microbes.

Beta-glucan has demonstrated a protective effect against *Candida albicans, Staphylococcus aureus, Escherichia coli, Pneumocystis carinii, Listeria monocytogenes, Leishmania donovani, Herpes simplex,* and *Ascaris suum*—which together represent a very broad spectrum of activity against fungi, parasites, bacteria, and viruses. Mice that were given glucans showed significant increase in candidacidal activity and reduction of growth in both candida and *Staphylococcus aureus.* It also had a synergistic effect when combined with amphotericin B.[12]

When added to an antibiotic protocol in animals carrying a variety of bacterial infections (e.g., *Staphylococcus aureus, Klebsiella pneumoniae, Escherichia coli,* and others) and viral pathogens (herpes), it decreased the amount of antibiotic or antiviral needed to handle the infection.[13] Beta-glucan can both activate and suppress immunity; that means it can help boost a weak immune system or calm down an overactive one as well as aid in autoimmunity.

Ironically, beta-glucan is one of the sugars that is found in both the cell wall and the biofilm of candida; it is a tool used by candida to manipulate the immune system of the host. It is this ability of beta-glucan that we are turning to our advantage to work *against* candida. However, if you have SIBO, you should be aware that beta-glucan can exacerbate this condition.

Numerous studies have demonstrated that beta-glucan can significantly reduce tumor cells and increase survival in people with cancer.[14] Studies by the U.S. Army found beta-glucan to be the preferred agent out of 440 against anthrax spores.[15]

When shopping for beta-glucan, look for form 1/3/1,6 to ensure it meets purification and potency standards for optimal effectiveness.

Colostrum

Colostrum is a naturally occurring substance found in the premilk fluid of all mammalian mothers in the first few days after giving birth. It is typically transferred to the infant during breast-feeding. It is chock full of immunoglobulins and has a powerful anti-inflammatory effect. Colostrum has been to shown to contain antibodies against more than nineteen different types of microbes, including candida, *E. coli, H. pylori,* rotavirus, staphylococcus, and salmonella. It contains polypeptides (chains of amino acids) that stimulate an underactive immune system or calm down one that is overactive. It has demonstrated a powerful ability to appreciably enhance immune-system activity against pathogens such as yeast, *H. pylori,* certain strains of the flu virus, and the common cold virus.

Colostrum also provides support for the thymus, a vital gland for immunity, as it is where some white blood cells go to mature. It contains lactalbumin, which defends against cancer and viruses, and lysozymes, which protect against bacteria. It also contains growth factors that support lean muscle mass and encourage normal growth and regeneration and accelerate repair of bones, cartilage, skin collagen, nerve tissues, and injured or aged muscles. It contains proline-rich polypeptides generated by macrophages and T cells to direct the actions of the communicatory cytokines. It can help regulate the inflammatory cytokines interleukin 1 and 6, interferon Y, and lymphokines, all chemical messengers involved in the immune system. For these reasons, colostrum can be beneficial for both enhancing an underactive immune system and slowing down an overactive one.

When we are first born, our gut is leaky by design because it is not yet fully matured. A leaky gut is needed to obtain passive immunity from our mothers. The gut becomes sealed and fully developed after the ingestion of colostrum through breast-feeding. (It contains growth factors for the epithelial and epidermal layers as well as other constituents needed for this task.) This is one of the reasons why breast-feeding is strongly encouraged. A child who is not breast-fed doesn't receive the substances needed to seal its gut. If leaky gut develops later in life, the consumption of colostrum can help seal the holes, repair tissue damage, and strengthen the gut barrier. Colostrum has been clinically proven to prevent and heal leaky gut in both humans and animals.[16] In summary, colostrum can boost the immune system's ability to kill candida directly, reduce inflammation involved in the process, and help heal the gut lining.

Lactalbumin has shown that it stimulates the release of serotonin and dopamine, two key neurotransmitters we've discussed. It also prolongs reuptake of the two substances, allowing them to linger and exert their effects for a longer period of time. At the same time, it has demonstrated the ability to lower cortisol levels.[17] Therefore, it can help reduce stress, improve the negative moods that commonly occur with candida overgrowth, and help alleviate cravings for sugar and carbs. However, do exercise caution here, as we have learned that excessive stimulation or artificial manipulation of neurotransmitters can contribute to disruption or depletion.

Transfer factors, compounds extracted from colostrum that enhance communication within the immune system, may be a promising way to boost immunity. In studies, one particular transfer factor product was found to increase natural killer cell activity by 437 percent.[18]

Bovine (cow) colostrum is identical to human colostrum but even more potent. Bovine colostrum can be purchased as a supplement to enhance immune function and heal the gut. There is a little bit of lactose in colostrum, but the amount is so minute that it shouldn't feed candida. Even many lactose-intolerant people can use colostrum without symptoms. Some lactose-intolerant people report they are less intolerant with the use of colostrum. However, if you are severely lactose intolerant, there are some options on the market that filter out the lactose.

When you purchase colostrum, you want it be 100 percent from the first milking and preferably within eight hours of the cow's having given birth. You also want it to be standardized to contain a high level of immunoglobulins, proline-rich peptides, lactoferrin, and growth factors. It should be obtained from free-range cattle so it will not be contaminated with hormones, antibiotics, and pesticides. Colostrum is activated by the saliva in the mouth; therefore, it should be consumed in powder form, not capsule, so that it comes in contact with the oral mucosa. Be sure to read the caution about colostrum on page 473, as it can be problematic for people who have issues with exorphins.

If you have an immune disorder, cancer, thyroid problem, or other endocrine disorder, you should consult with your doctor prior to using colostrum.

Lactoferrin

Lactoferrin is a protein that is present in very high numbers in colostrum. As discussed in previous chapters, it binds with iron and delivers it to the cells, which makes iron inaccessible to candida and other microbes that utilize it for their own survival and reproduction. It also prevents iron from being used in the formation of biofilms.

Lactoferrin also has a powerful effect on the immune system by stimulating phagocytes, macrophages, and neutrophils, and lymphocytes such as natural killer cells, all of which travel around the body and gobble up candida, bacteria, and other pathogens. Lactoferrin possesses cytokine-like abilities, which means it can enhance cell-to-cell communication within the immune system. It can also prevent pathogenic microbes from penetrating the gastrointestinal wall and getting into the bloodstream. It is exceptional at decreasing inflammation by regulating proinflammatory cytokines like interleukin-1 and interleukin-6, and tumor necrosis factor alpha. Like colostrum, lactoferrin can directly inhibit growth of candida and other microbes, reduce inflammation, and help heal the gut lining.

You will obtain a small amount of lactoferrin if you supplement with colostrum. However, higher doses of lactoferrin are typically needed for enhanced effectiveness, so it can also be supplemented as a stand-alone. Be sure to note that lactoferrin should be avoided by women who are pregnant as the immune-system stimulation could target the developing fetus. Lactoferrin is discussed in more detail in chapter 7, as it has antifungal capabilities as well.

Other Supplements for Immunity

When the immune system is engaged in battle with candida and other microbes, two results are oxidative stress and inflammation, which can perpetuate degradation of the gut and poor health. Inflammation may also occur as a result of the adherence of the organism to bodily tissue. High levels of antioxidants and anti-inflammatories can be used to control oxidative stress and inflammation. For this purpose, supplements like vitamin C, CoQ10, vitamin E, omega-3 fatty acids, or curcumin can be beneficial.

The mineral germanium is a potent inducer for the manufacturing of interferons (types of cell-signaling cytokines) and has also demonstrated some antifungal activity.[19] Interferons activate our natural killer cells, which then go after candida and other microbes. Cat's claw, another antifungal and antibacterial discussed in chapter 7, strengthens white blood cells, enhancing their abilities to kill candida and other pathogens. Echinacea increases production of white blood cells. However, echinacea loses effectiveness if taken for more than eight weeks and may actually lower white blood cells with long-term use. It can also cause liver damage if taken for more than eight weeks. Therefore, it should not be used long-term or combined with any other substance that can damage the liver. Nor is echinacea recommended for people with autoimmune disorders, HIV/AIDS, multiple sclerosis, tuberculosis, connective tissue disorders, seasonal allergies, white blood cell disorders, infants, or mothers who are pregnant or nursing.

Dr. Wayne Anderson has observed that when there are numerous coinfections (e.g., a combination of bacteria, viruses, and/or fungi), the immune system may prioritize. It may deal with one issue while ignoring another. You may need to address whichever issue your immune system is focused on at any given time.[20]

As you can see, the relationship between candida and the immune system is complicated. Supporting your immune system plays a vital role in the healing journey. The effectiveness of the treatment plan can be significantly increased by incorporating these steps. On the one hand, a weak immune system will leave you vulnerable to candida. On the other hand, the immune system is one of the systems most impacted by candida overgrowth. Work must be done to repair the damage that candida has inflicted on the immune system, and the immune system must be strengthened to help keep candida under control in the future.

CHAPTER 10

Paleo for Candida: How What You Eat Affects Your Health

D iet is the most fundamental component of the healing journey. The two chapters addressing this topic appear rather late in the book because I wanted to present the basic information beforehand so you could fully appreciate the importance of diet in treating candida.

This chapter reviews the ways that diet plays a role in candida overgrowth. Then it takes a look at many different types of food, examining how each one impacts candida and overall health. Chapter 11 focuses on strategies for implementing the diet.

THE OPTIMAL DIET: AN OVERVIEW

First and most important, the primary food sources for candida—sugar and anything that breaks down into sugar—must be eliminated from the diet in order to stop proliferation, prevent the organisms from morphing into the more aggressive hyphal form, and deprive them of resources for developing biofilms. Most people with candida are addicted to sugar and carbohydrates. If this issue is not addressed, cravings for these foods will sabotage efforts to remain compliant with the diet. The diet must remove all foods and substances that disrupt brain chemistry and the endocrine system; it must include more foods that restore balance to brain chemistry and the endocrine system—thus in turn eliminating cravings for sugar and carbs.

The food you eat also has a profound impact on the pH of your gastrointestinal tract, and keeping the gut from becoming too alkaline is vital for repelling candida and other harmful microbes and, again, for preventing them from morphing into hyphal form.

To give your immune system a fighting chance at controlling yeast organisms and other microbes, the food you eat must be void of substances that inhibit immune function and rich in foods that support immunity.

It must be rich in nutrients to replenish those that are often rendered deficient by candida overgrowth and void of foods and substances that cause or perpetuate nutritional deficiencies.

If SIBO or other bacterial overgrowth issues are present, then the diet must also reduce foods that contribute to proliferation of these organisms.

The diet must be rich in nutrients that support the adrenal glands and encourage parasympathetic nervous system activity and void of substances that drain the adrenals and fuel sympathetic nervous system activity.

The food you eat must be abundant in nutrients needed to form the neurotransmitters that are required to regulate gut health, motility, mood, appetite, and sympathetic dominance, and void of substances that deplete the neurotransmitters and inhibit their transmission.

Last but not least, the health of your gut is largely dependent on the foods you eat, and supporting a healthy gut is crucial for keeping candida under control. The diet must eliminate foods that degrade the integrity of the gut and include more of the foods that will be nourishing.

You most likely have run across a few products for eliminating candida overgrowth whose marketing materials claim there is no need to make any changes in your diet. You may have been treated by practitioners who did not suggest any dietary changes for candida. This is ludicrous and damaging advice. I urge you to see these statements for what they truly are—lies and manipulation—and resist trying to take the easy road out. As a way to hook you into buying their product or paying for their services, they are simply preying on the fact that human beings don't like change and are resistant to modifying their diet.

Changes in diet alone will not "cure" overgrowth of candida, but eating the right foods can help weaken biofilms, break candida's firm grasp, slow its spread by inhibiting its ability to morph into mycelial form, boost immunity, support gut health, reduce sympathetic dominance, and diminish overgrowth. Accomplishing these goals will reduce symptoms and enable your immune system and the antifungals you use to access the organisms more easily, making them more susceptible to treatment. Nothing else you do is likely to be effective if you do not correct your diet, because you will be unable to achieve those treatment goals. Stated bluntly, your diet will be the primary determining factor in how much improvement you make and how quickly that improvement is made.

In addition to candida overgrowth, there are numerous other serious conditions that researchers suspect may be linked to a high intake of sugar and high-carb foods, including insulin resistance, type 2 diabetes, obesity, cancer, heart disease, and Alzheimer's. Telling someone it is okay to eat a poor diet is irresponsible and lacking in common sense.

Before we get into specific recommendations, I'd like to make you aware that the first ingredient required for success is a change of mind-set. We have been socialized, programmed, and conditioned to believe that many unhealthy patterns, behaviors, and choices related to food are normal. These views must be abandoned and redefined in order to embrace a healthy diet. You will have to let go of all preconceived and well-established assumptions, ideas, and attitudes about the way you think your meals should look, taste, and be prepared. Be willing to approach the situation with a fresh and open mind and begin with a clean plate. It will take a little time to make this adjustment, but once you begin to see that your symptoms improve and you feel better physically and emotionally, this will help reinforce your new mind-set and commitment to change.

You may find many different versions of the candida diet on the Internet, in other books, or promoted by health-care professionals. The truth is that most of them contain foods that not only perpetuate candida and their biofilms but also ignite cravings for sugar and carbs, weaken immune function, contribute to deficiencies in nutrients, and promote inflammation and poor gut health.

Interestingly, a candida diet did not really need to be invented because it already existed. The diet that most successfully helps people manage chronic candida and overcome cravings for sugar and carbohydrates is a low-carb version of the paleo diet, also known as the caveman diet or hunter-gatherer diet. The paleo diet is the original diet consumed by all human beings, and it is naturally void of the foods that promote candida overgrowth, destroy the gut, weaken the immune system, deplete nutrients, stimulate sympathetic nervous system activity, and promote addiction to sugar and carbohydrates. It is based on anthropological research of what our ancestors ate prior to the agricultural revolution: animal protein, fat, fish, eggs, low-starch vegetables, and small amounts of nuts, seeds, and low-sugar fruit. It eliminates sugar, whole grains, legumes, and most high-carb foods.

You see, before the agricultural revolution, foods like potatoes, sugar, whole grains, legumes, and dairy were not part of the human diet. All the degenerative health conditions that plague our society today did not exist until we began to consume these foods. For millions of years, our ancestors lived and thrived on a diet that was high in animal protein and fat and low in carbohydrates because they simply did not have access to carbohydrates very frequently. When they did, they were nothing like the carbohydrates found on most plates today. The human body evolved running primarily on fat, protein, and ketones (a byproduct of fat metabolism), with only an occasional burst of glucose when extra energy was needed. This way of eating enabled us to grow bigger and smarter brains, develop strong bones and an impressive physique, enjoy good health, and become the supreme species at the top of the food chain that we are. Our ancestors could live well into their seventies unless they met with some type of tragedy like the attack of a rival tribe, a deadly accident, or an infectious disease, which were the leading causes of death at that time. They did not die from diseases like cancer, heart disease, type 2 diabetes, or obesity. They did not experience conditions like hyperactivity, depression, low blood sugar, and anxiety disorders. Candida overgrowth did not exist. A study at Cambridge University demonstrated that people became weaker, less active, and slower after agriculture became dominant, around seven thousand years ago.[1]

When the agricultural revolution took hold, humans exchanged animal protein and fat for high-carbohydrate foods, forcing the body to run on glucose as its primary fuel source and causing great damage to metabolism, brain, nervous system, endocrine system, immune system, gastrointestinal system, and cardiovascular system. The destruction has been so severe that the human brain is now shrinking, and our bodies are becoming smaller and weaker. Dr. Barry Groves states that the human brain is about 8 percent smaller since the advent of agriculture about 10,000 years ago.[2,3] Our genes today are programmed directly by the diet and behaviors of our ancestors. Genetically, we are still 99.99 percent the same as our Paleolithic ancestors, and we function most optimally when we mimic their diet and lifestyle habits. When you eat the way you were genetically designed to eat, yeast overgrowth is discouraged and you may be able to reverse many diet-related conditions.

The rest of the chapter takes a closer look at some of these dietary factors and how they apply to candida.

SUGAR

This section outlines the many reasons why eliminating sugar from the diet is the first and most important change to make in treating candida and related conditions.

Most people know that sugar feeds candida and that it should be avoided. Candida ferments sugar to create energy for its survival. What you may not know is that the cell wall of candida is made of sugar, sugar is the primary component used for the development of biofilms, and sugar enables candida to convert from a yeast organism into its more pathogenic hyphal form. Once in the hyphal form it can spread more quickly throughout the body. So not only does sugar make candida grow, but it also strengthens the biofilm, and allows the organism to disperse to a larger area. Candida digests most food substances externally by secreting enzymes, but it doesn't need any enzymes to absorb sugar, which it absorbs directly.

Besides candida, all the other microbes that may exist in conjunction with candida also prefer sugar (e.g., parasites and bacteria associated with SIBO and *H. pylori*). So do cancer cells. Elevated levels of blood glucose provide a glucose-rich environment for the bacteria that cause urinary tract infections. Long-term elevation of blood glucose can damage nerve tissue and lead to neuropathy, which can affect many different areas of the body, including hands, feet, and bladder. Neuropathy in the bladder can affect its ability to contract appropriately, resulting in only partial emptying and leaving pools of static urine where bacteria can grow.[4]

The higher the level of sugar in the body, the more opportunities that are present for yeast and bacteria to thrive. Additionally, sugar can block hormone receptors, possibly leading to hormonal imbalances which encourage more overgrowth of candida.

As discussed in chapter 9, elevated levels of glucose impair the body's ability to defend itself against infection and disease by inhibiting the activity of the white blood cells known as phagocytes. They typically gobble up invaders like candida, parasites, viruses, and bacteria. Elevated glucose also impairs neutrophils and diminishes the ability of the white blood cells to travel to the area where they are needed. Studies have found that the immune system is impaired for at least five hours after ingestion of sugar.[5] Thus, elimination of sugar is vital for building a strong immune system that is able to fight off candida and other microbes. An Australian study also suggests that consumption of sugar switches off the genes that protect us against heart disease and diabetes for two weeks, and continued consumption can result in damage that is passed through blood lines to our offspring.[6]

Sugar is void of any nutritional value. Metabolizing it requires drawing on the body's vitamin and mineral reserves, depleting nutrients that are needed for neurotransmitter production and function, gut health, immunity, the adrenal glands, and other systems.

The consumption of sugar and other carbohydrates leads to insulin and leptin resistance, resulting in cravings for sugar and carbs and increasing risk for a variety of health conditions such as obesity, heart disease, type 2 diabetes, and more. The cycle of craving goes like this: Consuming sugar and other carbs increases blood glucose levels significantly, prompting the release of high levels of insulin in order to lower blood sugar levels. The release of high levels of insulin lowers sugar levels too much, triggering symptoms of low blood sugar. Cravings for sugar and carbs kick in to increase blood sugar levels once again, perpetuating a vicious cycle of high blood sugar/low blood sugar and incessant cravings for foods that will feed candida and other microbes.

If sugar and carbs are eaten on a frequent basis, hormone receptors on the body's cells eventually become less responsive to insulin (a condition known as insulin resistance). At that point, the ability of glucose to enter the cell is hampered, leading to perpetual cravings for sugar and carbs. When glucose can't get into the cell, the cell sends hunger signals to the hypothalamus, and the hypothalamus sends out signals to make you want more sugar and carbs. However, no matter how much sugar you eat, you still feel hungry, because insulin is unable to deliver glucose to the cell. Further, the more carbs you eat, the less responsive to insulin the cells become. Your body's cells can be "swimming" in glucose but unable to access it.

Leptin is a hormone that tells you when you are full. It is often referred to as the satiety hormone. It works in harmony with another hormone, ghrelin, which tells you when you are hungry. They signal us to eat and to stop eating. Leptin also helps modulate our taste for sweets by targeting receptors on the tongue. Insulin causes an increase in ghrelin and a decrease in leptin; an elevation in insulin means hunger is never turned off and cravings for sweets and carbs are never satisfied. If this goes on every day, eventually leptin receptors become unresponsive (leptin resistance), and appetite and the desire for sweets remain switched on—all of which can snowball into cravings for other substances like caffeine, chocolate, alcohol, or other psychotropic drugs. Another vicious cycle develops: insulin resistance and leptin resistance lead to cravings for sugar and carbs, and consumption of sugar and carbs perpetuates the insulin and leptin resistance.

This blood sugar–insulin roller-coaster ride is perceived by the body as stress. When blood sugar rises too much, the stress response system is activated, and when blood sugar drops too low, the stress response system is activated. As discussed in several places in this book, stress encourages candida overgrowth, triggers cravings for sugar and carbs, weakens the immune system, and affects gut motility. A diet high in sugar and carbs encourages sympathetic dominance, and the cycle perpetuated by their consumption. All of this results in impairment to the endocrine system, metabolic damage, and carbohydrate intolerance. A hallmark of carbohydrate intolerance is cravings for sugar and carbs. Since the adrenal glands are called upon any time blood sugar spikes or plummets, this yo-yo effect can contribute to weakening of the adrenal glands. It is critical to keep blood sugar stable to support the adrenal glands. In order to break these cycles, sugar and carbs need to be removed and replaced with animal protein and fat, which will restore sensitivity to insulin and leptin.

High levels of insulin impact the thyroid by impairing conversion of thyroid hormone T4 to T3. It also increases the conversion of gamma linolenic acid into arachidonic acid. Higher than normal levels of arachidonic acid is converted into high levels of proinflammatory mediators known as prostaglandins and cytokines, which create inflammation. Insulin also causes excess sugar to be stored as fat in the body's fat cells, potentially causing weight gain and the associated risks of obesity, heart disease, type 2 diabetes, and cancer.

In his book *Grain Brain* (a must-read book for everyone), Dr. David Perlmutter states that high blood sugar is correlated with brain shrinkage, one of the primary symptoms of dementia and Alzheimer's. Studies indicate that even people who maintain blood glucose numbers at the high end of normal (90 to 100) have a much higher risk of brain shrinkage than those with lower numbers. Even a slight increase in blood sugar is directly associated with a higher risk of shrinkage of the hippocampus, our memory center. Higher levels of hemoglobin A1c, which provides an average for blood sugar over a three- to four-month period, is also linked to a higher degree of brain shrinkage. According to Perlmutter, insulin resistance "sparks the formation of those infamous plaques that are present in diseased brains like Alzheimer's."

Furthermore, sugar is an addictive, mind-altering drug. Brain scans indicate that the brain is impacted in the same manner by sugar as it is by alcohol and hard drugs like cocaine and heroin and that sugar is actually more addictive than cocaine.[7] Its biochemical makeup is almost identical to that of alcohol. The consumption of sugar creates a rush of excessively high levels in the brain of the neurotransmitters dopamine, serotonin, endorphins, and GABA. This is what produces the "sugar high." When neurotransmitter release is stimulated to excess, the brain is tricked into thinking it has too many. It reduces responsiveness or production and begins to utilize the artificial substance instead, which in this case is sugar. This results in depletion of one's natural neurotransmitters, plus tolerance of and addiction to the substance that replaces the missing neurotransmitters. Additionally, as we learned in the early chapters, candida itself can deplete dopamine reserves, which contributes to more cravings. In *Breaking the Food Seduction,* Dr. Neal Barnard explains that just the "taste of sugar touching the tongue" sends a signal to the brain that instantly triggers the release of our natural opiates (endorphins) and they "activate the dopamine system" and that combining sugar with fat in a 50/50 mixture (another substance that triggers endorphins) makes it irresistible.

Withdrawal from sugar addiction can be just as severe as withdrawal from drugs and alcohol. If someone who is addicted to sugar stops consuming it, the depleted neurotransmitters will not be available to perform their duties of regulating mood, thought, appetite, behavior, and emotion, and withdrawal is experienced. Cravings for sugar and foods that break down into sugar emerge from the body's unconscious attempt to replace the missing neurotransmitters.

Over time, tolerance develops, and more and more sugar is needed to produce the same effect. This often progresses to addiction to harder substances like alcohol and drugs, which provide a more intense boost in neurotransmitters. People recovering from an addiction to alcohol or drugs often experience relapse due to their consumption of sugar, because the sugar affects the brain in the same manner and provokes cravings for the substance of choice. Depleted or disrupted brain neurotransmitters are the root cause of addiction to all substances as well as of depression, anxiety, and other mental health and cognitive issues.

Although you may not observe any immediate repercussions from sugar consumption the way you do with alcohol, meth, cocaine, or heroin, in the long run the damage can be just as fierce. Sugar is a silent killer that takes years for its effects to accumulate and manifest as it slowly degrades organs and systems. The consumption of sugar is thought to be linked to numerous other health conditions like heart disease, cancer, liver and kidney damage, depression, insomnia, asthma, obesity, anxiety disorders, antisocial behavior (e.g., crime, violence, and delinquency), elevated triglycerides, and more. Even the American Diabetic Association considers sugar to be one of the three major causes of degenerative disease in America.[8]

Pretty much everyone with candida has cravings for sugar and carbs, and most people believe that these cravings are due to the fact that candida needs sugar to survive. Although it is true that candida can manipulate your appetite and make you crave the sugar it wants, the primary driving force behind an inability to refrain from sugar is because you are addicted to it in the same manner as an alcoholic or drug addict is addicted. Sugar addiction and candida overgrowth go hand in hand and perpetuate one another. The more sugar you eat, the more candida proliferates; the more it proliferates, the more sugar you eat. It is another vicious circle. You can break the cycle and overcome your cravings for sugar by making the necessary changes in diet. When you eat the right foods, your cravings for sugar and carbohydrates will cease to exist. Remaining compliant with your diet will not be a struggle, candida will diminish, and you will have fewer cravings.

We've looked at how candida and other microbes can induce cravings for their preferred food sources. It is also true that the foods you choose to eat influence your microbiome. Provide harmful microbes with a lot of the food they love and they will proliferate; restrict that food and they will decrease in numbers. As mentioned in chapter 6, evolutionary biologist and psychologist Athena Aktipis explains that "microbes have the capacity to manipulate behavior and mood through altering the neural signals in the vagus nerve, changing taste receptors, producing toxins to make us feel bad, and releasing chemical rewards to make us feel good."[9] However, we can just as easily influence our microbes by what we choose to put into our bodies. By becoming aware that microbes have this ability and saying no to them, we can put the power back in our own hands. If one is eating sugar and a lot of carbs, drinking alcohol, consuming caffeine, etc., then, yes, it will be extremely difficult to resist the signals from our microbes. But when you restrict their food choices, they will begin to diminish in numbers and send out fewer signals. You can also manipulate what microbes are present with the use of probiotics, prebiotics, and antibiotics, and by making other recommended lifestyle choices.

The following forms of sugar should be removed from the diet:

- alcohol (the most refined and potent form of sugar you can consume)
- white table sugar
- brown sugar
- high-fructose corn syrup
- cane sugar
- date sugar
- beet sugar
- maple sugar or syrup
- organic cane syrup, juice, or sugar
- lactose
- maltose
- dextrose
- maltodextrin
- fructose
- fruit juice
- barley malt
- rice syrup
- agave
- molasses
- honey
- coconut sugar
- coconut nectar
- anything else with the word *sugar* in it, or other forms of sugar that I may have missed

Many health-conscious individuals are under the false assumption that organic cane juice, organic cane syrup, organic cane sugar, maple syrup, honey, coconut sugar and nectar, and agave nectar are healthy. Although these types of sugar may be *slightly* less destructive than white sugar or high-fructose corn syrup, it is not by much, if any. Sugar is sugar in candida's eyes. Each of these forms causes candida and other microbes to proliferate, they are equally addictive, and each contributes significantly to the other sugar-related conditions we've discussed. It is an elevation in blood glucose that causes these issues, and an elevation in blood glucose is caused by any source of sugar or high carbohydrate food.

Honey is considered an acceptable sweetener on the standard paleo diet because it was consumed by our ancestors. However, honey was heavily guarded by bees; therefore, it was not easy to access and was consumed only on special occasions, not daily or even monthly. Honey affects neurotransmitters and blood sugar like any other sugar, which means it will incite more cravings for sugar and carbs. When it comes to paleo for candida, honey is a strong source of sugar that will enable candida to multiply profusely and should be avoided. Although a healthy individual can indulge in a little honey now and then, that is not the case for the individual with candida, bacteria, or parasites and sugar/carb addiction.

ALCOHOL

Alcoholic beverages are a potent source of sugar—the most refined sugar you can consume; it doesn't even have to be digested as a significant portion of it is absorbed directly through the gut wall. It is like hooking up your candida with an IV of sugar and will make it proliferate out of control. The same is true for bacteria. The consumption of alcohol disrupts and depletes neurotransmitters, triggering all the negative effects we have discussed, such as impairment in gut function, motility, appetite, mood, preventing sympathetic dominance, etc. Alcoholic drinks also cause a spike in blood glucose; then insulin is released, which results in a crash in blood sugar, which then leads to cravings for more alcohol or sugar and carbs and damage to the adrenal glands, as we discussed previously. Furthermore, alcohol is a toxin that impairs liver function, stresses the immune system, and destroys the gut lining—all of which can perpetuate candida and other microbes.

COMPLEX CARBOHYDRATES

Many people are unaware that any food that breaks down into sugar in the body will feed candida, provide raw materials for the biofilms, encourage yeast to change to the hyphae form and travel to more areas throughout the GI tract and body, weaken the immune system further, contribute to sympathetic dominance and all the other degenerative health conditions associated with sugar consumption. Foods that are high in starchy carbohydrates—for example, whole grains, potatoes, and legumes—as well as fruit and some nuts, are broken down into sugar.

Refined grains and whole grains (wheat, oats, rye, corn, barley, white rice, brown rice) are some of the worst offenders. They all break down into sugar very quickly in the body, increasing blood sugar by too much, feeding candida, and perpetuating cravings for carbs and sugar. A medium-size potato is equal to half a cup of sugar. Legumes are also very high in carbohydrates. As we discussed in chapter 9, grains and legumes contain antinutrients called lectins and phytates that destroy the gut lining, contribute to inflammation and leaky gut, inhibit digestive enzymes and absorption of nutrients, and impair immune function. Lectins also block leptin receptors, which means they can contribute to an increase in appetite, cravings for sugar and carbs, and compulsive overeating—sabotaging your ability to remain committed to your diet. They contain protease inhibitors, which impede the ability of digestive enzymes to break down protein. The amino acids that are produced by the breakdown of proteins contribute to production of antibodies and neurotransmitters. Protease inhibitors also cause a buildup of other enzymes like trypsin when they inhibit another, which results in the release of antibodies and proinflammatory cytokines, resulting in inflammation.

In some ways, whole grains are even more destructive than processed grains, because whole grains are higher in the antinutrients that degrade health and prompt an immune response, and they contain substances that convert quickly into sugar. For example, brown rice is more nutrient dense than white rice; however, it is loaded with antinutrients like phytates, lectins, and protease inhibitors, which make the nutrients unavailable for absorption. White rice is free of those substances, because the bran and germ, home to those substances, have been stripped away. The bran and germ in brown rice are themselves gut irritants. They can contribute to leaky gut, food sensitivities, mental health issues, and autoimmune disorders. White rice is actually a better choice than brown rice if one is going to indulge in rice. That said, once white rice is digested it produces a high glucose load in the body, which will feed candida, incite cravings for sugar and carbs, and can perpetuate the blood sugar/insulin cycle we've discussed.

Many grains contain gluten, which increases levels of zonulin, the substance that causes leaky gut and leaky brain. In *Grain Brain*, Dr. Perlmutter explains that antibodies that are created against gliadin (a component of gluten) can "directly combine with specific proteins found in the brain that look like gliadin protein found in gluten-containing foods," which "leads to the formation of more inflammatory cytokines."

As mentioned, complex carbohydrates quickly break down in the body into glucose, triggering the blood sugar/insulin cycle. In his book *Wheat Belly,* Dr. William Davis explains that two pieces of whole wheat bread or a bowl of oatmeal can increase blood sugar levels even more than table sugar or some candy bars. Dr. David Perlmutter writes in *Grain Brain* that "so-called 'complex carbs' may actually represent a more significant threat to health than simple sugar in that they may not only raise blood sugar, but keep it elevated for a more prolonged period of time." When you replace the sugar and high-carb foods with animal protein and fat, you interrupt this cycle, blood sugar levels balance out, and cravings disappear. Dr. Perlmutter also states "most grain foods, whether we're talking about quinoa, amaranth, the very popular grains of the day—the reality is they still are associated with a carbohydrate surge."

As discussed in chapter 6, a diet high in carbs encourages an increase in the microbes firmicutes, actinobacteria, and certain clostridia, but a decrease in bacteroidetes and other species of clostridia, resulting in less gut diversity. Furthermore, high blood glucose overworks the kidneys, reducing their ability to filtrate properly.

Some grains contain high levels of opiate-like substances called exorphins. These impersonate our natural brain neurotransmitters called endorphins and produce the same type of high as heroin or morphine: sedation, pain relief, euphoria, etc. Endorphins have many important functions such as moderating mood, relaxation, and emotional and physical pain, and promoting feelings of well-being and empowerment. Under normal circumstances, receptors for endorphins are stimulated naturally by dietary fats and fruit so that you will be motivated to eat those foods. They are also stimulated by activities like exercise, communing with nature, sex, and falling in love. Gluten gets broken down in the body into peptides called exorphins. The most well known of these is gliadorphin, but there are four others called gluten exorphin A5, B4, B5, and C; all of them have the same opiate-like characteristics that can alter thought, mood, energy, behavior, cognition, and even development, just like heroin or morphine.

The problem with exorphins is that they provide artificial stimulation to the endorphin receptors, and that stimulation is much higher than it would be through natural means. Your brain is tricked into believing there are too many endorphins, so it stops responding to or producing the natural endorphins and relies on the exorphins instead, because it can't tell the difference between the two. This results in depletion of your natural endorphins. As happens with morphine or heroin, one develops tolerance to the exorphins, requiring higher doses of grains to produce the same result. Eventually the brain becomes dependent on (addicted to) the grain to perform the duties of the missing endorphins. Thus, intense cravings for grains will ensue to keep exorphins around and you will not remain compliant on your paleo for candida diet. This is one of the primary reasons that much of our population is madly in love with all the grain-based foods like pizza, pasta, bread, cereal, pie, bagels, cake, and cookies. Most of our society is caught in this addiction to opiate-like substances. In some cases, as tolerance levels increase, severe depletion in endorphins caused by consuming grains can eventually lead to addiction to alcohol, heroin, or morphine. And, as touched on above, anyone who is recovering from addiction to alcohol, morphine, or heroin can be triggered to relapse by the consumption of grains, whose exorphin content can incite cravings for the drug of choice. Many people develop severe psychiatric or neurological symptoms in response to gluten exorphins, including OCD, compulsive overeating, schizophrenia, autism, hyperactivity, Tourette syndrome, depression, anxiety, attention deficit, multiple sclerosis, fatigue, fibromyalgia, and more. I discuss exorphins in more detail on pages 265–267.

High-glycemic foods, which include sugar and starchy carb foods (grains, legumes, potatoes, etc.), also trigger a sudden, powerful, and extreme increase in the levels of neurotransmitters in the brain in the same manner as alcohol and drugs. This is what provides the euphoric effect many people have when consuming carbs. This confuses the brain, because it now thinks it has too many neurotransmitters, so it downregulates their receptors. Downregulation results in depletion, which leads to cravings for (addiction to) more starchy carbohydrates. Furthermore, insulin surges caused by the consumption of sugar or carbs prevent tryptophan from crossing the blood-brain barrier for conversion into serotonin, leading to inhibition of serotonin production. As Nora Gedgaudas writes in her book *Primal Body, Primal Mind* (another must-read book for everyone), "The same sort of damage that is done to the brain in alcoholism occurs at a slow, but steady rate when consuming any form of a carbohydrate (sugar and/or starch) rich diet." Dr. Charles Gant explains in *End Your Addiction Now* that carbohydrates are addictive by nature. It is the way they are designed to propagate their species. So your cravings are partly due to a natural force beyond your control. He also states that a "carb is a carb." Complex carbohydrates have the same impact as refined carbs on the endocrine system and the brain. Cravings are eliminated by avoiding the foods that have the highest addiction potential.

For some people, grains can have an excitotoxic effect by increasing glutamate. Recall from earlier chapters that glutamate is our main excitatory neurotransmitter; when present in excess it becomes toxic to the brain because it overstimulates brain cells to the point of death, resulting in psychiatric symptoms like ADHD, OCD, anxiety and panic disorders, seizures, insomnia, autism and more, and often triggers cravings for sugar, high carbohydrate foods, caffeine, and/or drugs and alcohol.

Many people are under the false assumption that carbohydrates are needed for energy and are concerned about reducing complex carbohydrates in their diet, but this is not accurate and there is no cause for concern. The human body has actually preferred fat as its chief energy source through most of our evolution, and carbohydrates are a nonessential nutrient. Dr. Charles Gant explains that none of the top one hundred most reputable nutritional texts indicates that carbohydrates are an essential component of the diet.[10] There are essential amino acids, so the body needs dietary protein. There are essential fatty acids, so the body needs dietary fat. There are no essential carbohydrates, because the body can make the required glucose from protein and fat. If you provide your body with a bunch of carbohydrates, then it will be forced to downregulate its hardware designed for running on fat and protein and upregulate the hardware for running on carbohydrates. You will experience a drop in energy if you don't keep carbohydrates in your system, but this is not the body's preference. Reliance on carbohydrates is a dysfunctional state that results in deterioration of mental and physical health. It creates the illusion that carbohydrates are needed, because the equipment for running on protein and fat has been downregulated. If you remove carbohydrates from your diet, within a few weeks your body will return to its normal state by upregulating the mechanisms it uses to run on fat and protein, and carbohydrates will become unnecessary. At this point, your feelings of low energy, hunger between meals, and cravings for sugar and carbohydrates will begin to dissipate and you'll feel satiated with each meal.

While it is true that some of our cells can run only on glucose (red blood cells, certain brain cells, and kidney cells), most cells can run on fat *or* glucose. As long as you are consuming an adequate intake of fat and protein, the nominal amount of glucose that is needed can be produced by the liver through gluconeogenesis, wherein protein and a byproduct of fat called glycerol are converted into glucose.

Chapter 11 goes into more detail about recommendations for total carbohydrate intake and how to find your optimal carb threshold.

THE KETOGENIC DIET

Other byproducts of fat metabolism called ketones (or ketone bodies) can be used by most cells for energy instead of glucose. In fact, ATP (the body's primary source of energy) is produced more efficiently from ketones than it is from glucose. Many bodily cells (including many brain cells) actually prefer ketones over glucose and run more efficiently on them. The brain has often been described as a carbohydrate-dependent organ, but this is only true when one is eating a high-carb diet. When you remove the carbs, the brain becomes more dependent on ketones and may actually run better. In *Primal Body, Primal Mind,* Nora Gedgaudas explains that "ketones are a steady, long-burning, efficient fuel that we were designed to use as our primary source of fuel for most things (except in an emergency), which is when glucose gets released as a turbocharged supplemental source of energy." But, "we always pay a price for the use of glucose as an energy source, even in low amounts."

Ketones are a natural, normal, and healthy byproduct of fat metabolism. When you eat a low-carb diet (typically less than 50 grams of carbs per day) in combination with a high-fat diet and a moderate amount of protein, and your body returns to running on fat as its primary source of fuel, as it was intended, it enters a state called ketosis. During ketosis, the body generates byproducts called ketones. Ketosis should not be confused with ketoacidosis. Ketoacidosis is a dangerous state in which production of ketones are out of control due to a loss of insulin and the body's inability to utilize glucose. It affects primarily insulin-dependent type 1 diabetics, some late-stage, insulin-dependent type 2 diabetics, and chronic alcoholics. If you do not fall under one of those categories, you cannot end up in ketoacidosis by eating a low-carb diet.

A low-carb ketogenic diet is beneficial not only for candida overgrowth and overcoming sugar and carb addiction, but many studies indicate it is highly effective for weight loss, insulin resistance, type 2 diabetes, metabolic syndrome, depression, schizophrenia, obsessive-compulsive disorders, autism, Alzheimer's, Lou Gehrig's disease (ALS), Parkinson's, PCOS (polycystic ovary syndrome), heart disease, multiple sclerosis, migraines, epilepsy, and cancer. Ketosis activates a gene that generates a protein called brain-derived neurotrophic factor (BDNF), which helps protect existing neurons, encourages connection between neurons, and creates new neurons. That means it will also assist in keeping those all-important neurotransmitters working more efficiently. The ketogenic diet helps maintain balance between GABA and glutamate. It improves the detoxification system, increases antioxidants, decreases oxidative stress and free radical production, prevents cell death, increases growth of new mitochondria, lowers blood glucose levels, reduces amyloid (the protein that is present in brain plaque), and increases efficacy of metabolism.[11] In *Primal Body, Primal Mind,* Nora Gedgaudas writes, "The more you use ketones for energy in your lifetime as opposed to glucose the longer and healthier you will live." She also quotes Gary Taubes (who is quoting Dr. Richard Veech, a researcher at the United States National Institutes of Health), who asserts that ketosis is the "normal state of man." Not only is it natural, but it is healthy.

In *Keto Clarity* by Jimmy Moore and Dr. Eric Westman, they state that a study from 2014 in *Nature* magazine "found that ketogenic dieting increased microbes of the genus bacteroides and decreased firmicutes." You'll note from our previous discussions that the opposite is found in people with SIBO and related conditions like IBS and GERD. The firmicutes are the ones that prefer carbohydrates. Jimmy states the opposite is also associated with obesity and that "the microbial alterations induced by the ketogenic diets were associated with reduced levels of inflammation."

There is a belief in some people that a very low-carb or ketogenic diet may contribute to hypothyroidism or adrenal fatigue. I disagree. Most people have an adrenal and thyroid problem prior to eating the low-carbohydrate diet, and it gets worse from other factors as time goes on, not the lowering of carbs. However, if there is not sufficient intake of calories when going low-carb this could contribute. In *Keto Clarity*, research shows that when you are "on a well formulated low-carb, moderate protein, high-fat diet with adequate calories there has been no occurrence of low thyroid."

Additionally, according to Nora Gedgaudas in *Keto Clarity*, a lowered thyroid level on a thyroid test for someone who is eating ketogenic may be a sign of "improved efficiency of metabolic functions and a desirable longevity marker." There may be a lowered conversion of T4 to T3, but that doesn't mean there is a problem. And Dr. Chris Decker explains in *Keto Clarity*, "When we are burning ketones from fat as our primary fuel source, our thyroid just doesn't have to work as hard as it does when it's got to manage bodily metabolism on a less preferred fuel (glucose)."

Furthermore, I would assert that carbohydrates are much more stressful and harder on the adrenal glands than eating ketogenic. As explained by Dr. Eric Westman, also in *Keto Clarity*, "Being in a state of ketosis lowers the amount of stress on the body through the elimination of such culprit foods as sugar, white flour, grains, legumes and more. Switching over from the unnatural and stressful state of being a sugar-burner to the more relaxed state of being a fat-burner is arguably far less taxing on your adrenal glands." This issue is discussed in more detail on page 392.

Other studies cited in *Keto Clarity* have shown that the ketogenic diet improves many mental health issues including bipolar and schizophrenia. One of the other contributors to this book, neuroscientist Dr. Bryan Barksdale, points out that ketones have "neuroprotective properties"—they protect brain cells.

Keto Clarity is a very informative and easy-to-read book about the ketogenic diet. I began reading the book when I was almost finished writing this book and it quickly became one of my favorites. If I had found it earlier in the process, you would have seen many other references to this work. I encourage you to take a look at it if you want to learn more about the ketogenic diet.

Additionally, a ketogenic diet has been shown to increase the GAD enzyme, needed to convert glutamate into GABA, and neurons can use ketones as a precursor to GABA. Glutamate can become aspartate or GABA. Aspartate is excitatory and neurotoxic in excess, like glutamate. A ketogenic diet favors glutamate becoming converted to GABA instead of aspartate. Thus, the ketogenic diet is highly beneficial for increasing GABA levels and dealing with any conditions associated with excess glutamate that we have already discussed.

Some research suggests that after a period of adaptation candida may feed on ketones, and that the killing of candida by neutrophils (white blood cells that protect us from microbes) may be impaired in ketosis.[12,13,14] That has not been my personal experience, and no one I've worked with directly has made this report to me. However, that doesn't mean it can't happen. Some people writing in online forums believe they have had this experience with ketones. Many others report feeling best when maintaining a state of ketosis. These conflicting reports demonstrate how complex and adaptable candida is and how the experience may vary from person to person. Still, this does not mean that one should abandon a low-carb diet and start consuming a lot of starches. Considering the fact that sugar and carbs are candida's preferred foods and they enable candida to do its worst damage, and the fact that these foods are associated with so many other problems like cravings for more sugar and carbs, addiction, metabolic syndrome and dementia, and the fact that a ketogenic diet provides so many other benefits that we just discussed, it remains clear that maintaining nutritional ketosis is the better choice even if this circumstance does occur. Be aware of this potential for ketones to exacerbate candida, and monitor how your body responds. If you sense that a ketogenic diet is worsening your candida, the logical course of action would be to strike a middle ground: eat a diet that does not increase either glucose or ketones too much—that is, consuming a total of around 60 to 70 grams of carbohydrate per day. That would be total carbs, not net carbs.

Please also be aware that eating low-carb is not equal to maintaining a state of ketosis. Ketosis typically requires an intake of carbs below 50 grams every day, an adequate intake of fat, and avoiding too much protein. It is easy to eat a low-carb diet that can help reduce candida overgrowth without going into ketosis. When you eat low carb, you generate more ketones than people do who eat a high-carb diet, but you won't necessarily be in ketosis. Furthermore, since it takes time for candida to adapt to the presence of ketones, you may experience great benefit from a short-term engagement with ketosis before adaptation takes place, if it does at all.

Many people worry that they are missing critical nutrients on a low-carb diet. Again, that is not true. A low-carb diet is a well-balanced diet. Since carbohydrates are nonessential, you can get all the nutrients you need to support a strong mind and body without eating them. In the 1920s, a low-carb diet was the treatment of choice for conditions like diabetes and seizures. Chapter 11 discusses total carbohydrate intake in more detail and how to find your ideal threshold.

FRUIT

Although our paleo ancestors ate fruit, it was only available seasonally, so they did not eat it on a daily basis. There would be many months when the only food available was animal protein and fat. Furthermore, the fruit they did consume was much lower in sugar than what we consume today. Modern fruit is cultivated to be larger in size and higher in sugar than the wild fruit that was eaten by our ancestors. It is also much lower in fiber and nutrient content. Fruit is a staple on the paleo diet, but in sensible amounts. That said, the naturally occurring sugar, carbs, and fiber contained in fruit feed candida, bacteria, and parasites, and have the same effects on the body as other sources of sugar. Eating too much fruit may contribute to sugar and carb addiction, weaken immunity, and sabotage your dietary efforts if not managed properly. In addition, the fruit in sugar (fructose) gets stored as fat much more quickly than any other form of sugar, so it's important to minimize fruit intake if you are trying to lose weight. Fructose also increases ghrelin, the hunger hormone, and decreases leptin, the satiety hormone.

Since fruit contains fiber, water, and an abundance of micronutrients, and since fructose must be converted into glucose before being utilized by the blood, fruit has a less severe impact on blood sugar, insulin, and neurotransmitters than refined sugar (sucrose); however, fruit intake must still be minimized—and in some cases eliminated completely—depending on how it affects each individual. Some fruit is higher in sugar/carbs than others; choose fruits that have the lowest carb content. The greater the amount of carb in the fruit, the more it will feed candida and the more impact it will have on neurotransmitters, sympathetic nervous system activity, and blood sugar levels.

The fruits that are lowest in carbs include olives, apricots, lemons, limes, plums, kiwis, strawberries, raspberries, and blackberries. Next on the list are coconut, grapefruit, peaches, cherries, blueberries, pears, oranges, cranberries, and apples. The fruits with the highest carb content are bananas, pomegranates, melons of all kinds, pineapple, and mangoes.

Note that the ripeness of a banana affects its sugar content; an unripe banana contains less glucose than a ripe one. However, a green banana is much higher in resistant starch than a ripe one, which provides a feast for SIBO. Green apples are less sweet than other types of apples. Melons, cantaloupes, mangoes, grapefruit, and oranges are particularly high in mold, which can provoke a wide variety of symptoms, so they are best avoided. For example, melons cause blisters on my mouth. All dried fruit is exceptionally high in sugar and should only be consumed in small quantities on special occasions or used when cravings for sugar are uncontrollable. Some fruits taste sweeter than others even though the sugar content isn't very high, which may trigger cravings for more sugar.

Fruit should never be eaten on an empty stomach. Doing so will provide very easy access to sugar for candida and have more negative impact on blood sugar, insulin, and neurotransmitters. It should be eaten after a full-course meal that contains a significant amount of animal protein and fat, which will dilute its impact. Fruit should be ripe, as it is easier to digest and absorb and reduces the resistant starch that can feed SIBO organisms. In most cases, fruit should not be eaten more than once per day at most. Fruit juice should be avoided completely, because it is a concentrated source of sugar. The pulp has been removed, eliminating the fruit's fiber, which provides a feast for candida and a spike in blood sugar.

Most people with candida cannot eat much fruit without significant symptoms, but how much fruit one can tolerate varies widely. Sometimes adjusting the quantity can enable an individual to consume some fruit. Generally speaking, keep the serving size of fruit to no more than half a cup at a time; if that amount produces symptoms, make it smaller. You may have to stick with just a few bites. Fruit consumption should be determined by how many symptoms it produces. When you consume fruit, if you develop anxiety, genital itching, acne, depression, irritability, hyperactivity, attention deficit, gas, abdominal pain, or other symptoms of candida overgrowth, or if you experience cravings for more fruit or other carbs, then the fruit is probably feeding candida/bacteria and/or disrupting the endocrine system and brain chemistry. This is an indication that the amount consumed is too high and should be reduced.

If you have SIBO (see chapter 6) in addition to candida, fruit consumption will need to be limited even more, or it may need to be restricted all together. Fruit is also more tolerable when cooked when SIBO is present. Even more than candida, bacteria proliferate on fruit because they also feed on the fiber. Other tweaks to the diet are necessary with SIBO as well, and are presented in chapter 6.

COCONUT

Coconut in all its forms (oil, butter, cream, milk, flakes, kefir) is a very popular food in the paleo community and that of certain other diet philosophies. Some people suggest that everyone should consume coconut. It possesses some antifungal, antibacterial, and antioxidant characteristics, is low in omega-6 fatty acids, does not oxidize in high heat, and is a great source of saturated fat, particularly medium-chain fatty acids, also known as medium-chain triglycerides. These medi-um-chain triglycerides do not have to be acted upon by bile; instead, they are absorbed quickly through the small intestine and then con-verted into ketones by the liver. As mentioned previously, ketones can be used by our cells for energy, thus, they can provide a very rapid source of fuel. For this reason, coconut oil is used quite successfully for the treatment of patients with neurological disorders like Alzheimer's and Parkinson's, who have difficulty utilizing glucose. Furthermore, the sugar content of coconut is low, and what is there is accompa-nied by a high fat content, so its impact on insulin is minimal. These are great qualities for someone with candida and its accompanying complications.

However, coconut has a few downsides to consider. As discussed in the section on FODMAPs, further ahead, coconut can be problematic for the gastrointestinal tract due to its ratio of fructose to glucose. It contains a significant level of phytates, the antinutrient we discussed earlier that irritates the gut, obstructs absorption of vital minerals like zinc and iron, and inhibits digestive enzymes like trypsin, amylase, and pepsin. Coconut also contains a substantial amount of salicylates, an organic acid that is used by plants to protect themselves from infection and disease. In some individuals, salicylates can provoke a wide variety of symptoms, including gastrointestinal discomfort, nausea, itching, fatigue, hyperactivity, nasal congestion, and burning eyes. Coconut is quite high in fiber, which for some people can be irritating to the gut and bowel and can cause inflammation. This is especially true of coco-nut flakes. This fiber can also be a significant food source for SIBO.

From an evolutionary viewpoint, most of our ancestors did not eat coconut since it was found only in the tropics. Many of us may not be genetically adapted to consume it, potentially making us more vulnerable to gastrointestinal disturbance upon eating it and to devel-oping a sensitivity against it, which could then contribute to more digestive problems, inflammation, skin problems, autoimmunity, etc. Many people with candida have sensitive gallbladders. I have learned through my own experience and from clients and visitors to my web-site that coconut oil can cause substantial problems for the gallblad-der. Additionally, all forms of coconut are considered "concentrated" sources of fat, which can overstimulate some neurotransmitters (see pages 302–303 for more on this topic). Coconut's combination of fat and sugar may be a trigger for some food-addicted individuals. At the same time, be aware that a craving for coconut fat may occur because it provides such a rapid source of fuel. Coconut may provide your body with something it lacks, like energy or adequate dietary fat.

For all these reasons, coconut falls under the category of foods that should be assessed and adjusted accordingly. If it causes any of the aforementioned issues, then it should be eliminated or moderated, and your reaction may vary depending on the form you consume. For example, coconut oil may cause gallbladder distress, but other forms may not. Flakes may cause your IBS or SIBO to flare, but not butter or oil. Case in point: for me, coconut oil provokes a severe gallbladder attack and incapacitating nausea, but coconut flakes and coconut butter do not in small amounts. Before I developed SIBO, I found that if I ate a couple of tablespoons of coconut butter when I felt a migraine headache beginning to form, I could sometimes stop it in its tracks or substantially minimize its severity. However, coconut flakes cause inflammation in my small intestine and colon. If I eat too much coconut in any form, I just don't feel well and my GI tract is irritated. So I don't eat coconut daily or even weekly. I reserve it for special treats now and then—for dessert dishes on the holidays and for certain migraine days. I'm very cautious with flakes and oil and stick mostly with coconut butter, cream, or milk. Likewise, you need to find what works for you and your body.

COW'S-MILK DAIRY PRODUCTS

Dairy products are not an innate component of a true paleo diet. However, a significant portion of the paleo community will eat moderate amounts of certain forms of dairy, for example, full-fat yogurt, butter, ghee, cream, and some cheeses. Unlike grains and legumes, dairy falls within a gray zone, meaning it can be beneficial for some people and destructive for others. You will need to experiment to see how your body responds. People with candida must consider special circumstances when it comes to dairy.

Yogurt, milk, cottage cheese, and most other soft cheeses contain lactose. Lactose is a sugar, and like any sugar it feeds candida and biofilms, weakens immunity, and prompts spikes in insulin and neurotransmitters. Therefore, any forms of dairy that are high in lactose should be eliminated or restricted to use on special occasions. The fermentation process reduces lactose, so fermented dairy may be acceptable. Many brands of yogurt contain added sugar, even those found in the health food store; be sure to read the label and use only unsweetened brands. Greek yogurt is lower in lactose than other types. Hard, aged cheese does not contain lactose, so if you like to indulge in cheese now and then, a hard cheese like sharp cheddar or feta would be an acceptable choice in terms of its lactose content. However, hard, aged cheese is high in histamine and glutamate as discussed in those sections.

Butter, ghee, and cream are practically devoid of lactose or any other type of carbohydrate, so they do not contribute to this problem. Butter is a rich source of vitamin A, arachidonic acid, and cholesterol and is a good source of lecithin, and vitamins K, D, and E. These nutrients can be very beneficial for some of the conditions that often accompany candida, like adrenal fatigue, low blood sugar, neurotransmitter depletion, hormone imbalances, deficiencies in fatty acids, and low cholesterol. Butter is also rich in short- and medium-chain fatty acids, which can provide an instant source of energy and afford antimicrobial and antitumor capabilities. If the butter is obtained from grass-fed sources, as it should be, it is also rich in CLA (conjugated linoleic acid), a powerful anticancer agent that also helps to build muscle, burn fat, reduce circulating glucose, and improve insulin sensitivity. The omega-3 and omega-6 content of butter is low, but in grass-fed sources it is present in balanced amounts. Butterfat also contains generous amounts of other nutrients, including chromium, manganese, glutathione, iodine, and zinc.

If you consume dairy that contains lactose, select the full-fat version; to obtain the full nutritional value that dairy offers, skip the low-fat varieties. The presence of fat makes the lactose less accessible to candida, decreases its impact on blood sugar, insulin, and neurotransmitters, and assists in the digestion of lactose and dairy proteins. Furthermore, fat is important for a healthy brain and immune system (discussed below).

Kefir contains a significant amount of alcohol, which in my opinion counteracts the beneficial bacteria aspect in people with candida. It could also be problematic for individuals with addiction issues. Some clients with candida report that kefir makes them feel drunk, and it has led to relapse in some recovering alcoholics. I think it is best to get your healthy bacteria elsewhere. Kefir would also be high in histamine and glutamate.

Dairy is one of the most common foods to which people develop sensitivities, intolerances, or allergies. In people who are intolerant, it contributes to inflammation, leaky gut, autoimmune conditions, and possibly to cravings for dairy, sugar, and carbs. Cravings for the allergenic substance develop in the advanced stages of allergy or sensitivity. Naturally, dairy should be avoided if you fall within this group. However, it is believed that the real cause of lactose intolerance, allergies, and sensitivities to dairy may be the result of pasteurization, because vital enzymes that are needed for digestion and absorption are eliminated during the pasteurization process. Many individuals who are lactose intolerant can eat raw dairy without any gastrointestinal issues, because it contains those vital enzymes as well as more than one hundred different strains of beneficial bacteria and the prebiotics to keep them alive—all of which makes raw dairy products much more compatible with the human gut. If they can be obtained, raw dairy products are preferred over pasteurized.

Lectins, the problematic antinutrients discussed earlier, are present to some degree in all dairy products, but they are present in larger amounts in traditional factory-raised cattle than in grass-fed cattle due to the cows' consumption of lectin-rich grains. If you're eating dairy from grass-fed animals, as you should be, then levels of lectin may not be high enough to cause concern. It's important to note that the fermentation process reduces lectin content so levels will be lower in the fermented dairy products.

Like grains, dairy contains opiate-mimicking exorphins, with all the potential problems we discussed. In dairy, these substances are called casomorphins and are produced from casein and whey. The greater the amounts of casein and whey, the more casomorphins that will be present. Cheese is a concentrated source of casein, and whey powder is a concentrated source of whey; they contain more exorphins than other dairy products.

Dairy also contains small amounts of naturally occurring morphine itself, which may also contribute to addictive eating of the substance. This is true of the milk of all milk-bearing species, including humans. It is believed that morphine is present in mother's milk to provide a calming, drug-like effect that will ensure a bond between mother and infant so the infant will seek out the mother's milk that is needed for its survival. It also slows down intestinal transit time, which helps prevent diarrhea. If levels of opiates increase too much in the milk of a lactating woman, they can enter the bloodstream, travel to the brain, and result in postpartum psychosis. These peptides may also be passed on to the child and result in colic.[15]

Cheese contains PEA (phenylethylamine), an addictive amphetamine-like substance that is also found in chocolate and occurs naturally as a neurochemical in the brain. In high amounts, it affects the brain in much the same way as Adderall, Ritalin, and methamphetamine, causing an increase in pulse, blood pressure, alertness, and blood sugar. This may perpetuate addictive eating.

Some people are more susceptible than others to exorphins (both casomorphins in dairy and gluten exorphins in grains), a condition thought to be largely influenced by lack of the enzyme DPP-IV, which is needed to break down casomorphin or gliadorphin into a harmless substance. DPP-IV may be completely absent, partially absent, inactive, or not functioning optimally. In order for DPP-IV to work adequately it needs zinc and amino acids, so if these nutrients are not present in the diet in sufficient amounts, the enzyme may be unable to do its job. Candida can inhibit the DPP-IV enzyme, making people with candida much more likely to be vulnerable to problems with exorphins. DPP-IV may also be obstructed by a genetic polymorphism, other nutritional deficiencies, antibiotics, certain types of diabetic medications, vaccines, wheat and dairy products, interferon, gelatin in vaccines, pesticides, and heavy metals. Other factors that can make one more vulnerable to exorphins may include the amount of healthy bacteria that are present in the gut and people who already have low levels of endorphins or other neurotransmitters due to genetics, chronic stress, poor diet, environmental toxins, or an active addiction to drugs or alcohol. A lab test called the Gluten/Casein Peptides Test can assess whether a person is breaking down exorphins; however, not everyone who develops symptoms from exorphins tests positive—another example of the rule that "the absence of evidence is not evidence of absence." According to an excellent video presentation by Dr. James Greenblatt, other signs that suggest there is a problem with exorphins include "intense obsessions or intrusive thoughts that appear refractory to psychological interventions (failure of CBT or medications), excessive consumption of dairy or wheat to the exclusion of other food groups (eating nothing but), or intense feelings of sedation or calm after eating dairy or wheat." Dr. Greenblatt has had great success in treating people with OCD, autism, eating disorders, and schizophrenia by eliminating dairy or supplementing with DPP-IV.[16]

Some cows produce higher levels of casomorphins than others. Dr. Greenblatt explains, there are thirteen different genetic variations of beta-casein produced by cows. The two most common found in milk are known as A1 and A2. Incomplete breakdown of A1 results in casomorphins, making the person who consumes that type of milk much more vulnerable to the mental health symptoms that are associated with casomorphins. Cows that produce more A1 will result in higher levels of casomorphin. The A1 variation is also correlated with higher mortality rates from ischemic heart disease. Milk containing high levels of A2 is correlated with a lower prevalence of type 1 diabetes and cardiovascular disease. Another variation, known as BCM-7, is believed to be linked to sudden infant death syndrome, autism, schizophrenia, and other neurological disorders, as well as leaky gut, digestive problems, and inflammation in the joints.[17]

As you can imagine, if someone is vulnerable to both casomorphins and gliadorphins, they may experience profound neurological symptoms when consuming meals in which dairy and grains are combined—for example, pizza, lasagna, or a bowl of cereal. Symptoms caused by dairy may also involve an IgG response, IgE response, autoimmune disorder, or other unknown factors. Some people just feel better if they avoid dairy even if all the tests are negative. On the other hand, some dairy peptides may possess antihypertensive, antidiarrheal, antibacterial, and immunomodulatory characteristics. Some are opioid antagonists, which inhibit the heroin-like effects. It's not a black-and-white situation.[18]

Whey is high in glutamate, which can contribute to an imbalance in GABA and glutamate, especially in people who have excess glutamate naturally or in whom it is elevated due to candida. As we discussed in other chapters, glutamate is toxic to the brain when present in excess. This is especially true for whey powder, which is a concentrated source of whey. Anyone who tends to lean toward excess glutamate should avoid whey powder. Depending on the severity of your imbalance, whey in other forms can be problematic as well. Glutamate is also formed in the process of ultrapasteurization, the addition of enzymes, and the aging of cheese, making cheese potentially problematic for this reason as well.

Some health professionals, including Loren Cordain, believe that naturally occurring hormones in the cow that are present in dairy products may disrupt human hormones, and that a growth factor called betacellulin may cause cancer.[19] Others disagree, claiming that betacellulin is only carcinogenic when it is isolated from other compounds that are found in dairy and that have anticarcinogenic effects (e.g., CLA and saturated fat).[20] If the milk is full-fat and from grass-fed cows, this may not apply. Still, dairy does increase IGF-1, a substance in the blood that is known to aggressively promote cancer cells and that has been associated with prostate and breast cancer. Supplements containing casein and whey can also increase IGF-1. Other studies have found a variety of anticarcinogenic substances in dairy. It's worth noting that the fermentation process eliminates most of the IGF.

Dairy contains protease inhibitors, which, as mentioned in the discussion of grains, can impair digestion of proteins, play a part in gut permeability and inflammation, increase the mucus in the gastrointestinal tract (which may inhibit nutrient absorption and inflame the gut), and may have the ability to quell activation of vitamin D.

Some people are worried that they won't get adequate levels of calcium if they don't eat dairy, but that's not really true. The prevalence of thinning bones is much lower in countries that consume very little dairy than it is in the United States, where people consume a great deal of dairy. A twelve-year study from Harvard University that involved seventy-eight thousand nurses found that bone strength was not improved at all with dairy consumption. In fact, the incidence of hip fractures was nearly double in women who consumed a lot of dairy products in comparison to those who ate very little or none.[21] However, I would like to point out that this study involved pasteurized milk and not raw milk. Pasteurized dairy removes the enzyme phosphatase that is needed to absorb calcium, so unless one is consuming raw dairy, the calcium in dairy isn't absorbable anyhow.

Dark green leafy vegetables such as collard greens, turnip greens, kale, Brussels sprouts, and broccoli contain high levels of calcium that is readily absorbable because it is also accompanied by vitamin K, which is needed for absorption of calcium. Salmon, sardines, Brazil nuts, sesame seeds, sunflower seeds, figs, and almonds are also good sources of calcium. Almonds actually contain more calcium than dairy. I'm not trying to say you should never eat dairy; I'm just pointing out that if you choose not to eat dairy, or are incapable for one reason or another, you don't have to worry about a calcium deficiency, because it can be obtained in sufficient amounts from numerous other sources.

Even though dairy can provide a variety of health benefits for some people, it clearly was not part of our Paleolithic ancestors' diet. However, it is thought to have been part of the diet of many native cultures that came later. I am hesitant to say one way or another whether it should be included in the diet. There is not a clear-cut answer, and it varies from person to person depending on the issues they are addressing. Your decision may also be based on which issues you have with dairy, and just because one form of dairy has to be eliminated doesn't mean all forms have to go. The primary substances in dairy that people have problems with are lactose, casein, and whey. However, the severity of those problems can vary widely. Butter, ghee, and heavy cream are almost pure fat so they may still be enjoyed by many. For example, if a person is only mildly intolerant of casein, they may be able to eat ghee since it contains only minute amounts of casein, even if they must avoid all other forms of dairy. If your only problem with dairy is lactose, then you may still be able to eat butter, ghee, heavy cream, and hard cheese since they contain little to none. On the other hand, if you are gluten intolerant, you will typically need to avoid all dairy because cow's milk is a gluten cross-reactor. That means you may produce antibodies toward dairy in the same manner as you do toward gluten. Even ghee, which contains minute traces of casein, can be problematic in the gluten intolerant. So don't assume you need to eliminate all forms of dairy just because you have a problem with one; and sometimes it is a matter of frequency or quantity. You may be able to eat cheese or yogurt once in a while, but not on a regular basis, or you may be able to enjoy a small amount but not a large amount. Experiment and assess how your body responds to each dairy product.

Your decision about whether to include dairy should also be gauged by the health of your gut, the level of healing you've achieved, whether you're insulin resistant or type 2 diabetic, the severity of symptoms dairy produces, and whether it incites cravings for sugar and carbs or a bout of compulsive overeating. You should also take into account whether you're dealing with an autoimmune condition, adrenal fatigue or exhaustion, OCD, Tourette syndrome, or other mental health issues. But, again, the form of the dairy will still come into play; cheese and yogurt may trigger you to binge on carbs, but butter and ghee may not—and even this state of affairs may change from time to time. You must also be careful of the ingredients that are added during the manufacturing process and that may cause symptoms. For example, I permit the use of butter daily, and heavy cream or ghee weekly, but I only indulge in yogurt or cheese once in a while. If I eat raw and sharp cheddar I have fewer problems, but other forms are not tolerable at all. I can't eat butter that contains any lactic acid. I can eat Organic Valley butter with no problems, but some other brands give me bizarre brain symptoms. As you can see, my reaction varies from brand to brand; yours may as well, so be sure to try different brands if you have symptoms with one.

I encourage you to use discretion with dairy and limit its use according to your needs, especially if one of the aforementioned issues applies. As mentioned, any dairy you consume should always be obtained from cows that have been organically raised and grass-fed. It is void of the antibiotics and hormones that can perpetuate a candida problem, weaken immunity, disrupt the brain and the endocrine system, and cause hormonal imbalances. It's also richer in nutrients. Dairy should never take the place of meat as an alternative source of protein as it can't compare to meat nutritionally. It should only complement the meal.

GOAT'S MILK AND CHEESE

Goat's milk is generally considered to be easier to digest and less allergenic than cow's milk because it is more like human milk than cow's milk, its fat molecules are smaller, and it doesn't contain agglutinin (a substance that causes the fat to separate and coagulate). When a food is easier to digest it moves through the gastrointestinal tract quicker and is less likely to cause problems. However, like cow's milk, goat's milk contains the common allergens beta-lactoglobulin and casein, so those who have a true allergy to cow's milk may also react to goat's milk.

Cow's milk is considered to be an acidic food but goat's milk is considered more alkaline. Goat's milk does not create mucus or phlegm so it's better for people with allergies or asthma. The smaller, more easily digested proteins are better tolerated by those with compromised liver functioning, which is common in those suffering with candida. Goat's milk is higher in a variety of vitamins and minerals, including vitamin A, calcium, niacin, copper, vitamin B6, potassium, manganese, and selenium, but it is lower in folic acid, zinc, and vitamin B12. It is slightly higher in fat than cow's milk, but again the fat particles are smaller in size and don't contain agglutinin so they're easier to digest. Because goat's milk does digest quicker, some people who are lactose intolerant or have a milk allergy are able to tolerate it better than cow's milk; other, more sensitive people don't do well with either. Like most things, tolerance of goat's milk varies from individual to individual.

Goat's milk contains almost the same amount of lactose as cow's milk so those who are lactose intolerant or who have candida overgrowth are likely to still have a problem with consumption. The amount of lactose contained in goat's milk is *slightly* lower than in cow's milk, so it may feed candida a little less than cow's milk, but it will still feed it. Goat's-milk cream, cheese, and yogurt contain only minuscule amounts of lactose. If you're not lactose intolerant and you have no sensitivity to cow's milk, or your cow's-milk sensitivity is mild, then you may get away with adding goat's milk to your diet now and then. Like cow's milk, it is not inherently part of the paleo diet.

MOLDS AND FERMENTED FOODS

People with candida typically need to avoid fermented foods and moldy foods. These foods don't actually make candida grow, but they provoke an allergic-like reaction because they are similar to candida in their biochemical makeup and many of them release mycotoxins. This reaction may also contribute to an immune response, inflammation, and leaky gut. People who are genetically impaired in their ability to eliminate toxins, as discussed on page 209, may have more problems with these foods. Foods that fall under this category include vinegar (including apple cider vinegar), mushrooms, truffles, melons (including cantaloupe), mango, grapefruit, oranges, sauerkraut and other fermented vegetables, kefir, kombucha, and anything else fermented.

It may also include dried fruits (pineapple, raisins, dates, etc.). Coffee, which should be avoided for other reasons mentioned on pages 293–294, is very high in mold as well. As mentioned in the nut section, below, nuts can be moldy too. However, some mushrooms, like shiitake and reishi, afford a variety of health benefits such as a boost in the immune system; sun-dried mushrooms are very high in vitamin D.[22]

Vinegar is made by fermenting alcohol into acetic acid. So there are trace amounts of alcohol in vinegar. This can be problematic for someone who is very alcohol sensitive. It can also be an issue for the alcohol addicted in recovery, potentially triggering cravings for an alcoholic drink. Washing the brine off of foods bathed in vinegar will not resolve the problem, because it is absorbed systemically into the food.

Additionally, fermented vegetables, kefir, and kombucha contain alcohol, which can feed candida and trigger cravings for sugar, carbs, or alcohol. As mentioned previously, I have heard reports of people feeling drunk on kefir and other reports of people relapsing in their recovery from alcohol addiction after eating cultured vegetables. I once purchased some freshly cultured vegetables because they are supposed to be so good for the gastrointestinal tract and I was unaware they contained alcohol. After my first serving, I was craving them like I would an alcoholic drink. They were so good I wanted to eat the entire jar in one sitting, and I couldn't quit thinking about them. After a few days, I began to feel addicted to them. I thought, "Something isn't right here" and did a little research. I discovered that cultured veggies contain alcohol, which explained my experience. (I am a recovered alcoholic, so I am more vulnerable to foods' alcohol content than others may be.) I quit eating them, because I felt that doing so put my sobriety at risk. My point is that if you have a history with addiction, you want to be cautious with fermented foods. Anything fermented has a small amount of alcohol and many people with candida have an alcohol addiction. Fermented foods are also very high in glutamate and histamine, which can disrupt the GABA and glutamate balance in people who are susceptible and contribute to excess histamine. As discussed previously, this is a common problem for people with candida, and it can cause severe neurological and gastrointestinal distress and perpetuate sympathetic dominance.

Dried herbs, herbal teas, and spices also accumulate mold; these products should be used fresh when possible. Keep all herbs stored in the refrigerator to discourage mold growth. Be careful with left-overs, because they, too, accumulate mold. Leftover foods, particularly protein-containing foods, can accumulate histamine. Generally, leftovers should be eaten within twenty-four hours, but you can gauge how you respond. Depending on your level of sensitivity you may not have a problem until the third day. Adjust accordingly. As mentioned in the section on dairy, most cheeses contain some amount of mold, yeast, or fungi, which can be problematic. Sprouts (e.g., alfalfa sprouts) are also very moldy and incite symptoms in many.

NUTS AND SEEDS

Nuts and seeds can be problematic for the individual with candida in a number of ways. First, some contain a significant amount of carbohydrate, which will feed yeast and trigger cravings for sugar and carbs. Cashews, chestnuts, pistachios, and chia seeds are the highest in carbs so they should be restricted more. Walnuts, Brazil nuts, macadamia nuts, pecans, pumpkin seeds, sunflower seeds, and pine nuts are the lowest in carbohydrates. Nuts and seeds contain significant levels of fiber, which can make SIBO proliferate greatly. Therefore, if SIBO is present, they may need to be greatly restricted or avoided altogether.

Nuts and seeds tend to be a little moldy, which can aggravate yeast since the two are closely related. They may trigger allergic-like symptoms. The macadamia nut is less moldy than others, and it is richest in fats that are good for your brain and body. Pistachios are particularly high in mold and also in a toxin emitted by mold called aflatoxin, so they can be more problematic than others and are best restricted. Be sure to note that peanuts are not nuts, they are legumes. Peanuts should be eliminated completely. Peanuts are even higher in aflatoxins than pistachios.

Some people do better if they roast their nuts, which reduces mold content. Roasting nuts and seeds makes them more tolerable for people with SIBO as well, as it reduces the food source available for the bacteria. However, do note that heating a nut or seed oxidizes its polyunsaturated fatty acids (PUFAs), which turns them rancid and consequently produces a variety of toxins that increase free radicals. The higher the amount of PUFAs, the more vulnerable they are to oxidation. This means the macadamia nut would be less vulnerable and the walnut would be highly vulnerable. Other factors that can influence the degree of oxidation in roasted nuts include the amounts of vitamin E and flavonoids that are present in the nut, the temperature to which the nut is heated, and how long it is exposed to the heat. When nuts or seeds are roasted, they should be only lightly roasted. Dry-roasted nuts and seeds are less vulnerable to oxidation than those roasted in oil.

One must also limit nut consumption because most nuts and seeds, with the exception of macadamias and chestnuts, are higher in omega-6 than omega-3 polyunsaturated fatty acids. If they are eaten frequently they will cause an imbalance in a person's ratio of omega-3s to omega-6s. Too much omega-6 results in inflammation and its attendant health problems, which can include gut problems and overgrowth of candida and other microbes. While it is true that walnuts are high in omega-3 fatty acids, they are even higher in omega-6s. Additionally, even too much omega-3 is not healthy. It is linked to an increased risk in colitis and changes in immune function that may impair the body's ability to fight off microbes like candida and bacteria.[23] Furthermore, the omega-3 in walnuts is in the form ALA, which has to be converted into DHA and EPA for use by the body. Many people do not make this conversion very efficiently. Only a small fraction of ALA is converted into DHA or EPA, and saturated fat needs to be present to enhance the process. DHA and EPA are two omega-3 fatty acids that are critical for the brain, other parts of the nervous system, and the cardiovascular system. They do not exist in the plant world. The same problem exists in flaxseeds and chia seeds, which are falsely believed to meet one's needs for DHA and EPA. Therefore, nuts and seeds are a very poor source of omega-3 fatty acids. Sunflower seeds, walnuts, and pine nuts are all significantly higher in PUFAs than MUFAS (monounsaturated fats) and most of it is in the form of omega-6.

Flaxseed is an acceptable seed on the paleo diet. However, flax contains high levels of phytoestrogens, naturally occurring substances that mimic estrogen in the body. People who are estrogen dominant, which is very common in individuals with candida, don't want to eat foods that increase estrogen even more. As we learned in the early chapters, excess estrogen fuels overgrowth of candida and can lead to a wide array of symptoms. For these reasons, it is my opinion that flax should be avoided.

That said, as paleo expert Mark Sisson points out, nuts and seeds are rich in protein, fat, and a variety of micronutrients that supply some level of protection against oxidation and decrease the effects of their high levels of PUFAs. Eating them in their whole form is not the same as eating plant oils such as corn oil, soybean oil, or even the oil from the nut itself. They shouldn't be too big a concern as long as you consume them in moderation. The biggest problems occur when the nut or seed oil is isolated and refined.[24]

Nuts and seeds also contain considerable amounts of phytates, the antinutrients that can impair absorption of minerals and impede digestive enzymes. Recall that if phytates are eaten too frequently or in large quantities, they can cause inflammation in the gut and contribute to deficiencies in minerals, leaky gut, and autoimmunity in people with gut problems. Some people are more sensitive to phytates than others, and the body can deal with them in small quantities (about 100 to 400 mg per day), so as long as you eliminate other foods high in phytates (grains, legumes, chocolate) and don't eat excessive quantities of nuts and seeds, the phytates they contain should not cause too much concern. Most nuts are high in histamine and tyramine, so they can trigger symptoms from this angle as well.

Phytate content can be substantially reduced through the process of soaking nuts and seeds. This is a practice that you should adopt. Cover them with water and let them sit for about twelve hours. Pour the water off, pat them dry, and store them in the freezer or the fridge. Or process them in the food processor and turn them into nut butter. If you're too busy for all this, a great company called Blue Mountain Organics carries an entire line of soaked nuts and seeds and their respective butters. Nuts and nut butters should always be stored in the refrigerator to inhibit mold growth and prevent oxidation.

The bottom line with nuts is that whether or not they should be included in the diet varies based on how an individual responds to them. If they trigger cravings and bingeing, set off a flurry of symptoms, or cause irritation and inflammation to the gut, they should be eliminated. If not, they can be eaten with restriction. Like fruit, your tolerance of nuts may be a matter of quantity; you may be able to eat a small serving of nuts or nut butter without symptoms, but a larger serving may produce symptoms. Regardless, they should only compose a very small percentage of your meal and should not be eaten every day, especially when you are trying to heal your gut. Choose nuts that are higher in MUFA than PUFA as often as possible, and eat those that are higher in omega-6 less frequently. With all things considered, the macadamia nut is usually the best choice for the person with candida and/or sibo.

EGGS

Eggs are embraced by most people on the paleo diet as a good source of protein, fat, and a variety of micronutrients like choline, lecithin, sulfur and other minerals, B vitamins, vitamins A, D, and E, and cholesterol. They do not feed candida. On the flip side, the egg white contains a variety of antinutrients to safeguard the embryo. These are difficult for some people to digest, and they can attach to nutrients and prevent them from being absorbed. They can cause inflammation, leaky gut, and an immune response in some people. Our early ancestors did not have access to eggs year-round, so in an evolutionary context, they weren't eaten every day. For these reasons, most informed paleo health-care professionals suggest that eggs should not be consumed daily but rather should be limited to around six eggs per week at most.[25] If one has an autoimmune condition, it is typically recommended to remove eggs. Avidin, a naturally occurring antimicrobial found in egg white, binds to biotin and can make it unavailable to the body. Cooking the egg white denatures avidin, disrupting this process, but raw egg white can be problematic for this reason. Since the problems with eggs typically reside in the white portion, one option is to discard the egg white and eat only the yolk. Still, the person with a severe autoimmune condition may have a negative response to the minute traces of white left behind.

NIGHTSHADES

Foods in the nightshade family, which include potatoes, tomatoes, eggplant, cayenne, chili peppers, red pepper, jalapeno, bell peppers (also known as sweet peppers), and paprika contain a variety of naturally occurring pesticides, such as alkaloids, lectins, and saponins.

They protect the plants from predators and can be problematic when consumed by humans. They may need to be eliminated or restricted by some people with candida, food sensitivities, autoimmune disorders, or leaky gut. Other, less commonly eaten nightshades include tomatillos, pimentos, habeneros, ashwagandha, goji berries, cape gooseberries (but not normal gooseberries), ground cherries (but not Rainier or Bing), garden huckleberries (but not regular huckleberries), and tobacco. Some of these may not be true nightshades but share the same alkaloids.

Alkaloids like solanine are difficult for some people to excrete. They can build up in the body and result in a wide array of symptoms, including joint and muscle pain, fatigue, muscle tremors, stomach pain, heartburn, and other gastrointestinal discomfort. Alkaloids are a common underlying cause of arthritis-like symptoms and conditions. The inability to excrete them is generally linked to inefficiency of the liver, and since the liver of individuals with candida is already dealing with an overload of toxins, they may be even more susceptible to alkaloids. Any other condition that affects liver function or detoxification would compound this issue.

Lectins, as already discussed, can contribute to inflammation, leaky gut, insulin resistance, leptin resistance, and autoimmune disorders.

Like lectins, saponins, bitter substances with detergent-like qualities, damage the gut lining and prompt an immune response, thus contributing to leaky gut, inhibited nutrient absorption and transportation, and autoimmune disorders. If saponins are present in a high proportion in the bloodstream, they can injure the membranes of red blood cells and generate proinflammatory cytokines (messengers used by the immune system to tell white blood cells to attack), contributing to widespread inflammation. Saponins can impede an enzyme called acetylcholinesterase from performing its duties of breaking down acetylcholine, one of the main neurotransmitters (and which I've discussed in earlier chapters). As with phytates and lectins, the body can deal with a small amount of saponins; they only become problematic when ingested frequently or at concentrated levels. They are more problematic for someone who already has leaky gut, which is usually the case in a person with candida or SIBO. Saponin content is not reduced with sprouting or soaking.

Most processed tomato products found in the can or jar are

preserved with a manufactured source of citric acid that is derived from yeast, which can destroy healthy bacteria in the gut and encourage yeast overgrowth. Therefore, the consumption of canned or jarred tomato products should be limited. Additionally, tomatoes and eggplants contain small amounts of naturally occurring nicotine, which can potentially trigger cravings for a cigarette in individuals who are trying to quit smoking, and possibly snowball into cravings for sugar, carbs, or other addictive substances.

As mentioned previously, the sugar content of a medium potato is equal to half a cup of sugar. That means potatoes provide a significant food source for candida and SIBO and could potentially contribute to all the previously listed problems triggered by consumption of high-carb foods. Potatoes should be restricted for this reason in addition to restricting them for any issues they may cause as members of the nightshade family.

Some people are more sensitive than others to the effects of alkaloids, lectins, and saponins; symptoms caused by these substances vary widely from person to person. Some may eat them with little problem, while another may be unable to eat them at all, and yet another may be okay if they are consumed once in a while or in small servings. For example, if I eat tomatoes too many days in a row, or even eat too many in one day, I will develop arthritic-like pain all over my body. But if I eat only a small serving once in a while, then I don't notice too much discomfort. You should experiment and monitor these foods to assess how your body responds and adjust accordingly. Even for a healthy individual, ingesting too great a quantity of nightshades can be toxic. Consumption should always be moderated, and they should not be consumed on a daily basis.

LEGUMES

Although I have already discussed legumes in several places throughout the book, I want to be certain to drive home the point that legumes should be completely avoided because they contain high levels of the carbohydrates that feed candida and SIBO and perpetuate cravings for sugar and carbs. They also contain antinutrients like lectins, phytates, and saponins, which cause and perpetuate inflammation, leaky gut, food sensitivities, autoimmune disorders, overstimulation of the sympathetic nervous system, and nutritional deficiencies.

Please note that green beans are technically a legume, but they are significantly lower in lectins, phytates, and carbs, so most people can include them on the paleo diet or the paleo for candida diet. That said, some paleo experts, such as Loren Cordain, exclude them.

ARTIFICIAL SWEETENERS

All artificial sweeteners should be avoided. They are chemicals, not real foods, and they disrupt the endocrine system and vital brain neurotransmitters, both of which can result in cravings for sugar and carbohydrates, a larger appetite, bingeing, weight gain, and a wide variety of other side effects like panic attacks, hyperactivity, depression, nervousness, attention deficit, headaches, irritability, seizures, dizziness, joint pain, inhibit the migrating motor complex, and much more. They also lower healthy gut bacteria and cause numerous digestive disturbances such as abdominal pain and cramping, diarrhea, and nausea. Everyone knows that saccharin causes cancer, but other artificial sweeteners also potentially cause problems.

At one time, aspartame, the artificial sweetener known as Equal, NutraSweet, Canderel, or AminoSweet, was registered by the Pentagon as an agent of biochemical warfare. Aspartame weakens the immune system, and it's an excitotoxin that increases glutamate levels and perpetuates sympathetic dominance.[26] Aspartame may produce a high similar to that created by psychotropic drugs, which means it is altering other neurotransmitters and may be an addictive drug in and of itself. Sucralose, the sweetener known as Splenda, which is often promoted in many of the low-carb diets, is derived from a pesticide formula and has been shown to increase levels of zonulin. As you learned earlier, zonulin increases gut- and brain-barrier permeability. Splenda also causes a decrease in friendly bacteria in the gut of animals, and increases fecal pH, all of which encourage overgrowth of candida or other microbes. It also alters cytochrome P450 detoxification and contains the sweeteners maltodextrin and glucose.[27,28] In *A New IBS Solution,* Dr. Pimentel states that bacteria can feed on Splenda as well.

Acesulfame potassium, known as Sunett or Sweet One and found in many sodas, is believed to cause neurological damage, influence prenatal development, affect the thyroid gland, and be carcinogenic.[29,30,31] Both sucralose and acesulfame potassium prompt an insulin response, leading to cravings for sugar and carbs and can contributing to insulin resistance, type 2 diabetes, and the other problems described earlier.

These substances do not belong anywhere on the menu for the numerous reasons discussed, but the bottom line with artificial sweeteners is that they will impede your ability to refrain from other foods that make candida proliferate by perpetuating the craving cycle. Your objective when designing your diet is not to replace sugary foods with something else, but to eliminate your desire for them altogether. This cannot be achieved if you exchange your addiction to sugar with one to artificial sweeteners. When you eat the right foods, you'll restore balance to your endocrine system and brain chemistry, and then you'll no longer have a need for either sugar or artificial sweeteners because you'll come to appreciate the flavors that are inherent in your food. In my work helping people overcome their addictions, I have witnessed repeatedly that consumption of artificial sweeteners is a primary cause of relapse on their diet.

STEVIA

Stevia is a naturally sweet herb that does not contain any sugar or carbs; therefore, it does not feed candida or SIBO, and in most cases it does not have an impact on blood sugar and insulin or trigger cravings for sugar and carbs. However, in some people whose metabolism is very damaged, the body may respond to stevia by producing insulin because it gets confused by the sweet taste on the palate, which can then lead to cravings for more stevia. I occasionally work with people who've become addicted to stevia. So although stevia can be used safely in regard to candida, it should be done so with moderation. If you discover that you exhibit addictive tendencies with stevia, eliminate it for a period of time. After a while, once brain chemistry and the endocrine system have been restored to balance, you may try it again to see if it remains a trigger. Still, keep in mind that you don't want to replace sugar with another substance, so stevia should always be used sparingly. When you eat a diet of whole foods, you should have very little need for stevia because you shouldn't be making foods that require it as an ingredient. Stevia has also been shown to exert an inhibitory effect on organisms in biofilms.

Be sure that you use only a pure and organic form of stevia from a reputable company. Truvia, which can be found in mainstream grocery stores, is not true stevia. It is about 0.5 percent Rebiana, a highly refined extract (steviol glycoside) from the stevia plant, and about 99.5 percent erythritol, a sugar alcohol. Mainstream erythritol is frequently procured from genetically modified corn and was found to have a potent pesticide action against fruit flies due to the presence of the herbicide Roundup used on the crops. The more Truvia the fruit flies consumed, the quicker they died.[32] As discussed previously, pesticides have a profound impact on neurotransmitters in your brain, your gut, and your endocrine system and can lead to cravings for sugar and carbs, compulsive overeating, depression, anxiety, and other problems. Genetically modified crops that have been sprayed with Roundup destroy the healthy bacteria in the gut. Additionally, erythritol is under the FODMAPs category (see the next section) and therefore exacerbates SIBO symptoms. Not only that, Truvia has a third ingredient listed as "natural flavors," which can mean just about anything, since the term is not regulated and may not be natural at all. The main takeaway point: this form of unnatural stevia should be avoided.

FODMAPS

People with candida frequently have problems with FODMAPs. FODMAPs are foods that contain naturally occurring substances called fermentable short-chain carbohydrates that are poorly absorbed by some people; thus, they travel through the gastrointestinal tract partially digested, where they become a food source for any bacteria that are present, as well as candida. *FODMAP* is an acronym: *F* stands for *fermentable,* *O* stands for *oligosaccharides* (e.g., fructans, galactans), *D* stands for *disaccharides* (e.g., lactose), *M* stands for *monosaccharides* (e.g., fructose), *A* stands for *and,* *P* stands for *polyols* (sugar alcohols).

Since the individual with candida has an imbalance between the friendly/unfriendly bacteria in the gut, he or she tends to have high levels of bacteria besides candida that feed on these substances. Other people who are susceptible to FODMAPs include those with SIBO, IBS, or other functional gut disorders, which are commonly experienced by people with candida as well.

Bacteria generate large amounts of waste products when they feed on FODMAPs—as candida does when it feeds on sugar and carbs—and the waste products induce an array of symptoms including flatulence, bloating, abdominal pain and cramping, nausea, anxiety, depression, fatigue, and brain fog. Some of them pull water into the GI tract, which causes diarrhea and may either increase or decrease the transit time through the gastrointestinal tract, which can produce either diarrhea or constipation (or both).

A large number of studies have confirmed a great deal of success in reducing the symptoms of IBS by decreasing consumption of foods that are high in FODMAPs. Other studies have shown that about 75 percent of individuals who have functional gut disorders can attain substantial relief of their symptoms by following a diet low in FODMAPs.[33,34]

A low-FODMAPs diet was first designed by Dr. Susan Shepherd and Dr. Peter Gibson at Monash University in Melbourne, but it fails to eliminate many other substances that are detrimental to our health, so it needs to be combined with the paleo diet principles. It is also higher in resistant starch, which, as discussed on pages 475–484, can have the same negative effect on the gut.

FODMAPs generally do not *cause* IBS, SIBO, or other functional gut disorders, but they magnify a condition that is already present: an abundance of pathogenic organisms in the GI tract or insufficient enzymes necessary to break down the specific substances. For example, SIBO obstructs the production of enzymes that are required for digestion and absorption of nutrients found in the FODMAPs fructose and lactose. Studies have found that everyone experiences at least some degree of gas when they eat foods that are high in FODMAPs, but people with IBS experience excessive gas, as well as fatigue and a variety of other disruptive gastrointestinal symptoms that people who don't have IBS do not experience. This suggests that the level of pathogenic organisms in the gastrointestinal tract is what determines the severity of one's intolerance to FODMAPs. Additionally, deficiency in the enzymes lactase and fructase can develop from damage to the brush border caused by candida, SIBO, or other factors. On the flip side, eating a diet that is high in FODMAPs provides the intestinal microbes with a large food source, which can incite overgrowth.

As you can see, many of the symptoms generated when bacteria eat FODMAPs are very similar to those produced by candida, which means not all the symptoms one may attribute to candida are necessarily from candida. They may be caused by the combination of both candida and bacteria feeding on FODMAPs. If you limit your consumption of these foods, you may be able to achieve significant improvements in more of your symptoms. Again, as with candida, the more food you provide for bacteria, the more they will proliferate. High numbers of pathogenic bacteria cause a lot of fermentation, which produces the uncomfortable symptoms. The greater the number of bacteria, the more fermentation, the more bacterial byproducts, and the more symptoms. Likewise, fewer bacteria mean fewer byproducts and fewer symptoms.

Here is an overview of each type of FODMAP.

Fructans

Fructans are chains of fructose molecules with a glucose molecule at the end. In people who lack certain enzymes in the small intestine, fructans may not be absorbed at all. Foods that are high in fructans include wheat, barley, rye, chicory, artichokes, onions, scallions, leeks, garlic, cabbage, snow peas, Brussels sprouts, shallots, watermelon, okra, pistachios, fennel, radish, broccoli, lettuce, beets, butternut squash, and asparagus. The supplements FOS and inulin also contain fructans. If you can't bear the thought of going without garlic on some of your favorite dishes, don't despair; garlic oil does not contain any fructans, so it can be used freely. The green tops of scallions don't contain any either, so they can be used as well.

Galactans

Galactans are present in all beans (legumes), including lentils, kidney beans, black-eyed peas, and garbanzos (chickpeas), as well as in broccoli and soy-based products. They consist of chains of a sugar called galactose that are fused to a fructose molecule. They cannot be broken down by the human body because we are missing the required enzymes. These substances remain completely unabsorbed, which is why we all develop flatulence to some degree when we eat beans. However, some people (e.g., those with candida or overgrowth of bacteria) experience more severe gastrointestinal difficulties than others after consuming foods containing galactans.

Lactose

Lactose is a naturally occurring sugar that is present in the milk of cows, goats, and sheep. Some people are deficient in the enzyme lactase, which is necessary to digest lactose properly, resulting in lactose intolerance. The enzyme may be completely or partially missing, which affects the severity of the intolerance.

Lactose is most plentiful in milk, cottage cheese, soft cheese, ice cream, yogurt, and custard. Butter and heavy cream contain only minute traces, so many people who are lactose intolerant can eat butter and heavy cream with no problem. Ghee does not contain any lactose. Raw dairy products contain the enzymes needed to break down lactose; therefore, as mentioned in the section on dairy, many people who are lactose intolerant have no problems with raw dairy. The test to diagnose lactose intolerance is called the hydrogen breath test.

Fructose

Fructose is a predominant sugar found in fruit. As discussed previously, fruit should be minimized in the diet due to its ability to feed candida. However, if one has a condition known as fructose malabsorption, then even small amounts of certain fruit can compound the problem. Fructose malabsorption arises in people who are deficient in the fructose transporter known as GLUT5. It is normally present in the small intestine, and its absence results in an inability to absorb fructose completely.

Not all fruits trigger fructose intolerance equally. Fruit also contains the sugar glucose. If a particular fruit contains a glucose/fructose ratio of 1:1, it will have less negative impact than fruits that contain more fructose than glucose. The individual with fructose malabsorption typically must be cautious with all fruit, but more so with varieties that have a higher ratio of fructose to glucose. Also be aware that ripe fruit is lower in fructose than unripe fruit, so fruit should always be consumed when ripe.

Foods that are high in fructose include honey, agave, high-fructose corn syrup, some wines like sherry and port, all dried fruit, fruit juices, apples, peaches, cherries, grapes, mangoes, pears, coconut, watermelon, artichokes, eggplant, sweet corn, and asparagus.

Please note that fructose malabsorption is a different condition from hereditary fructose intolerance. Heredity fructose intolerance is a very serious and somewhat rare genetic disorder in which a defective gene leads to a deficiency in the enzyme aldolase B, which is necessary to break down fructose. In this case, all fructose must be eliminated. The hydrogen breath test can diagnose whether you are subject to fructose malabsorption.

Polyols

Polyols, which you probably know as sugar alcohols, are made of molecules that are too large for anyone's small intestine to break down. They pull water into the colon, generating a laxative effect called osmotic diarrhea and can be consumed by bacteria, but not candida. Erythritol, xylitol, mannitol, sorbitol, maltitol, isomalt, and the supplement inositol are all types of sugar alcohols. Polyols also exist naturally in a variety of fruits and vegetables such as cherries, peaches, apples, plums, nectarines, apricots, pears, blackberries, persimmons, watermelons, prunes, avocados, celery, cauliflower, green bell pepper, button mushrooms, snow peas, and sweet potatoes.

Not all polyols create the same effect; it depends on the size of their molecules. The ones that are smaller in size are absorbed better than larger ones and have less negative impact on the gastrointestinal tract. Typically, xylitol and erythritol are the best tolerated, and maltitol, mannitol, and sorbitol are the least tolerated.

It's important to note that some foods like cherries, pears, and apples contain both polyols and fructose. Therefore, you could experience a negative impact from both substances rather than just one, significantly increasing the severity of symptoms. Additionally, fructose has an additive effect when united with fructans, lactose, galactans, or polyols, meaning the impact of each builds on the other, increasing the impact on the gastrointestinal tract and resulting in more severe symptoms. Generally, the more types of FODMAPs that are combined, the more symptoms one is likely to experience. For example, say you have eaten a meal that contained polyols, fructose, fructans, lactose, and galactans; the severity of your symptoms may be much worse than if the meal had contained just one of these substances. Research indicates that the FODMAPs that tend to be the least tolerated are those contained in wheat, onions, apples, and pears.

Although polyols are called sugar alcohols, they are neither sugars nor alcohols. Polyols (especially xylitol, which is believed to have some antifungal properties), are often encouraged on a variety of candida diets and are used as an alternative to sugar in the low-carb community. They do not feed candida, and they may be able to help break down some types of biofilms, so from that standpoint they are safe to use. But due to their potential to cause the other problems I've discussed, and because your goal is to lose interest in sweet foods rather than replacing them with something else, they should be limited to special occasions. Most professionals believe that polyols do not have a significant impact on blood sugar and insulin, but at this time we are not certain. However, they may stimulate cravings for sugar and carbs in some people due to the sweet taste on the palate affecting the endocrine system and the brain, and if that is the case, then they should be eliminated completely until brain chemistry and the endocrine system have stabilized to some degree.

The majority of xylitol on the market is obtained from corn, which is a grain. As described in the section on stevia, most traditionally grown corn is genetically modified and contaminated with Roundup. To avoid this danger, only purchase xylitol whose label states it is derived from birch. Additionally, as already mentioned, most erythritol is also created from GMO crops tainted with Roundup, so be sure your erythritol is organic and pure.

Identifying Your FODMAPs Threshold

Once you transition to a low-carb paleo diet to address candida overgrowth, you will eliminate many of the high-FODMAP foods—for example, legumes, high-fructose corn syrup, agave, rye, barley, wheat, soft cheese, and cottage cheese. You will also be strictly limiting the fruits and high-starch vegetables that fall under this category. However, several high-FODMAP foods are nutrient dense, can enrich health, do not encourage yeast overgrowth, and are eaten freely by many people who follow a paleo diet.

You don't want to sacrifice the nutrients and health benefits these foods offer by eliminating them unnecessarily. If a particular FOD-MAP food is permitted on the candida diet, and if you don't have SIBO, IBS, GERD, or some other functional gut disorder, and if you do not experience any negative effects from such foods, then you don't need to be concerned about them. However, if you are being compliant with your paleo for candida diet and are still having significant gastrointestinal symptoms or unresolved psychological symptoms (e.g., OCD, fear, anxiety, or panic), then you will want to look into whether you are having issues with some of the FODMAPs. Additionally, you don't want to eliminate all fermentable carbohydrates because they are utilized as a food source by your healthy gut bacteria. Furthermore, the fermentation process generates short-chain fatty acids that provide a variety of health benefits in moderation—for example, improving responsiveness to insulin and reducing inflammation.

Even if you are intolerant of FODMAPs, not everyone has the same threshold, which means the degree of intolerance and the severity of the symptoms can vary widely from individual to individual. Your own threshold may vary for each type of FODMAP. For example, one person may not tolerate any of the FODMAPs while another person only has problems with one or two of them. One individual may be completely incapable of eating a particular FODMAP while another is only mildly intolerant. Or perhaps you have a serious intolerance to fructose, fructans, and galactans but only a mild intolerance to polyols and no problem with lactose—or vice versa.

The presence and severity of symptoms can be further affected by the quantity and combination of FODMAPs consumed. A quarter cup of cherries, a few slices of a pear, a small piece of cheese, or a small quantity of xylitol may fail to produce symptoms, whereas a half cup of cherries, a whole pear, a large piece of cheese, or a greater quantity of xylitol may result in significant distress. You may experience mild symptoms when you eat broccoli, but unbearable symptoms if that broccoli is combined with onion or garlic, or if you have simultaneously eaten apples. Whether the food is raw or cooked can also influence the degree of the intolerance; raw foods are more likely to provoke more symptoms of greater severity. In another possible scenario, you may exceed your threshold if you eat lactose, fructans, and galactans all at once, but you may not if you eat just lactose or fructans. For example, in my own life, I can eat small amounts of erythritol or xylitol without any symptoms, but a little too much will give me severe abdominal pain and diarrhea. I can eat a little cabbage as long as it is cooked soft, but if it is raw or undercooked then I develop abdominal pain, cramping, and diarrhea. If I combine that cooked cabbage with another food that contains a small amount of a polyol, the two of them together produce distress and diarrhea, but separately they do not.

Your threshold and the severity of your symptoms can go up and down in response to a variety of other factors such as the degree of inflammation in your GI tract, the overall health of your gut, how many bacteria or fungi are present and what type they are, exposure to environmental toxins, and stress. A healthy gut has fewer pathogenic bacteria that may feed on FODMAPs. Environmental toxins can get lodged in the gastrointestinal tract and inhibit digestion and absorption. Stress basically shuts down the digestive system and directs all bodily resources to dealing with the stressor. Stress also inhibits a transporter in the small intestine that is essential for carrying glucose, and it decimates friendly gut flora—all of which combine to create the perfect environment for the flourishing of pathogenic organisms that thrive on FODMAPs.

Therefore, your tolerance for FODMAPs can change at various points in your life depending on these issues. Your intolerance may be very severe in the early stages of your healing journey because your gut is extremely damaged, but in six months or one year, as your gut health improves, your tolerance may increase. When you follow the candida diet as presented in this book and also remove FODMAPs, inflammation in the gut will decrease and gut flora will become more balanced, so there may be fewer pathogenic organisms to feed on the FODMAPs, and intolerance to them could decrease. Tolerance may improve for all FODMAPs, or it may improve for one or two only. On the other hand, if you experience a significant stressor or are surrounded by a lot of toxins, a more severe intolerance may develop. When I experience high stress, my tolerance for FODMAPs decreases, and when the stressful event ends, my tolerance increases.

You can assess your FODMAP intolerances and their severity by eliminating FODMAPs from your diet for four to six weeks. During that time, monitor whether you experience any improvements. Keep a food and symptom journal to track your results. After a period of elimination, add back one FODMAP at a time, and observe how you respond. It's important to test only one food at a time for about a week before trying another; otherwise you won't know which one is problematic. Symptoms may occur shortly after eating, hours after eating, or the next day. If symptoms are provoked, then play around with quantities and combinations to see if they are affected by other factors. Then adjust accordingly. Keep in mind that your tolerance and the severity of your symptoms may change from time to time.

The primary point for you to take away is that even if you have an intolerance to FODMAPs that are permitted on the candida diet, it may not be necessary to remove all FODMAPs. Nor does the food always have to be completely eliminated; it may only need to be moderated or reduced. As with all the other factors that come into play when you create your diet, you need to refine and personalize consumption of FODMAPs according to your individual biochemical needs. Don't remove a food and assume that it's necessarily gone forever. Use the list of high-FODMAP foods as a guideline, not as a rule set in stone. Challenge yourself periodically to test for changes, and then adjust accordingly. Because many of the vegetables that are high in FODMAPs offer health-enhancing benefits, you want to continue consuming them if possible. Finally, note that FODMAPs are much more problematic for individuals who have SIBO in addition to candida (see chapter 6).

CAFFEINE

Caffeine is an addictive mind-altering drug; it affects the brain in a manner similar to other psychotropics like amphetamines and cocaine,[35,36,37] which means it disrupts neurotransmitters, resulting in the perpetuation of the assorted problems discussed in earlier chapters. Like other addictions, caffeine withdrawal is now listed as a mental disorder in the DSM-5 Diagnostic and Statistic Manual of Mental

Disorders.[38] I would disagree that it is a mental disorder, but I mention this to demonstrate that it is considered by the mental health world to be a legitimate condition.

A study published in the *Journal of Caffeine Research* in 2013 coauthored by Laura Juliano, PhD, a psychology professor at American University in Washington, DC, "indicates that more people are dependent on caffeine to the point that they suffer withdrawal symptoms and are unable to reduce caffeine consumption even if they have another condition that may be impacted by caffeine—such as pregnancy, a heart condition, or a bleeding disorder. The negative effects of caffeine are often not recognized as such because it is a socially acceptable and widely consumed drug that is well integrated into our customs and routines. There is misconception among professionals and lay people alike that caffeine is not difficult to give up. However, in population-based studies, more than 50 percent of regular caffeine consumers report that they have had difficulty quitting or reducing caffeine use."[39,40]

According to NIDA (National Institute on Drug Abuse), "chronic caffeine use produces greater tolerance in adolescents compared with adults, suggesting that caffeine may cause greater brain changes in young people. Caffeine consumption is also known to be correlated with increased risk for illicit drug use and substance use disorders. Caffeine use by adolescents may prime the still developing brain for later use of other illicit drugs."[41]

Recall the importance of GABA and serotonin, which play a vital role in many aspects of health, including gut health, regulating sympathetic dominance, and modulating appetite. Caffeine disrupts normal metabolism of GABA and suppresses serotonin. Acetylcholine is vital for cognitive functions and regulating the autonomic nervous system. At first, caffeine floods the brain with acetylcholine, which is one of the reasons why it makes you feel alert, focused, and energized. But remember that excessive amounts of a neurotransmitter eventually lead to tolerance and then a heightened need for more of the addictive substance to replace the missing neurotransmitter. The same is true of dopamine and serotonin, critical for brain function, mood, and appetite. Initially there is a boost in dopamine and serotonin from caffeine, but over time the brain responds by reducing receptor sensitivity or downregulating production. The more often caffeine is consumed the more these neurotransmitters will become depleted and the more depleted they become the greater the cravings for caffeine. Dr. Al Sears explains, if acetylcholine is unavailable, this sets the brain off on a desperate search to find some, and it will extract it from your brain cell membranes. In more simple terms, your brain literally begins to destroy itself—this is called auto-cannibalism, because the body is destroying one part of itself to provide for another. The auto-cannibalism will be effective as a short-term solution, providing your brain with the acetylcholine it needs to perform its functions. However, in the long run, it creates a bigger problem, because it will impede your neurons' ability to fire as efficiently as they should, thus compromising brain function even more and creating more cravings.[42]

The consumption of caffeine prompts the liver to release its stored sugar (glycogen) into the bloodstream. Blood glucose levels rise, as if you had eaten sugar, feeding candida. Then insulin is released, and blood glucose levels drop, resulting in symptoms of low blood sugar. When blood sugar drops too low, you crave more caffeine, sugar, or carbs, and have difficulty remaining committed to your diet. It is impossible to maintain the crucial stability in blood sugar levels if one consumes caffeine.

Caffeine triggers the stress response system, potentially leading to sympathetic dominance and damaging the adrenal glands when consumed on a daily basis. If adrenal fatigue and/or sympathetic dominance are already present, caffeine consumption will impair one's ability to make improvement in these areas. As discussed, supporting the adrenal glands and reducing sympathetic dominance is an important step in the process of healing candida and managing cravings for sugar and carbs.

In your brain you have another neurotransmitter called adenosine, which has the primary role of dampening or slowing down firing of neurons. In Caffeine Blues, nutritional biochemist Stephen Cherniske explains that when you consume caffeine, it blocks adenosine receptors (also found in the gastrointestinal tract, kidneys, cardiovascular system, and respiratory system) so that adenosine is not able to do its job. This results in continuous and uncontrolled firing of neurons, which results in a feeling of alertness experienced with caffeine. This creates an emergency situation which triggers the classic stress response system, "affecting virtually every cell in the body." "A single

250 milligram dose of caffeine has been shown to increase levels of the stress hormone epinephrine by more than 200 percent." An eight-ounce cup of coffee may contain anywhere from 95 to 200 mg of caffeine.[43] In about an hour or so, your stress hormones will begin dissipate, and then you start to feel tired, fatigued, hungry, irritable, and get a headache, so then you reach for more caffeine or sugar or some other self-medicating substance. It is this vicious cycle that can deplete the adrenal glands over time and lead to sympathetic dominance.

Caffeine inhibits absorption of a wide array of the critical nutrients that are needed for a strong immune system and to keep neurotransmitters in balance and support a healthy gut, including zinc, potassium, iron, calcium, vitamins D and B1, biotin, and inositol. If you drink a cup of coffee with your morning supplements, you are throwing your money away, because caffeine impedes their absorption.

Additionally, caffeine increases kynurenate, which is a neurotoxin when present in excess. Normally, tryptophan is converted into serotonin, but some substances encourage tryptophan to convert into kynurenate instead. Caffeine consumption may lead to excessive levels of kynurenate.

If your favorite source of caffeine is coffee, coffee (both caffeinated and decaf) also contains a substance known as cafestol, which is a potent morphine-like compound, affecting the brain in a similar manner as other opiates. Which means it depletes your natural opiates (endorphins) and leads to addiction to coffee for the morphine effect.[44] Coffee is also high in mold toxins, increases histamine levels, and causes inflammation in the gut, all of which encourage yeast overgrowth, degrade the health of the gut further, and may contribute to food sensitivities and autoimmune disorders.

All forms of caffeine should be avoided, including coffee, tea (even green tea), chocolate, raw cacao, soda pop, energy drinks, and even "decaffeinated" coffee. Decaffeinated coffee has a lower level of caffeine, but it is not truly caffeine-free. Any amount of caffeine will keep the addiction cycle active and perpetuate sympathetic dominance.

Yes, I know you may be confused, because every time you turn around somebody is telling you about a benefit you can derive from drinking coffee. It does not matter if we have a thousand studies that make some kind of health benefit claim for coffee, none of these assertions change the fact that caffeine is an addictive mind-altering drug that sets off the stress response system and incites the long list of negative effects on health associated with these issues. Also, please be aware that combining your coffee with some form of fat, which is commonly promoted as healthy within the paleo/primal community, does not change these facts either. When determining whether something is truly healthy for consumption, we must look at the entire nutritional picture, not just one particular aspect.

The consumption of coffee and other caffeinated beverages is one of the biggest triggers for relapse when trying to remain on a low-carbohydrate diet (and in recovery from drug and alcohol addiction) and it is often one of the most difficult addictions to overcome because it is so deeply ingrained in and accepted by our society. Caffeine has been reported to be "the most widely used drug in the world. In the United States, more than 90% of adults use it regularly, and, among them, average consumption is more than 200 mg of caffeine per day—more caffeine than is contained in two 6-ounce cups of coffee or five 12-ounce cans of soft drinks."[45] In 2013, coffee was a "$30 billion-a-year national industry."[46] I work with people on a frequent basis who are true caffeine junkies and struggling as severely as a heroin addict to get clean. But, unlike other addictions, they have no one in their corner (not even their health-care practitioner) who believes their addiction is serious and supports their recovery. To be successful in this area, you must see caffeine for what it truly is (an addictive mind-altering drug) and let go of the need to fit in and conform socially.

SALT

Salt (sodium chloride) is absolutely essential for the human body. It supports hydration, assists with adrenal function, regulates blood pressure, maintains cell membranes and balance in pH and blood volume, prevents insulin resistance, helps prevent the formation of arterial plaque, helps one cope better with stress, and may even increase life expectancy. It is needed to support strong muscles and to assist the body in absorbing other vital nutrients. It is critical for transmission between nerve cells (firing of neurons), which means it plays an important role in neurotransmitter function and consequently in managing cravings for sugar and carbs and in good mental health. A true deficiency in salt would lead to brain swelling, coma, and heart failure.

In *The Art and Science of Low Carbohydrate Living* (another essential read for all low-carbers), Drs. Volek and Phinney explain that the amount of carbs present in the diet heavily influences one's need for salt. When you eat a high-carb diet, the kidneys retain salt; this may be one of the reasons why many people believe that salt may be bad for you. But when you eat a low-carb diet, such as the one presented in this book, within a week or two the kidneys will begin to excrete salt and water more rapidly. According to Phinney and Volek, if you consume less than 60 grams of carbs per day, an additional 2 to 3 grams of sodium are required daily to compensate for this loss, unless you are taking diuretic medication for blood pressure or fluid retention. If one is planning to exercise hard or for a prolonged period (produce sweat), then 1 of those grams of sodium needs to be consumed within the hour before exercise. Even if your carb intake is above 60 grams per day and exercise leaves you feeling faint, light-headed, or fatigued, they suggest that your salt intake may need to be increased. If one does not increase salt intake on a low-carb diet, then the loss of sodium will "compromise circulation," which can result in a wide variety of unpleasant symptoms such as light-headedness upon standing up quickly, feeling faint, weakness, fatigue (worse after exercise), headaches, and constipation.

Adequate sodium in the diet is very important to support the adrenal glands, which as described are typically very taxed in the individual with candida. Sodium helps regulate aldosterone, a hormone produced by the adrenals that manages blood pressure, potassium and sodium levels, and kidney function. When adrenal function is impaired, aldosterone levels may drop, resulting in a loss of sodium through the urine and the retention of potassium—an imbalance in sodium and potassium levels. Some individuals may have a genetic polymorphism that impairs aldosterone function and that can be improved with salt intake as well. Furthermore, without ample levels of salt, vitamin C, which is critical for the adrenal glands to produce their hormones, cannot be delivered adequately to the adrenals.

When aldosterone is low, blood pressure is low, and when aldosterone is high, blood pressure is high. That is why many people with adrenal fatigue have low blood pressure. Ironically, when the diet is too low in salt, the body increases release of aldosterone and also of an enzyme called renin, which increases blood pressure. Several very large studies have found that reducing salt intake does not decrease the risk of stroke, heart attack, or death in people with normal or high blood pressure. As a matter of fact, some of them demonstrated that lower levels of sodium were associated with higher risk of dying and heart disease, and that the more salt a person consumed the less likely she or he was to die from heart disease.[47] Turns out that the advice to reduce salt intake was based on questionable, flawed, and unsubstantial data and observations. Studies also demonstrate that removing salt from the diet decreases blood pressure only slightly. The long-held belief that salt causes high blood pressure, strokes, and heart disease may not be true at all.

A small percentage of the population may be hypersensitive to salt; for them, salt causes an increase in blood pressure. These individuals do need to be more cautious with their salt intake. Still, other factors can impact the effect salt has on the body—such as fructose consumption, potassium and magnesium levels, processed foods, stress, and alcohol consumption. Consumption of fructose increases the kidney's absorption of sodium and increases blood pressure. Potassium and magnesium both help keep sodium in balance, so if they are present in insufficient levels blood pressure may rise. (Most people eating a standard American diet do not consume enough potassium or magnesium.) Many people acquire their salt from processed food, not natural sources, and it is this combination that may be at the root of the problem. A higher level of stress and alcohol consumption, which are both well known to increase blood pressure, may make one more sensitive to salt. Based on these considerations, ensuring that the diet has adequate levels of potassium and magnesium, managing stress, avoiding alcohol, fructose, and processed foods—all of which you should be doing to address candida—may be just as important for reducing your risk of high blood pressure, heart attack, and stroke.[48,49,50]

In an evolutionary context, our Paleolithic ancestors did not mine salt to sprinkle on their food as we do today. Evidence suggests that their diet may have contained a substantial amount of naturally occurring salt from seafood such as shellfish, which was a common staple. Coastal dwellers often dipped their food into salty seawater and made salt from dried seawater. Aboriginal cultures drank the blood from freshly killed animals, a rich source of sodium, and followed animals to their salt licks. Salt has been a part of the diet for a long time in one form or another.

Conventional table salt should be avoided. All its vital nutrients have been removed, leaving nothing but sodium chloride. Additives such as bleach, aluminum, and ferrocyanide are added during the refining process. All of these are toxic chemicals that can inhibit neurotransmitter function, trigger cravings for sugar and carbs, weaken the immune system, alter pH, and degrade the integrity of the gut. Furthermore, sugar is often added to salt as a flowing agent. It is refined conventional salt that can lead to disease and make the body too acidic; not pure, unrefined salt. Pure and unrefined salt is rich in health-enhancing minerals, which give the salt a pink or gray color. It is also much coarser than refined salt. My favorite brand is Real Salt, which is obtained from salt beds in Utah. Himalayan salt, rock salt, and Celtic salt are other healthier choices. Even many types of sea salt have been refined and polluted with chemicals, so you must be cautious when choosing your brand. If salt is fine and white in color, it should be avoided.

As with most aspects of the diet, the amount of salt that is best for one individual may not be for another, and too much or too little may lead to problems. If you are eating a paleo for candida diet, then you will have removed all the foods that contain refined salt and will acquire your sodium from natural sources. Therefore, salting food to taste should not put you at risk of excess intake. A bare minimum of 500 mg of sodium per day is required to sustain life, but the research suggests that in most cases health is supported best with an intake of somewhere between 3,000 and 6,000 mg of salt per day (salt is 40 percent sodium).[51] If you eat a low-carb diet (less than 60 grams per day), have adrenal fatigue, are really active, or sweat a lot, then your need may be greater. If, on the other hand, you have a sedentary lifestyle or are sensitive to salt, your need may be on the lower end. Sodium intake should be gauged according to the unique biochemical needs of each individual.

CHOCOLATE AND RAW CACAO

Chocolate (including dark chocolate and raw cacao) contains hundreds of naturally occurring chemicals, many of which are addictive psychotropic drugs. These substances affect the brain in the same manner as marijuana, cocaine, alcohol, amphetamines, and heroin all at the same time, which is why so many people are addicted to chocolate. It is less potent than these hard drugs, but has the same effects on the brain. Consuming chocolate basically gets you high. It floods the brain with neurotransmitters (dopamine, endorphins, GABA, serotonin, endocannabinoids), which, as discussed, can lead to depletion of these vital brain chemicals over time. With depletion comes tolerance and cravings for more chocolate, to mimic the effects of the depleted neurotransmitters.

In *Breaking the Food Seduction,* Dr. Neal Barnard states "the truth is that chocolate is, in essence, an addictive drug. It targets the same spot on your brain as heroin or morphine." This is demonstrated partly by the fact that chocolate contains a substance called epicatechin that has potent opiate-like activity.[52] Studies have found that Naloxone, an opiate-blocking drug that is used to reverse the effects of a heroin overdose, also eliminates cravings and desire for chocolate, to the point of rendering it completely unappealing. Barnard states, chocolate does not stimulate opiate receptors to the same degree as narcotics, but it is a similar effect and this is the driving force of what keeps us coming back for more chocolate. According to Barnard, cravings for chocolate can also be eliminated with some other drugs that target neurotransmitters like wellbutrin and topamax, again demonstrating chocolate's influence over neurotransmitters. Dr. Barnard goes on to explain that chocolate also contains a chemical called theobromine (a stimulant similar to caffeine) in hefty amounts, and another stimulant called phenylethylamine (PEA) that we discussed previously, as well as trace amounts of THC (a substance similar to one of our endocannabinoid neurotransmitters called anandamide, also present in marijuana). Additionally, other chemicals in chocolate decrease the breakdown of our neurotransmitter anandamide, which prolongs the euphoric effects of chocolate. Barnard explains, "chocolate is not just a single drug-like compound, it's basically the whole drugstore, traces of mild opiates, caffeine, amphetamine-like components, and the equivalent of a slight whiff of marijuana," all wrapped into one. However, just as the "taste of sugar touching the tongue appears to send a signal to the brain that triggers a virtually instant opiate effect, chocolate likely does the same in addition to the effects of its chemical cornucopia." If chocolate is combined with a 50/50 mixture of sugar and fat (substances that also affect neurotransmitters) it "reaches its point of maximal irresistibility." Dr. Barnard explains one of the ways chocolate consumption is "pushed" in our society is because the Chocolate Manufacturers Association attends hearings every five years when a federal panel is redrafting the Dietary Guidelines for Americans and makes a case that this food should be included in the diet, with press releases claiming chocolate "contains healthy antioxidants."[53]

In a review of the literature published in the *Journal of the American Dietetic Association*, researchers concluded that "chocolate may evoke similar psychopharmacologic and behavioral reactions in susceptible persons" as drugs and alcohol. They point out that "chocolate contains several biologically active constituents (methylxanthines, biogenic amines, and cannabinoid-like fatty acids), all of which potentially cause abnormal behaviors and psychological sensations that parallel those of other addictive substances. It may be used by some as a form of self-medication for dietary deficiencies (e.g., magnesium) or to balance low levels of neurotransmitters involved in the regulation of mood, food intake, and compulsive behaviors (e.g., serotonin and dopamine)." They warn dietetics professionals that they "must be aware that chocolate cravings are real. The psychopharmacologic and chemosensory effects of chocolate must be considered when formulating recommendations for overall healthful eating and for treatment of nutritionally related health issues."[54]

Chocolate is high in caffeine and in phytates, and some brands contain high levels of heavy metals. Problems with all these substances have been outlined in earlier pages. Many of these chemicals like caffeine and theobromine can be very detrimental to the adrenal glands and fuel sympathetic dominance if consumed frequently.

All chocolate is produced through fermentation, and any food that is fermented is high in glutamate and histamine, which can contribute to elevated levels in people with high histamine or glutamate and all the associated symptoms and consequences we've already discussed earlier. It is also high in mold and in mycotoxins like aflatoxin and ochratoxin, which can lead to a wide array of neurological symptoms and candida-related complications.

For all these reasons, consumption of chocolate (or raw cacao) perpetuates an addiction to sugar and carbs; contributes to symptoms like depression, anxiety, mood swings, attention deficit, fatigue, hyperactivity, insomnia, and irritability; weakens the adrenal glands; and perpetuates sympathetic dominance—all of which can sabotage your efforts to remain on the diet and can limit your healing. Chocolate in all forms should be avoided. Even if it is rich in antioxidants or magnesium, we can obtain those nutrients from other foods that do not impair our health. Again, it doesn't matter if there are thousands of studies that claim some kind of benefit for chocolate or raw cacao; this does not change any of the issues we have discussed in this section. Remember, when accessing whether a particular food is really healthy for consumption, we must look at the complete nutritional picture, not just one component. The negative health effects of chocolate far outweigh the positive. If we are talking about raw cacao, the negative effects can be even more pronounced as the mind-altering chemicals are even more potent. Some chocolate on the market claims they are healthy because it removes the mycotoxins. Please be aware that this only removes one of the issues. This does not change any of the other facts we have mentioned.

SEAFOOD

Seafood is an integral component of the paleo diet and is a good source of vitamins D and A and omega-3 fatty acids. However, it is very difficult to acquire seafood that is not polluted with the numerous toxins that are present in our waterways, including mercury and other heavy metals, pesticides, and petrochemicals. Most fish is treated with formaldehyde when processed. These toxins can encourage candida overgrowth, fuel sympathetic nervous system activity, weaken immunity, and disrupt neurotransmitters. Therefore, you must be very careful about where you purchase your seafood, and consumption may need to be limited if it produces symptoms for you.

The cleanest fish that can be found is wild Alaskan or Pacific; of these, salmon is your safest choice. Salmon is high in a powerful antioxidant called astaxanthin. Be sure to avoid the salmon available in your local grocery store as it is likely to be genetically modified, voiding all these benefits and adding the risks of GMO. Farmed fish should be avoided completely as well because it is loaded with toxins and does not contain the proper ratio of omega-3 to omega-6 fatty acids. Shark, swordfish, king mackerel, tilefish, marlin, and tuna are exceptionally high in mercury. Other fish, such as walleye, large-mouth bass, halibut, lobster, and mahi mahi, also contain significant levels of mercury. Shrimp, tilapia, Pacific sole, and anchovies have lower levels.

You can help your body eliminate the toxins found in seafood more efficiently by eating lots of sulfur-containing foods like garlic, cabbage, broccoli, eggs, and cauliflower. Sulfur attaches to heavy metals and other toxins and carries them out of the body via elimination. It is critical that other minerals such as iron, zinc, and selenium be present in your body in sufficient amounts because they counteract the effects of these toxins. Deficiencies in any of these minerals allow toxins to attach to receptor cites. Since candida and other microbes may deplete the body of some of these minerals, individuals with candida may be more vulnerable to the toxins in seafood.

ALTERNATIVE GRAINS

The alternative grains (spelt, amaranth, kamut, teff, buckwheat, millet, quinoa, wild rice) should be avoided because they are all very high in the carbohydrates that feed candida, spike insulin, lead to low blood sugar, and perpetuate cravings for sugar and carbs. None of the foods in this category are considered to be paleo. However, you may find that some paleo adherents occasionally permit some of the ones that aren't true grains if they want to boost their carb intake. For example, quinoa is part of the chenopod family, wild rice is a marsh grass, and buckwheat is a seed related to rhubarb. From the viewpoint of treating candida, they should only be used on special occasions, if at all. Note that quinoa is high in saponins, the bitter, naturally occurring substances that are also found in nightshades. They can destroy the gut lining, promote inflammation, contribute to autoimmune disorders, and disrupt the autonomic nervous system. Quinoa also contains lectins and phytates. Wild rice contains significant levels of antinutrients like phytates and may become infected with a toxic fungus called ergot, distinguished by purple or pink blotches. Amaranth contains phytates, and buckwheat contains saponins and phytates. Spelt, kamut, teff, and millet are grains, so they shouldn't even be considered for all the reasons already discussed.

FAT

As you have learned, your diet should contain sufficient levels of fat for numerous reasons. First, fatty acids are critical for the formation and repair of neurons (brain and nerve cells) and the proper transmission of neurotransmitters. Fat helps maintain flexibility in cell membranes and is essential in the formation of myelin, the protective sheath that surrounds a section of some neurons called the axon. Neurotransmitters travel through the axons. Myelin also amplifies the strength and speed of neurotransmission.

Dietary fat is crucial for a healthy immune system and for the construction of hormones. It helps to maintain stable blood sugar levels, and it assists in digestion and in the prevention of constipation. It prevents food from being absorbed too rapidly, prolonging satiation, and provides the body with energy. Short-chain and medium-chain fatty acids don't have to be acted on by bile salts; they are absorbed directly from the small intestine into the liver to be used as an immediate source of energy. Fat assists in the absorption of minerals and the conversion of beta-carotene into vitamin A, and it is a transporter of the fat-soluble vitamins E, D, A, and K. Some fat, like DHA, activates BDNF (brain-derived neurotrophic factor), a substance critical for neurogenesis. BDNF also protects existing neurons by encouraging synapse formation and enhances the detoxification system. Higher levels of BDNF are associated with a decrease in appetite. Omega-3 fats are critical for managing inflammation.

Do be aware that concentrated sources of fat can overstimulate the neurotransmitters dopamine, endorphins, and endocannabinoids in a similar manner to that accomplished by sugar, drugs, or alcohol, which can result in compulsive overeating and bingeing in some people. Concentrated fat is found in cream, butter, cheese, ghee, coconut oil, coconut cream, coconut butter, coconut flakes, certain cuts of fatty meat, and some nuts. A person may crave fat and binge on it when he or she is deficient in fatty acids, the adrenals are weak, dopamine and endorphins are low, or if he or she harbors some type of parasite infection, all of which are very common in the candida population. Once you have been eating adequate fat and protein for a period of time to address these issues, cravings often subside. When a concentrated source of fat is combined with a concentrated source of sugar (especially in a fifty/fifty ratio) the result is a powerful, addictive drug, intensifying cravings and making them irresistible.[55] If concentrated sources of fat trigger uncontrollable cravings or binges, then they need to be moderated or eliminated accordingly. Please note, I am only speaking of "concentrated" sources of fat here. Fat that is less concentrated does not have this overstimulating effect.

The type of fat that you consume is critical to your health; it should be obtained primarily from saturated fats and monounsaturated fats, and there should be a balance between omega-3 and omega-6 fatty acids. Avoid hydrogenated fats, partially hydrogenated fats, artificial trans fats, and high levels of omega-6 polyunsaturated fats (otherwise known as PUFAs), such as those contained in margarine, safflower oil, cottonseed oil, canola oil, shortening, soybean oil, or any other vegetable or seed oil. These are the types of fat that contribute to inflammation, heart disease, and cancer. Healthy saturated fat is hard or semihard at room temperature; it occurs naturally in animal foods such as chicken, buffalo/bison, beef, turkey, lamb, venison, duck, pheasant, and fish, and egg yolks, coconut, and other tropical oils. Good sources of monounsaturated fat include olives and avocados (and their respective oils), macadamia nuts, and to a lesser degree other nuts. Do remember that most nuts (except the macadamia and chestnut) are also high in omega-6 polyunsaturated fats, so they should be eaten in moderation. If one can tolerate dairy and doesn't have issues with the dairy exorphins or concentrated sources of fat discussed earlier, then some forms of dairy can be good sources of fat, for example, butter, ghee, heavy cream, and cream cheese.

Contrary to popular belief, the consumption of saturated fat does not lead to heart disease, type 2 diabetes, cancer, or other degenerative health conditions, so it should not be feared. Again, saturated fat provides integrity to the body's cells, protects the liver, enhances immune function, and is essential for healthy bones. According to many health-care professionals, including Drs. Volek and Phinney, biomarkers for diabetes and metabolic syndrome such as CRP (C-reactive protein), IL-6 (interleukin-6), palmitoleic acid, serum triglycerides, as well as the size of LDL particles and the levels of HDL cholesterol, all show striking improvements on a well-formulated high-fat and low-carb diet. "The strongest correlation between a major dietary nutrient and blood levels of saturated fat is with dietary carbohydrates not with saturated fat intake."[56] The more carbs one eats, the higher the level of saturated fat that is present in the blood. Dr. Al Sears explains that "studies have shown that the plaque in arteries that causes heart disease is mostly made of unsaturated fats, especially polyunsaturated ones (in vegetable oil), not the saturated fat of animals."[57] A very large study on heart disease conducted by Russell Smith demonstrated that mortality rates decreased when the consumption of animal products increased.[58]

Fat intake should be gauged in a manner similar to how you gauge carb intake: based on how it makes you feel. The amount and types consumed should make you feel satiated without triggering a binge. One person may need more fat than another depending on each person's unique personal needs, so each individual must find the balance that works for them. The fewer carbs you consume the more fat you will need because the body will be using fat for energy instead of glucose the majority of the time. You will most likely notice that after you lower your carb intake you are drawn toward fat when you are hungry, especially if you are consuming less than 50 grams of carbs per day. This indicates that your body is running on fat, as it is supposed to, so it is nothing to be concerned about. It will also depend on other factors—for example, how long you've been eating low carb and the amount of body fat that you are carrying. If you begin eating a low-carb diet and you are quite thin and have very little body fat, your fat intake will need to increase immediately since the body will begin using fat for fuel. If, on the other hand, you are carrying a great deal of extra body fat, once you lower your carb intake your body will begin to burn the stored fat for energy. During this time, an increase in fat intake is not required. Once you have burned off the excess bodily fat, dietary fat intake will need to be increased to provide the necessary fuel. In *The Art and Science of Low Carbohydrate Living,* Drs. Volek and Phinney explain that when the body is using fat for fuel, as it does on a low-carb diet, it prefers saturated and monounsaturated fats. You will find it very unpleasant and difficult to sustain a low-carb diet in the long run if fat intake is not increased accordingly.

It appears that some microbes use fat in the development of biofilms; some practitioners recommend cutting fat out of the diet for people with candida, SIBO, or another microbial infection. This is a really bad idea. Fat is not the same as carbohydrate. As mentioned previously, carbs are completely nonessential in the diet, so they can be sacrificed without any harm to the body; you will be better off without them. That is not the case with fat. To repeat, fat is vital for brain health, the endocrine system, the immune system, gut health, regulating appetite, adrenal function, managing sympathetic dominance, and other functions. Without adequate fat in the diet, you are not going to make much progress in the healing journey. Cutting fat would do more harm than good despite the fact it may be used in biofilm formation. If you have a need to moderate fat (due to SIBO or gallbladder issues), allow as much as you possibly can comfortably.

ANIMAL PROTEIN

Each meal of the day, including breakfast, should include between 4 and 8 ounces of animal protein. Adequate animal protein helps to maintain balanced blood sugar levels, prevents muscle loss, supports the immune system, and provides the brain with the nutrients it needs to produce neurotransmitters. It is animal protein and fat that will prevent hunger between meals and eliminate cravings for sugar and carbs.

Protein is also needed for the thyroid to convert T4 into T3. T3 is what controls metabolism of most nutrients, so the more T3 you have available the more efficient your metabolism. The infrastructure of every cell in your body is constructed of protein, and it's used in the formation of the muscles, hormones, nerves, and enzymes that are responsible for normal organ functioning. The antibodies generated by the immune system to help fight off candida and other microbes are made from proteins. Animal protein is the superior source of protein. Protein from any other source either is incomplete, because it does not contain all the essential amino acids, or contains insufficient amounts of the essential amino acids.

When it is from organic, grass-fed, hormone-free, antibiotic-free, and cage-free animals, as was intended by nature, animal protein does not cause heart disease, cancer, or any other deterioration in health. It was the consumption of animal protein that propelled development of the human brain and advancement of our species. A great deal of energy is required to run the human brain, and in the caveman days, animal protein was the most attainable source of fuel. By consuming animal protein our early ancestors were able to obtain greater amounts of nutrients and calories with a lot less labor. They traded a bigger digestive tract for a larger brain and were enabled to move into climates where vegetation was not broadly obtainable—all of which encouraged us to progress as a species.[59] Researchers who have analyzed the diet of our hunter-gatherer ancestors found that "whenever and wherever it was ecologically possible, hunter-gatherers consumed high amounts (45–65% of energy) of animal food. Most (73%) of the worldwide hunter-gatherer societies derived > 50% (> or = 56–65% of energy) of their subsistence from animal foods, whereas only 14% of these societies derived > 50% (> or = 56–65% of energy) of their subsistence from gathered plant foods."[60]

Unlike what is commonly believed, a high-protein diet does not lead to kidney damage in someone with healthy kidneys. The studies that found protein harmful to the kidneys were performed on subjects who already had kidney damage. If a person has existing kidney damage, eating a lot of protein can be problematic, but not if the kidneys are healthy. Nor does protein cause weak bones. Although it is true that the consumption of a lot of protein causes a slight increase in excretion of urinary calcium, at the same time more protein in the diet also prompts greater calcium absorption, which balances everything out.[61]

There is a popular belief in the paleo/keto community, as well as other diet philosophies, that if you consume more protein than your system needs for basic repair and maintenance, the liver will convert any excess into glucose through gluconeogenesis. If this is correct, that means that over consumption of animal protein could increase blood sugar levels and provide fuel for candida and contribute to other issues we've already discussed associated with elevations in glucose. It may also interrupt ketosis. So even if you are eating a low-carb diet, excess protein could increase candida overgrowth. However, it is unclear whether this is actually true. Paleo expert Amber O'Hearn has presented a variety of studies that call this theory into question. These studies suggest that gluconeogenesis is driven by demand, not by supply.[62] At this time I have not made a final decision, but I lean toward agreeing with this line of thinking. Regardless, production of glucose through gluconeogenesis is moderated and occurs at a slower rate than production of glucose from dietary sugar and carbs, so it does not tend to cause the large spike in insulin that occurs after eating carbs. With moderate consumption of protein, the body will only generate as much glucose as is needed, and nothing more. How much protein is needed for basic repair and maintenance varies from person to person and depends on many different factors like current health status, age, and carb and fat intake. Your needs may change over time. Typically, one should be safe if they remain within the 4 to 8 ounces of animal protein per meal regardless of what is true. As with everything else, your needs for fat and protein may change over time as you go through the healing process and through different phases of life.

If you have a high histamine issue, make sure your meat is fresh or frozen. Meat accumulates histamine the longer it sits without being frozen. Check the expiration date on your meat products when buying fresh. Frozen is a better option, but this can vary from manufacturer to manufacturer depending on how the meat was handled when it was processed. If it was frozen immediately after processing, or if there was a longer period before the meat made it to the freezer, its histamine content will be affected. You may be able to eat meat from some producers but not others, depending on their procedures. You may have to experiment with many different brands to find one that is tolerable for you.

CHOLESTEROL

Contrary to popular belief, you don't really need to worry about having high blood cholesterol. Your bigger worry is low cholesterol. But how does *dietary* cholesterol (cholesterol contained in the foods you eat) affect *blood* cholesterol (the cholesterol numbers that are checked when your doctor orders blood work)? There are no reliable studies that prove dietary levels of cholesterol are connected to disease. Furthermore, the lower your blood cholesterol, the more health problems you are likely to experience. The Framingham study, which has been ongoing since 1948 and has studied the dietary habits of fifteen thousand subjects, has found no correlation between dietary cholesterol levels and blood cholesterol levels.[63] Not only that, the subjects in the study who consumed the most saturated fat, cholesterol, and calories had the lowest weight. Individuals with low blood cholesterol are found to experience higher rates of depression, suicide, and acts of violence,[64,65,66] as well as cancer, impaired cognitive functioning and memory loss, lower attention spans, and a shorter life span than those with higher cholesterol. Unbiased studies have demonstrated that the plaque in arteries that causes heart disease consists primarily of unsaturated fats, particularly polyunsaturated fats, not saturated fat from animals. As mentioned previously, other studies have demonstrated that mortality rates decrease when consumption of animal products increases.

Cholesterol is used by the body in a variety of important ways. It is so vital that about 75 percent of it is made by the liver and the remaining 25 percent is acquired through dietary sources. Astrocytes (specialized cells in the brain and central nervous system) can make cholesterol for the brain. The sun interacts with cholesterol to create vitamin D, which is critical to strengthen the immune system and to produce the peptides that fight off candida and other microbes. Vitamin D also assists in the management of enzymes in the brain and the cerebrospinal fluid that are needed for activating nerve growth and producing neurotransmitters. It protects neurons from the damaging effects of free radicals and decreases inflammation. Vitamin D can boost serotonin production up to thirtyfold.[67] A variety of studies have demonstrated that individuals experience significantly more cognitive decline if they are deficient in vitamin D. In one study, the subjects with the highest level of vitamin D experienced a 77 percent decrease in their risk for Alzheimer's.[68] Vitamin D also plays a vital role in blood sugar regulation and insulin sensitivity, which means it is needed for managing cravings for sugar and carbs. Some vitamin D can be obtained from cold-water fish (e.g., salmon) and mushrooms, but the best way to get it is through exposure to sunshine (see pages 403–406; 461–462). Please read more about vitamin D in chapters 13 and 14. Additionally, with the help of vitamin A, cholesterol is converted into the hormones estrogen, progesterone, and androgen, as well as cortisol, aldosterone, and DHEA, which are vital for addressing the adrenal fatigue that so often accompanies candida. If you lack sufficient cholesterol, your adrenal glands will be unable to make their hormones.

Cholesterol acts as an antioxidant, repairs damaged tissue in arteries, is converted into bile salts by the liver (needed for the absorption of fats and fat-soluble vitamins), and is critical for healthy and normal brain function. It is the basic building block of the cell membrane. It serves as a fuel for neurons and aids in the formation of synapses (spaces between neurons that enable communication) and many other neuron functions. Without cholesterol, thought process and memory will fail to operate correctly. According to Dr. William Shaw, there is a direct correlation "between the concentration of cholesterol in the brain, particularly the myelin, and how well the brain functions." Nearly 60 percent of the autistic population is found to be deficient in cholesterol. Without adequate levels of cholesterol, "gene expression, neurotransmission and hormone synthesis are all impaired."[69] The Framingham study found that brain function plummets when cholesterol levels are low. Participants with cholesterol levels below 200 mg/dl performed worse than those with borderline high or high levels in areas of attention, concentration, word fluency, abstract reasoning, and executive functioning. Subjects with the highest cholesterol levels performed best. The brain obtains the cholesterol it needs via LDL (low-density lipoprotein), which carries it through the bloodstream. In *Grain Brain*, Dr. Perlmutter explains that "sugar molecules attach themselves to LDL," which changes its shape, making it less usable and increasing free radicals, rendering it unable to transport cholesterol to the neurons. It is *oxidized* LDL that causes disease, not normal LDL, and LDL becomes oxidized through a diet that is high in sugar and carbohydrates.

As you can see, ensuring that you have adequate levels of blood cholesterol is critical for many aspects of healing candida, including immune function, brain function, inflammation control, gut health, and adrenal health. It plays a vital role in keeping cravings for sugar and carbs under control so that you may remain compliant with the diet. According to a seminar presented by Dr. Charles Gant, a cholesterol level below 160 is actually dangerous, and you'd better "get to eating some butter real quick."[70] Recall from other studies that even people whose cholesterol is at the recommended 200 mg/dl may experience a decline in health, which indicates that a number over 200 is most likely better.

FIBER

Many people are concerned that they won't consume enough fiber if they eliminate grains and other starchy foods from their diet, but this is the result of misinformation. Although it is true that grains help the bowels move because they move stool more quickly through the digestive tract, consuming grains is an unnatural way to attain the desired result. Contrary to what you have been led to believe, fiber is not the determining factor for the health of your gut and the elimination process. It is the healthy bacteria in the colon that control the water content, soften the stool, and increase bulk, so the elimination process will be smooth, comfortable, and operating sufficiently. That is to say, it is the presence or absence in the gastrointestinal tract of healthy or unfriendly bacteria that causes constipation and other intestinal disorders, not the lack of fiber or roughage.[71] Many pathogenic microbes inhibit peristalsis as a way to prevent their removal. There would be no need for grains to keep the bowels moving if friendly bacteria levels are sufficient and unfriendly organisms were not present. Adequate fat and water intake and regular physical activity are also needed for intestinal motility.

Whole grains, or too much fiber from any other source, actually feed the unhealthy microbes and make them multiply rapidly, causing more constipation and bowel distress and perpetuating the problem. Additionally, byproducts of excessive fiber fermentation can kill friendly bacteria. Nor is fiber the critical factor in cholesterol levels, cancer, or type 2 diabetes; as discussed, it is the presence of sugar and carbohydrates that increases risk for these conditions.

Excessive amounts of insoluble fiber can bind to the minerals zinc, calcium, magnesium, and iron, making them inaccessible for use. Some types of fiber, such as pectin, when present in excess, can inhibit pancreatic enzyme activity and the digestion of protein. The bacteria in the gut ferment soluble fiber into the short-chain fatty acids butyrate, propionate, and acetate. Butyrate enhances sensitivity to insulin and has an anti-inflammatory effect; it can also be found in high-fat dairy foods. So some amount of soluble fiber is necessary for digestion and gut health. However, the presence of too many short-chain fatty acids can cause symptoms such as depression, anxiety, and migraines.

This doesn't mean that fiber plays no role in your health or that it should be avoided completely. Soluble fiber is a food source for the healthy bacteria in your gut and consequently enhances elimination and gastrointestinal health. But again, too much soluble fiber can overfeed even the good guys, which can lead to problems. Fiber is a primary food source for SIBO, so it must be regulated closely in people with SIBO. All the fiber you need can and should be acquired primarily through low-starch vegetables (cabbage, broccoli, cauliflower, all leafy greens, green beans, etc.) and to a lesser degree from nuts, seeds, and fruits that are low in sugar. Sufficient healthy fats (not artificial trans or hydrogenated fats), adequate water intake, and regular physical activity are also important for the elimination process.

YEAST

The diet should eliminate all foods that contain yeast (baker's yeast, brewer's yeast, yeast extracts, autolyzed yeast, etc.) because yeast is fermented in the gut and feeds candida. Yeast extract or autolyzed yeast also contains free glutamic acid, which can contribute to excess levels of glutamate in people who have that problem.

PORK

Pork is a popular food for most people following a paleo diet. However, I am not an advocate of eating pork because it harbors several types of parasites and retroviruses that are not destroyed in the cooking process. These pathogens can destroy the gut and health and make reducing candida overgrowth more difficult. I just don't feel there is any reason to take this unnecessary risk. If you aren't concerned with this issue, then pork is acceptable from other angles that affect candida.

WATER AND OTHER BEVERAGES

Water is really the only beverage that your body needs and that you should consume. Ensuring that you keep your body hydrated every day is vital for the delivery of oxygen and nutrients to the cells and for the proper functioning of your organs and systems. It is also important for detoxification—both everyday detoxification and the increased detoxification required when you're dealing with the toxic byproducts of candida and other microbes, especially during their eradication. The body eliminates water more effectively during a low-carb diet, boosting the need for water intake. Water aids in the transition from sugar burner to fat burner. Thirst can actually be experienced as hunger or cravings, so water plays an important role in managing cravings for sugar and carbs. As mentioned in chapter 8, adequate water intake is also essential for the colon and elimination process.

Tap water should be avoided because it contains chlorine, fluoride, and other potential toxins like pesticides, pharmaceutical drugs, and parasites. Earlier chapters have discussed the problems associated with these harmful substances. As mentioned in chapter 2, the water supply in most cities is treated with chlorine to kill bacteria, and it does precisely the same thing in your gastrointestinal tract: eliminates your healthy bacteria. Therefore, your water should be obtained from a purified source.

Sparkling mineral water (e.g., Gerolsteiner, Mountain Valley, Pellegrino, Perrier) is permitted. Enhance it with a splash of lemon or lime now and then for a little added flavor. However, if you have SIBO, be aware that carbonated water can increase acid reflux and gas. Since herbal teas consist primarily of water, they are an acceptable beverage (as long as they don't contain caffeine). However, as mentioned, dried herbs often accumulate mold and may trigger symptoms in those who are sensitive to mold. Coconut milk and almond milk may be acceptable in small amounts on occasion, but do keep in mind their carb and fiber content, as well as the other issues discussed in the sections on nuts and coconut. Be especially mindful of the fact that they can feed candida and SIBO.

OILS

Acceptable oils include olive oil, coconut oil, walnut oil, macadamia oil, avocado oil, sesame oil, red palm oil, and high-oleic sunflower oil. Avoid consuming any oils in large amounts because their higher content of omega-6 fatty acids can increase inflammation. As mentioned in the nut section, the macadamia nut has higher levels of MUFAs and lower levels of PUFAs than any other nut, and so does its oil. Remember that the walnut is exceptionally high in PUFAs, and most of it is omega-6, so don't go overboard.

The common sunflower oil that you will find in most grocery stores is too high in the omega-6 fat called linoleic acid. High-oleic sunflower oil, which can be found in most health food stores, is low in omega-6 and rich in oleic acid, the same healthy monounsaturated fat that is present in olive oil. Avoid conventional sunflower oil, but high-oleic is acceptable. Be sure to look for the phrase *high-oleic* on the bottle; it will be displayed prominently. Olive oil should be first pressed only and extra virgin.

All oils are subject to oxidation and free-radical production when heated, so none of them except coconut oil should be used for frying. Oils should always be cold pressed so they are not exposed to heat and expeller pressed so they are not exposed to chemicals. Keep them refrigerated after opening because exposure to light and air can cause them to oxidize and turn rancid. Light can also decrease their polyphenol (an antioxidant) content. You can add a vitamin E capsule to the bottle to help preserve an oil that's been opened.

BONE BROTH

Bone broth is rich in several highly absorbable nutrients such as glycine, arginine, proline, chondroitin, glucosamine, magnesium, calcium, potassium, and phosphorus. It has been consumed by humans for millions of years and is very popular among paleo devotees and followers of many other diet philosophies because it is believed to help heal and seal the gut, oppose inflammation, encourage healthy digestion, support the immune system, inhibit infection by microbes, reduce joint pain and inflammation, promote strong and healthy bones, hair, and nails, and balance the nervous system.

As you can see, the benefits derived from bone broth can target many of the issues associated with candida overgrowth. However, it's important to be aware that bone broth is quite high in free glutamate, which increases the body's glutamate levels. This can be very problematic for anyone who has issues with excess glutamate, which, as discussed earlier, is quite often the case in individuals with candida, and sugar and carb addiction, as well as anxiety and panic disorders, OCD, autism spectrum disorders, migraines, hyperactivity, ALS, Parkinson's, Tourette's, PANDAS, seizures, multiple sclerosis, fibromyalgia, multiple chemical sensitivity, chronic fatigue, SIBO, and more. I've also outlined other problems with high levels of glutamate, including its toxicity to the brain. Please refer to chapters 1 and 13 for more information on the glutamate and GABA balance. Additionally, bone broth is very high in histamine, which makes it a bad choice for people with histadelia (high brain histamine) or histamine intolerance also very common in the individual with candida and SIBO. Please refer to pages 444–449 to learn more about these issues. In summary, both excess histamine and excess glutamate perpetuate sympathetic nervous system activity, degrade the gut, impair immunity, and promote cravings for sugar and carbs, all of which fuel overgrowth of candida and other microbes.

That said, problems with glutamate and histamine have a variety of contributing factors; therefore, if some of these factors are eliminated, one's glutamate levels may be lowered enough that one may be able to enjoy the benefits bone broth has to offer. Still, some people have a genetic predisposition to a higher number of glutamate receptors than others, and some of the aforementioned issues may be hard to resolve. Such individuals will always be inclined toward excessive levels of glutamate and will always need to moderate substances that increase glutamate, like bone broth. The same is true for histamine. Some people who have problems with high-histamine foods like bone broth can lower their levels enough to be able to consume such foods comfortably. For others, limiting high-histamine foods may remain a lifelong endeavor.

The process of making bone broth pulls mucopolysaccharides from the animal's joint and cartilage tissue. Mucopolysaccharides feed small intestinal bacterial overgrowth (SIBO). Experts on SIBO recommend making broth from meat, not bone.[72] If you try this method, make sure that no bone at all is connected to the meat; any amount of bone will also increase the broth's histamine and glutamate content.

For these reasons, consumption of bone broth for people with the aforementioned issues can be downright harmful and should be avoided. Ironically, under these circumstances, bone broth can cause or exacerbate some of the very conditions it is publicized as healing. It will undermine your ability to stay committed to your diet. I frequently work with clients who have experienced a very significant setback in their health from following diets that encourage the consumption of bone broth because nobody educated them about the potential risks and contraindications. I learned about these issues through my own personal experience, when a very tiny sip of bone broth immediately made my lips and tongue numb, produced severe heart racing, and gave me a migraine instantaneously. I can't even cook food that has a bone present; I must remove the meat from the bone or the meat will do the same thing. I am high in both histamine and glutamate.

If you have no issues with excess glutamate or histamine and are sure you don't have SIBO or any disorder that may be associated with SIBO (e.g., IBS, GERD, heartburn, autoimmune disorders), then bone broth might be a healthy addition to your diet. If you can consume it without experiencing headaches, migraines, cognitive impairment, a flare in OCD, anxiety, or cravings for sugar, carbs, or other mind-altering substances, then you can use it as a tool to help you heal your gut and improve immunity. If you're not sure, then pay close attention to your symptoms when you consume it, and monitor your response. In most cases, negative symptoms will develop quickly, and it will be apparent that the bone broth is causing the problems. Sometimes, however, symptoms may develop gradually, as the histamine or glutamate load builds up over time. Many people are instructed to keep drinking the broth despite a worsening of symptoms because their practitioner or a website may claim that they are undergoing a healing crises. I disagree with this stance; the most likely cause of negative symptoms is a histamine, glutamate, or SIBO issue, and continuing to consume the bone broth will lead to serious problems. Since candida can cause an elevation in both glutamate and histamine, the chances that you will have problems with bone broth are high, but it depends on how many other contributing factors you are dealing with as well.

Chicken bones are higher in glutamate than beef bones, so some people who can't drink broth derived from chicken bones can drink it when it's made from beef bones, but not always. If your only issue with bone broth is high glutamate and not high histamine, then this may work, but it will have no impact on the histamine issue. In my own situation, it doesn't matter what type of bones they are; they all cause problems.

Bone broth is made by simmering animal bones submerged in water over low heat for twenty-four to forty-eight hours, depending on the type of bones used (beef, chicken, turkey, duck, buffalo). It is best to make your own, but a variety of reputable online vendors sell it premade. Be sure it is derived from organic, grass-fed, pastured, free-range animal sources so it will be free of the toxins commonly found in CAFO (confined-animal feeding operations) meat. See chapter 11 for more on the importance of organic and free-range foods.

CAROB

Carob is a legume—and legumes, as you know by now, are eliminated from the paleo for candida diet—so carob should not be included as part of your daily diet. However, for a special occasion, it is a much better choice than chocolate because it doesn't contain caffeine or the hundreds of other harmful, mind-altering chemicals that are present in chocolate that we discussed earlier in the chapter. It is acceptable to have a little unsweetened carob if you want a treat on holidays that traditionally focus on chocolate, like Valentine's Day, Easter, Christmas, or Halloween. Carob may also work to stave off an uncontrollable craving for sweets or chocolate. Cooking legumes reduces some of their antinutrient content, so always use roasted carob, or cook or melt it yourself before using. Carob can be used in any way that chocolate may be used—for example, added to nut butter to make a fudge, or melted and poured over cherries or strawberries. You can find some recipes using carob in the companion to this book, *Healing Chronic Candida Cookbook.*

So, now you should have a good foundation for what should and should not be eaten when addressing candida overgrowth and its related conditions and for overcoming your cravings for sugar and carbs. In the next chapter we will go into more detail about moderating carbohydrate intake, various levels of the candida diet, how to put it into action, coping with adjustment and transition, the importance of organic, grass-fed, and cage-free, preparation, other foods that can be troublemakers (e.g., oxalates, glutamate, histamine), individualizing the diet for your specific needs and more.

CHAPTER 11

Implementing the
Paleo for Candida Diet

N ow that you have a sense of the best foods to include and those to steer clear of in your dietary plan for candida, we turn our attention to the many strategies and considerations that will help you implement the paleo for candida diet. First we'll look at principles that apply to everyone, and then we'll discuss how to individualize the diet for your needs.

TOTAL CARB INTAKE

To reduce overgrowth and its accompanying symptoms, most people with candida should generally aim for a maximum daily carbohydrate intake of 60 to 70 grams. This includes the carbs contained in vegetables, fruit, nuts, and seeds, and dairy if it is permitted. However, the healing process will be most enhanced and you will likely feel the best staying under 50 grams a day, and most optimal at somewhere around 25 to 30 grams of carbs per day, at least in the early phases of recovery. Those who make the most progress stick primarily to eating animal protein and low-starch vegetables. If you're dealing with SIBO or related conditions like IBS or GERD, then carb intake needs to remain below 50 grams and in many cases around 25 to 30 grams or even less. Be sure to read pages 140–146 for more details on the diet for SIBO.

Please note that when I speak of carb consumption, I am referring to total carbs, not net carbs (total carbs minus fiber content). Although calories cannot be obtained from insoluble dietary fiber and it is not absorbed and therefore has no impact on blood sugar and insulin, that is not true of soluble dietary fiber. For one, calories can be acquired from soluble fiber. Soluble dietary fiber is fermented by bacteria into short-chain fatty acids that can be used in gluconeogenesis. One particular type of fatty acid (propionate) is converted into glucose, while another fatty acid (acetate) is partially converted to glucose, which means soluble fiber can contribute to the glucose load. Furthermore, the soluble fiber encourages proliferation of bacteria if overgrowth is involved. Soluble fiber can also disrupt ketosis, if you're trying to adhere to a ketogenic diet. Therefore, for our purposes, it is best to count total carbs.

Optimal carb intake will vary from individual to individual; as with anything else, assess what is right for you by gauging how many symptoms are provoked. If you still experience significant candida symptoms, that means the candida is being fed. The more carbs you eat, the more you feed candida. The more you feed candida, the higher your level of overgrowth. The higher your level of overgrowth, the more toxins that are released. The more toxins that are emitted, the more symptoms you will experience and the sicker you will feel. Additionally, remember that consuming high volumes of carbohydrate will disrupt your brain chemistry and endocrine system—triggering cravings for more carbohydrates. The higher your level of carbohydrates the more disrupted your brain chemistry and endocrine system will be and the more you will crave carbohydrates. Your cravings for carbohydrate will be directly influenced by your consumption of carbohydrate. The less you consume, the less you want them. If you still crave carbohydrates, it means your blood sugar and insulin are being spiked and neurotransmitters are disrupted and you need to further reduce your carb intake.

If you are not too severely metabolically damaged, you may be able to consume more carbs comfortably, but please note, if you suffer with alcoholism, sugar and carb addiction, compulsive overeating, bingeing, or food addiction, these are clear signs that you have significant metabolic damage. Your body does not handle glucose well. These problems would not exist otherwise, because metabolic damage is a primary factor contributing to the cravings or addiction. As discussed in earlier chapters, people with candida have issues with carbohydrates not only because carbs feed candida but also because most candida sufferers are "carbohydrate intolerant," meaning they have a problem metabolizing carbohydrates. For such individuals, consumption of carbohydrates contributes to weight gain, insulin resistance, type 2 diabetes, heart disease, cancer, anxiety, depression, brain disorders like Alzheimer's, compulsive overeating, bingeing, and cravings for sugar and carbs. Carbohydrate intolerance is similar to gluten intolerance or lactose intolerance. As Drs. Volek and Phinney explain in *The Art and Science of Low Carbohydrate Living,* when one is intolerant of carbohydrates, the logical course of action is to reduce one's intake of the problematic substance below the threshold that produces symptoms in the same way that one would eliminate gluten or lactose if they were intolerant of these substances. Although Phinney and Volek are discussing carb reduction to address conditions such as type 2 diabetes and heart disease, the same principle applies here. People with candida are addicted to sugar and carbs, and the root of the addiction is impairment of the endocrine system and disrupted brain chemistry, both of which are addressed by minimizing intake of carbohydrates. However, there is a wide variance in individuals' severity of intolerance to carbohydrate. Some people may be completely intolerant, and others may be mildly or moderately so. Determine your degree of intolerance by assessing the symptoms and cravings produced when you consume carbs, and find the carb intake (or carb threshold) that resolves the most symptoms for you and eliminates your cravings. I don't typically advocate a zero-carb diet, which would provide no food for your healthy bacteria and would require you to avoid vegetables altogether, possibly making the body too acidic and eliminating nutrients from the diet that could be health enhancing. However, some people with severe SIBO feel they have no choice but to eliminate the carbs completely to find some relief.

Your intake of carbohydrate will also be influenced by where you are in the healing process. Carbohydrates typically must be restricted to a much greater extent in the early phases of recovery. Once you've made some progress in reducing your level of overgrowth, improved the health of your gut, and restored some stability to your brain chemistry and endocrine system, you will likely tolerate more carbohydrate. When you first begin your recovery process, for example, you may only tolerate 25 to 30 grams per day, but later you may be able to consume 40 or 50 grams. If you make significant progress in reducing overgrowth you may be fine at 60 or 70 grams per day. Consumption should always be monitored by how you feel. Even a person who is in perfect health should not consume more than 100 to 150 grams of carbs per day. A person who has had candida can usually never increase to that level or overgrowth will return.

How many carbohydrates a person can consume comfortably is also influenced by how long she or he has had candida, whether it is systemic or local, the severity of overgrowth and biofilms, the species and strain of candida, the health of the gut, the presence of other microbes, other health conditions, stress levels, adrenal health, the presence of insulin resistance, and age. Most of us become much less tolerant of carbohydrates as we grow older. If SIBO and related conditions like IBS, GERD, and autoimmunity remain unresolved, carb intake must be minimized to avoid feeding the microbes that lie at the root of these problems. Even if someone is 100 percent successful in eliminating SIBO or candida, they must continue to eat low carb to keep the conditions at bay. Additionally, once carbohydrate intolerance develops, it typically does not go away. I discuss this issue in more detail on page 341.

Sometimes people may require a higher carbohydrate intake than what we have discussed. These include women who are breast-feeding, women who are pregnant or trying to become pregnant, and athletes or other people who exercise a lot. Even under these circumstances only paleo-approved carbs should be consumed—that is, all the low-carb vegetables, fruit, nuts and seeds, sweet potatoes and other tubers, and winter squashes. Still, these needs must always be balanced with the need to reduce candida. Furthermore, once an individual has been eating low carb for a while, their body is well adjusted to functioning on fat and ketones (see the applicable sections in chapter 10), which will affect their carbohydrate needs even under the special circumstances mentioned above. In other words, if you are new to eating low carb, eliminating too many carbs under these circumstances is not the best scenario. However, once you become adapted to running on fat and ketones, your needs for carbs will change.

Even still, pregnant or breast-feeding women should always consult with their doctor before undertaking any significant dietary changes. Additionally, if you are on medication for diabetes or heart disease, and are going low carb for the first time, then an adjustment in medication may be needed. So it is important to discuss these changes in diet with your physician before implementation and continue to be monitored.

FOOD SENSITIVITIES

Most people with candida have numerous food intolerances or sensitivities because yeast and bacteria cause leaky gut and allow undigested proteins to get into the bloodstream, where the immune system sees them as invaders. And as you learned in chapter 10, many foods and substances themselves lead to the development of leaky gut. Symptoms of food sensitivity can overlap with symptoms of yeast or bacterial overgrowth, making it difficult to distinguish between the two.

Once you have adopted the proper candida diet as presented in this book, you will have eliminated some of the most common offenders for sensitivities. However, it is possible to have intolerances to a wide variety of foods that are an acceptable part of the diet, including things like eggs, garlic, onion, tomatoes, chicken, or beef. If you continue to eat a food to which you have a sensitivity, it will perpetuate the immune response, inflammation, and leaky gut, encouraging candida to travel and contributing to symptoms such as depression, anxiety, irritability, gastrointestinal distress, headaches, autoimmune disorders, and cravings for sugar and carbs. Furthermore, some people may experience a psychotropic effect from food sensitivities, which can result in cravings for sugar and carbs or other mind-altering substances.

It is important to identify any food intolerances that you may have and remove those foods from the diet for a period of time. This can be achieved with an elimination diet: eliminate the foods for a month, and then add them back to the diet, one at a time, to see what kind of response you have. You can also undergo food sensitivity testing. In my opinion, not all food sensitivity testing is created equal; I prefer the Alcat test, which is more sophisticated and accurate than standard IgG testing. However, there are other good ones out there and new technology is always evolving. Keep in mind that food sensitivity is a symptom of gut permeability, not a condition in and of itself.

ORGANIC, CAGE-FREE, AND GRASS-FED: AN OVERVIEW

It is critical that all your meat sources be organic and hormone-free, your poultry and eggs come from cage-free or pastured birds, and your beef, bison, and dairy products come from grass-fed or pastured animals. Be aware that the label "free-range" can be deceptive. The

FDA (shamefully) allows a manufacturer to use this label if the chicken coop has a door, but the birds may not actually ever go outside the cage. Conventional factory-farmed meat is loaded with hormones, antibiotics, GMOs, and other toxins that impair the immune system, endocrine system, gut, and brain and contribute to bacterial resistance. Plus, grain-fed cattle are too high in omega-6 polyunsaturated fats. Omega-6 is critical for health, but too much leads to inflammation and all the associated diseases (heart disease, obesity, etc.). The human body needs preferably a 1:1 ratio of omega-6 to omega-3 fatty acids, or at most a 2:1 ratio. The omega-6 to omega-3 ratio in meat from grain-fed cattle is around 20:1. It is this imbalance in omegas that can be a primary contributing factor to inflammation, heart disease, mental health disorders like depression, hyperactivity, and schizophrenia, and degradation of health—not the red meat itself.

Meat from grass-fed cattle has an omega-6 to omega-3 ratio ranging from about 0.16:1 to 3:1. It provides a healthy balance that supports the heart, the brain, and our overall health. Cattle are supposed to eat grass, not grains. The grass contains chloroplasts that the cows convert into omega-3 polyunsaturated fatty acids. If they aren't eating grass, they aren't producing many omega-3s, which is what causes the skewed ratio of omega-6s to omega-3s. Furthermore, it is common practice in commercial farming to feed cattle things like chicken manure, cardboard, chicken feathers, newspapers, and bubblegum in the wrapper to fatten them up and cut costs, which leads to poor health in the animals. Meat from grass-fed cattle is leaner and much richer in a variety of nutrients such as conjugated linoleic acid, a natural trans fat that provides protection against free radicals and is a powerful cancer fighter. CLA content in grass-fed cattle is two to three times higher than in grain-fed. It is CAFO (concentrated animal-feeding operations) meat that causes disease, not meat itself. Eggs acquired from organic cage-free chickens that are permitted to eat insects and plants have a 1:1 omega-6 to omega-3 ratio, while conventional store-bought eggs may be 19 percent higher in omega-6 than omega-3.[1]

On the same note, all the foods you consume (vegetables, fruits, nuts, seeds, etc.) should be organic as well. Besides the fact that our early ancestors never consumed pesticides, herbicides, fungicides, fertilizers, and other toxins, as discussed earlier, these chemicals disrupt the endocrine system and autonomic nervous system, disrupt neurotransmitters, weaken immunity, set off the stress response system, damage the gut, and cause birth defects. They can perpetuate candida overgrowth, trigger cravings for sugar and carbohydrates, and sabotage your dietary efforts. For the same reasons, the diet should also be free of preservatives, additives, nitrates, artificial flavorings and dyes, and MSG.

Additionally, organic vegetables and fruits have been shown to contain higher amounts of many nutrients like iron, magnesium, vitamin C, and other antioxidants.[2] When left to fend for themselves, fruits and vegetables produce substances called phenolics (types of antioxidants) to defend themselves from pests.[3] This action is inhibited when pesticides and herbicides are used. Taste tests have demonstrated that organic food tastes better. Organic farming preserves soil and the ecosystem (insects, frogs, microorganisms, birds, wildlife) and reduces air and water pollution. Furthermore, your choices in food influence the health of future generations by their impact on epigenetic factors (factors that affect how genes will be expressed) that can be passed from generation to generation.

Microwave use should be avoided. Many studies suggest that the nutrient content of food cooked in the microwave is significantly reduced,[4] not to mention the radiation exposure generated by microwave use.[5]

COOKED VS. RAW

Although fresh food is typically considered to be the highest in nutritional value, it's important to note that the longer it sits on the shelf, or on a truck or plane to be delivered to its destination, the more nutrient content it loses. Unless you have access to recently harvested food, in many cases frozen food may be higher in nutritional value because its nutrients are locked in when it is frozen, which typically occurs shortly after harvesting. A study at South Dakota State University discovered that freezing blueberries actually increased availability of antioxidants, and that frozen blueberries were just as nutritious as fresh ones even after six months of being frozen.[6] Usage of canned foods should be limited because the food can pick up toxins from the can. When you do use canned food be sure to choose brands whose cans are free of BPA (bisphenol A), an endocrine-disrupting toxin that is correlated with insulin resistance, birth defects, early puberty, miscarriage, damage to DNA, testosterone deficiency, and cancer.[7]

It is commonly believed that raw foods are healthier than cooked foods, but that is not always the case. Cooking fruits and vegetables that are high in the fat-soluble vitamins (E, D, A, and K) doubles their nutritional value.[8,9] Water-soluble vitamins can be lost due to cooking, but that is typically only an issue when the food is overcooked. Astaxanthin, lycopene, lutein, and beta-carotene (all powerful antioxidants) are made bioavailable to the body only by being released through heat. Absorbability of other types of antioxidants found in fruits and veggies called phenolics and flavonoids is also increased when they are cooked.

In an evolutionary context, humans have been cooking their food for at least two hundred thousand years. In addition to the consumption of meat, some researchers believe that cooking food was one of the chief elements that gave human beings the means to grow larger and superior brains and to thrive as a species.[10] Brain size is dependent on how many neurons are present, and the number of neurons is dependent on how much energy (calories) is accessible to provide nourishment to the brain. Human brains have a higher number of neurons than the brains of other primates, because cooking our food enabled us to ingest and utilize more energy on a daily basis. A study by Suzana Herculano-Houzel and Karina Fonseca-Azevedo, at the National Institute of Translational Neuroscience in São Paulo, Brazil, demonstrated that we would have to eat for 9.3 hours every day to supply our brains with the calories needed to operate sufficiently with raw food.[11] Research by Dr. Richard Wrangham, from Harvard University, indicates that our taste receptors are hardwired to favor softer foods because they are easier to break down, which means it takes a lot loss energy to access nutrients. Wrangham also found that cooked food is 50 to 95 percent more absorbable than raw food.[12]

The process of cooking appreciably reduces the content of oxalic acid and goitrogens in many foods. Oxalic acid is a naturally occurring substance in kale, chard, collards, parsley, and spinach; it is generated by the plant to protect itself from predators. It can cause a variety of problems in the human body by getting deposited in the kidneys, muscles, or extremities and leading to kidney stones, gout, or muscle pain. Or it attaches to calcium, rendering it unavailable to the body.

Goitrogens are naturally occurring substances found in the cruciferous family (cabbage, broccoli, cauliflower, Brussels sprouts, kale), most leafy greens, sweet potatoes, and cassava. When eaten in excess or by individuals who are already low in iodine, it can interfere with thyroid hormone production and iodine metabolism by inhibiting iodine uptake and utilization. This can lead to the development of goiters and other symptoms such as brain fog, fatigue, weight gain, depression, and impaired cognitive function. These problems are very bad for someone with hypothyroidism, which commonly occurs with candida. Raw smoothies are not a good idea for anyone with a thyroid issue.

Cooking your food also reduces amounts of any antinutrients (lectins, phytates, etc.) that may be present. Recall that they can inhibit mineral absorption; cooking therefore makes the minerals in foods more available. Furthermore, individuals who have inflammation in the gut and colon, as is typical in candida or SIBO, generally find the roughage provided by raw food to be a serious irritant. Food sensitivities are often much more severely triggered by food in its raw state than by cooked food. Raw fruits and vegetables are also higher in the fiber and resistant starch that can feed SIBO.

Based on all these factors, a person who eats a diet that consists primarily of raw food is at high risk of calcium and iodine deficiency, thyroid disorders, osteoporosis, gout, kidney stones, and muscle pain. Other problems associated with a raw-food diet include excess tooth decay and other dental problems, gastrointestinal disorders, deficiencies in other nutrients such as vitamins K, D, and B12, selenium, zinc, iron, essential fatty acids DHA and EPA, higher levels of homocysteine, and lower levels of HDL (putting them at greater risk for cardiovascular disease). As you can see, eating food cooked is the best choice for the individual with candida, leaky gut, SIBO, IBS, or other gut issues. Consuming cooked food helps to prevent nutritional deficiencies, reduce antinutrient content, and avoid other potential problems. Furthermore, digesting raw food requires more energy than digesting cooked food, a critical issue for the individual with adrenal fatigue; processing too much raw food is a burden for weak adrenals.

With all that being said, I don't intend to imply that you should avoid all raw foods. Nuts and seeds are healthier and more nutritious in their raw state, and so is dairy. You may want to delight in avocados, berries, salads, or a fresh apple. A healthy, individualized paleo for candida plan will contain a combination of both raw and cooked foods. How much raw food you permit in your diet should be gauged by the severity of your conditions and symptoms. If you have only mild adrenal fatigue and make great progress in reducing your candida overgrowth, you may be able to eat raw food a lot more freely than someone who has a significant load of candida and advanced-stage adrenal fatigue. Some people may feel best if they don't touch any raw food until a degree of healing has occurred. If you have SIBO in addition to candida, then raw food consumption should be little to none.

The method that is used for cooking food is critical. Overcooking food, boiling it to death, or charbroiling it can deplete vital nutrients or in some cases produce cancer-causing substances. Boiling should be avoided because it extracts nutrients. The first choice is steaming, which does not reduce alkalizing properties and retains most of the food's nutrient content. You can drink the water that is left in the bottom of the pan after steaming to obtain any of the nutrients that were drawn out. However, if you are trying to avoid oxalate or goitrogens, don't do this as they will be present in the steam water. It is also acceptable to sauté or stir-fry now and then, as long as you use an appropriate oil (see chapter 10). Baking in a covered dish or a Crock-Pot is another good option. Meat should never be burned and is best baked or slow roasted. If you fry, the only oils you should use are coconut oil, ghee, or butter; all other oils turn rancid and into trans fat when heated.

Although advocates of a raw-food diet assert that enzymes in the food are destroyed in the cooking process, this point is irrelevant because the same enzymes are destroyed by hydrochloric acid in the stomach. The purpose of these enzymes is to provide an advantage for the plant, not humans. In the history of humankind there has never been a culture that has sustained itself with a raw-food diet alone. To do so without considerable nutritional supplementation would lead to degradation of health.

So why do many people claim that they experienced improved health on a raw-food diet? Because in most cases they probably exchanged the standard American diet, which is high in sugar and processed foods, for a raw diet. Making that change will most likely lead to better health, at least to some degree. However, any improvements will be short term and will eventually be replaced with more deterioration in health.

Losing weight on a raw-food diet is common, but the weight loss is the result of nutrient deprivation, which is not healthy in the long run and will inevitably cause bigger problems down the road.

pH AND DIET

As discussed in chapter 2, the pH of the gut needs to be acidic, but the pH of the blood and body tissue should be alkaline. The body has several built-in systems to maintain balance in body and tissue pH. If you become too alkaline, it will dump minerals and if you get too acidic it will take calcium and other minerals from the bones and teeth. Many people are concerned that a diet high in animal protein is too acidic, but the paleo for candida diet provides the right combination of foods to promote optimal pH in the gut and the rest of the body. Yes, it is true that animal protein is acidic. However, when it is combined with liberal amounts of alkaline vegetables, then the acid is neutralized. If the diet consisted of nothing but animal protein, then it could be too acidic, and if it consisted mostly of vegetables and fruit and little to no meat, then it could be too alkaline. Fat is neutral, so it has no impact one way or another. There need to be both acidic and alkaline foods in the diet to balance one another out. Problems arise when we go too far in either direction. A body that is too acidic is vulnerable to osteoporosis, muscle loss, high blood pressure, kidney stones, and more, but a gut that is too alkaline is susceptible to invasion by microbes. On the other hand, too much acid in the gut can contribute to things like acid reflux, gastritis, and ulcers. Again, balance is the key.

Although some health professionals believe that many people are too acidic, the problem is not caused by eating meat. It is caused by consuming caffeine, alcohol, processed foods, carbonated drinks, artificial sweeteners, sugar, grains, and legumes, and not eating enough alkaline vegetables. Pharmaceutical and recreational drugs and cigarettes also play a role. Because the individual healing from candida will be removing these other contributing factors and eating whole foods, there is no need to be concerned about the acidity of meat—as long as you eat enough vegetables to buffer the acid and promote a healthy balance in pH. Our kidneys become less able to handle acidity as we age, so age may contribute as well.

The paleo for candida diet will encourage the correct pH for your stomach, small intestine, colon, and vagina. However, to prevent excess alkalinity it may also be necessary to supplement with acidophilus and other healthy bacteria, avoid antibiotics, supplement with vitamin C, and avoid acid blockers, antacids, and chlorinated water. You will be doing all these things anyway to address candida overgrowth. Supplementation with hydrochloric acid may be needed in some cases, which is discussed in more detail on pages 89–91.

AUTOIMMUNE CONDITIONS

If you have an autoimmune disorder of any kind, which is common in people with candida, eggs, nightshades, nuts, seeds, dairy, quinoa, and sometimes coconut are eliminated from the diet as well, due to the issues we discussed about each of these foods having the ability to prompt an immune response. Review the applicable sections in chapter 10. Many people have had great success putting their autoimmune disorders into remission by following what is referred to as a paleo autoimmune protocol, which is basically the diet presented in this book minus the consumption of eggs, nightshades, nuts, seeds, dairy, and possibly coconut.

INTERMITTENT FASTING

Intermittent fasting is very popular in the paleo community, but please be aware that it is not right for everyone. Intermittent fasting is highly counterproductive for the person with adrenal fatigue and the many associated conditions like blood sugar regulation impairment, sympathetic nervous system dominance, candida overgrowth, SIBO, sugar and carb addiction, or anyone in the process of trying to replenish neurotransmitter levels associated with anxiety, depression, addiction, insomnia, eating disorders, or other mental health or cognitive conditions.

Yes, it is true that intermittent fasting was a natural part of our ancestors' lives, but our ancestors weren't living with microbial overgrowth, adrenal fatigue, disrupted brain chemistry, and impairment of the endocrine system, as much of society is today. The adrenal glands must be strong to handle the hormonal and metabolic changes that take place during intermittent fasting and the brain must not be depleted in neurotransmitters. If they are not, intermittent fasting can exacerbate the aforementioned issues and cause more degradation in health.

WITHDRAWAL AND ADJUSTMENT

As discussed, caffeine, sugar, chocolate, and carbohydrates affect the brain in the same way as drugs and alcohol. Excess sugar and carbohydrates are also toxic to the liver. When people initially give up these foods, they go through a withdrawal period similar to that experienced by a newly sober alcoholic or drug addict. The withdrawal can be just as serious, debilitating, and disruptive, including headaches, shaking and trembling, brain fog, lethargy, insomnia, irritability, restlessness, anxiety, weakness, fatigue, inability to cope, and feeling like one is losing one's mind.

You may feel like you have a cold or the flu, your blood sugar levels may fluctuate, you may experience skin irritations, pimples, or full-blown acne, your moods may swing wildly, you may suffer from diarrhea or constipation, and you may lose weight. You may doubt yourself and your decision to change your diet. You may feel impatient and overwhelmed, wonder if this will ever end or get easier, and think you won't survive. You may feel hungrier than normal, and that's okay. It's important that you don't deprive yourself of food. Eat as much as you need to feel satiated, even if it's a lot more than normal, but always choose foods from the paleo-approved list and stick with animal protein and fat. You may experience only a few of these symptoms, or you may experience all of them, or somewhere in between. It's different for everyone.

When you eat sugar, carbs, and other garbage food, the liver has to work overtime to clear them from your system. This means it cannot devote as much time and energy to detoxing substances like environmental toxins. The detoxification system may become impaired, leaving toxins stored in the body. When you start eating healthy foods, toxins that have been stored will start being eliminated, adding to the detox symptoms you may experience from giving up sugar, carbs, and caffeine and the toxins emitted from the microbes.

The brain, endocrine system, and the rest of the body will go through a huge adjustment as they transition from running on carbs (glucose) to running on protein and fat. One of my mentors, Dr. Charles Gant, has described the process of restoring balance to the endocrine system as "turning around a battleship."[13] It takes place very slowly, and it requires consistency and repetition. It involves significant discomfort and time. For most people it takes between two and three weeks to complete the most difficult part of the transition, but it may take up to six weeks.

Remaining compliant with the diet is the key not only to reducing candida overgrowth but also to overcoming cravings for sugar and carbs. If sugar and carbs are kept out of the diet, then your body will switch from running on carbs to its preferred source of fuel (fat), and candida will be starved. When that occurs, symptoms and cravings will begin to subside. Without a change in diet, however, neither of these things can happen. Eating sugar or too many carbohydrates will cause setbacks every time. Overgrowth will be perpetuated, and the endocrine system and brain chemistry will be impaired. (Recall that healthy endocrine and nervous systems are necessary to overcome cravings.) The more carbohydrates that are present in the diet, the longer it takes to overcome cravings and get through the transition.

You may be able to get away with cheating once in a while without a significant setback, but the more often you cheat the more candida will grow and the more difficult it will be to eradicate. And the more disrupted your brain chemistry and endocrine system will be, which means greater cravings for sugar and carbs. The more often you cheat, the greater the setback. Your level of compliance is the primary factor that will influence how quickly and to what degree your overgrowth and cravings are reduced. The more compliant you are, the more quickly and comfortably you will get through the transition process.

However, during the transition period it is difficult to remain compliant. Cravings for sugar and carbs will be intense and possibly uncontrollable at times. An occasional indulgence of the right kind can be helpful in remaining compliant. Resist giving in as much as possible, but if you have periods when you can't take it anymore, stick with paleo-approved carbs (listed below) to satisfy those cravings. These foods are much less damaging than sugar, grains, and legumes and may actually help you move forward—as long as you don't cheat too frequently. This means you don't give yourself permission to indulge all the time, only when it becomes unbearable. As you refrain from consuming sugar and carbs, cravings that seem overwhelming or out of control will begin to diminish in frequency. The longer you remain on the diet, the less often you will feel the need to indulge.

Paleo-approved carbs that can be indulged in occasionally include fruit, dried fruit, nuts, seeds, sweet potatoes, chestnuts, yams, winter squash, taro, cassava, or other tubers. Indulgences that aren't "paleo approved" but can still be used occasionally may include cheese, yogurt, carob, wild rice, and quinoa. Anytime you indulge in carbs, accompany them with protein and fat (e.g., nut butters, butter, whipped cream, coconut cream, coconut butter), and eat them after your main meal, which lowers their glycemic index, causing them to have less impact on blood sugar, insulin levels, and neurotransmitters and making the sugars less accessible to candida. Eating nothing but carbs triggers a large spike in blood sugar, insulin, and neurotransmitters and provides an infusion of sugar for candida to feast upon. When cravings arise, try to go for a food high in fat instead of sugar and carbs; doing so will help train the body to use fat instead of glucose as its primary source of fuel. In addition, when you stop overstimulating your taste buds with sugar and artificial substances, they will also adjust and begin to appreciate the taste of real and nutritious food.

One of the best food combinations to satiate overwhelming cravings is to dip dates or a banana in nut butter, or combine coconut butter with your favorite nut butter, or combine unsweetened homemade whipped cream or coconut cream with fruit and nuts. Again, I'm not saying these treats should be eaten frequently. In fact, they should be avoided if you are capable of doing so. I am saying they can be used in the beginning of your transition when you can't control yourself and you're about to head to the bakery or the ice cream shop. Or they can be used on a special occasion like a birthday or holiday.

How often a person can indulge and what foods he or she can indulge in vary greatly from individual to individual depending on the level of overgrowth, the severity of imbalance in brain chemistry and the endocrine system, and the degree of carbohydrate intolerance. One person may be able to indulge once a week; another may indulge once a month. Some people are incapable of indulging at all without totally sabotaging their dietary efforts. One individual may be able to indulge only in fruit and nothing else, while another can indulge only in sweet potatoes and nuts, but not fruit. If your indulgence incites you to completely blow your diet and eat everything in the house and then go out for more, then either you are indulging in the wrong foods or you may be in the category of people who are unable to indulge. Coming to understand and be aware of your unique patterns around eating and then adjusting accordingly will be critical to your ability to remain compliant.

Not only is healing a process, but so is change. It may take time for you to become as compliant as you need to be, and you may fall on your face a few times before getting there. This is a natural part of the process. Although not very pleasant, falling on your face will remind you of why you're doing what you're doing. It will motivate you to get back on track. Understand that the transition process is erratic, and it is normal to go up and down. You may be on top of the world one day and think you have it conquered, and feel awful and struggle with temptation the next. This is also normal.

If you give in and fall down, do not beat yourself up or be harsh or critical; doing so will only perpetuate the problem by increasing feelings of guilt, shame, self-hatred, and low self-esteem, all of which can trigger another binge in an attempt to self-medicate the uncomfortable feelings. Get back up, show yourself kindness, brush yourself off, forgive, reflect on the reasons you are making the changes, pick up where you left off, and keep moving forward. Don't allow a weak moment to become an excuse to indulge in a full-blown carb fest or abandon your goal completely. Yet be aware that there is a very fine line between forgiveness, patience, and acceptance and giving yourself permission to engage destructively with food. You will have to find the middle ground. You must also be self-disciplined and consistent.

Try to stay focused on the prize: freedom from cravings for sugar and carbs, a reduction in symptoms of candida overgrowth, and feeling better. Reassure yourself that this is a normal and natural part of the transition process and that it will subside. Take note of improvements you have made so you can review them when temptations arise again. Once you begin to understand how sugar and carbs affect your body and mind, and once you see improvements in your physical and mental health, you'll become more motivated to remain compliant. In time, symptoms will start to diminish, your brain will start to feel clearer, you'll have more energy, you'll sleep better, and you'll begin to take pride in your accomplishments and feel excited about the process.

After the initial transition period, staying on your diet won't be nearly as difficult. It may take six months to a year or more for the brain and endocrine system to be "completely" restored to balance, but once the initial transition and withdrawal period are over, the process becomes a whole lot easier and more comfortable. The longer you remain compliant with the diet, the easier it becomes. Eventually, once your brain and endocrine system regain balance, you will no longer be drawn to sugar and carbs at all, and you will prefer fat and protein. You'll appreciate and value your new diet, and you'll be amazed at how delicious and gratifying a food like a berry or a nut can be. Sugary or high-carb foods will become unappealing.

The severity and duration of withdrawal and adjustment will also depend on how much damage has been done to one's brain chemistry and endocrine system, other conditions that may exist because of or in addition to candida, the quality of one's earlier diet, and previous use of other mind-altering substances. A junk-food addict or someone who is insulin resistant is likely to experience more severity than someone who has already cleaned up their diet to some degree and has managed to hold on to some insulin sensitivity. If one was addicted to or using caffeine, nicotine, alcohol, marijuana, or other drugs (including both recreational drugs and pharmaceutical drugs like antidepressants and benzodiazepines), the process will be more difficult and prolonged due to the greater level of damage to the brain and body.

Frankly, withdrawal and adjustment are just something one has to be willing to endure to achieve the goal; there is no other way out but to go through. So strap on your seat belt and hold on; it's going to be a rocky ride. To make the transition as comfortable as possible, make sure to consume adequate salt, fat, water, and calories, because failing to get enough of any of these can make the journey more challenging and result in more complications. Too few calories can also lead to problems with the thyroid and adrenals.[14] A low-carb diet should not be low in calories. You should eat as much animal protein and fat as you need to feel satiated. Drinking plenty of water, as Dr. Charles Gant explains, is important because our cells need to stay wet during detoxification and to diffuse toxins.[15] Nora Gedgaudas, author of *Primal Body, Primal Mind*, suggests that adding a little lemon juice to your water can help alkalize you if you feel too acidic. A variety of supplements may assist with this process, including L-carnitine, 5-HTP, glutamine, magnesium, DLPA, CoQ10, chromium, CLA, taurine, tyrosine, vitamins B6 and B3, and digestive enzymes. Their effectiveness will vary from person to person. However, some of them can be contraindicated and are discussed further in chapter 14. L-carnitine may be of the most value as it helps carry fat into the cells to be burned for energy.

Many people feel a desire to reward themselves at the end of a long week or when they have been compliant with the diet. This often involves eating carbohydrates, which usually leads to eating more carbohydrates. Celebrate your successes and reward yourself with non-food rewards such as taking a hot bath, getting a massage, enjoying a day at the lake, buying new paleo cookbooks or cooking utensils, or going to a concert, the theater, a movie, or the spa.

Plan ahead when beginning the diet so you can rearrange your schedule, minimize distractions, and reduce unnecessary stress as much as possible. Line up some friends or other supportive people whom you can reach out to for help in running errands, doing household chores, or providing child care. Taking time off work, if possible, would be ideal. I suggest you do everything you can to free up at least one week (preferably two) to devote entirely to the transition period. People who have serious drug or alcohol addictions often have to go into rehab for thirty days or so to begin their recovery. Think of coming off sugar, carbs, and caffeine in the same way. You must make yourself a priority during this period and take time to rest, nurture, pamper, and heal, just like you would if you had cancer or heart disease. As someone who has recovered from drug and alcohol addiction, as well as from a variety of food addictions and compulsive overeating, I can tell you with certainty that addiction to sugar and carbs is no different from addiction to drugs and alcohol. Just like drug and alcohol addiction, addiction to food is chronic and progresses when left untreated. Although it happens at a slower pace, it can destroy lives and kill people and should be taken just as seriously.

Be sure to eat three full meals per day, no more than five hours apart, to keep blood sugar stable. If blood sugar drops, cravings for sugar and carbs will increase, and you will have trouble remaining committed to your diet. If you get shaky, tremble, become irritable, get headaches, become nervous, nauseated, weak, or moody, or if you develop ravenous hunger between meals (signs of low blood sugar), then consider eating five meals per day or adding a snack that consists of animal protein with fat. Otherwise, snacking should be avoided. After you've been on the diet for a while, you'll find you no longer need to snack, and going five hours without food will be a breeze.

If it feels too frightening or overwhelming to give up everything at once, you can do it in baby steps. First get rid of the worst offenders—sugar, caffeine, chocolate, white flour, junk food—then work on eliminating whole grains, complex carbs like potatoes, and so on. However, do be aware that the process takes longer with this method, and you will have to go through withdrawal and adjustment numerous times rather than just once.

YOUR INDIVIDUALIZED PALEO FOR CANDIDA DIET

As you can see, some basic diet principles apply to everyone. However, many factors will be highly individual, based on your unique biochemical needs. The candida diet is not a one-size-fits-all program. What works best for you may look very different from what works for John, Jane, or Nancy. One person may need more fat while another needs more protein. Fruit and nuts may be off limits for one individual, but another may eat them comfortably. You may reap many benefits from eggs and coconut, but they may cause a deterioration in health for someone else. Dairy can be a super food for one individual and a poison for another. Each person needs to tune in to his or her body, listen to what it is saying, and customize his or her diet. I call this designing your individualized paleo plan. It is achieved by experimenting with different foods, monitoring your response physically and emotionally, and adjusting accordingly. Use the paleo for candida diet as a guideline, and then personalize it for your particular needs.

Dietary needs are influenced by many factors, including age, sex, phase of life, individual food sensitivities, genetics, heritage, stress levels, toxin load, degree of candida overgrowth, species and strains of candida involved, level of physical activity, gut health, sleep, carbohydrate tolerance, how much body fat one is carrying, other health conditions, and stage of healing. Furthermore, it's important to be aware that your dietary needs change over time in response to any of the aforementioned influences, so fine-tuning and revising as needed is an ongoing and lifelong process. For example, a person with severe over-growth will eat a diet that is different from the diet of a person who has mild overgrowth. The diet that makes you thrive in young adult-hood is very different from the one that promotes optimal health at age fifty. Your food choices in the early phases of healing candida will be more restricted than they are in the later stages. Your dietary needs can even fluctuate on a day-to-day basis in response to hormones, stress, emotions, menstrual cycle, physical activity, or how much sleep you had the night before. For example, many women are less tolerant of carbohydrates when they are menstruating, or a person may have a greater need for fat on a high-stress day.

If you are dealing with a variety of health conditions such as SIBO, adrenal fatigue, or an autoimmune condition, your dietary needs may conflict and you may have to make compromises. Butter may be a super food for someone with adrenal fatigue or whose cholesterol is too low, for example, but in the presence of severe leaky gut or an autoimmune disorder, butter could contribute to inflammation and launch an immune response. Sometimes you must weigh the benefits against the drawbacks of a particular food to determine whether or not you should include it in your diet. One health issue may take precedence over another for a period of time. Be sure to assess and adjust the high-FODMAPs, high-glutamate, high oxalates, and high-histamine foods as described in chapter 10 and later in this chapter.

Even within the paleo for candida diet, there is no one size that fits all. You must play around with each of the macronutrients (fat, protein, carbohydrate) and find the ratio that best fits you. This is determined by how many of your symptoms are resolved. When your diet is working well, your symptoms will begin to diminish, you'll feel satiated after eating, you won't get hungry between meals, crav-ings for sugar, carbs, or fat will disappear, anxiety and depression will dissipate, you won't gain weight, your mood and mental health will be more stable, and overgrowth of microbes will decrease. If these improvements aren't happening for you, then you need to reassess and modify. You do this by learning to listen to your body, which will guide you to exactly what you should and should not eat.

In the beginning, you may find it difficult to recognize your body's true "voice." You must learn to distinguish between its true voice and the voice of a disrupted brain chemistry and endocrine system.

Disrupted brain chemistry and impairment in the endocrine system will scream for sugar, carbs, chocolate, caffeine, nicotine, alcohol, or drugs. They may also drive you to get too little sleep, exercise too hard, or engage in other behaviors that undermine health. Your internal wiring gets jumbled up and sends out bad messages in a misguided attempt to correct the problems that occur because of poor diet, chronic stress, exposure to environmental toxins, overgrowth of microbes, drug or alcohol use, or other unhealthy lifestyle choices. Acting on those messages only throws fuel on the fire.

The true voice of your body, by contrast, will never lead you to do anything that is counterproductive. It will consistently guide you toward what is most beneficial for your health. For example, your body is speaking when you experience undesirable symptoms like depression, anxiety, fatigue, irritability, or impaired cognitive skills in response to consumption of sugar, carbs, caffeine, or chocolate. It's saying that those foods should be eliminated. If you're exhausted after exercising, your body is telling you to slow it down. Disrupted brain chemistry makes excuses for why you can't follow the diet, while the body's true voice encourages you to make your diet the top priority in your life. Your body's true voice will impart a healthy dose of skepticism and will be accompanied by a discerning eye, but excessive skepticism is the result of an impaired endocrine system or disrupted brain chemistry that prevents you from reaching your goals. That said, the messages from your disrupted brain chemistry and endocrine system should not be ignored; they are telling you something very important. Acknowledge those messages, but don't act on them. In most cases, you should do the opposite of what they say or the urges they provoke.

The voice that comes from disrupted brain chemistry and an impaired endocrine system can be much louder and more powerful than your true voice when you first begin the healing journey. It may be difficult to resist. Know that the more often you act on it, the stronger it becomes, because the behaviors it promotes disrupt those systems even further, causing them to send out more misguided messages. If instead you begin listening and acting on the guidance provided by the true voice of your body, you will slowly begin to strengthen that voice and eventually create a positive-feedback loop, whereby the disrupted brain chemistry and endocrine system will regain balance and stop sending misguided messages. At first you must approach these unbalanced bodily systems as you would a two-year-old: as someone who needs strong discipline accompanied by love, acceptance, and support. Small children must be forced to do what is best for themselves, even when they throw temper tantrums, but eventually they grow up and do it for themselves.

The messages of your true inner voice at one moment in your life may differ somewhat from its messages at another stage of life, based on your age, health status, and the other factors listed earlier. You must develop an intimate relationship with your body so that you can remain in tune with those changes and modify as you go along. As is true in any successful relationship, you must become a good listener.

EATING MINDFULLY

As you will learn in chapter 12, the regular use of mindfulness techniques can offer great benefit to one's physical and emotional health. Applying these techniques to the act of eating is another must-do practice. Take your time, and be present with your food and with the experience of eating. Pay attention to and appreciate each food's unique characteristics: its color, shape, smell, texture, how it sounds against your teeth, how it feels against your lips and in your mouth, how it tastes, its temperature. Be aware and engaged with each bite and sensation, as if nothing else in the world exists in that moment. Be with your food and the experience of eating as if you were meditating or engaged in tender lovemaking with the love of your life for the first time. Close your eyes intermittently, and revel in the entire eating experience. Don't wolf food down without thought or awareness. After you're finished eating, sit and reflect on the experience for a moment—on how enjoyable or delicious it was and how it looked, and experience gratitude for the meal and the experience—before getting up and moving on to another activity.

Eating in a more mindful manner enriches the experience. Your meals will seem much more flavorful, gratifying, and satiating. Eating mindfully allows time for neurotransmitters and hormones to convey information to your body and brain that will turn off your appetite, helping to prevent overeating and discouraging cravings for sugar and carbs. Eating mindfully also enhances the digestion process, helping your body absorb and utilize more nutrients and enhancing immunity.

It also boosts mood, feelings of well-being, and connectedness. Use it as a guide to help individualize your diet as well, by being mindful of how your body responds to the food you eat and adjusting accordingly.

WHAT'S FOR BREAKFAST?

Our caveman ancestors (and even your grandparents) thrived on animal protein for breakfast, which was often left over from the kill the night before. This is what works best for us as well. A paleo breakfast should look pretty much the same as the meals you eat at lunch and dinner (animal protein, fat, and low-starch vegetables). It is the consumption of animal protein and fat in each meal and the elimination of carbohydrates that will keep blood sugar stable, put a stop to your cravings for sugar and carbohydrates, and remove the food source for candida. As an added bonus, a breakfast that is rich in animal protein and fat will provide you with energy throughout the morning, enhance cognitive functioning, prevent anxiety, depression, brain fog, and mid-morning hunger, and activate your fat-burning metabolism, which will help you drop excess weight.

One of the easiest and most nutritious meals to make for breakfast is to heat leftovers from dinner the night before. Examples might include meatloaf, stew, baked chicken breasts, roast beef, buffalo burgers, or lamb chops. Just add steamed vegetables and you're set. Other possibilities include steak and eggs with a side of steamed vegetables, baked salmon with scrambled eggs and kale, hard-boiled eggs and avocado, nitrate-free and sugar-free sausage with cabbage. Although such a breakfast may seem weird at first because you're going against long-held beliefs and habits, it won't be long until it feels like second nature and you can't imagine eating anything else.

MORE THAN A DIET

Eating paleo is about much more than being on a diet. You aren't making a temporary change in food choices; you are developing a new lifestyle and new values that should remain with you for the rest of your life. Changing your diet is not just something you do ("I'm eating healthy paleo foods"). It's something you become ("I'm a healthy paleo eater").

Additionally, your individualized paleo plan will be most effective when you also mimic other lifestyle behaviors of our early ancestors: communing with nature on a regular basis, spending time in sunshine, engaging in regular physical activity, getting adequate sleep, managing stress, and living "green." All these behaviors support a stronger immune system and a healthier gut that can help fight off candida and other microbes, encourage more parasympathetic nervous system activity, balance the endocrine system, and promote healthy functioning of the neurotransmitters that regulate appetite and help eliminate cravings for sugar and carbs. I have written about each of these issues in more detail in chapters 12 and 13.

LEVELS OF THE CANDIDA DIET

The candida diet has three distinct levels, which for simplicity's sake we will call levels one, two, and three. There is no set time frame for each level, and you may not always move through them sequentially. The phase you are in at any particular time should be determined by how many symptoms you experience with that particular level of carbohydrates and whether that level of carbohydrates produces cravings for sugar and carbs. It is not determined by the number of weeks, months, or years you have been following the diet. One person may remain in the first level for years, while another sprints to the third level within months. Either way, it's contingent upon one's severity of overgrowth, level of healing, other conditions that may exist, and degree of carbohydrate intolerance. Individuals may shift back and forth between levels at different points in their healing depending on the current state of affairs at that time.

For example, one may have been eating comfortably at level three for a significant period of time and then may experience some type of setback (e.g., a bout with a cold or the flu, an exceptionally stressful life event, hormonal fluctuation, pesticide exposure, a condition that demanded the use of an antibiotic, overindulging on carbs during the holidays). The setback may require him or her to move back to level two or even level one. After a few weeks or months, depending on the degree of damage that was done, he or she may return to level three. It's even possible to vacillate between levels on a daily or weekly basis in response to changing circumstances. If in level two or three you experience a lot of symptoms or intense cravings for sugar and carbs, then you need to return to level one until you're improved. In each level you continually assess how you feel and whether symptoms and cravings are improving or getting worse, and you adjust accordingly.

Level One

In this level, carbohydrates and other food choices are most restricted. Foods like nuts, seeds, fruit, yogurt, and cheese may need to be eliminated completely until overgrowth is reduced and the gut, brain, immune system, and endocrine system are healed to some degree. Even high-carb foods that are paleo approved, such as sweet potatoes and winter squash, should be avoided. Carb intake is restricted to 25 to 30 grams per day. Basically, level one consists of nothing more than animal protein, fish, eggs, low-starch vegetables, acceptable oils, and possibly ghee and butter. Many people do a short period at this level and then move on to level two, while other people remain here indefinitely. People with severe SIBO in addition to candida often do best at this level until the issue is improved.

Level Two

After symptoms and cravings begin to improve and you start to feel better, restrictions can relax a little. An occasional serving of fruit, nuts, seeds, yogurt, or cheese may be permissible. Carb intake may be comfortable between 30 and 50 grams per day. You may spend most of your time in this level, as it is a nice middle ground for most people. Cravings for sugar and carbs, sugar and carb addiction, and compulsive overeating are often best managed in this zone.

Level Three

After reaching a significant level of healing, an individual may be able to eat much more freely. Small servings of fruit, nuts, seeds, cheese, or yogurt may be acceptable on a daily basis, and an occasional indulgence in a sweet potato or winter squash may not result in problems. Again, what works differs from person to person. One individual may be fine with cheese and yogurt but not nuts, seeds, and fruit—or vice versa. Another person may be fine with a sweet potato but not fruit, nuts, or seeds. Carb intake stays around 60 to 70 grams per day, with an occasional splurge between 70 and 100 grams. Rarely, someone may be able to stay in the range of 70 to 100 grams daily if metabolic damage is not too severe or if overgrowth was mild or does not grow rampant again. I don't believe that staying at a carb intake over 70 grams for the long term or indulging too frequently is wise because with time both candida and cravings for carbs are likely to return (as well as SIBO, if applicable). Generally speaking, maintenance should stay between 60 and 70 grams per day at most.

Please be aware that alcohol, caffeine, grains, legumes, chocolate, refined or processed foods, or any other non paleo-approved items are never brought back into the diet. They will only cause the brain, endocrine system, immune system, and gut to become compromised again, which will lead to the return of candida and cravings for sugar and carbs. The basic changes in diet are permanent and lifelong. Additionally, once someone has become carbohydrate intolerant they typically remain that way for life. Their intolerance may improve a little, or it may get worse. For example, when I was in my twenties and thirties, I was carbohydrate intolerant, but I managed my condition by staying away from all refined sugars and foods and most grains. I could get away with a fair amount of cheating on complex carbohydrates. When I was in my forties this started to change, and the older I got the more intolerant I became. By the end of my forties and in my fifties I had to reduce my daily intake of complex carbohydrates to below 50 grams most of the time or I gained excessive weight. I hear a similar story from many of my women clients. Metabolism changes after we go through menopause and as we age.

Sometimes it's the quantity of a particular food that produces symptoms and cravings, and simply moderating consumption or identifying the right portion size for your body, rather than complete elimination, may resolve the issue. As always, listen to your body and adjust accordingly. A half cup of fruit, for example, may incite anxiety, IBS, genital itching, and cravings, but a few pieces or a quarter cup may produce no symptoms. You may be unable to eat an entire peach, but you are fine with a few slices. Bananas or oranges may be entirely off limits, but berries may be no problem. You may be unable to eat fruit, nuts, or seeds every day, but once or twice a week may be fine. A large serving of nuts and seeds or their respective butters may generate symptoms, but a small serving may not. Indulging in a cheese plate or in a bowl of yogurt may incite symptoms, but you may remain symptom free with one or two pieces of cheese or a half cup of yogurt. A whole sweet potato or winter squash may put you in bed or send you on a carb fest, but half of one may be comfortable.

Or maybe the form or type of a particular food is the problem. Whole nuts, chunky nut butter, coconut flakes, or raw cabbage may inflame your gut, but smooth nut butter, coconut butter, and cooked cabbage may not. Yogurt and cheese may produce cravings or symptoms, but butter and ghee may not. Cashews and pistachios may be off limits, but almonds, walnuts, pecans, or macadamias may present no problems. Pineapples and bananas may trigger uncontrollable cravings, but a small serving of berries may not. For me, nuts in their whole form, nut meal, raw cabbage, and coconut flakes all inflame my GI tract, but coconut butter, nut butter, and cooked cabbage are okay in moderation. It can also be related to timing: some people can't eat fruit at night but can in the morning.

Be wary of moving into the second or third level too quickly after experiencing improvement; rushing things can lead to a setback. Don't be hasty, and always use your body as a guide. If symptoms or cravings return when you try to increase carb intake, go back to the previous level. You choose the appropriate level according to which one produces the least symptoms and alleviates cravings. Even when overgrowth is diminished and even if you've been on your healing journey for years, you may find that you feel best if you keep your carb intake below 50 grams per day, so don't feel that you *have to* move to a higher level. There is no harm in keeping your intake below 50 grams for the long term. As discussed in chapter 10, your body is designed to function perfectly with very few carbohydrates. Even though I've been addressing candida for more than twenty-five years, I feel best if I stay at level one the majority of the time. I may allow myself to go to level two a couple of times a week, and I only splurge in the third level on holidays. Again, everyone is different. Someone else may do just fine remaining in the third level once they have achieved a certain level of healing. As another factor, a genetic polymorphism in the VDR Fok (vitamin D receptor) gene can inhibit one's ability to adequately regulate blood sugar, which may contribute to a lifelong need to moderate carbohydrate intake.

If you follow the paleo community, you may notice that many people adhere to the 80/20 rule recommended by Mark Sisson or the 85/15 rule recommended by Loren Cordain. Basically, those guidelines state that as long as you're compliant 80 percent (or 85 percent) of the time, you can afford to be flexible 20 percent (or 15 percent) of the time. Although this may be acceptable for the general population, it is not typically the case for the individual with sugar and carb addiction, compulsive overeating, candida, and related conditions. Under these circumstances, it really is necessary to remain compliant about 98 or 99 percent of the time, and some people may need to be compliant 100 percent of the time. In this population, consumption of carbs or other non-paleo foods leads to cravings for carbs, which can lead to complete abandonment of the diet. You can get away with an occasional indulgence, but anything more than that is likely to sabotage your efforts. Additionally, 80 or 85 percent compliance will not keep microbial overgrowth under control.

HIGH-GLUTAMATE FOODS

As mentioned on page 29, candida can cause glutamate storms, increasing the body's overall level of glutamate. Excess glutamate is toxic to the brain, can result in an array of neurological symptoms, may encourage overgrowth of candida, SIBO, and other microbes, and may perpetuate sympathetic dominance. Consumption of foods high in glutamate can worsen the problem; likewise, reducing their consumption can help alleviate many of these symptoms and maintain balance between GABA and glutamate.

Most foods that are high in glutamate are already eliminated on the paleo for candida diet, including MSG, aspartame, gluten, hydrolyzed yeast, hydrolyzed protein, hydrolyzed oat flour (or anything hydrolyzed), sodium caseinate, calcium caseinate, disodium caseinate, autolyzed yeast, yeast extract (or any other autolyzed substance), any malted foods, maltodextrin, soy extract, soy protein, soy protein concentrate, soy protein isolate, soy sauce, textured protein, bouillon, protein-fortified foods, ultrapasteurized foods, vitamin-enriched foods, corn syrup, caramel flavoring or coloring, flowing agents, dry milk, egg substitutes, cornstarch, some brands of corn chips, citric acid if it is processed from corn, certain brands of cold cuts, hot dogs, and sausages (even the ones from health food stores), many canned foods, pickles, processed foods, many mainstream meats, tofu, and other fermented soy products.

In addition, the following foods that are often considered paleo/primal friendly increase glutamate:

- bone broth

- fermented foods (kefir, cultured vegetables, kombucha, apple cider vinegar, balsamic vinegar, etc.)

- whey protein, whey protein concentrate or isolate

- milk casein (any dairy product that contains casein has the potential for problems, but particularly cheese, which contains a concentrated form of casein)

- gelatin

- carrageenan or vegetable gum

- guar gum

- kombu extract

- xanthan gum

- certain spices and seasonings (many contain unidentified additives that increase glutamate)

Some commonly eaten foods that are particularly high in glutamate include parmesan cheese, Roquefort cheese, tomato juice, grape juice, and peas. You should already be avoiding these foods. However, walnuts, mushrooms, broccoli, tomatoes, and oysters are moderately high as well. Chicken and potatoes to a lesser degree. If you eliminate all the other high-glutamate substances, you may not need to reduce consumption of the health-enhancing foods like broccoli, walnuts, and chicken. However, if your glutamate levels are really elevated, then these foods may prove problematic as well, at least until you reduce glutamate levels somewhat. Even slow-cooking meat for a long time, particularly braising, can increase glutamate. Chicken skin and chicken bone are high in glutamate, so chicken should be boneless and skinless. I've noticed that I have a glutamate reaction if I eat chicken thighs even with the bones and skin removed, but I can eat chicken breasts as long as I don't eat them two days in a row. Apparently chicken thighs are higher in glutamate.

A note about ghee (clarified butter). Ghee technically should be low in glutamate as it consists almost entirely of fat. However, I've observed that I can sometimes eat ghee with no problems at all, but every now and then a batch from the usual brand I buy triggers a migraine and neurological symptoms. I must throw that batch away and wait for a new batch to hit the store. I can't say with certainty what is happening, but I believe that sometimes a particular batch is less thoroughly clarified of its proteins than other batches. On the other hand, it could have something to do with butyrate levels or amines. Either way, the problem must be related to the clarifying process, because I do not have these symptoms when eating butter from the same brand, which contains more proteins. I've heard reports of other people getting migraines from ghee. It's something to consider.

As discussed early in the book, the balance between GABA and glutamate may be disrupted by a variety of factors. Additionally, the body may have problems regulating the balance between the two because of a deficiency in an enzyme called GAD (glutamate decarboxylase), which is needed to convert glutamate into GABA. GAD can be inhibited by viruses, candida, other microbes, problems with methylation, impairment of the Krebs cycle, pancreatic insufficiency, deficiency in vitamin B6 (which is needed as a cofactor with the GAD enzyme to create GABA), and genetic polymorphisms. Your level of intolerance for foods high in glutamate will be influenced by how many of these other factors you may be dealing with. Please read pages 435–444 (also 29–32) for more detail on issues related to GABA and glutamate.

It isn't possible to remove every potential dietary source of glutamate, and nor should you. Glutamate is a neurotransmitter that, at the right concentration, is critical for a properly functioning brain. The objective is to prevent a surplus, which can lead to overstimulation, cell death, and neurological symptoms. In most cases, you are moderating accumulation. The more sources of glutamate you consume, the more glutamate your body accumulates. Limiting consumption prevents accumulation. It may also be a matter of potency. Some foods have higher concentrations of glutamate than others. You may get away with eating foods that contain less but have problems with foods that contain more. For example, I have no glutamate symptoms when I consume yogurt and butter, but I have severe and unbearable glutamate symptoms if I consume whey protein powder. The glutamate present in whey protein is much more concentrated than it is in butter or yogurt. Any food with a higher concentration of glutamate will raise bodily glutamate levels higher than a food with a lower concentration.

Many nutritional supplements also increase glutamate; they are listed on page 442–443.

HIGH-HISTAMINE FOODS

As described in chapters 1 and 6, leaky gut, candida (and SIBO) increases histamine, excessive levels of which can result in debilitating symptoms and perpetuation of candida and SIBO. By moderating consumption of foods that are high in histamine, you can help reduce levels and alleviate many of the associated symptoms.

Many foods that are high in histamine are already eliminated from the paleo diet. These include alcoholic beverages (which also inhibit the enzyme DAO, needed to break down histamine), cured meats, coffee, chocolate, cocoa, soy products, peanuts and certain other legumes, and wheat. And, other foods that release histamine like wheat germ, food additives and preservatives like nitrates, food dyes, benzoate, sulfites, and yeast; or substances that inhibit DAO like green tea, black tea, mate tea, and energy drinks.

However, quite a few foods that are considered paleo/primal friendly may be high in histamine or may stimulate the release of histamine, including the following:

- kefir
- cultured vegetables
- yogurt (depending on the bacteria present)
- any other food that utilizes microbial fermentation
- bone broth
- sour cream
- vinegar-cured foods (e.g., mayonnaise, olives, and pickles)
- anything cured
- dried fruit
- citrus (oranges, tangerines, mandarin, lemon, lime, grapefruit, kumquat, tangelo)
- grapes
- aged cheese

- walnuts

- cashews

- avocados

- eggplant

- spinach

- tomatoes

- olives (However, olive oil contains less, so they might be tolerated by some. Additionally, olive oil can increase the DAO enzyme, so not a black and white situation. Can test and see how you do.)

- pork

- chicken liver

- beef liver

- bananas

- pineapple

- papaya

- strawberries, raspberries, blueberries, most other berries

- pumpkin and its seeds

- nuts

- Anything with benzoates or sulfites

- cinnamon, chili powder, cloves, anise, nutmeg, curry powder, thyme, and cayenne

- egg white (raw)

- smoked fish or smoked meats

- leftovers (Particularly meat. The longer meat is left over, the more histamine it accumulates.)

- fish (Some species of fish are more prone to histamine, including mackerel, mahi mahi, tuna, anchovies, herring, sardines, shellfish, or any fish that is stored for an extended period of time [including those in a can]. However, most other forms of fish have the potential for high histamine as well, depending on how they are handled and processed. See below.)

Amounts of histamine present in each type of food can vary dramatically depending on how the food was processed. Some foods are more prone to histamine buildup than others. For example, bacteria colonize the gut of a fish as soon as it dies. If the fish is not gutted soon after the catch, it will have higher levels of histamine. It will continue to build until the fish is cooked or frozen, especially if it is not kept cool enough before cooking. Reactions to fish that are believed to be allergies are often reactions to histamine.

Make sure your meat is fresh or frozen when purchasing. Check the date on packages of fresh meat, and don't eat any that has an impending expiration date; it will accumulate histamine unless it is frozen. How meat is handled varies from manufacturer to manufacturer. The longer it sits out after processing and before freezing, the more histamine it will develop. This issue is discussed in more detail on page 314.

Be sure to read page 203 to learn about probiotics that increase histamine.

Histamine Threshold

Histamine intolerance can vary in severity from one individual to another depending on a variety of factors—for example, how much of the enzymes DAO and HMT the body is producing (that are needed to break down histamine), the level of bacterial overgrowth involved, whether genetic polymorphisms or autoimmune disorders are present, the health of the gut, methylation function, and how much histamine was ingested. The biggest problems arise when histamine levels are elevated and the body's ability to eliminate histamine is taxed. Furthermore, one's threshold for histamine can waver from day to day depending on the above factors as well as others, such as stress, exposure to pollens or sunshine, and exercise. You may be able to eat a particular high-histamine food at certain times of the year, but you may be incapable of doing so if the weather is hot and you are in the sun, or you've been exposed to pollens, or you're experiencing a high-stress event. Please read about other contributing factors for high histamine on page 446.

One person may have problems only with foods that are exceptionally high in histamine, while another may be unable to tolerate any of them. Sometimes it's a matter of accumulation; you may have no problems with one high-histamine food, but you may be pushed over your threshold if you eat three in one day. Or you may be able to consume a high-histamine food by adjusting the serving size. Case in point, I can't eat kefir, bone broth, or chicken liver due to their histamine and glutamate content. I can, however, eat a little strawberries and yogurt on occasion. Eating half of an avocado gives me a migraine, but I can eat a quarter of an avocado without symptoms. As you can see, just because a person has high histamine does not mean she or he will have problems with all the foods in the list or must completely avoid each food. I've also found that if I eat a little more carbohydrate than I typically consume (e.g., fruit and nuts and high-carb vegetable) with a high-histamine food that it can counteract the effects of the histamine. Not something you want to do on a regular basis, but it may allow you to enjoy a high-histamine food now and then.

Consuming animal protein could potentially contribute to the problem of high histamine if there is bacterial overgrowth in the GI tract. Histamine is produced naturally in the body from the amino acid histidine, which is present in animal protein. Bacteria can also convert histidine into histamine, and, of course, SIBO results in an abnormally high bacterial count. If a person's histamine levels are high from bacterial overgrowth or foods high in histamine, then the body's natural conversion of histidine to histamine could contribute to the problem. If that is the case, he or she could experiment with reducing the serving sizes of animal protein, but I certainly wouldn't recommend removing animal protein from the diet. In most cases, reducing candida and bacterial overgrowth and anything else that damages the gut, improving DAO enzyme function and avoiding high-histamine foods will be sufficient, and those areas are where most of one's focus should be directed.

Since many of the high-histamine foods can be beneficial for health, test your body's response before eliminating all of them, and adjust accordingly. Furthermore, conditions can change over time, so reassess periodically to see if some of the foods can be reintroduced.

Most people who are sensitive to histamine are also sensitive to tyramine, a byproduct of tyrosine breakdown, which produces similar symptoms as histamine. Many of the foods that are high in histamine are also high in tyramine. These include all fermented, pickled, or cured foods, aged cheese, fish, aged meat, nuts, seeds, avocado, and citrus fruits. Other foods high in tyramine include olives, yeast extracts, sweet potato, potato, and pineapple. Grilling increases amines and so can slow cooking.

HIGH-OXALATE FOODS

As you learned on page 36, candida produces high levels of oxalates, which can result in undesirable symptoms and degradation of health. Consuming foods that are high in oxalates will increase levels even more, potentially worsening symptoms. According to Dr. William Shaw, founder of Great Plains Laboratory, about 50 percent of the oxalates present in the body come from within the body, and the other 50 percent come from food.[16] A diet that is high in oxalates can increase bodily levels, especially in the presence of candida or another issue that may impair your ability to eliminate oxalates. Eating a low-oxalate diet can help lower the levels.

Oxalates are present in many foods to varying degrees, but the following foods contain the most:

- spinach
- beets
- Swiss chard
- collards
- parsley
- chocolate/cocoa
- peanuts
- wheat bran and germ
- tea
- cashews
- pecans
- almonds
- berries
- rhubarb
- sweet potato
- soy protein
- tofu
- leeks
- okra
- lemon peel, lime peel, and orange peel
- quinoa
- black pepper
- instant coffee
- sesame seeds
- kiwi
- figs
- potatoes
- tangerines
- carrots
- summer squash
- celery

Cooking your food can reduce oxalate content; by how much depends on the method of cooking. One study found that boiling reduced oxalate content by 30 to 87 percent, and steaming reduced it by 5 to 53 percent.[17] Cooking also helps reduce phytic acid, which can inhibit absorption of minerals. I typically recommend steaming over boiling, because boiling results in a greater loss of nutrient content than steaming. However, if one is trying to lower a really high oxalate level, then a brief period of boiling food would be acceptable. Something I've noticed in my own life that you may want to note is that I get a migraine if I eat green beans that were boiled, but I do not if they were steamed and reheated. I can't eat them immediately after cooking. They need to be kept in the refrigerator overnight and eaten the next day. I'm not sure what is the culprit of the migraine in the green bean, but steaming and reheating eliminates the problem. Green beans contain a moderate level of oxalates. Additionally, I tolerate some brands of green beans better than others. In contrast, raw foods contain much higher levels of oxalate and should be restricted in the individual trying to bring numbers down.

Oxalate Threshold

If you are already following the low-carb paleo for candida diet, as I hope you are, you will have eliminated many of the foods listed above, such as chocolate, soy, coffee, wheat bran and germ, peanuts, tea, and potatoes. Still, many paleo-friendly foods that provide nutritional value are on the list—foods that you may want to keep in your diet. Once again, addressing high oxalate levels is about finding your own threshold and moderating accordingly. Whether or not you should remove a particular food depends on how high your oxalate levels are, the severity of your symptoms, and how much oxalate content in foods you can tolerate comfortably. One person may tolerate more than another. Some foods may be completely off limits, while others may be acceptable in small amounts or for a certain period of time. It's a matter of accumulation, ability to eliminate, and the presence of other health conditions.

Since candida produces oxalates, your level of yeast overgrowth is another factor influencing your oxalate levels. As discussed in chapter

13, oxalate levels are also affected by inflammation, insufficient levels of vitamin B6, genetic problems with the AGXT enzyme (needed to break down oxalates), leaky gut, fructose, malabsorption of fatty acids, excessive omega-6 fatty acids, a vegetarian diet, and surgery in the small intestine or pancreas. Please read pages 432–435 for more on oxalate levels.

For example, prior to a histamine problem with spinach, I could eat spinach with no problem for a day or two, but if I ate spinach for three or more consecutive days, I began to develop severe pain in my eyes from what I assume were oxalate crystals. My reaction varied depending on the brand of spinach. Some were completely intolerable for me and others weren't.

MANAGING WEIGHT LOSS

In the early stages of the paleo for candida diet, a person may experience weight loss due to the lower carb consumption which encourages the burning of fat, the elimination of sugar, and a reduction in common food sensitivities that disrupt metabolism and encourage weight gain. People who are carrying extra weight appreciate this aspect of the diet, but those who have no weight to lose may find it disturbing. Most weight loss is experienced at the beginning of the diet, and then it levels off after a while, but for some it may continue.

It's important that you consume enough calories. I would like to emphasize again that a low-carb diet should not be low in calories, and you should not feel hungry. Eat as much animal protein and fat per meal as you need to feel satiated. If three meals a day is not enough, then eat more often.

When you reduce carbs and your body starts burning fat for fuel instead of glucose, you need to provide it with lots of fat. If fat is lacking from the diet, what gets burned is the fat stored in the fat cells. If sufficient fat is present in the diet, what gets burned is dietary fat instead of bodily fat. If you're trying to lose weight, don't increase your fat intake too much until after you have lost the desired weight.

Other strategies that may help include the following:

Increase your serving sizes of meat and fat in each meal.

Choose fattier cuts of meat.

Include high-calorie foods such as coconut oil, olive oil, avocado oil, butter, ghee, heavy cream, olives, and avocados as often as possible.

Full-fat yogurt can be used once in a while if tolerated.

Add liberal amounts of butter, ghee, or permitted oils to your vegetables and meat.

If you tolerate nuts and seeds, use them occasionally to boost calorie intake, but exercise caution because these foods feed candida and SIBO.

Increasing salt intake will cause a retention of water, which results in weight gain. Although this is not a true gain of fat, it gives the appearance of gaining weight.

Adding protein powder to meals may help, but be cautious if you have high glutamate.

If you must eat carbs, stick with chestnuts, sweet potatoes, yams, or winter squash. Again, be aware that these foods feed candida and SIBO, so they must be consumed in small portions. Quinoa and wild rice are not true grains, so they can be consumed occasionally. Be sure to add liberal quantities of fat to these foods in the form of butter, ghee, or oil. But, beware of the potential problems for quinoa and wild rice already discussed in chapter 10.

Eat shortly before going to bed so you don't have time to burn it off.

Have testosterone levels checked. Inability to gain weight can be related to low testosterone.

Weight loss may be the result of bacteria or parasites consuming your nutrients or impairing absorption, so taking the other steps presented in this book should help address the issue over time.

Be sure you have discussed any weight loss concerns with your health-care practitioner to rule out other potential causes.

PALEO FOR CANDIDA AT A GLANCE

Foods to Eat Freely

animal protein (grass-fed, pastured, hormone- and antibiotic-free, organic, and cage-free):

- beef
- buffalo (bison)
- chicken
- turkey
- duck
- ostrich
- lamb
- venison
- other wild game

low-starch vegetables

Foods to Assess and Moderate Accordingly

olives

avocados

seafood

nuts and seeds

coconut

eggs

nightshades

fruit

apple cider vinegar

bone broth

salt (only rock salt or Himalayan salt, not table salt)

stevia

butter, ghee, heavy cream, cream cheese, hard cheese

high-histamine foods

high-FODMAP foods

high-glutamate foods

high-oxalate foods

Occasional Paleo-Friendly Indulgences

sweet potato

yam

dried fruit

winter squash (e.g., butternut, acorn)

beets

chestnuts

parsnips

plantains

tapioca

taro

cassava

lotus root

tomato sauce

Occasional Non-Paleo Indulgences

carob

yogurt

soft cheese

potato

wild rice

quinoa

buckwheat

Foods to Avoid Completely

alcohol

all forms of sugar (including fructose, white sugar, powdered sugar, brown sugar, date sugar, beet sugar, organic sugar, organic cane juice, organic cane syrup, coconut sugar, coconut nectar)

high-fructose corn syrup

refined/processed foods

soda pop

whole grains

refined grains

legumes

honey

maple syrup

agave

rice syrup

molasses

barley malt

artificial sweeteners (acesulfame potassium, aspartame, sucralose, and others that might enter the market)

fruit juice

chocolate

coffee

tea (black and green)

microwaved foods

In general, your paleo for candida plate should be composed of animal protein, fat, and low-starch vegetables, in that order. Unless you prefer keto; then it would be fat, animal protein, and carb. It should always be low-carb.

CHAPTER 12

Beyond Diet and Antifungals:
Managing Stress, Reducing Sympathetic Dominance, and Supporting the Adrenal Glands

It is probably clear to you by now that healing from chronic candida is a complex process that consists of addressing each of the many related conditions that may develop, not just the overgrowth.

As I've stated, the first and most important element of the healing plan is the diet. It should be in place prior to taking any other steps. Ignoring the dietary guidelines will prevent you from seeing any significant or lasting results, no matter what other steps you put into action. The paleo for candida diet is the foundation on which everything else is built. If a person continues to eat foods that make candida and other microbes proliferate, perpetuate cravings for sugar and carbs, and that trigger the related conditions, other healing methods won't have a fighting chance.

That said, once the diet is in place, and a regimen of antifungals has been introduced, other actions need to be taken to improve the effectiveness of those steps and to enhance overall healing.

THE EFFECTS OF STRESS: A REVIEW

Throughout this book I've emphasized that stress can play a critical role in the development and perpetuation of candida, bacterial overgrowth, and other gut disorders. To review, stress increases blood sugar and insulin levels, weakens the immune system, kills friendly bacteria in the gut, depletes nutrient levels, inhibits stomach acid (and thus digestion and gastric emptying), impairs digestive enzymes (and thus nutrient absorption), and impedes gut motility and the migrating motor complex. Stress disrupts communication between the brain and the gut via the vagus nerve, suppresses serotonin and other vital neurotransmitters, inhibits transportation of glucose, disrupts hormone balance and thyroid function, impairs and burdens the detoxification system, weakens the adrenal glands, and inhibits impulse control. Remember: all these effects can foster overgrowth of candida and other microbes and lead to cravings for sugar and carbs that will sabotage the diet. When stress becomes chronic, it may lead to an imbalance in the autonomic nervous system wherein the sympathetic nervous system becomes dominant and the body remains in a perpetual state of stress.

Recall, too, that dealing with candida and other microbial overgrowth is a form of stress in itself. Other forms of chronic stress—including trauma endured as a child or as an adult—can also permanently upregulate the stress response system, leaving a person vulnerable throughout his or her lifetime to sympathetic dominance, functional gastrointestinal disorders, and affective disorders. One of the primary consequences of candida overgrowth or sympathetic dominance is adrenal fatigue, and once adrenal fatigue occurs it perpetuates overgrowth of candida and other microbes. What results is a self-perpetuating cycle of microbial overgrowth, sympathetic dominance, and weak adrenals that encourage more overgrowth . . . and on and on.

Chronic stress also depletes vital neurotransmitters (e.g., serotonin, dopamine, GABA, endorphins), which are needed for gut function, brain function, modulation of the stress response system, and regulation of mood, thought, and appetite. Neurotransmitters may also be depleted by nutritional deficiencies, candida, environmental toxins, drug or alcohol use, or a poor diet. As you can see, depleted neurotransmitters can be both a cause and a result of sympathetic dominance. On the flip side, any activity that increases these neurotransmitters helps to downregulate the sympathetic nervous system; that's because they oppose norepinephrine, the excitatory neurotransmitter that ignites the stress response.

For all these reasons, activities that reduce stress and sympathetic dominance and support the adrenal glands need to be ongoing components of the healing plan. The higher one's level of stress or the more severe one's sympathetic dominance, the more frequently these methods should be utilized. If you endured trauma in early childhood or acute stress in adulthood, you may have a lifelong need for extra attention to this detail.

Furthermore, many people with candida have such severe reactions to even the smallest level of intervention that attempts to eradicate the problem due to an imbalance in the autonomic nervous system caused by candida itself, that they are unable to proceed with treatment. They get caught in an unfortunate catch-22. For such individuals, a significant amount of time must be spent on reducing sympathetic response and increasing parasympathetic response before they are capable of taking antifungals, probiotics, or nutritional supplements. At the very least, the two aspects of treatment need to occur in conjunction with each other.

This chapter introduces a handful of basic daily tools for addressing stress and its related conditions: sympathetic dominance and adrenal fatigue. Chapter 13 gets into this issue a littler deeper by focusing on the lifestyle factors that should be addressed.

DEEP BREATHING

The easiest and most effective technique to manage stress and sympathetic dominance and to strengthen the adrenal glands is the regular use of deep-breathing exercises. When utilized properly, the breath can stimulate the vagus nerve, which turns on the parasympathetic nervous system. Directly turning *on* the parasympathetic nervous system turns *off* the sympathetic nervous system, providing an immediate reduction in stress and its associated symptoms and promoting a heightened sense of calm and relaxation. In his CD *Breathing: The Master Key to Self-Healing*, Dr. Andrew Weil explains that when the sympathetic nervous system is dominant the breath is fast, short, and shallow, but when the parasympathetic nervous system is activated the breaths are slower, deeper, and longer. Therefore, if we *intentionally* breathe slower, deeper, and longer, we can turn on the parasympathetic nervous system. The more often we do so, the more often we put the parasympathetic nervous system in the driver's seat and calm the sympathetic nervous system. If we do it consistently and repetitively, we can train our breathing to naturally become slower, deeper, and longer on its own, the benefits of which will increase over time.

Dr. Weil also explains that since breathing can be an unconscious or a conscious act, the breath is the link between the conscious and unconscious minds and the bridge that connects mind and body. Many cultures believe that breath is where the spirit resides. When we are focusing on our breath, we are focusing on the nonphysical (spiritual) essence of who we are. It is the breath that connects us to all other living things, including the earth and the universe, because all beings share the rhythmic expansion and contraction of breath.

Some of the greatest benefits of deep-breathing exercises are that they cost absolutely nothing, they require no prescription, supplements, equipment, or trip to the doctor's office or health food store, and they can be practiced anywhere, anytime, by anybody. In addition, they have the astonishing ability to provide numerous benefits besides reducing stress and sympathetic dominance—benefits that can simultaneously enhance all levels of health, including the physical, emotional/psychological, cognitive, and spiritual. On the physical level deep breathing can increase oxygen supply, boost immunity, improve detoxification, decrease heart rate and blood pressure, promote better sleep, create more energy, improve digestion and circulation, stimulate melatonin (the primary sleep hormone), and increase the release of beta-endorphins, which can provide relief of physical and emotional pain. On the emotional/psychological level, deep breathing can quiet internal chatter and increase release of inhibitory neurotransmitters. (Recall that these neurotransmitters enhance feelings of well-being, stabilize emotions, help maintain relationships, regulate appetite, prevent depression and anxiety, generate a better outlook on life, reduce internal conflict, and create a more centered state of mind.) On the spiritual level deep breathing can increase inner peace, intuition, insight, and creativity, provide a deeper and more meaningful connection with self, others, and one's spiritual source, and confer higher states of consciousness and spiritual awareness. On the cognitive level deep breathing can improve focus, attention, and memory.

For decades I have used deep-breathing exercises in combination with mindfulness techniques (discussed below) to relieve migraine headaches and other types of pain. Migraine is one of the severest forms of pain one can experience. Its relief through breathing and mindfulness demonstrates the amazing power of those techniques. I also experience very high levels of creativity when I practice my breathing exercises. Words, sentences, and paragraphs, as well as new ideas and insights for books, webpages, newsletters, and other projects, flow like a river and send me running for my pencil and paper after I'm done. Sometimes I have to stop in the middle of my practice to jot everything down because I get so excited. Breathing exercises also stimulate my memory. I can't tell you how many times I've remembered something during my practice that I was unable to recall on a previous day. Suddenly, in the middle of the breathing exercise, the memory I was trying to access percolates out of nowhere.

There are many different types of deep-breathing exercises, each of which can provide different results. People who have excess sympathetic nervous system activity—as is most often the case for individuals dealing with candida, other microbes, and adrenal fatigue—must use a specific type of breathing. I describe it below. If it's not done properly, the breath can produce an effect opposite of what we are trying to achieve. It can actually stimulate the sympathetic nervous system.

Here are the basic principles of how to breathe to address sympathetic dominance and to support the adrenal glands. Specific steps are listed further below. Shut your mouth and breathe through your nose. Breathe from the abdomen. Avoid using breaths that are shallow and fast, and avoid holding the breath for too long, both of which actions can stimulate the sympathetic nervous system. Your breath should flow in and out through your nose in a long, slow, deep, steady, and controlled pattern. Positioning your eyes in certain ways can also activate the sympathetic nervous system. When practicing with your eyes shut, don't shut them too tightly. Don't roll your eyes around, look too far to either side, or strain them in any way. Let your eyelids rest comfortably and gently on top of your eyes. Deep breathing can be done without closing the eyes, but closing the eyes enhances the process. The very act of closing your eyes immediately activates alpha brain waves, which promote instant relaxation. There may be times when you want to practice your breathing exercises when closing the eyes would be impossible, for instance, when you're driving your car or in a meeting. If breathing with your eyes open, apply the same principles of relaxing the eyes and the eyelids.

Employ what is called abdominal breathing. The belly, not the chest, should protrude when you inhale. Place your hands on your belly; if they rise and fall with each breath, you are breathing correctly. Most of us have been taught that the chest should expand when we breathe in and that the belly should remain flat at all times. This is an unhealthy practice and a primary contributor to overactivity of the sympathetic nervous system.

When you inhale, breathe in slowly through the nose, not the mouth, until the lungs are almost full. Exhale slowly through the nose, not the mouth, until almost all the air is expelled. Each breath in and out should feel comfortable. If you feel uncomfortable, then you are inhaling or exhaling for too long.

Basic Breathing Exercise

Here's a list of steps to help you put the above principles into action.

1. Close your eyes if possible. If not, begin with the following step.

2. Close your mouth.

3. Take a long, slow, full, and controlled breath in through your nose, expanding your abdomen as described above.

4. Pause only for a second.

5. Keeping your mouth closed, breathe out through your nose in a long, slow, and controlled manner until air is expelled comfortably.

6. For added effect, when you breathe out, imagine that your breath is flowing out of your body through your fingers and toes like a slow moving stream, carrying your stress away with it into the universe.

7. Pause for a second or two.

8. Repeat.

Remember, each breath should be inhaled and exhaled through the nose, and should be deep, complete, long, slow, and controlled.

For the purpose of reducing sympathetic nervous system activity and supporting adrenal function, practice deep-breathing exercises for six to ten minutes at a time every morning before you get out of bed and each night right before going to sleep. Repeat the exercise for as many minutes as you prefer anytime throughout the day when you feel challenged, stressed, or overwhelmed. No matter where you are or what you're doing, it is easy to stop and take a couple of minutes to breathe. Each time you breathe in and out constitutes a complete cycle. If you are in a hurry, one simple cycle will provide some relief. However, three cycles is better, and eight or more is optimal.

For the purpose of alleviating chronic pain, practice for 10 to 15 minutes. If you wake up in the middle of the night, use the breathing exercise to help you get back to sleep because it stimulates the release of melatonin. As soon as you wake up, begin breathing—before your brain can start thinking about anything. Don't get up, turn on a light, or do anything but breathe. In a few minutes or less, you'll be sleeping again.

Additional Breathing Exercise

I learned the following exercise, which I love, from the Gupta Amygdala Retraining Programme. They borrowed it from the Art of Living Foundation.[1] I like to do this one in the morning when I wake up and the basic technique when I go to bed and throughout the day. I also prefer this one when I have a migraine because it is very powerful for relieving pain.

1. Close your eyes.

2. Close your mouth.

3. Place the thumb of your right hand over your right nostril and close off the airway to that nostril.

4. Through the left nostril, take in a slow, long, deep, and controlled breath.

5. Remove your thumb from the right nostril, and close the left nostril with the fingers of your right hand.

6. Exhale through the right nostril.

7. Inhale through the right nostril.

8. Remove your fingers from the left nostril, and close the right nostril with your thumb.

9. Exhale through the left nostril.

10. Inhale through the left nostril.

11. Remove your thumb from the right nostril, and close your left nostril with your fingers.

12. Exhale through the right nostril.

13. Repeat.

When you first start practicing deep-breathing exercises, you may feel a little resistance. If you are experiencing a very high-stress event when you're about to practice, the resistance may be even stronger. If you push yourself a bit to move forward despite feeling resistance, you will very quickly begin to relax, and the resistance will fade. Ease into the regular practice of deep breathing slowly, with just a minute here and there, and gradually work up to more minutes. Eventually it will become a habit, and as you begin to experience and appreciate its positive effects you'll become more responsive, which will motivate you to practice more often. The more often you practice, the more effective deep breathing becomes, which creates a positive-feedback loop that motivates you even more. Still, a little resistance may reappear now and then. If it does, just kindly acknowledge it, give yourself a little push, and do your practice anyhow. It will dissipate again.

MINDFULNESS-BASED MEDITATION

The second most effective and simple way to manage stress and sympathetic dominance and support the adrenals is with the daily practice of mindfulness-based meditation. A vast amount of research demonstrates that mindfulness meditation is a highly effective stress-management tool. Neuroimaging studies conducted on the brain during mindfulness demonstrate that it stimulates the areas of the brain that help regulate the autonomic nervous system. Like the breath, it can be used to directly turn off the sympathetic nervous system and turn on the parasympathetic nervous system, resulting in an immediate reduction of stress and its associated symptoms and an increase in relaxation. Mindfulness meditation also stimulates areas of the brain associated with regulating pain, mood, memory, sense of self, empathy, compassion, and introspection, and it increases the neurotransmitters serotonin, dopamine, GABA, and endorphins. It has the capacity to enhance health on the emotional, psychological, cognitive, and spiritual levels, as well as the physical. Mindfulness has been shown to actually change the structure of the brain.[2]

At the Stress Reduction Clinic at the University of Massachusetts, Jon Kabat-Zinn has shown that individuals with backaches, headaches, and migraines were able to use mindfulness to reduce their level of pain by more than 50 percent, and also to achieve long-term improvements in anxiety and depression and in the ability to carry out day-to-day activities.[3,4] In a study at the University of North Carolina, with the regular practice of mindfulness individuals with IBS were able to decrease symptoms by 38 percent and significantly reduce psychological distress and increase quality of life.[5]

Other studies have demonstrated that participants with fibromyalgia, multiple sclerosis, arthritis, cancer, Parkinson's, AIDS, and other conditions can significantly reduce pain, stress, fatigue, anxiety, and depression. They also report a higher tolerance for pain, better coping skills, a more positive outlook, increased immune function, better sleep, and a greater sense of well-being. Additionally, mindfulness has been shown to be useful in the treatment of insomnia, most mental health disorders, behavioral disorders, violent tendencies, heart disease, and high blood pressure. Mindfulness is highly effective as an adjunct treatment in the prevention of relapse for alcoholism, addiction, or substance abuse, so it can be a great tool in reducing cravings for sugar, carbs, caffeine, and chocolate. People who use mindfulness on a regular basis report a variety of other benefits, including more inner peace, self-awareness, empathy, compassion, creativity, intuition, insight, joy, happiness, pleasure, improved memory and cognitive function, a higher level of consciousness, and a richer, more meaningful life. Other types of meditation have been shown to reduce oxidative stress and increase glutathione levels.[6]

The more often you practice mindfulness, the more effective it becomes, so consistency and repetition are needed here as well. However, mindfulness meditation does not have to be time consuming or difficult. According to Dr. Dan Siegel, associate clinical professor of psychiatry at the UCLA School of Medicine and author of *The Mindful Brain,* just three minutes of mindfulness meditation per day can be beneficial, and repetition is more important than duration. Repetition strengthens neural connections that will make it easier to achieve the goal and reinforce the benefits.[7]

Although mindfulness meditation originated in Buddhism, the basic principles are free of any religious code and can be practiced within the context of any belief system. You don't have to become a formal student or study ancient Buddhist secrets. It's very simple to learn, and you can put it into action and begin experiencing the benefits immediately. The simplicity of mindfulness and its powerful impact on the autonomic nervous system help many people overcome the barriers (feeling antsy, distracted, unable to focus) that often prevent them from committing to a regular meditation routine.

Here are a few simple techniques to get you started.

Breathing Meditation

One of the easiest ways to learn mindfulness is with the breath.

1. Stand, sit, or lie down in a quiet space.

2. Close your eyes.

3. With your mouth closed, take in a long, slow, and deep breath through the nose and from the abdomen. (Refer to the basic breathing exercise above.)

4. Exhale through your nose in a slow and controlled manner.

5. Repeat for several minutes, or as long as you desire.

6. During this process, stay completely focused on nothing but your breath and the breathing process. Follow your breath in and out.

7. Let go of all thoughts, and think of nothing but your breath.

8. Be one with your breath.

9. If thoughts intrude, as they will, just acknowledge them and release them without judgment. As Jon Kabat-Zinn says about thoughts cropping up during meditation, "This is what minds do."[8] Gently and persistently bring the mind back to following the breath.

In a mindfulness seminar, Dr. Charles Gant explained that in the depths of mindfulness, there is no distinction between the breather and the breath, the feeler and the feeling, the experiencer and the experience; they are one and the same.[9]

As you can see, in this particular meditation we are combining mindfulness meditation with a deep-breathing exercise, so we can accomplish both tasks at once and reap the benefits of each simultaneously. However, once the basic principle is mastered, we can use many other focal points or anchors for our mindfulness meditation instead of the breath, including silence, music, walking, the sound of rain or crickets, a tree, the sky, a particular body part, pain, the sun or wind against your skin, your footsteps while walking, dance, a focal point behind the eyes, a mantra, or the self.

Silence Meditation

Here's a technique using silence as the focal point.

1. Stand, sit, or lie down in a space that has complete silence.

2. Close your eyes.

3. Latch onto the silence with your mind.

4. Tune everything else out, and zero in on the essence of silence.

5. Become completely aware of how still it is—how it sounds and feels.

6. Feel the stillness.

7. Focus on nothing but the sound of nothingness.

8. Go into the silence.

9. Be one with the silence.

10. If thoughts intrude, as they will, gently bring the mind back to the silence.

11. Sit with the silence for a few minutes or however long you desire.

Relieving Pain with Mindfulness

As I mentioned, I have been using mindfulness as a pain-management tool for many years. Here is how you put mindfulness into action to alleviate pain.

1. Stand, sit, or lie down in a quiet space.

2. Close your eyes and breathe in and out slowly as you learned previously.

3. Go inward and locate the source of your pain.

4. Become aware of nothing but your pain.

5. Don't judge or label your pain with words like *awful* or *terrible*. The pain is not bad or good; it just is.

6. Just allow your pain to exist as it is in its entirety. Feel it completely.

7. Use the source of your pain as your focal point for the meditation.

8. Sit with your pain, embrace it, explore it, go into it, and become one with it.

9. If thoughts intrude, as they will, gently bring your mind back to the pain.

10. Breathe in as you learned on page 362, and when you breathe out, imagine that your breath is flowing into the area where the pain resides and washing through it. Imagine that as the breath flows out like a slow-moving stream, it carries the pain away.

11. Do this for a few minutes. You'll most likely begin to feel your pain diminish.

Although it may seem counterintuitive, when we fully accept and experience our pain and let go of resistance to it, we are able rise above it and live a less painful life.

The same principle can be applied to emotional pain. Use the full force of the emotional pain as the focal point of the meditation.

Although I've stated that benefits can be derived with as little as three minutes of mindfulness meditation, greater relaxation and other benefits can be achieved with sessions of ten to twenty minutes. You can mix it up throughout the day by doing three minutes here and there when you are busy, but try also to fit in a longer session of fifteen or twenty minutes daily, or at least on most days of the week.

DAILY MINDFULNESS

Meditation is only one method of putting mindfulness to use. The simple act of being more mindful in your daily life is a great stress-management tool that can also enhance your physical, emotional, and spiritual health. The essence of mindfulness entails being completely present with and aware of the current moment without judgment or labels. Judgment and labels cause stress and unhappiness. An emotion, feeling, thought, or experience is not bad or good, right or wrong. It just is. Focus only on what is happening right now with acceptance, which could mean focusing on your breath, your footsteps, your surroundings, your emotions or thoughts, washing the dishes, making love, listening to music, taking a walk, gardening, baking, eating a meal, drinking a glass of water, or engaging in conversation. To simplify the concept, I often tell people to think of mindfulness in the following way: approach each situation, experience, and activity as if you were engaging in a deep and passionate lovemaking session with the love of your life for the first time.

You can essentially be mindful in every area of your life, and when you are, eventually mindfulness will stop being a practice and become more a way of being and living. I think the following quote from Henry Miller sums it up beautifully.

The moment one gives close attention to anything,
even a blade of grass, it becomes a mysterious,
awesome, indescribably magnificent world in itself.

Applying this concept to any chronic health issue, including candida overgrowth, is highly beneficial. It can increase your ability to cope and your quality of life despite the challenges, peaks, and valleys you will withstand during the healing process. Much of the misery that is associated with dealing with a chronic health condition comes from our mind-set and preconceived ideas about how we think our lives are supposed to be, not from the condition itself. Many of us constantly judge and compare our lives to society's ideals, and when we can't measure up, that mind-set drags us down even further. We live by judgments like "This is bad," "This shouldn't be happening," "I have to get rid of this immediately." Stop judging or labeling your symptoms, your condition, your losses, your limits, and just let them be with a mindful attitude.

At one end of the spectrum, there are a lot of people who don't take care of their health; they eat poorly, live recklessly, or take drugs. At the other end of the spectrum is the mind-set that we should have perfect health and a perfectly fit body. It is almost a sin or shameful if you cannot overcome all health limitations and achieve this perfection. Many people judge or look down with scrutiny on those who are unable to heal. This creates a lot of pressure on those with chronic health conditions, lowers their self-esteem and self-worth, and encourages feelings of shame, guilt, helplessness, hopelessness, franticness, and desperation. But if you frantically and desperately try to attain better health, you are succumbing to another form of stress, which of course becomes counterproductive. Anything that you resist seems to grow bigger and stronger. When you embrace your discomfort, it loses its power over you. Yes, we should pursue good health, but we should do so gently and with acceptance of where we are on the healing path at any given moment. Adopting this attitude will enable you to live a full, productive, and joyful life no matter what phase of healing you are in. Mindfulness is the tool that can help you achieve this frame of mind. Being mindful should also be applied to the act of eating, which is discussed in more detail in chapter 11.

Along the same lines, the language you use internally or externally can either reinforce your suffering and symptoms or reduce them. If you frequently use phrases like "This is so horrible," "This is a nightmare," "This is unbearable," "I can't take it," or if you constantly talk about your symptoms and suffering, you will reinforce them. If, on the other hand, you avoid those kinds of statements or replace them with more empowering phrases like "I am strong and capable," you will reinforce that outlook. You can encourage the parasympathetic nervous system by talking to yourself in a positive way. Give yourself reassurance and support. Talk to yourself in the same manner as you would talk to a friend in need: "You'll be okay." "You're incredible."

"We can do this." "There's nothing to be concerned about." "We'll get through this."

Do not keep your focus on your symptoms or on how bad things are; doing so only perpetuates the stress response system, burdens the adrenal glands, and lowers your quality of life. Whatever you put your focus on becomes bigger and more powerful. If all your focus is on your symptoms, pain, and complaining, those things will become worse. Keep your focus on the healing process and what you have rather than on the condition and what you don't have. If you focus on the good things in your life, you will be happier and less symptomatic.

Yes, indeed, it is not fair, it is unjust, and it may be sad and horrific that you have to endure this condition. These are valid feelings that should be mindfully acknowledged as well, and you should allow yourself to grieve and be angry. You may need to express those feelings from time to time, but don't allow yourself to wallow there indefinitely. Get it off your chest now and then, and get back to focusing on how to heal and on the good things in your life. The neat thing is that the less you focus on the bad things, the less you will feel the need to vent. And don't surround yourself with other people who are completely focused on their symptoms and suffering all the time; their attitude will drag you down.

The mind-set that we aren't supposed to experience any type of discomfort is a driving force for more stress. Some stress and anxiety is normal and healthy, and there is no way to avoid it completely. We must accept discomfort to some degree and learn how to live with it to minimize its impact on our lives. You must learn to find peace, happiness, and gratitude in the midst of the storm.

Embracing your condition with mindfulness does not mean that this is the way it will be forever or that you are resigning to defeat. Quite the opposite—acceptance gives you the strength and resilience to keep moving forward and make changes. It means you accept the way things are right now, and you work toward changing them in the future.

SMILING

You may be surprised to learn that a simple smile can have a very powerful effect on the mind and body. This basic human expression that we all posses, even in the womb, can help reduce stress, boost the immune system, improve mood, increase energy and stamina, and contribute to a deeper level of life satisfaction. A smiling face stimulates release of dopamine, serotonin, GABA, and endorphins, which, as discussed throughout this book, regulate mood, cognitive functions, sleep, pain, anxiety, thoughts, appetite, and feelings of well-being, and downregulate the sympathetic nervous system.

A study has discovered that a lone smile can generate the same level of brain stimulation as two thousand chocolate bars. The reason chocolate makes you feel good is because it stimulates neurotransmitters like a drug. However, a smile is not associated with any of chocolate's negative side effects (see pages 297–300). The same study also found that a smile has the same effect on neurotransmitter release as receiving twenty-five thousand dollars. That means if you smile a lot on a regular basis, you can feel like a millionaire.[10] In addition, smiling generates a disease-fighting protein called gamma interferon and increases the production of B-cells and T-cells, two white blood cells that create antibodies and play a vital role in immune function, protecting us from pathogens like candida (see chapter 9).

As explained in the facial-feedback hypotheses, a person's brain takes cues from his or her facial expressions, and when the brain senses a smiling face it generates an emotion to match. As a bonus, the brain cannot tell the difference between a real smile and a fake smile, so a fake smile can be just as effective. In other words, if you smile even though you don't feel happy, your brain will think you are happy and will generate corresponding neurotransmitters. A person's smiling face has the ability to change his or her own negative mood into a positive one, creating a positive-feedback loop. The smile reduces stress and increases happiness, relaxation, and inner peace, all of which elicit a more powerful smile that further promotes relaxation and happiness.

All you have to do is plant a big fake smile on your face as often as you can, and the wider the better. In my experience, I have found a wider smile stimulates a greater release of neurotransmitters, increasing the benefits. To start reaping the benefits now, smile while you're cooking, washing the dishes, exercising, watching TV, at your computer, taking a walk, watching the sunset, cleaning the house, driving, or shopping. Psychologist Dr. Robert Zajonc found in a study from 1989 that participants who looked at themselves in a mirror while smiling experienced a higher level of positive emotions than those who couldn't see their faces while smiling.[11] So look at yourself in the mirror while smiling when you can. And smiles are contagious, which means you can help other people reduce their stress and have more happiness and inner peace. In a fantastic TED talk, Ron Gutman describes research demonstrating that an evolutionary mechanism suppresses control over our facial muscles when we see another person smiling.[12] We can't help but smile when we look at another smiling face. Seeing someone else smile stimulates our mirror neurons, which allow us to sense the emotions of others and reproduce that same chemistry in our brain. Mirror neurons are what enable us to feel empathy. Our brain's neurons will start firing in the same manner as what we are observing. A smile begets a smile, and a frown begets a frown. That's why we feel uplifted when we are around happy people and feel pulled down by negative people.

Smiling is another simple but powerful health-enhancing strategy that costs you nothing, is available for use twenty-four hours a day, and requires no trip to the doctor's office. Yes, I know that when you don't feel good you do not feel like smiling. But smiling even though you don't feel like it will improve how you feel. So smile all the time, for no reason at all, and you will find that you feel happier and more relaxed.

If you have a hard time remembering to smile, provide yourself with some kind of prompt. Place a smiley face near your bed, computer, or work space, on your car visor, refrigerator door, and bathroom mirror. You can't help but smile when you look at a smiley face; it happens automatically, due to mirror neurons.

COMMUNING WITH NATURE

The human species evolved living in the great outdoors, so from an evolutionary standpoint we are hardwired to spend time with nature. From birth to death, the lives of our early ancestors took place in the wild. They bathed in streams, took shelter near rocks, climbed trees, swung on vines, chased down their dinner, got warmth by basking in the sun, ate meals outdoors, and procreated under the stars. It is no wonder studies indicate that communing with nature provides us with a variety of health benefits—physically, emotionally, cognitively, and spiritually. To do so is in our genes. A growing body of research indicates that mimicking our ancestors by spending more time in nature can significantly decrease stress and sympathetic nervous system activity, increase parasympathetic nervous system activity, lower blood pressure and heart rate, decrease depression, anxiety, ADHD, and the need for pain medication, promote faster healing time, assist in recovery from drug and alcohol addiction, aid in coping with trauma and disability, improve self-esteem and self-discipline, increase anticancer protein expression and natural killer cells, and foster inner peace, joy, feelings of well-being, and transcendental connectedness.[13,14,15,16]

How can spending a little time in the elements provide so many incredible benefits? There are probably a variety of different mechanisms in place (e.g., exposure to sunlight which stimulates vitamin D production) and others that we don't fully understand, but the most important action related to the topic of this chapter is that it boosts those all-important calming neurotransmitters.

In one study, just twenty minutes of looking at a forest lowered cortisol levels an average of 13.4 percent. When the subjects went into the forest for a three-day trip, they experienced a 50 percent increase in the activity of their natural killer cells as well as an increase in the actual number of natural killer cells.[17] Another study found that touching metal provoked a stress response in the brain, but touching a leaf produced a calming effect.[18] Spending time with nature is so effective that many health-care practitioners, including medical doctors, now prescribe it as part of the treatment plan for a wide variety of health conditions. Some health professionals even partner with park professionals to make it happen. Journalist and author Richard Louv calls it vitamin N (nature) and chronicles the consequences of a nature deficit in his book *Last Child in the Woods*.[19]

Although modern civilization has enhanced our lives in many ways, it has also ripped us away from our primal roots and increased our stress level tenfold, which is one of the primary causes of the decline in mental and physical health that plagues our society. As would any animal that is removed from its natural habitat, we experience negative consequences that can have a profound impact on emotional and physical well-being. Nature is not something that is separate from us; it is part of us and we are part of it. We emerged from the natural world. Simply returning to our native environment to regularly commune with Mother Nature can help counteract some of the side effects of modern living and nourish us back to health. It is an innate need that should not be ignored.

Ideally, we should all live where we are surrounded by nature on a daily basis so that all we have to do is look out the window or step out the door to return to our natural home. If you have the ability to make that happen, I highly encourage you to do so. It will greatly enhance your life. Regardless of where you live, however, immerse yourself in nature as much as you can in any way you can. Try to spend at least a little bit of time outside each day, and more than a little, if possible. Exercise outside, take a break from work and go outside, have a picnic lunch or evening dinner under the trees, conduct meetings in the park, plant a garden or just a few flowers, feed the birds, relax on the porch, walk your dog, go hiking, read in the recliner in your backyard, play with the children, and gaze at the stars. You don't always have to spend extended periods of time outdoors. Just go out and stand in the sun or the wind for a couple of minutes, or walk around the yard or parking lot, and then go back to what you were doing. Sit in your backyard and watch the sunrise, sunset, approaching storm, or cloud formations. The great outdoors is a fantastic place to meditate and do your deep-breathing exercises. Don't just sit with nature; interact with it and get intimate. Touch the rocks, snowflakes, raindrops, flowers, or leaves with your fingers, or brush them against your cheek. Lie on the ground, lean against a tree, sit on a rock, let an insect crawl across your foot or hand. Take a walk in the rain or the falling snow.

Put mindfulness into action here as well; be completely aware of and one with the breeze or the sun against your skin, the sound of your footsteps against the earth, the song of a bird or chirp of the crickets. Tune everything else out and be completely absorbed in the nature moment.

In addition, try to get out for longer periods a couple of times a week. Spend a whole day with nature weekly if possible, but at least a couple of times a month. Plan your vacation in a beautiful natural setting. If long vacations are not an option, take occasional day trips to the lake, the mountains, the ocean, the forest, or the desert.

When you can't get outside, bring nature to you. Open the doors and windows and listen to the birds, the wind, the rain, or the silence. Try to live in a home with lots of windows. Look out the window frequently throughout the day, just a minute here and there if that's all the time you have, and appreciate the sky, clouds, sunshine, birds, flow-ers, and trees. Place your desk with your computer and your favorite recliner next to a window so that you can look up and nurture yourself for a few seconds occasionally throughout the workday, or spend a half hour in your recliner observing wildlife behavior, changes in the weather, the clouds rolling by, snowfall, or the rising or setting sun. Bring plants, rocks, seashells, acorns, and pinecones into your home. Take advantage of every opportunity you can find to spend more time in nature.

I find that spending time with nature is as critical for me as eating my three paleo meals per day. I build it into my life naturally. I grew up in a small rural town, so I was surrounded by nature as a child. I rode my bike under the trees, snacked on wild berries on a regular basis, dug in the dirt, swung on vines in the woods, and ran around barefoot for most of my childhood and teenage years. I have scars on my knees from bike crashes on gravel roads that launched me into the bushes and on my feet from numerous barefoot injuries. Once I got my driv-er's license, I took long drives in the country to observe the fall leaves, spring blooms, and winter snowfall. I have always been drawn to a natural environment. As an adult, I moved to the city for a few years and then returned to a country setting, and that is where I've remained. Although I have lived in a variety of different terrains over the years, I currently live in the high-desert mountains, where am I surrounded by coyotes, birds, jackrabbits, bunnies, and squirrels, all of which befriend me on a regular basis. When I step out my door I enter their world, and I am caressed by the loving arms of nature. I work from home, and my desk sits in front of a window where I am surrounded by wide-open blue skies and mountains. I don't think I could survive in any other setting, and I wouldn't think of trying. Although I may move to a different community at some point, it is inconceivable to me that I would ever live anywhere besides an area that provides me with constant intimacy with nature. It nurtures, sustains, and entertains me and provides me with solace.

STRESS MANAGEMENT: WRAP-UP

Work toward using all the stress-management tools discussed in this chapter—not just one—on a daily basis. You can even combine them and perform them simultaneously. For example, you could do your deep breathing exercises and mindfulness meditation while sitting outside and end the routine with a big smile on your face. You want to throw as many soothing activities as you can at your autonomic nervous system on a repetitive and consistent basis. When you have a condition like candida or SIBO that regularly triggers the sympathetic nervous system, you must counteract it as frequently as possible. This is even more important if you suffered trauma as a child or acute stress as an adult. You will need to make yourself and your healing a priority. Utilizing these techniques needs to become a way of living, not something you do once in a while. You must make a commitment to take time daily to rest, relax, and nurture yourself. As the insightful John Lennon once said, "I'm just sitting here watching the wheels go round and round."[20] Live by that motto frequently.

If you have high levels of stress and need more maintenance than time allows, you can simply stop whatever you're doing throughout the day and close your eyes for thirty seconds. As mentioned earlier in the chapter, closing the eyes activates alpha brain waves, triggering neurotransmitters that in turn activate the relaxation response.

Dr. Herbert Benson found that inducing the relaxation response through meditation, yoga, tai chi, and similar techniques changed gene expression in about two thousand different genes. Many genes associated with stress, inflammation, or cell death could actually be turned off. However, the effects did not appear to be permanent. In order to sustain the benefits, the relaxation techniques had to be practiced daily on an ongoing basis. Some changes in genes were noted in as little as eight weeks, but the longer the subjects practiced, "the greater the effect." A 2015 study coauthored by Dr. Benson found that people who elicit the relaxation response with these activities can reduce the cost they spend on health care by as much as 43 percent.[21]

It's worth repeating that deep-breathing exercises, mindfulness meditation, or any of the other tools for managing stress and sympathetic dominance are less likely to be effective if they are not done in conjunction with the dietary changes presented in chapters 10 and 11 and the strategies for green living presented in chapter 13. If you continue to eat substances like caffeine, chocolate, grains, high-starch foods, and sugar while failing to provide the body with essential nutrients, or if you are regularly exposed to high levels of environmental toxins, then mindfulness, deep breathing, smiling, and other stress-reduction techniques won't stand a chance. You'll be swimming upstream, limiting your potential benefits. Combining these stress-moderating techniques with the proper diet and green-living principles, however, optimizes the advantages provided by each.

Many other tools have the potential to moderate stress and reduce sympathetic dominance. The ones discussed in this chapter are my favorites because they are so easy and practical that everyone can use them. Other good options include biofeedback, walking, yoga, tai chi, qigong, listening to music, creating art, dancing, and spending time with your pet. If any of these activities resonate for you, adopt them as well.

The field of neuroscience is growing rapidly, and new discoveries are being made all the time. It is likely that many other programs will exist in the future to help moderate the sympathetic nervous system. Perhaps even individuals who've suffered permanent damage to the autonomic nervous system will be able to reverse the condition someday. I encourage you to be on the lookout for other possible strategies and to be open to exploring their potential benefits.

In addition to the daily techniques discussed in this chapter, numerous other lifestyle changes should be made as well to manage stress, reduce sympathetic dominance, and support the adrenal glands. That's the topic of the next chapter.

CHAPTER 13

Going Deeper: Addressing Other Lifestyle Factors

The previous chapter presented specific techniques that can be used to manage stress, reduce sympathetic dominance, and consequently support the adrenal glands. Now we will take a look at lifestyle factors that are equally important for achieving those goals and they will enhance many other aspects of the healing journey as well. Again, you don't want to engage in just one or two of these suggestions; you want to adopt as many of them as possible and build a new lifestyle. You want to intentionally live in a manner that encourages health and more parasympathetic nervous system activity on a daily basis.

LIVE GREEN

As discussed in chapter 2 and elsewhere, environmental toxins of all kinds, including those contained in everyday household and personal-care products, can trigger the stress response system, disrupt the endocrine system, and deplete or inhibit neurotransmitters—keeping one stuck in sympathetic dominance and triggering overwhelming cravings for sugar and carbs. The autonomic nervous system simply cannot be restored to balance if it is constantly exposed to high levels of environmental toxins. In *An Alternative Approach to Allergies,* Dr. Theron Randolph explained that some people are biochemically susceptible to experiencing a pleasurable, euphoric, addictive high when exposed to environmental toxins.[1] These toxins can stimulate the reward pathway in the brain in a similar manner as alcohol and/or drugs, which means they will deplete neurotransmitters in the same manner as well, thus contributing to all the issues we have discussed in regard to neurotransmitter depletion. Once the toxin leaves the system, the individual can experience the same type of physical and emotional crash that is experienced with drug or alcohol use, where they feel depressed, fatigued, anxious, confused, or hyper, and then develop cravings for more psychotropic substances (e.g., sugar, carbs, caffeine, alcohol, or drugs). Toxins can also impair the immune system (discussed in more detail on page 63), contribute to blood sugar imbalance, overload the detoxification system, cause anxiety and depression, kill friendly flora, and get lodged in the small intestine, where they can exacerbate nutritional deficiencies and damage the already vulnerable gut. Pathogens thrive in a toxic environment. For these reasons, reducing your exposure to toxins by living a green and environmentally friendly lifestyle is a critical component of healing. It should be at the top of your priority list going hand in hand with diet.

As discussed in chapter 2, there are few things more damaging (if any) to the brain and body than pesticides, so protecting yourself from these chemicals should be the first place you start. Avoid the use of insecticides or herbicides in your home or on your property. If your neighbors use them, ask them to notify you before use so you can be sure to shut your windows and doors. Take your shoes off at the door to avoid tracking them into your house; pesticides and herbicides are everywhere—at the grocery store, bank, local park, highway shoulders, post office, golf courses, schools, athletic fields, and most businesses. When pesticide residue enters the house, it concentrates at a higher level, which makes it more potent and toxic than it was outdoors. They also persist longer inside than they do outside, because they aren't exposed to sunlight and rain, which helps break them down. Pesticide concentrations indoors can be 10 to 100 times higher than concentrations outdoors.[2] Be mindful of where your pet walks, as they can bring it in the house on their paws. Avoid living in industrial or agricultural areas; toxic drift is responsible for great deterioration in health. Don't use insect repellent on your skin and avoid living in areas that spray for mosquitoes. At the very least, know the spray schedule and keep your windows shut during that time and stay indoors for at least several hours afterward. Being exposed to airborne mosquito repellent is a serious risk in and of itself, but to directly apply it to the skin is just absurd. All the harmful ingredients are absorbed directly into your body. The repellent known as DEET inhibits acetylcholinesterase,[3] the enzyme needed to break down acetylcholine, leading to the associated problems we discussed in chapter 1. Additionally, DEET has been shown to be associated with death of neurons in regions of the brain that control muscle movement, learning, memory and concentration, and with toxic encephalopathy. Within six hours 48 percent of the application is absorbed.[4] It is absorbed by the gut as well. The combined exposure to DEET and permethrin (another common pesticide discussed in chapter 1) can lead to motor deficits and learning and memory dysfunction and disruption of the blood-brain barrier. Researchers found that exposure to both DEET and permethrin experienced by service personnel in the Persian Gulf War has played an important role in causing the symptoms of Gulf War Syndrome like headache, loss of memory, fatigue, muscle and joint pain, and ataxia, which causes an inability to coordinate muscular movements.[5]

Switch your personal-care products and household-cleaning products to green and environmentally friendly ones. These can be found at your local natural health store or online. You can save a fortune by simply using baking soda and hydrogen peroxide or lemon and vinegar for all your household cleaning needs. There really isn't any job that baking soda and hydrogen peroxide cannot do just as adequately as harsher chemicals, including the laundry. Get rid of your cologne, perfume, and cosmetics, and learn to love yourself the way you were born—au naturel. True beauty is a reflection of the inner self, which is largely influenced by your diet and lifestyle choices, not by the amount of eyeliner, blush, concealer, or lipstick that is caked on your skin. Mother Nature did not intend for you to cover up the face you were born with and hide behind a façade, and you should not need makeup to feel beautiful. Learn to appreciate and embrace your natural look and imperfections, dare to be bare, and stand proud.

Throw away your air fresheners; a clean house does not have a smell. If you need to remodel, be sure to use green construction materials. Use a filter on your shower or bath water to remove toxins. Seek environmentally friendly employment. Buy clothing and bedding that is organic and made from natural fibers. Polyester is made from petroleum. Traditional cotton crops use more pesticides than any other single crop.[6] More than 600,000 tons of pesticides, herbicide, fertilizer, and other chemicals are used on cotton crops per year in the U.S.[7] At the very least, be sure to wash your new clothes several times before wearing as they are processed with formaldehyde and other toxic chemicals.

This doesn't mean you have to go out and buy everything in one day. If you're just beginning your green lifestyle, the next time you run out of a particular item simply replace it with a natural, nontoxic, environmentally friendly version. Continue this pattern with all the products in your home until you have completed the transition and all your products are green.

Electrosmog (electromagnetic radiation fields discharged from wireless and electronic devices) has been found to cause pathogens like bacteria, mold, candida, and viruses to multiply in numbers and release higher levels of toxins. Dr. Klinghardt writes that research from Europe has shown that the release of mycotoxins from molds may increase by as much as six hundred times when the molds are exposed to high levels of EMFs.[8] Exposure to EMFs may also alter cells within the brain, other parts of the nervous system, and the immune system, and disrupt cell-to-cell communication. Electrosmog triggers the stress response system. All of these effects can activate uncontrollable cravings for sugar and carbohydrates and thus abandonment of the diet, weaken the immune system, fuel sympathetic dominance, and impede one's ability to make improvements.

In *Primal Body, Primal Mind*, Nora Gedgaudas writes, "The human body is a bioelectrical system; we are 'electric' beings. Our bodies and even our DNA transmit and receive frequencies like any other antenna. Our brains are extremely vulnerable to any technology that emits EMFs because the brain immediately starts resonating to the outside signal by a kind of tuning-fork effect. EMF pollution affects us all in insidious ways that we've barely begun to recognize. It is known to generate or exacerbate damaging (even mutating) excitatory activity in the brain." Nora also quotes Dr. Siegfried Othmer, physicist and chief scientist at the EEG Institute in Woodland Hills, California, as saying "Recent neurobiology research has revealed that small voltage fluctuations imposed on neuronal populations can drive them to alter their firing properties."

Electromagnetic fields are pervasive in our environment and very difficult to escape from completely, but you should attempt to limit your exposure. Don't carry your cell phone on your body. Use a headset instead of holding the phone to your head. Don't sleep with your cell phone or any other electronic device next to you. Turn off your wifi while sleeping. Set limits on how often you are exposed to items that have high levels of electromagnetic radiation such as cell phones, cordless phones, and computers, and never live near a cell phone tower or high-power electrical lines.

Be sure to opt out from the "smart meters" that many electric companies are using to replace analog meters. Some researchers believe that electromagnetic radiation from smart meters causes severe dysfunction to the autonomic nervous system. "What is particularly concerning about Smart Meters is they put out both electromagnetic fields (EMF) and radio frequency radiation (RFR). RFR comes from the signals between meters, poles, and the station. The meters will transmit pulses of microwave energy at various rates, around the clock, and may repeat the signals from neighboring meters in what's called a 'mesh network'; additional antennas will be installed on light and power poles. This kind of microwave pulsing works differently than more continuous cell phone radiation, and is more dangerous as it is stronger (though shorter duration). It particularly affects the brain, nervous system, and hormones, disrupting the functioning of body systems and causing leakage of your blood-brain barrier."[9] Some people are so sick from the effects of the smart meter, they are forced to move out of their homes.[10] Not only that, they violate your rights. No one should be permitted to force you to install toxic equipment on your own home. Dr. David Carpenter, a public health physician and Harvard Medical School graduate, who worked for the New York State Department of Public Health for eighteen years where he was responsible for administering a program on electromagnetic fields and subsequently became the dean of the school of public health and currently serves as a faculty member in the school of public health and the director of the institute for health and the environment at the University of Albany made the following statement in an interview:

There is no evidence that proves that the smart meter is safe or has no adverse health effects. In fact, while no one has actually done human health studies in relation to people living in homes with smart meters, we have evidence from a whole variety of other sources of radio frequency exposure that demonstrates convincingly and consistently that exposure to radio frequency radiation at elevated levels for long periods of time increases the risk of cancer, increases the damage to the nervous system, causes electrosensitivity, has adverse reproductive effects and a variety of other effects on different organ systems. It should be up to each individual to identify whether or not they want to be continuously exposed 24/7 to elevated levels of radio frequency radiation. The smart meter is for the benefit of the utility, it saves them money because they don't have to then have people going out and reading the meters and it's at the expense of the consumer who has to live in the house that has this constant exposure. So, an informed person should demand that they be allowed to keep their analog meter.[11]

"Unplug" yourself from all electronics periodically. Some products are designed that claim to deflect electromagnetic radiation. They are worn on the body or fitted to an electronic device. I don't know whether they are truly effective, but they offer a possible solution you can explore.

Many people are susceptible to the mycotoxins that are released by mold, and people with candida tend to fall into that category because of mold's similarity to yeast. They are both a type of fungi. Mycotoxins can have the same type of impact on the brain, neurotransmitters, autonomic nervous system, immune system, and endocrine system as any other toxin. They are thought to contribute to excessive sympathetic nervous system activity, weakened immunity, anxiety and depression, obsessive-compulsive behaviors, headaches, cancer, asthma, hives, sinusitis, rashes, impaired cognitive functioning, fatigue, hyperactivity, gastrointestinal distress, irritability, and heart palpitations. They may make it difficult to remain on the candida diet due to their triggering of ravenous cravings for sugar and carbs or other mind-altering substances. As discussed on pages 29–30, mold toxins can also lead to surges in glutamate, contributing to neurotoxicity.

Mold in the house prompts an immune response, which may be exhibited as sinus inflammation, fatigue, or respiratory problems. Ongoing exposure weakens the immune system, which allows candida to develop a stronger foothold. It may also result in a hypersensitivity to fungi, rendering one more vulnerable to candida and causing more severe symptoms. In turn, the fact that you have candida may make you more vulnerable to any mold present in your home—creating another vicious circle. Many physicians notice a connection between people living in moldy environments and their experiencing candida overgrowth. They observe that treatment for candida is much more difficult if a patient continues to live in a moldy environment.[12,13]

As discussed in chapter 8, some people may have a genetic polymorphism that impairs the body's ability to effectively recognize and eliminate mycotoxins of all kinds, including toxins produced by mold.[14] The first step for addressing this issue is to remove the source of mold. Everything we discussed in chapter 8 for minimizing die-off of candida would also be beneficial for improving one's ability to deal with mold toxins. Many of the antifungals discussed in chapter 7 would be effective if mold colonization has taken place in the body (in the gut, vagina, sinuses, lungs, bladder). However, if you have a serious impairment of health due to a mold exposure related to a genetic predisposition, then it would be advisable to work with a practitioner who has expertise in this area. Please refer to work by experts such as Dr. Ritchie Shoemaker, Dr. Neil Nathan, Dr. Wayne Anderson, Dr. Jill Carnahan, and Dr. Marvin Sponaugle.

To assess whether you are mold sensitive, take note of whether your symptoms or your cravings for sugar and carbs increase on rainy or humid days, or when you go into the basement, rake the leaves, or enter any moldy environment. If you do, it's an indication that mold toxins are problematic for you.

If you're mold sensitive, humidity in your home should be kept below 50 percent, which can be achieved with a dehumidifier if necessary. Be sure there are no undetected leaks in your plumbing, and keep moist areas like the bathrooms, shower curtains, under the kitchen sink, closets, refrigerator drip trays, garbage pails, and laundry areas as dry as possible and well lighted. Tents are very vulnerable to mold proliferation, so be sure to store them in a dry area and bake them in the sun periodically to air them out. Avoid damp, musty areas like the basement, piles of leaves, barns, attics, and old buildings. Restrict consumption of moldy foods, which are discussed in chapter 10. Mold accumulates in dust, so keep up on your dusting, and use a damp rag or mop when dusting or mopping to prevent dust from spreading. Open the windows when you dust or sweep to help minimize symptoms. Clean the coils of air conditioning units on a regular basis. Maintain good air circulation throughout the house and good drainage around the house.

All furniture items should be placed a few inches away from the wall so that air can circulate around them to prevent mold growth. Avoid carpeting; it harbors mold. Use throw rugs that can be washed instead. Use a dehumidifier in damp rooms like the basement or bathroom. Don't place clothes you have worn back in the closet or drawer; once they have been worn mold begins to grow on them. Put washable covers on pillows, furniture, and mattresses. Hydrogen peroxide or baking soda is excellent for cleaning any mold that does develop.

If you are highly sensitive to mold, you may need to consider moving to a dry climate. This may seem like a drastic step, but it can lead to significant improvement in health. I had to move to the desert due to my extreme sensitivity to mold and humidity, and I can tell you that it made a world of difference in my health. I would never even consider living in an environment that is not arid or semiarid. People who are mold sensitive may also need to avoid foods like nuts, cheese, and spices (see chapter 10).

While it isn't possible to elude all harmful toxins because they are so pervasive in our environment, you can appreciably lower your exposure—and thus minimize the negative effects on your health—by living a green and environmentally friendly lifestyle. Of course, a large part of living green involves eating an organic diet, which is discussed in more detail on pages 321–323.

DISCONNECT FROM TECHNOLOGY

MRIs of the brain indicate that the constant and excessive stimulation produced by Facebook, Twitter, and social media in general is as addictive and bad for your brain as methamphetamine and cocaine.[15] Use of social media overstimulates the neurotransmitter dopamine in the same manner as those hard drugs do, which results in dopamine depletion and then an increased need for stimulation. Dopamine, as you may recall, is needed to keep sympathetic stress in check, and it is responsible for enabling us to feel pleasure, joy, motivation, energy, mental clarity, and focus. In addition, the constant stimulation of technology is another form of stress that keeps the body in fight-or-flight mode.

Disconnect regularly from your cell phone, laptop, tablet, e-book reader, computer, and other electronic devices. Make a conscious effort to get completely away from technology for at least a period of time each day. Aim for one or two days a week when you avoid electronic devices completely or as much as possible. Don't use instant notifications from e-mail, Facebook, or other social media; they keep you in a perpetual state of overstimulation.

Yes, technology and the Internet bring many benefits to our lives, but we must maintain balance.

SLOW DOWN

The stress response system is hardwired to go into action when we are in a rush or hurrying. Earlier in our evolution, when the autonomic nervous system was developing, if we were running or rushing, it was because we were trying to escape a rival tribe or wild animal. We needed the sympathetic nervous system to kick in under such circumstances. Nowadays, anytime we rush or hurry, the brain thinks we are trying to escape danger, and it goes into stress-response mode. Make a mindful effort to slow down in all your activities.

PAY ATTENTION TO YOUR THOUGHTS

An impaired autonomic nervous system influences your thoughts. On the flip side, the way you think affects your autonomic nervous system. In order to restore balance to your autonomic nervous system, you must change the way you think. Let go of perfectionistic demands, unrealistic expectations, and negative self-talk. Silence the inner critic, and work on focusing on the positives in your life instead of on your symptoms, worries, fears, and problems. Whatever thoughts you pay the most attention to are the ones that will be dominant. Choosing to focus on love, relaxation, appreciation, gratitude, and peace encourages the parasympathetic nervous system, while fear, worry, demand, and criticism encourage the sympathetic nervous system. Likewise, if you focus on thoughts about how stressed you are or on your symptoms, your stress levels and your symptoms will become stronger. To some degree, we can minimize the impact of stress on our lives by adjusting the way we respond to it. Granted, if you have excess sympathetic nervous system activity, changing your thoughts may at first feel impossible, but as you practice it will become easier and more effective.

I don't want to imply that healing candida or any other chronic health condition is as simple as changing your thoughts. It is not. I'm not in the camp that believes that anything can be healed by thought alone, but I do believe it can be a contributing factor that should be addressed.

HAVE A GOOD CRY

On the flip side, if you're feeling sad or heavy-hearted with grief, let it out. Crying helps decrease stress hormones, promoting more relaxation and less sympathetic nervous system activity. It also triggers the release of our natural pain-killing, mood-enhancing endorphins. If you suppress your tears, it will have the exact opposite effect, increasing stress and dampening mood.

RETRAIN YOUR LIMBIC SYSTEM

The autonomic nervous is controlled by an area of the brain called the limbic system. Recent research has discovered that some dysfunction in the autonomic nervous system is the result of pathways built by neurons that keep things stuck in sympathetic dominance. These pathways can sometimes be rewired to turn off sympathetic dominance.

Several books teach rewiring of the brain, but they are mostly focused on habits. In addition, two programs that I am aware of were designed for people with chronic fatigue and multiple chemical sensitivity. One is Gupta Amygdala Retraining and the other is Dynamic Neural Retraining. The basic principles taught in these programs can be applied to any symptom or condition. Both use a combination of neurolinguistic programming, mindfulness, and deep breathing to rewire the brain to lessen reactivity of the sympathetic nervous system. I used both the programs faithfully but did not find them to be cure-alls. I was able to rewire some pathways permanently, but not the majority. In most cases I can temporarily turn off the sympathetic response, but it always returns and the technique has to be repeated, despite using the programs for years. Some symptoms and triggers don't respond at all, like pesticides. However, I do feel that these programs significantly improved the quality of my life, by lowering the threshold of my sympathetic dominance. I, as well as some of my clients, have found them to be great management tools. Keep in mind that I fall under the category of people who lived with extreme physical, emotional, and sexual abuse, neglect, and loss of the primary caregiver when I was a child, which means my limbic system is greatly damaged and may inhibit the effectiveness of the programs. A small percentage of people report complete cures or very significant improvements using these two programs. Others report none. I continue to use the basic principles of the programs heavily on a day-to-day basis. I consider them among my top six management resources, along with diet, breathing, mindfulness, green living, and communing with nature. They can be used to turn off symptoms from candida or other microbes, food sensitivities, or sympathetic dominance. I suspect there will be more programs like these developed, so that is something to watch for in the future. One relatively new treatment that shows promise is neurofeedback. It's a type of biofeedback that attempts to rewire the brain.

I've also found another simple program, Trauma Releasing Exercises, designed by Dr. David Berceli, to be highly beneficial. Immediately after doing the first exercise routine I felt very calm and relaxed, and had an enhanced sense of well-being. I wanted to go to sleep, but I couldn't because I had things to do. When I went to bed that night I had one of the best nights of sleep I'd had in years. In the morning I felt better rested than I had in years, and the enhanced sense of well-being was still with me.

HAVE FUN

Make time to play, laugh, and have fun on a regular basis. Research suggests that many health benefits are derived from play, including an enhanced perception of one's quality of life, higher levels of self-worth, self-reliance, and self-confidence, greater adaptability and resilience, stronger connections with those whom you play with, greater productivity, less stress, and stronger immunity. One study found that engaging in enjoyable leisurely activities can enhance immune function even "more powerfully than stress can suppress it."[16] Go to the park and ride the swings or seesaw, play board games or outdoor games with your children or pet, allow yourself to be silly for no reason, or simply color in a coloring book. Studies have found that coloring is an excellent stress reliever for adults. It also stimulates areas of the brain associated with the senses, creativity, and motor skills. There's a whole market that creates coloring books for adults.[17]

MAKE TIME FOR SOLITUDE

Spending at least a little time each day completely alone and in silence is vital to help the brain and the autonomic nervous system rest and rejuvenate. Quiet solitude can also provide profound relief from stress and tension. Go inward, contemplate, reflect, and just enjoy the peace, quiet, and stillness. Make some time in each day for silence and solitude.

EAT TO ENCOURAGE MORE PARASYMPATHETIC NERVOUS SYSTEM ACTIVITY

What you eat has a profound impact on your autonomic nervous system and the adrenal glands. Sugar, grains, high-carb foods, food additives, preservatives, dyes, caffeine, chocolate, and pesticides all trigger the fight-or-flight system and keep the sympathetic nervous system on high alert. Such foods should be eliminated. These substances also deplete the neurotransmitters that regulate the autonomic nervous system, appetite, and gut. Foods that are high in starches—for example, whole grains, potatoes, and legumes—break down into sugar in the body and should be avoided as they, too, trigger fight or flight and deplete neurotransmitters. Even too much fruit or high-carb vegetables can stimulate sympathetic stress, burden adrenals, and drain neurotransmitters.

Additionally, if the diet lacks the right amount of nutrients that the body needs to produce hormones such as cortisol or that the brain needs to produce neurotransmitters, then hormones and neurotransmitters will not be available in sufficient amounts to regulate the autonomic nervous system.

The diet should be high in animal protein and contain a moderate amount of fat (or high in fat and moderate in protein if you want to do keto), and be low in carbohydrate. If you tolerate dairy, then butter, ghee, heavy cream, and full-fat yogurt can be good for the endocrine and nervous systems. The diet is the foundation for supporting the adrenals and reducing sympathetic dominance (just as it is for supporting healing from candida). The paleo for candida diet (presented in great depth in chapters 10 and 11) is best not only for restoring balance to the autonomic nervous system but for optimal health overall. It should also moderate high-histamine and high-glutamate foods as discussed in those chapters as well, if there are elevations. However, there are a few other things to note with regard to diet and the adrenals.

Many people with adrenal fatigue have problems with foods that are high in potassium because the adrenal glands produce a hormone called aldosterone that regulates balance between sodium and potassium. When the adrenals are not functioning properly, aldosterone may be produced in insufficient quantities, resulting in a loss of sodium in the urine and a retention of potassium. Just like the hormones DHEA and cortisol, aldosterone can become depleted. Classic symptoms of this imbalance include dizziness and lightheadedness when standing up, increased thirst, and low blood pressure. For these reasons, people with adrenal fatigue may have a much greater than average need for salt. There is also a genetic polymorphism that can affect aldosterone levels. Therefore, many practitioners recommend that individuals with adrenal fatigue restrict potassium intake. However, one's ability to regulate potassium and sodium can vary widely depending on one's phase of adrenal fatigue. Not everyone with adrenal fatigue is low in aldosterone. The solution is to be careful with potassium foods and monitor how you respond.

As mentioned in chapter 14, the three most critical nutrients for the adrenals are pantethine, vitamin C, and vitamin B6. Pantethine and vitamin C directly enable the production of cortisol and other adrenal hormones, and B6 helps modulate them. However, vitamin C cannot be delivered to the adrenals without adequate salt, so there needs to be sufficient salt in the diet for this purpose as well. Some people improve the adrenals by taking $1/4$ or $1/2$ teaspoon of salt stirred into a glass of water, in addition to salt in the diet. Doing so helps regulate aldosterone-related functions. However, it's important to be aware that aldosterone also regulates blood pressure, so the extra salt can make a person's blood pressure shoot up if it is not needed, and it can be too stimulating for some people. Please be sure to read more about salt on pages 294–297. You should consult with your doctor before supplementing with salt, but salt should be used liberally on your food. Adequate levels of other minerals are also important, but be sure to read about possible complications from supplementing with minerals in chapter 14.

Cholesterol is needed for the synthesis of the steroid hormones. If you don't have enough cholesterol, you can't produce the life-sustaining hormones progesterone, estrogen, aldosterone, testosterone, and—most importantly in regard to adrenal fatigue—cortisol and DHEA. One of the quickest ways to increase cholesterol is to eat a lot of organic butter from grass-fed cows (if you can tolerate butter). As mentioned on page 307, true vitamin A from animal fat is also critical for cholesterol to be converted into cortisol; butter is rich in vitamin A, so you can kill both birds with one stone. The importance of cholesterol is discussed in more detail in chapter 10.

Keeping blood sugar levels stable is absolutely critical for the adrenals. Do this by eating three low-carb paleo meals per day, no more than five hours apart. The adrenals are called upon anytime blood sugar rises or plummets, because each of these events is perceived by the body as stress. The consumption of carbs, which causes a quick rise and then a dip in blood sugar, keeps the adrenals on a roller-coaster ride that depletes them further. Each time carbs are consumed it stresses the adrenals. The more carbs you consume, the harder the adrenal glands have to work. Animal protein and fat are what will stabilize blood sugar and support your adrenals (see chapter 10).

There is a belief within the paleo/keto community that gluconeogenesis (converting protein or fat into glucose), which occurs when eating low-carb, is stressful and puts excess burden on the adrenals, because it requires cortisol for the process. However, that is not completely accurate. The hormone that is called into action to prompt gluconeogenesis is glucagon (not cortisol), which is produced by the pancreas. This typically happens before blood sugar gets low enough to trigger cortisol and epinephrine.[18] When blood sugar first begins to drop, it is glucagon that regulates blood sugar. If for some reason glucagon does not perform the job of stabilizing blood sugar or gluconeogenesis is impaired for some other reason, then blood sugar levels drop even further and hypoglycemia is experienced. At this point then cortisol and epinephrine would be elevated.

There are a few rare genetic disorders that can impair gluconeo-genesis. However, most people do not have a problem with glucagon production. People with "true" hypoglycemia have lost their ability to make glucagon. But you can experience symptoms that mimic true hypoglycemia simply because you are not eating enough animal protein and fat or you're eating too many carbs. Additionally, candida itself (as well as bacteria) can impair gluconeogenesis because of its ability to impair ATP production (needed for gluconeogenesis), which is often the culprit of the low blood sugar.

In either case, my personal experience has shown that the solution to all these problems is to keep carb consumption low and ensure there is adequate animal protein and fat in the diet and that you don't go too long without eating. No more than four to five hours in between meals. This will prevent blood sugar from dropping too low that would prompt elevations in cortisol and epinephrine. If you are experiencing the drop in blood sugar and the cortisol/epinephrine surge, then you aren't eating enough animal protein or you are going too long between meals. We discovered way back in 1936 that one of the best ways to control hypoglycemia is with a diet high in protein and low in carbohydrate.[19]

In my own life, it appears I have a problem with glucagon production. I have been eating low-carb paleo for decades and eating keto for about five years, but I will still experience severe low blood sugar if I do not eat every four to five hours like clockwork or if I do not eat enough animal protein and fat in each meal. The ratio of animal protein to fat is vital. If I don't eat the right amount of animal protein in each meal I will have hypoglycemia, regardless of how much fat or carb I eat. And, if I don't have enough fat with that animal protein I will get hypoglycemia as well, regardless of how much protein or carb is eaten. You need to find the ratio that works best for your body.

GET LOTS OF REST

Unfortunately, our society tends to frown upon people who rest and take naps. We are expected to be doing something all the time, and if we aren't we may be labeled as lazy or lacking in motivation. This attitude contributes greatly to conditions affecting the autonomic nervous system, because basically the norm is to run yourself into the ground. Taking time to rest and nap is very healthy, and getting plenty of rest is a crucial part of recovery for an overactive sympathetic nervous system. This includes ensuring that you get eight or nine hours of sleep each night. The adrenal glands, as well as the body in general, regenerate while we sleep.

There should be lots of resting, napping, and taking it easy as much as possible. Take frequent breaks throughout the day. At the same time, however, don't stop engaging in life, and don't become too sedentary. If you completely stop taking on difficult activities, you will send a message to your brain that you are incapable, which in turn will cause you to become even less capable. As discussed in more detail on page 407, research has found that being too sedentary can cause changes in brain neurons that encourage sympathetic nervous system activity, potentially perpetuating adrenal fatigue. On the other hand, too much physical activity, including overdoing the exercise, can overstimulate the sympathetic nervous system. The key is to find a fine balance.

Be gentle and don't push yourself too hard, but don't withdraw altogether. Break up large tasks into smaller tasks when they feel insurmountable or overwhelming. For example, wash one third of the dishes and rest, wash the second third and rest, and then wash the final third. When cleaning the bathroom, clean the toilet and take a break, clean the sink and take a break, then clean the tub. Don't do too many things in one day. Limbic system retraining, as discussed above, is an excellent tool for this purpose. If reading a book is a challenge for you, then read one or two paragraphs, or whatever you are capable of, and then take a break. It may take a long time to get through the book, but it will happen eventually. Engage in physical activity, but not too much (see pages 407–413).

Try to keep stressful people out of your life as much as possible. Choose your battles carefully, and don't engage in useless arguments, debates, or attempts to make people see your point of view. Don't watch the news very often; it's stressful. Get your headlines and keep up with current events online or in the newspaper. Don't use an alarm clock, which immediately sets off the stress response system.

DETERMINE WHERE YOU ARE ON THE SPECTRUM

Adrenal fatigue and sympathetic dominance occur on a spectrum that runs from mild to completely incapacitating. Where you are on the spectrum affects how quickly your adrenals will recover, how hard you have to work to lower sympathetic dominance, the supplementation program you require, and other steps you may need to take. A person on the milder end of the spectrum is likely to have an easier time than someone at the more severe end. People with advanced-stage adrenal fatigue and sympathetic dominance suffer worse symptoms. The longer the adrenals function at suboptimal levels, the more problems that develop as other organs and systems begin to break down as they try to compensate for the worn-out adrenals. You can measure the severity of your condition by the number and severity of your symptoms. You may move back and forth along the spectrum during different phases of healing or stages of life in response to changes in any of the factors I have written about that affect these conditions. Where you are on the adrenal spectrum can differ from where you are on the sympathetic dominance spectrum, but they often coincide.

Be aware that some treatment approaches that might be helpful for a person with early-stage adrenal fatigue can be harmful for someone who is in a more advanced stage. For example, supplementing with glandulars, adaptogens like ashwaganda, or herbs like ginseng and licorice may be too stimulating for some individuals, leading to further depletion of the adrenal glands. Ginseng is an amphetamine so it shouldn't even be considered. One should be very careful when experimenting with natural remedies for adrenal fatigue. It is my opinion that these methods should be avoided both because they can cause quite a significant setback, and because they do not actually regenerate the adrenal glands. They work as a temporary Band-Aid, which eventually falls off, triggering further deterioration. The goal should be enabling the adrenal glands to return to producing their hormones at optimal levels, which is best achieved with the nutrients discussed on page(s) 455–457 (vitamin C); 457–458 (pantethine); 460–461 (vitamin A) and reducing sympathetic dominance.

Both the adrenal glands and the autonomic nervous system can become compromised following a one-time stressful event, or as the result of many little stressors that build up over time. Remaining mindful of all the stressors that may affect you is important throughout your healing journey.

UNDERSTAND THE RELATIONSHIP BETWEEN HYPOTHYROIDISM AND ADRENAL FATIGUE

Hypothyroidism can be primary or secondary. If it is primary, it should respond well to thyroid-hormone replacement. If low-thyroid symptoms (fatigue, weight gain, dry skin and hair, constipation, low body temperature, depression, hair loss) continue despite treatment, that means the hypothyroidism is secondary and one must consider possible underlying factors. If the underlying cause is adrenal fatigue, then treatment of hypothyroidism without adrenal support is not only ineffective; it can be highly counterproductive.

As described in chapter 1, when the adrenal glands fail to function properly, they have difficulty handling the naturally occurring stress associated with normal bodily functions and energy production. Production of energy and all metabolic functions are downregulated, including the thyroid, in order to conserve energy, leading to chronic fatigue and low thyroid function.

Adrenal expert Dr. Michael Lam explains that when the thyroid is downregulated, production of the hormones T4 and T3 is reduced, but TBG (thyroid-binding globulin) increases, resulting in less free T4 and free T3 if measured in the blood, while total T3 and T4 may remain normal. Some T4 is also directed toward making the inactive rT3 (reverse T3), which works as a "braking system" to oppose T3 functions. Both the reduction in T3 and the increase in rT3 can persist long after the stressful situation has ended and cortisol levels have normalized. Reverse T3 also inhibits conversion of T4 into T3 and perpetuates production of itself. If levels of rT3 are higher than levels of T3, a condition called rT3 dominance may result, producing symptoms of hypothyroidism despite the presence of sufficient levels of T3 and T4. When this occurs, standard lab tests that measure T4 and T3 may be normal despite hypothyroid symptoms. On the other hand, free T4 and free T3 may be low on lab tests while TSH (thyroid-simulating hormone) is normal or high. Administering thyroid medication may normalize lab tests, even while the individual continues to experience low body temperature and continued deterioration in health associated with hypothyroidism.

This whole series of events is directed by the adrenal glands to intentionally slow things down so the body can rest and ensure survival. Under such circumstances, replacing T4 or T3 without first addressing the adrenal glands can lead to further deterioration in the adrenals. The body wants to slow down and rest, but the medication, which increases metabolic function and energy production, speeds things up. Increasing T4 and T3 directly opposes the adrenal glands' attempts to do what is best for the body. You are essentially trying to jump-start the system while the system is applying the brakes. As Dr. Lam says, it is "analogous to pouring oil onto a fire." The weak adrenal glands will be unable to handle the stress associated with stimulation of these functions, which is why they downregulated the system in the first place.[20] Forcing them to do so only depletes them further, potentially resulting in a mild case of adrenal fatigue being pushed to the more serious, exhausted phase. For someone who is already in an advanced stage of adrenal fatigue, pushing them beyond their capacity can lead to an adrenal crash and severe impairment in their ability to function.

Lam explains that under these circumstances, thyroid medication may initially provide some relief from fatigue and other symptoms, but it won't last long. As the adrenal glands become more burdened and weakened by the medication, they downregulate the system further, and symptoms worsen. At this point many practitioners may increase medication or switch to a different one, once again providing some initial relief but ultimately further weakening the adrenals and worsening both conditions (adrenal fatigue and thyroid malfunction). A vicious cycle ensues: the adrenal glands reduce the body's response to the medication, exacerbating the symptoms and increasing the need for medication.[21]

As discussed in chapter 1, thyroid hormones are needed for every cell in the body. When the thyroid slows down, all other organs and systems decelerate as well, including gut motility. Contraction of the muscles that move food and stool through the gastrointestinal tract are weakened, leading to slow transit time and constipation. Impaired motility creates an environment that encourages overgrowth of candida and SIBO, which in turn perpetuates reduced thyroid and adrenal function, which again perpetuates overgrowth of candida or bacteria.

You may also recall from chapter 1 that weak adrenals inhibit the conversion of T4 into its active form, T3. They also hinder the actions of the hypothalamus and pituitary glands, which produce thyroid hormones. Weak adrenals decrease thyroid-receptor sensitivity and produce insufficient levels of cortisol and DHEA, which are needed for modulating thyroid function. Toxic byproducts of candida or SIBO can overwhelm the liver, inhibiting conversion of T4 to T3. Candida can impede communication between all hormones and can bind with adrenal hormones, rendering them inaccessible for use by the body.

If you have failed to respond to thyroid treatment or have observed the aforementioned events in yourself, you should consider the possibility that adrenal fatigue is at the root of your thyroid problem. When the adrenal glands are supported and are regaining their vigor, they will stop downregulating the system. Hypothyroidism symptoms often improve naturally as the thyroid is permitted to restore normal function. As adrenal function improves, thyroid medication may no longer be needed or it may need to be reduced. According to Dr. Lam, a classic lab "picture" of someone who has low thyroid caused by poor adrenal function consists of high levels of thyroid-binding globulin (TBG), low free T4, low free T3, high TSH, slow ankle reflex, and low body temperature.[22]

Thyroid function can be affected by a variety of other factors, including insufficient iodine, selenium, or tyrosine, exposure to pesticides, halides, other problems with the pituitary or hypothalamus, neurotransmitter depletion, insulin resistance, heavy metals, candida toxins, and genetic mutations. Thyroid inhibition can lead to constipation, cravings for sugar and carbs, and other issues that could contribute to candida overgrowth or SIBO, possibly triggering further impairment of adrenal and thyroid function. Traditional testing for thyroid hormone is not very reliable. The most reliable way to test for hypothyroidism is with the Barnes Basal Temperature Test. Work with a practitioner who uses this method and you can find instructions on my website if you want to look into this deeper. If hormone replacement is required, the best source is natural porcine-derived hormone that contains both T3 and T4. The body has a difficult time converting T4 to T3, and most synthetic drugs contain T4 only.

A similar scenario is true for the sex hormones. Dr. Orian Truss explains that if sex hormones (e.g., progesterone, estrogen, testosterone) are out of balance due to candida overgrowth (see pages 37–39), then "attempting to correct hormone problems by administering hormones not only fails, but may make it worse." The problem does not actually lie in an integral inability to produce hormones; it lies in interference with responsiveness.[23]

GET ADEQUATE SLEEP

It's kind of astounding to realize that we spend about one-third of our lives sleeping. Research demonstrates that sleep is critical to all aspects of health; we are only beginning to understand its impact. One study found that lack of sleep is as bad for your health as smoking.[24] Another showed that sleep deprivation is as dangerous as driving when drunk.[25] With regard to candida and related conditions, we learned in chapter 9 that sleep plays a vital role in the immune system and in chapter 6 that it is involved in gut motility and the migrating motor complex. Sleep is also essential for proper neurotransmitter and hormone function, management of appetite and cravings for sugar, carbs, and other addictive substances, regulating the stress response system, and moderating blood sugar levels.

Lack of sleep increases ghrelin (the hunger hormone) and decreases leptin (the satiety hormone). High levels of ghrelin and low levels of leptin lead to an increase in appetite and cravings for sugar and carbs. Additionally, insufficient sleep causes neurons to be less responsive to neurotransmitters, which impedes cell-to-cell communication. Failure to get enough sleep is a form of stress, producing all the related consequences I've written about in this book. Lack of sleep activates areas of the brain that make us seek out rewards (like indulging in junk food) and deactivates areas of the brain related to executive function, which would normally help us resist unhealthy choices.[26] Each of these issues can sabotage one's efforts to remain compliant with the diet and impair one's ability to handle stress.

The body heals and regenerates during sleep. The brain flushes itself of toxins and debris such as amyloid-beta proteins, which are linked to Alzheimer's when present in excess. The adrenal glands do most of their repair work on the body between the hours of 10:00 P.M. and 1:00 A.M., so sleeping during that time is absolutely essential for dealing with the adrenal fatigue that is so often present alongside candida. Staying up past 10:00 P.M. causes the adrenal glands to kick into high gear to keep us going. This means they will be producing cortisol and other stress hormones in higher numbers than they typically do in the evening, all of which puts them under high stress.

Many people with candida suffer bouts of insomnia or disrupted sleep patterns. These can be caused by the toxins released by candida (which, as you recall, affect brain neurotransmitters) or by candida-caused autonomic nervous system dysfunction, or other factors that disrupt the sleep/wake cycle. Another big contributor to sleep problems is the consumption of substances such as caffeine (including green tea), chocolate, alcohol, sugar, grains, and other high-carb foods. High-histamine foods and high glutamate foods may be involved, if one is dealing with excess. So is exposure to environmental toxins. All these substances overstimulate the brain. Therefore, when one begins the path of healing for candida—reducing microbial overgrowth, changing the lifestyle and diet as suggested in this book—this should, with time, improve the ability to sleep. The tools presented in the preceding chapter—for example, mindfulness meditation and deep-breathing exercises—can provide great assistance with sleep as well. Both increase melatonin release and turn off stimulatory neurotransmitters. Supplementing with magnesium may be helpful for some because it stimulates GABA receptors and reduces sympathetic nervous system activity, but be sure to read about potential contraindications in chapter 14.

However, sleep problems can also develop because your body's clock, otherwise known as its circadian rhythm, has become disrupted because of poor sleep patterns. You must set your body clock to work properly by engaging in the right sleep habits. If you regularly stay up late and deprive yourself of time for sleep, your clock will not be set properly. Most adults need somewhere between seven and nine hours of sleep a night. Newborns and toddlers may require up to eighteen hours of sleep, and adolescents generally call for nine or ten. Need for sleep can also be influenced by other factors, such as level of physical activity, cognitive demands, and health status. People who exert themselves a lot throughout the day, people who have jobs that demand a high degree of cognitive activity, and people with chronic health conditions like candida may have a greater need for sleep.

As you can see, your sleep requirements will vary throughout your life cycle. The rule of thumb for determining how much sleep you need is that you should sleep until you wake up in the morning without using an alarm clock. When your alarm clock goes off in the morning, it sets off your stress response system. You're beginning your day with an excess of sympathetic nervous system activity. Additionally, being forced to wake up before your body is ready disrupts your circadian rhythms. We should wake up naturally. Even if you don't feel refreshed after sleeping, which is sometimes the case for the individual with candida, you should still get the amount of sleep that enables you to function optimally.

Pretty much everyone is short on time in this day and age because of too many demands on their schedule. Many people cut down on sleep to make room for everything else. This habit must stop. You need to respect the fact that sleep is a basic need like food, water, and elimination. Make sleep a high priority. Go to bed around the same time each night, and get up about the same time each morning. Following a regular routine that allows for sufficient sleep will reset your body's clock.

We are hardwired to rise and retire with the rising and setting of the sun. Light and darkness trigger the hormones and neurotransmitters that regulate our sleep/wake cycle. Arrange your sleeping schedule as closely to this natural built-in rhythm as much as possible. Be sure your sleeping area is dark, or wear a sleep mask over your eyes; light prevents the production of melatonin (the primary sleep hormone). Darkness incites the conversion of serotonin into melatonin.

Establish a routine that allows you to wind down a little each night before bedtime. Avoid digital stimulation, turn off the lights, don't engage in vigorous exercise or other stimulating activities, and refrain from talking on the phone during this time. Create a calm, relaxing, and quiet environment that allows you to transition slowly from wake to sleep. Don't allow the temperature in the room where you sleep to be too hot or too cold; either one can wake you up.

Eat adequate animal protein and fat for dinner, and avoid carbs. A nighttime dip in blood sugar, caused by consuming carbohydrates, can incite the stress response and wake you up. Eating animal protein and fat will prevent this dip. Some people may need to eat a small serving of animal protein and fat shortly before bedtime to keep blood sugar stable overnight. Additionally, insulin release from carbohydrate consumption interferes with melatonin production.

Make note that drug-induced sleep (from prescription or over-the-counter drugs) is not natural or healthy. It disrupts stage-four sleep, so it should be avoided. Although drugs may provide you some short-term relief, in the long run they will disrupt the brain chemistry and hormones that are needed to regulate the sleep/wake cycle, ultimately disturbing circadian rhythms even more. This would be true of herbs used to induce sleep as well. Circadian rhythms are also disrupted by jet lag and working the graveyard shift.

Cortisol secretion is modulated by the sleep/wake cycle. So while it is true that high cortisol will keep you awake, failure to retire at an appropriate hour or to make time for sleep can increase nighttime secretion of cortisol, keeping you awake.

If you don't get enough sleep at night, or if you feel tired or sleepy at anytime throughout the day, you should take a nap. Research demonstrates that a nap can be a powerful and effective way to boost alertness, productivity, energy, memory, creativity, and mood, and to lower cortisol and reduce stress. A nap may be used to make up for lost sleep or as a reboot to the system that provides you with a fresh start.

Some believe that we may be hardwired by evolution to take a nap. As you may have noticed, most individuals feel a little sleepy in the afternoon. This is part of our natural circadian rhythm, built into us biologically by the napping behaviors of our ancient ancestors. For much of our evolution, our ancestors had biphasic sleep patterns, consisting of a large chunk of sleep time at night and a midday siesta. It is thought that the midday siesta was needed because nighttime sleep was often interrupted by security or family issues.[27] By resisting the urge to nap, we are actually fighting against our natural rhythms. Instead of reaching for a candy bar or cup of coffee to keep you going in the afternoon, what you really need is a nap. Some of the world's greatest thinkers, like Thomas Edison, John F. Kennedy, Winston Churchill, Eleanor Roosevelt, Napoleon Bonaparte, Leonardo da Vinci, and Albert Einstein, were avid nappers, so don't feel guilty for allowing yourself to indulge in this health-promoting behavior.

Circadian rhythms govern not only your sleeping patterns but also your eating patterns, brain wave patterns, the precise timing of neurochemical and hormone secretions, and cellular repair and regeneration. They play a vital role in all aspects of health.

FIND SOURCES OF EMOTIONAL SUPPORT

The changes in diet and lifestyle demanded by the healing journey can be a difficult adjustment at first. There is often a grieving period for foods and activities that must be given up, and you may feel overwhelmed. The healing process itself and the amount of learning you must undertake to address the issue effectively can also be overwhelming. All of this can become a counterproductive source of stress if it is not handled with care.

Getting some kind of emotional support by utilizing the services of a health coach, a health-oriented mental health professional, clergy, or a support group can help you cope more effectively, adjust more smoothly, keep things in perspective, and stay on track with your goals. Furthermore, it is hard for most people to stay committed to changes in diet when they are surrounded by people with poor dietary habits. Therefore, it is also critical to bring other like-minded people into your life who can support you in your goals.

SPEND TIME IN THE SUN

Contrary to popular belief, the sun is not your enemy. Exposure to the sun is our primary source of vitamin D, which as discussed in other chapters (9, 10, and 14) plays a vital role in immunity, killing candida and inhibiting biofilms, neurotransmitter production and function, insulin sensitivity, and blood sugar regulation. Cholesterol is converted into vitamin D when the skin is exposed to ultraviolet rays from the sun, which most likely explains why much of the population is deficient in vitamin D[28] (e.g., not enough sunshine and low levels of cholesterol). Sunshine also stimulates the release of serotonin, dopamine, and endorphins. Additionally, "sunlight helps your body to detoxify, speeding up the elimination of harmful chemicals. Studies have shown that sunlight helps animals expel lead, mercury, cobalt, manganese, cadmium, fluoride, pesticides, and dusts from their system 10 to 20 times faster than those without light."[29] The sun also activates minerals in the body and increases their activity and cofactor effect.[30]

404   Healing Chronic Candida

In *Your Best Health Under the Sun,* Dr. Al Sears states, "any evidence that exposing yourself to the sun is harmful evaporates under scrutiny. It's nothing more than conjecture and slivers of evidence blown out of proportion for commercial interests. What's worse; if you follow this no safe level of sun exposure dogma, you'll put yourself at greater risk of numerous deadly cancers, depression, bone loss, heart disease, diabetes and more." He states, "Our natural environment is the outdoors. Since the beginning of time until only recently we have lived and worked in harmony with the sun. The move from outdoor to indoor living began with the invention of the light bulb in 1879. It was soon after that cancer, heart disease and other degenerative diseases (that our ancestors never experienced) became prevalent. Sunlight is as natural to your body as breathing. As with oxygen, if you go without sunlight for long enough, your body suffers. The damage of living without your native sun is more gradual, but in the end, just as deadly. We are designed, cell by cell, as creatures of the sun. Virtually every organ system in your body is dependent on sunshine for optimal performance."

Dr. Sears goes on to explain that we have been deceived by the sun lotion industry to believe the sun is bad for us for their commercial gain. Sunscreen was initially created to allow people to get a suntan without getting a sunburn, not because we needed protection from the sun. When they realized how profitable it was, the sun suddenly became our enemy.

He expounds that skin cancer has increased in the last thirty years, not because of sun exposure, but because of the unhealthy foods we eat (more specifically, over-consumption of sugar and carbs, an excess of omega-6 fatty acids, and insufficient levels of antioxidants), chemicals we are exposed to, and the use of sunscreen. After the development of sunscreen, cases of melanoma skyrocketed. Most traditional sunscreen products contain as many as five carcinogenic chemicals. An SPF above eight blocks your vitamin D production by more than 95 percent, which can lead to vitamin D deficiency. An SPF of 15 decreases vitamin D production by more than 99 percent. Most sunscreens contain harmful endocrine/hormone disruptors, thus damaging your endocrine and hormonal systems that can result in a vast array of debilitating health conditions, and the endocrine system is responsible for creating vitamin D from the sun/cholesterol interaction. Sunscreen also blocks the body's production of melanin, a naturally occurring substance that protects you from sunburn. Furthermore, most sunscreens only protect you from UVB rays, the ones that cause sunburn and trigger vitamin D synthesis. But they offer no protection for UVA rays, the ones that penetrate deeper into the skin and are associated with skin cancer. Therefore, many people spend excessive amounts of time in the sun falsely believing they are protected. Even chemical sunscreen products that claim they have UVA protection only have an SPF of about 4. Sears feels "sunscreen could very well be the primary cause of the increase in skin cancer."

Other research revealed by Sears includes a study from the *Journal of the National Cancer Institute* in 2005, confirming "that exposure to the sun reduces the risk of skin cancer. Additional studies have shown that lifeguards in Australia have the lowest rates of melanoma," while "office workers have higher rates of malignant melanoma than construction workers, lifeguards and farmers." "Dozens of studies, including one review of more than 50 research papers, show that people whose occupations keep them indoors have a much higher incidence of melanoma than do those who work outside." "Rates of melanoma are higher in Minnesota than Arizona." "An overview of all of the published research reported in the *International Journal of Cancer* revealed that multiple studies show that people with 'heavy occupational exposure' to the sun have significantly lower risk of melanoma." Other studies carried out at the British Columbia Cancer Agency "confirmed that the higher your lifetime recreational sun exposure, the lower your risk of melanoma," while another study demonstrated that those who had the lowest incidence of melanoma were sunbathers. A 2002 study by the National Cancer Institute found "women whose jobs require consistent sun exposure are much less likely to die of breast cancer." Studies have also shown "that men with high exposure to the sun have half the risk of prostate cancer." A study published in the *Lancet* in 1989 "demonstrated that colon cancer is less prominent among people with regular exposure to the sun."

Yes, it is true: "over exposure" to the sun is harmful. It can cause skin damage and lead to two kinds of superficial skin cancer (basal cell carcinoma and squamous cell carcinoma), but it does not lead to the most dangerous form of skin cancer: melanoma. The sun actually prevents melanoma and aids in the healing process if it is acquired. Basal cell carcinoma and squamous cell are rarely fatal and easy to treat. A large study from Harvard concluded that "basal cell carcinoma comes from 'blistering sunburn' and is proportional to lifetime sunburn accumulation." Squamous cell carcinoma is associated with cumulative sun exposure, intermittent sunburns, and people who have fair skin and it usually develops in old age." No, you should not sunbathe for an entire day and you should avoid sunburns; however, complete avoidance of the sun is even more dangerous. Dr. Sears says use the common sense we've been using for eons and "get out of the sun before you burn."

Additionally, Sears points out, "the sun regulates a number of hormones in your body, including those that work as part of the stress response, and those that control your endocrine system, biological clock, and immune system. The 24-hour cycle of light and dark is vital in the production and regulation of hormones. It's not your willpower or your occupation that controls your circadian rhythm—it is your hormones. The sun regulates these hormones, stimulating them with light."

Dr. Sears tells us that fair skinned people should have about 10–20 minutes of sun exposure daily, while those with moderate pigmentation should get 20–40 minutes, and those with darker pigments may need up to 2 hours. Make sure that at least your head, face, neck, and arms are exposed. Don't wear sunscreen or sunglasses during this time. Howeve,r Dr. Sears also says that "for 97 percent of the time that we have lived on this planet, we lived naked in the sun, near the equator. Try to get naked in the sunshine . . . at least occasionally!"[31] Your body can store vitamin D for later use, so it averages out if you spend a lot of time in the sun one day but can't get any sun on another day. Open the curtains and let the sunshine into your living space; you won't get vitamin D this way because the glass impairs this process, but you can get a boost in neurotransmitters that will enhance mood, decrease stress, and regulate appetite.

If you can't avoid being out in the sun for long periods of time, Dr. Sears recommends using an umbrella, wearing a wide-brimmed hat, shielding yourself with clothes, and taking cover now and then in a building or shaded area. If you must use a sunscreen, then look for a brand that is natural and free of cancer-causing chemicals.[32]

ENGAGE IN PROPER PHYSICAL ACTIVITY

Of course, getting regular physical activity is another vital component for health. Exercise is needed for healthy immune and endocrine systems, gut function and motility, hormone function, maintenance of blood sugar levels, detoxification, a healthy brain, and improved sleep. (I have touched on some of these topics already; see pages 235 [immune system], and 215 [microbial die-off].) Exercise enhances insulin sensitivity as demonstrated by its lowering of hemoglobin A1c and glucose levels. It activates genes that produce antioxidants, suppress inflammation, and boost detoxification. Exercise can increase the brain's memory center and enable neurons to be more agile and more efficient with multitasking. It activates BDNF (brain-derived neurotrophic factor), which helps construct new neurons and neuronal networks and control appetite. All of these effects on the brain play an important role in modulating candida overgrowth and cravings for sugar and carbs. When done properly, exercise can help reduce excess sympathetic nervous system activity. A study of rats has shown that being too sedentary changes the shape of neurons in a manner that increases activity of the sympathetic nervous system.[33] All this to say that physical activity should be built into your healing plan.

At the same time, however, it is critical to be aware that too much exercise, or the wrong type of exercise, is just as bad as not enough. Most of the recommendations made by mainstream exercise experts are counterproductive and sometimes destructive. Many people find that having a trainer like Jillian Michaels snarling and barking at you like a drill sergeant is abusive and not conducive to long-lasting healing. You may make some weight-loss goals by being shamed into submission, but the results probably won't last. Follow-up with the contestants who participated in the *Biggest Loser* television show has demonstrated that the majority of these individuals (13 out of 14) gained back most, if not all, of the weight they lost.[34] Exercise that is good for you does not have to be so difficult or involve browbeating.

Some modern fitness experts now warn that doing traditional cardio and aerobics, running marathons, spending an hour at the gym doing nonstop repetitive movement, or performing any type of endurance exercise is unnatural and a form of severe stress on the body that sets off the stress response system. According to Mark Sisson, former elite endurance athlete, fitness expert, and author of *The Primal Blueprint*, "chronic cardio places excessive and prolonged physical stress on your body, leading to fat, injuries, compromised immune function and burnout. Sometimes less is more." In *P. A. C. E. The 12-Minute Fitness Revolution*, Dr. Al Sears presents research that demonstrates prolonged duration exercise of any kind (e.g., traditional aerobics, cardio, or long-distance running) reduces bone mass and increases risk of osteoporosis, increases LDL cholesterol and triglycerides, shrinks muscle mass, and sets off a cascade of inflammation and LDL oxidation that causes artery-hardening plague to form in your blood vessels, which can lead to heart disease and a wide variety of other chronic degenerative health conditions. In regard to repeated sessions of cardio, Dr. Sears states, "this type of continuous challenge simulates episodes of prolonged stress from our once-native hunter environment. It induces short-term survival strategies. But if you stay in survival mode too long it's very destructive." Dr. Arthur Siegel states "the 'inflammatory storm' triggered by the stress of running a marathon creates all the symptoms of heart disease." Marathon runners have an increased risk for heart attack, blood in urine, hardening of the arteries, lower back pain, repetitive stress injuries, permanent bone injury, stress fractures, and sudden cardiac death.[35] As we have established on numerous occasions throughout this book, severe stress leads to depletion of neurotransmitters, disrupted hormones, an increase in blood sugar levels and insulin response, weakened immunity, an increase in free radicals, an increase in appetite and cravings for sugar and carbs and off-limit foods, and perpetuates sympathetic nervous system dominance. High-intensity exercise also releases histamine, which can contribute to excess histamine in the individual with this problem, so this needs to be monitored as well.

Our early ancestors never engaged in physical exercise for the sake of exercise; instead, their exercise came from the demands of their lifestyle. Survival required that they engage in frequent physical activity while building shelter, hunting, gathering, preparing food, making tools, and moving from one location to another. They were very active, but the majority of the time they were moving slowly. Occasionally they engaged in short bursts of intensity—for example, when they ran from a predator or chased down their meal—but anytime they engaged in hard labor or intense physical exertion it was followed by rest and recovery.[36,37,38] They did not run marathons or engage in hours-long intense workouts or perform continuous exertion.

Because this is the manner in which human beings lived for millions of years, we evolved genetically to need this type of physical activity. To achieve optimal health we should mimic these patterns. Since we no longer have to design and construct our own homes, hunt for and gather food, and escape predators, we need to build similar activities into our days. We should move a lot, but the majority of the movement should be low intensity (e.g., walking, yoga, tai chi), and it should be interspersed with occasional short bursts of high-intensity movement and heavy lifting (e.g., sprints, weight lifting, swimming).

Recent research suggests that simply being more physically active throughout the day is much more important than engaging in a formal exercise routine. A study appearing in the *Annals of Internal Medicine* looked at the results of more than forty other studies that assessed the risk of disease and early death in people from two different groups—those who sit for long periods of time and those who don't—and the effect of exercise on each group. The researchers discovered that the people who sat for long periods of time, even if they exercised vigorously, were about 16 percent more likely to die from any cause than people who didn't sit for long periods of time.[39] Another study from the National Cancer Institute followed 240,000 people, ages fifty to seventy-one, for eight and a half years. None of the subjects had cancer or heart disease when they entered the study. At the end of the study, it was found that the people who were sedentary over seven hours per day, even if they exercised daily, had a "61 percent higher risk of dying from cardiovascular disease and a 22 percent higher risk of dying from cancer" in comparison to people who were sedentary for less than an hour per day. If they didn't exercise at all, then the risk of dying from all causes increased 47 percent and the risk of developing cardiovascular disease increased 100 percent.[40] This suggests that sitting, regardless of whether you exercise regularly, increases your risk of disease and death, and a vigorous exercise routine does not counteract the effects of sitting all day. Several other studies have confirmed the same.[41,42]

Dr. Joan Vernikos, former director of NASA's Life Sciences Division and author of *Sitting Kills, Moving Heals*, says there is an easy solution to this problem. In an interview with Dr. Joseph Mercola, she states, "The key is to make sure you move your body frequently throughout the day." The simple act of standing up from a seated position and then sitting back down has been found to be particularly effective at counteracting the detrimental health effects of sitting for too long. Dr. Vernikos explains that the human body deteriorates much more quickly in an antigravity environment, which is imitated by sitting for long periods of time. Physical activities such as bending down and standing up increase "the force of gravity on your body." By frequently standing up and moving around you alter the antigravity environment that causes cellular degeneration.

That said, standing up over and over at one time is not nearly as effective as standing up intermittently throughout the day. Even standing up once per hour is more effective than walking on a treadmill for fifteen minutes. Repeatedly sitting down and standing up for thirty-two minutes was not as beneficial as standing up thirty-two times throughout the course of the day. (Other research has backed this up.) The standing up (interruption of sitting) needs to be spread out over the entire day. The "key to counteract the ill effects of sitting is to repeatedly interrupt your sitting—frequent intermittent interactions with gravity."

Dr. Vernikos also points out that sitting isn't bad for us in and of itself; it is "uninterrupted" sitting that is bad for us. We aren't designed to sit continuously. However, standing all the time wouldn't be good for us either. Remaining on one's feet for long periods can cause negative health consequences as well. It is the "interruption" of the sitting and the change in posture that is good for us.[43]

Structure your life so that your exercise is naturally built into your day. Be more physically active by increasing your daily "nonexercise" activities. Walk to the mailbox, get up to change the channel on the TV, take the stairs instead of the elevator, park farther away from the store, wash the dishes by hand instead of loading them in the dishwasher, use the bathroom upstairs. Again, it's not exercise that is important; it is intermittent movement performed continuously throughout the day. You can add some form of structured exercise to your active routine if you like, depending on your needs. Any formal exercise that you engage in should be enjoyable and pleasant, not something you dread. Some good types of low-impact exercise include walking, tai chi, yoga, and qigong. Jumping on a mini trampoline for a short period of time is a great high-intensity option that will boost the immune and lymphatic systems, enhance elimination of toxins, and improve metabolism.

All exercise routines and physical activity should be gauged according to your body and your health status at any given time. A healthy person has different abilities than an individual with a chronic health condition, and your abilities will vary depending on where you are in the healing journey. This is especially true if you have adrenal fatigue. Exercising too often, for too long, or too intensely can prevent your adrenals from healing and possibly cause further deterioration. Do not push yourself too hard. If you are incapable of doing any structured exercise, that is okay; just stay active as described. Do what your body feels capable of and nothing more. As your health improves, you can increase the amount of exercise you engage in as you see fit. If you feel worse after exercising, then you have pushed too hard. Cut back as far as you need to feel comfortable.

Adrenal fatigue becomes even more common in menopausal and postmenopausal women, largely because the adrenals have taken on the job of producing sex hormones, which used to be the job of the ovaries. Since many women have adrenals that are overworked due to the demands in their lives, this hormonal change often pushes the adrenals over the edge. In addition, the adrenals naturally put out fewer hormones as we age.

Hormonal changes may affect a woman's insulin sensitivity, even if she is eating a good paleo/primal diet. A woman who has no problem with insulin resistance prior to menopause may suddenly develop it in response to hormonal changes. Her ability to handle carbohydrates may change with menopause, causing weight gain. For example, in my younger years I could get away with frequent cheating on carbohydrates without any consequences to my weight, but now I can't consume more than 50 grams a day or I gain weight at an alarming rate. A woman who experiences this change might increase her exercise, only to find that exercising harder and more often drains the adrenal glands and drives more fat storage. Instead, exercising properly and maybe less often, cutting carbs, and supporting the adrenal glands is what is needed.

An excellent source for learning how to exercise properly (as well as learning more about primal living) can be found in the book *The Primal Blueprint,* by Mark Sisson. He writes, "Best results come when your exercise routine is unstructured and intuitive and workout choices are aligned with your energy and motivation levels. Always allow for sufficient recovery and pursue goals that are fun and inspiring." Exercising properly helps to support immunity, encourage weight loss, balance blood sugar, eliminate cravings for sugar and carbs, prevent buildup of toxins from candida and other microbes, and reduce sympathetic dominance.

I will describe my own routine to illustrate how to put these principles into action. I start each morning with deep-breathing exercises, mindfulness-based meditation, and neurolinguistic programming designed for the limbic system to ignite more parasympathetic nervous system activity and downregulate sympathetic dominance. I also engage in these activities numerous times throughout the day, whenever I feel sympathetic dominance mounting.

I work from home, so I go to work at my desk. Every fifteen minutes or so I get up from my desk and do one or more of the following activities for thirty seconds to a minute or two, and then immediately return to work:

- squats

- knee lifts

- push-ups

- stretching

- bending over

- walking back and forth across the room

- marching in place while swinging my arms

- going outside and walking a lap around my yard

- standing in the yard and stretching in the sunshine or feeling the wind against my face

If I'm talking with a client on the phone, I will simply stand up and walk to another room and come back and sit down.

Sometimes I get wrapped up in my writing and forget to stand up, or sometimes I get up every five or ten minutes, rather than fifteen, but for the most part I stay pretty consistent.

Three or four times a week I take a gentle walk that lasts anywhere from twelve to twenty or so minutes depending on how busy I am or how I feel that day. Once or twice a month I engage in a longer, more strenuous activity, like a thirty-minute hike in the mountains. Once or twice a month I do a full-out sprint through the yard and lift some heavy rocks.

Doing too many squats at one time triggers histamine and my stress response, and I develop a migraine. So I only do five at a time, but, again, I do them several times throughout the day. If I walk for too long, I get exhausted and my brain doesn't work, so I keep it to no more than twenty minutes or so. If I walk too briskly for too long it releases histamine and triggers my stress response, so I avoid getting too worked up. You should adjust for these types of issues as well if needed.

AVOID EXPOSURE TO HEAVY METALS

In my opinion, the role of heavy metals (particularly mercury) in relation to feeding candida may be overrated, but heavy metals can cause significant health issues in numerous other ways. Metal toxicity can impair gut function, brain function, and immune function, and perpetuate sympathetic dominance, all of which can fuel cravings for sugar, carbs, or other mind-altering substances and perpetuate overgrowth of candida and other microbes. For these reasons, it's important to determine whether heavy metal exposure is or is not a factor. Within this category it is equally important to look at copper levels. Although copper is an essential nutrient, when present in excess it is toxic and can be a major contributor to sympathetic dominance and a wide array of neurological symptoms. On the other hand, low copper can contribute to a variety of problems, including hair loss, fatigue, anemia, and reduced white blood cell count. Balance is important. There is a fine line between too much and too little copper. Excess copper may also contribute to overgrowth of both candida and bacteria. On the other hand, low copper could also contribute to microbial overgrowth, because it is a natural antimicrobial. Again, balance is important with this nutrient.

The good news is that heavy metal toxicity testing can be used to help identify excess accumulation of metals in the body rather easily and affordably. You have several different options to choose from. If you want to take matters into your own hands, the easiest and most affordable option is a hair analysis. This is a test you can perform in the comfort of your home. A hair analysis tells you the level of toxic metals that are being stored in your tissues. However, it does not tell you about recent or ongoing exposures. An RBC (red blood cell) mineral test will tell you about recent and ongoing exposures, but it won't tell you what is being stored in the tissue. Hair analysis and RBC mineral should be used together for a complete picture. The RBC mineral test will also provide you with the status of your nutrient metals (calcium, magnesium, zinc, molybdenum, copper, potassium, selenium), another important piece of information. Both tests are available directly to the consumer through a variety of online labs. Be aware that hair analysis is not the best way to assess copper.

A chelation challenge test is often used by medical doctors and alternative health clinics. It is a reliable method of assessment that will tell you both toxic metals and nutrient metals, but it requires a visit to the doctor and is often associated with a variety of side effects.

According to Dr. Charles Gant, eliminating heavy metals can be achieved quite successfully without costly intravenous chelation. With the right nutritional supplements, a bathtub, and lifestyle changes, heavy metals can be addressed safely and naturally within the comfort of your home and at your own pace. Supplementation with the nutrient metals will help drive out the toxic metals. You can combine mineral supplementation with Epsom salt baths or clay baths and supplementation with chlorella. Chelation and far-infrared saunas are other options. Other supplements commonly used in this process include NAC, glutathione, vitamin C, vitamin E, MSM, and alpha-lipoic acid. However, according to Dr. Gant, cilantro, NAC, and alpha-lipoic acid should not be used in high doses until later in the process. If they are used too early in the process, they can drive the toxins into the brain.[44]

The key to eliminating heavy metal toxicity is to reduce the input and increase the output, so it is critical to find the source of your heavy metal toxicity and eliminate it so accumulation does not continue. Common sources for contamination include seafood, pesticides, dental work, fertilizers, tattoos, CFL light bulbs, tap water, cigarettes, and industrial or agricultural pollution.

USE ENEMAS AS NEEDED

A simple enema can be one of the most powerful tools you use on your healing journey. Since the colon is where candida is often found in very high numbers, overgrowth can be significantly and immediately reduced by physically flushing the microbes out of this area, which can result in almost instant relief from many symptoms. Furthermore, the body's detoxification system shuffles many toxins—both those produced by candida and those from other sources—into the colon to be transported out of the body through the stool. An enema physically removes these toxins as well, alleviating the symptoms associated with the toxins, preventing their reabsorption and redistribution, and improving liver function. It is critical that dead and dying yeast and their toxins be eliminated, and if the bowels are not working properly or transit time is slow, as is often the case with candida, the enema can perform this function. As mentioned in chapter 8, an enema is one of the most effective ways to quickly reduce the symptoms of die-off. It can also provide rapid and easy relief if you have overindulged in carbohydrates and experience an increase in candida overgrowth as a result. For the same reasons, enemas can be beneficial for the individual with parasites or bacterial overgrowth, and they can significantly lower methane levels associated with SIBO. All of these benefits of the enema can consequently help reduce excess sympathetic nervous system activity and take some burden off the adrenal glands.

Although a plain-water enema can be highly beneficial in itself, you can increase its effectiveness significantly by adding nystatin powder to the water, which will kill the yeast on contact as it travels through the colon. Food-grade hydrogen peroxide can also be used in this manner. Adding probiotics to the enema solution can help recolonize healthy bacteria. In this case, instead of expelling the solution, you retain it, allowing the microbes to colonize. This is referred to as a retention enema. As mentioned in the chapter on SIBO, it can be a great way to bypass the small intestine and implant directly in the colon. Other substances (e.g., coffee, antifungals) may also be used in a retention enema. When performing a retention enema, a plain-water cleansing enema is done first to cleanse the colon and allow space for retention.

Professional colonics are an option instead of enemas, but the home enema is much more convenient and affordable. A colonic can reach farther into the colon than an enema, so it is not a bad idea to use colonics occasionally, in conjunction with enemas.

Coffee enemas can provide a variety of other benefits and are often recommended for people with candida, parasites, or bacteria. Recall that the liver can become overwhelmed with toxins released by candida or other microbes or environmental toxins. When that happens, the detoxification system is impaired, which can intensify symptoms and further degrade health. The liver is the chief organ involved with detoxification, and bile is one of the substances used to carry toxins into the colon and out of the body through the feces. A coffee enema can open up bile ducts and stimulate the liver to produce more bile, thereby improving the detoxification system. Palmitates, substances found in coffee, when absorbed through the colon wall can stimulate production of the liver enzyme glutathione S-transferase, which increases production of glutathione. Glutathione is one of the key conjugating substances used by the detoxification system to bind to a toxin and prepare it to be transported out through bile. Each of these actions enhances the liver's ability to cope with incoming toxins in a more effective and efficient manner, thereby preventing toxins from getting backlogged in the system. Furthermore, naturally occurring alkaloids in a coffee enema provoke blood vessels to dilate, increasing the blood supply to the gastrointestinal tract, reducing inflammation, enhancing digestion and muscle tone, improving peristalsis and elimination, and enhancing the overall health of the gastrointestinal tract. Additionally, a coffee enema can be viewed as a mild form of liver dialysis since the coffee enema is retained for fifteen minutes and the blood travels through the liver every three minutes.

Some people with severe overactivity of the sympathetic nervous system may not tolerate the effects of a coffee enema very well. In some individuals the caffeine contained in a coffee enema can set off the stress response system in the same manner as if it were consumed. If this is the circumstance, then they should be avoided or only used with great caution. For example, in my own life, if I do a coffee enema it makes me shake and tremble so severely that I can't get off the floor and I feel like I'll pass out. Some individuals may be able to work around this problem by keeping the enema bag no more than eighteen inches above the head, which slows the flow of water and may reduce the systemic effect of the caffeine. Decreasing retention time or the amount of coffee used may also work, as may using decaffeinated coffee. However, it is the caffeine that stimulates the liver and gallbladder, so caffeine is an essential ingredient if you want to reap the full benefits of a coffee enema. That said, decaffeinated coffee is not completely free of caffeine; it merely contains a lesser amount, so a hypersensitive individual may still benefit. It's also possible that the smaller amount of caffeine may trigger the sympathetic nervous system, so one should still exercise caution.

Without exception, organic coffee should always be used for an enema. Traditional coffee is loaded with pesticides, which should not be inserted into the colon or absorbed by the liver under any circumstance. A coffee enema should not be done in the evening, as the stimulating effect may disrupt the sleep cycle. Of course, this doesn't mean you should drink coffee. As discussed on pages 289–293, caffeine consumption degrades the gut and perpetuates sympathetic dominance and microbial overgrowth. The only time coffee can be beneficial is when it is used in an enema. Additionally, it's important to note that coffee is high in mold and mycotoxins, which as discussed previously can have a wide array of negative effects on the brain and body. Be sure to purchase a higher-quality brand that advertises it is low in mycotoxins. You should also be aware that decaffeinated coffee is higher in mycotoxins because caffeine inhibits their growth.

The water you use in an enema should be free of chlorine and other contaminants that are found in tap water. They will be absorbed through the colon wall, which would obviously be counterproductive for the liver and colon. Individuals with an inflammatory bowel disorder like Crohn's or colitis may experience negative effects from an enema, so they should exercise caution. Enemas should be used in moderation; do not use them excessively. Too much of any good thing can be a bad thing. Always consult with your primary health-care provider before using an enema to confirm it is a good course of action for you.

How to Do a Basic Enema

Materials

- an enema bag, hose, and tip, preferably one that is free of BPA and PVC (I prefer stainless steel)
- filtered water that is free of chlorine, fluoride, etc. (not plain tap water)

Instructions

1. Fill the enema bag with plain (pure) water.

2. Hang the enema bag about eighteen to thirty-six inches above you. It needs to be higher than you are, to allow water to flow down naturally, but not too high or the water will flow too fast.

3. Lie down on the bathroom floor on a towel or in the bathtub.

4. Insert the tip gently into your rectum, open the clamp, and release the water slowly. You can lubricate the tip with a little coconut oil if you wish.

5. Fill the colon with as much water as you can take in without expelling it, then close the clamp. If you feel the urge to evacuate, close the clamp for a moment, take a few slow, deep breaths, and resume.

6. Gently massage your lower abdomen with your fingers, making your way around the entire length of the colon.

7. Expel the water in the toilet.

8. Repeat two or three times until bag of water is empty.

9. Wash your equipment thoroughly.

Variations

1. Add nystatin powder, food-grade hydrogen peroxide, or another antifungal to the water.

2. Add probiotics to the water, and retain the enema for as long as possible instead of expelling it. You must first cleanse the colon with plain water before doing a retention enema.

3. Do a coffee enema (instructions follow).

Coffee Enema Instructions

1. Stir 1 to 4 tablespoons of organic coffee grounds (depending on the strength you want) into a quart of water, bring it to a boil, and boil for about three minutes. Cover the pan with a lid, and let simmer for about fifteen minutes. Don't use instant coffee. Replace any water that was lost through boiling, so that there is still one quart.

2. Let the coffee cool. Strain the liquid from the coffee grounds.

3. After you have done a cleansing enema as described above, fill the enema bag with the coffee you've prepared.

4. Lie down again.

5. Insert the tip and release the liquid slowly until the enema bag is empty. If you feel the urge to evacuate, close the clamp for a moment, take a few slow, deep breaths, and resume.

6. Remain lying down for fifteen minutes. During that time, turn onto your left side for a few minutes, then lie flat on your back for a few minutes, then lie on your right side for a few minutes, then flat on your back again. This will help move the liquid to different parts of the colon.

7. After fifteen minutes, get up and expel the liquid.

8. Wash your equipment thoroughly.

ADDRESS METHYLATION ISSUES

Methylation is a vital biochemical process that is involved in detoxification, hormone balance, neurotransmitter function, conversion of serotonin to melatonin, immune function, inflammation, breakdown of histamine, elimination of estrogen, sympathetic nervous system activity, and energy production to name just a few. If the process doesn't occur properly, two of the results may be increased microbial overgrowth and sympathetic dominance.

Toxins released by candida (e.g., acetaldehyde) and other microbes may impair the methylation cycle. Other factors that affect methylation can include nutritional deficiencies, heavy metals, environmental toxins, stress, and genetic polymorphisms.

Methylation is needed to convert norepinephrine into epinephrine, which is then burned off. Norepinephrine is the neurotransmitter that triggers the sympathetic nervous system. When it is present in excess, a person remains in sympathetic dominance, which as we have learned fuels the overgrowth of candida and bacteria. And because of methylation's role in detoxification, problems in the process cause toxins from candida and other microbes to accumulate.

This book isn't the place for an in-depth discussion of this topic, but I wanted to make sure you are aware it is something that should be explored and addressed. Methylation is a very complex issue and my current understanding of it is elementary. To learn more, I recommend that you work with someone who has a great deal of expertise in this area. Addressing this issue without a well-rounded knowledge base can do more harm than good.

DON'T SMOKE

Smoking triggers the liver to release its stored sugar into the bloodstream, which, among other things, feeds candida and increases cravings for sugar and carbs.[45] This, of course, incites an insulin response, the long-term consequences of which I've detailed elsewhere in the book. The lowered blood sugar that results from an insulin dump makes a person irritable and nervous, impairs cognitive function, and incites cravings for sugar, carbs, and more cigarettes to boost blood sugar levels. It's another vicious cycle that perpetuates cravings and yeast overgrowth. Additionally, cigarettes contain up to 75 percent sugar, because tobacco is cured with sugar.[46] So, you're getting a double whammy.

In other words, nicotine use equals sugar, which feeds candida and fuels cravings for sugar and carbs. The reason smoking works so well as an appetite suppressant is because of its ability to quickly increase blood glucose levels. It takes about twenty minutes for food to increase glucose levels, but it happens in a matter of seconds after smoking. This is one of the reasons why people experience an increase in appetite when they first quit smoking. Once they quit, it takes a while for the body to regain its ability to manage blood sugar on its own. Furthermore, the cycle of nicotine use, blood sugar release, and insulin response is experienced by the body as stress, which fuels the stress cycle that we've discussed at length.

Nicotine is an addictive mind-altering drug that affects the brain in a manner similar to cocaine, heroin, or alcohol, including their effects on neurotransmitters. It leads to depletion of dopamine, serotonin, and acetylcholine. Nicotine has also been found to incite a biological urge for alcohol and impede the brain's ability to recover from alcohol addiction in someone in recovery. Smoking inhibits the ability to absorb many vital nutrients, including vitamin A, vitamin E, selenium, zinc, and calcium. It increases bone loss and is associated with higher levels of copper and beta-hemolytic streptococcus.

Additionally, nicotine is a neurotoxin that is so powerful it has been utilized as a pesticide. You may have seen an old episode of *The Andy Griffith Show* in which the gardener used nicotine to kill bugs on a bush. One cigarette contains about 10 milligrams of nicotine, of which only about 1 or 2 milligrams are inhaled. One drop of pure nicotine would kill an adult. Nicotine suppresses many different aspects of the immune system, including production of some types of white blood cells and their ability to seek and destroy. Cigarettes are loaded with heavy metals, pesticides, fertilizers, herbicides, fungicides, and ammonia—more than four thousand chemicals total, all of which can impair immunity, disrupt neurotransmitter production and function, increase sympathetic nervous system activity, disrupt the endocrine system, damage the adrenals, fuel cravings for sugar and carbs, and encourage overgrowth of yeast and other microbes. One of those primary toxins is acetaldehyde, which we discussed on pages 26–27 in terms of how it affects the brain and body and perpetuates the addiction cycle.

Studies have demonstrated that when candida is exposed to cigarette smoke, morphogenesis from blastospore to hyphal form is increased, resistance to osmotic and heat stress is increased, chitin production is increased, the organism's ability to adhere to cells is increased, and proliferation is increased by a factor of three.[47]

For all these reasons, then, nicotine can both cause and perpetuate cravings and overgrowth. If a person smokes, he or she will simply find it impossible to keep blood sugar levels stable, remain committed to the diet, and reduce candida overgrowth.

The new e-cigarette (electronic cigarette), marketed heavily by the infamous R. J. Reynolds Tobacco Company and other firms, is not any healthier for you. Nicotine is a neurotoxin and an addictive drug no matter how you consume it, be it through electronic means or traditional tobacco products. The commercials for e-cigarettes are repulsive, disturbing, disgusting, and insulting to the intelligent mind. I mean, really, there is nothing smarter or more sophisticated about this cigarette. In some ways using it makes a person look even more foolish for falling for the companies' deceptive marketing.

"We're all adults here," they say in the commercial. Well, then, it is time to act like an adult and quit trying to find a way to continue an addiction. The need to hold a cigarette in one's hand, move it to one's lips, and have it in one's mouth (which amounts to oral stimulation; think baby pacifier or thumb sucking) is an immature and infantile need. There is nothing freeing about being addicted—to an electronic product or otherwise.

Pretty much everything I've discussed here in relation to cigarette smoking applies to the electronic cigarette as well. Proponents of e-cigs claim they are healthier for you because they don't produce tobacco smoke. What they fail to mention is that you are exchanging the tobacco smoke for a variety of other harmful and cancer-causing agents.

The electronic cigarette consists of a stainless steel tube that resembles a cigarette and generates heated nicotine-infused water via a lithium battery to produce an odorless vapor, designed to simulate the smoking experience. Using e-cigs may allow you to avoid yellow teeth and smoker's breath, but you will still be exposed to toxic additives, emulsifiers, artificial flavors, diethylene glycol (known more commonly as antifreeze), nitrosamines (carcinogenic compounds), tetramethylpyrazine (a substance that can result in brain damage), and fluoride (if you use tap water and live in a place that adds fluoride to its water).

E-cigarettes have also been found to contain high levels of tin, nickel, silver, and copper nanoparticles; in some cases, intake of these substances is higher than one would get from a traditional cigarette. Nanoparticles can easily enter the bloodstream and other bodily tissues.[48]

The amount of nicotine contained in an electronic cigarette is higher (and thus more toxic) than that contained in a traditional cigarette— sometimes by double or triple. Mistakes made in manufacturing may even result in a lethal dose; as mentioned previously, nicotine is a neurotoxin and can kill you. This is of grave concern for children, whose bodies cannot handle the same-sized dosages as adults' bodies. In addition, users must be very careful not to inhale too strongly to avoid sucking in the nicotine liquid itself, which can't always be achieved.

Unlike with tobacco, at this time there are no federal regulations governing the sale of e-cigs, including no age restrictions, which means children can access them, potentially leading to addiction at an early age. (Some states, municipalities, and counties are imposing their own restrictions on the sale of e-cigs.) They are marketed not only to adults but also to teens and children; they can be purchased quite easily online or at many malls, where children frequently hang out. The false image being peddled that electronic cigarettes are cool and harmless is very dangerous for the mind of a child and should be criminal. I wonder, how do the people who sell these products sleep at night?

Since e-cigarettes are not universally regulated, nonsmokers may be subjected to a variety of toxins against their will. (Research on the effects of secondhand e-cig vapor is still in its early stages. Furthermore, many private businesses, but not all, restrict the use of e-cigs on their premises in the same way that they restrict the use of traditional tobacco products.) Some electronic cigarettes are subject to explosion. A man in Florida lost his front teeth and part of his tongue and was severely burned when his e-cig blew up in his face.[49] As I see it, e-cigs are not going to help you overcome nicotine addiction; they are going to make you even more addicted. They will have the same, and maybe even a more potent, impact on your brain chemistry as traditional tobacco products, which means they will contribute to addiction to harder substances, depression, anxiety, loss of motivation and focus, nervousness, and a host of other mental health issues.

AVOID MARIJUANA AND OTHER MIND-ALTERING DRUGS

All mind-altering drugs (psychotropics) deplete the vital neurotransmitters that I've discussed throughout the book, including the recreational drugs like cocaine, heroin, alcohol, and meth, as well as prescription-based antidepressants (e.g., Zoloft, Prozac), benzodiazepines (e.g., Xanax, Ativan), and stimulants (e.g., Adderall). Psychotropics initially relieve stress and many symptoms, but that is because they mimic natural neurotransmitters that turn off the sympathetic nervous system. As soon as the substance leaves the system, however, the user returns to an even more stressed-out state than before, and with ongoing use, neurotransmitter production gets suppressed by the drug. In *End Your Addiction Now*, Dr. Charles Gant explains that when neurotransmitters are mimicked by artificial substances, the brain responds by reducing production of or responsiveness to the natural neurotransmitter. The user becomes dependent on the mind-altering substance to fill in for the depleted neurotransmitter. This is called addiction, and it results in the same vicious cycle described earlier in the book.

When neurotransmitter levels drop, the user becomes dependent on the psychotropic substance to increase them again. The more a person turns to the psychotropic toxins, the more her or his neurotransmitters are depleted. Psychotropic drugs become a way of anesthetizing the excess sympathetic nervous system activity. Addicts of all kinds are unconsciously trying to restore balance to their brain chemistry, soothe their autonomic nervous system, and find inner peace. They're seeking the equilibrium that has been disrupted by toxins, a poor diet, or stress, and the use of psychotropic chemicals to artificially stimulate neurotransmitters.

Like other toxins, the psychotropic toxins must be removed in order to return to the parasympathetic state. There cannot be improvement in psychiatric or physiological health if one remains dependent on psychotropics. Dr. Charles Gant also states that psychotropics take the brain, which is the captain of the ship for the autonomic nervous system, out of the ball game.[50]

With the unfortunate and dangerous surge in the use of medical marijuana, many people are under the false impression that marijuana is safe. Nothing could be further from the truth. Marijuana is no different from any other mind-altering drug. It is highly addictive, results in significant changes in perceptions, moods, and behavior, stunts psycho-spiritual growth and maturity, diminishes a person's ability to function optimally in the world, and depletes neurotransmitters. It does not matter if you are using it for medical purposes or recreationally; the brain does not distinguish the difference between the two. Marijuana use is marijuana use.

Marijuana contains THC, which is a cannabinoid that resembles the endocannabinoids occurring naturally in the human brain. It occupies the cell receptors that would normally be occupied by our natural endocannabinoids. In other words, marijuana in any form mimics your natural endocannabinoids.

Both endocannabinoids and cannabinoids from exogenous (outside the body) sources affect sensory and time perception, pleasure, appetite, pain, coordination, concentration, memory, thought, movement, judgment, and decision making—which is why marijuana has such a wide range of effects on the mind and body. Unlike other neurotransmitters, endocannabinoids achieve their effects by dampening the effects of other neurotransmitters, so they have the ability to affect many other neurotransmitters. Like all psychotropic substances, marijuana causes a surge in dopamine initially (responsible for addiction, mood, cognitive function, and energy), but over time the brain responds to this artificial stimulation by downregulating production of or responsiveness to dopamine, and you now have lower than normal levels of dopamine.

The effects of the exogenous cannabinoids in marijuana are much more powerful than those of our natural endocannabinoids. They can practically stop the stream of consciousness, which is what provides the feelings of inner peace and "mellowing out" that makes the marijuana high so enjoyable. The more THC present in marijuana, the more potent its impact, and the amount of THC in marijuana has been increasing since the 1970s. Marijuana that is on the market today is much more powerful than what people were smoking in the 1960s and 1970s and consequently more addictive and destructive.

Remember that artificial stimulation leads to reduced production and responsiveness of our natural neurotransmitters, an effect known as tolerance. As tolerance increases, you need more of the substance to get the same effect. That means if you use marijuana on a regular basis, eventually your brain won't produce enough of its own endocannabinoids and dopamine, leading to addiction to the substance that can provide artificial stimulation since your natural neurotransmitters are not around to do the job. Additionally, since marijuana exerts its effects on all other neurotransmitters, then all neurotransmitters are potentially affected. If neurotransmitters are not available in sufficient amounts for whatever reason, they cannot perform the jobs that are so critical for healing from candida: reducing sympathetic nervous system activity, managing cravings for sugar and carbs, and regulating gut function.

Endocannabinoids are found in higher concentrations in certain parts of the brain, specifically, the cerebral cortex, hippocampus, basal ganglia, and cerebellum. Any functions associated with these areas can be impaired by marijuana use. The cerebellum maintains balance and coordination, the basal ganglia are involved in controlling movement, the hippocampus is critical for memory and learning, and the cerebral cortex plays roles in vision, problem solving, decision making, language, memory, processing information, and perception. Because of marijuana's effects on these functions, long-term users often experience low energy, cognitive decline, loss of focus and attention, anxiety, depression, low energy, loss of motivation, decreased reaction time, listlessness, apathy, and dulled or flat emotions and reactions. As mentioned, marijuana impedes emotional and spiritual growth and maturity.

Depending on where and how the marijuana is cultivated, it may be contaminated with heavy metals like cadmium, mercury, lead, and arsenic. These substances can come from the soil it is grown in or from the application of fertilizers and pesticides. Heavy metals and tobacco may be added intentionally to increase weight. THC can linger in the brain long after it is consumed, possibly taking months for the brain to return to normal. In addition, marijuana contains more than four hundred chemicals besides THC that have the potential to disrupt brain function and impair immunity. As with any psychotropic, marijuana use in children and adolescents is even more damaging. The brain is still developing during these years, which makes it more vulnerable. Marijuana can inhibit the neuronal communication network and neuroplasticity, resulting in profound and long-term effects on brain growth and development and leading to emotional and intellectual impairment. It can inhibit neuroplasticity in the adult as well, but the effects are more significant on the developing brain of a child or adolescent.

Marijuana use doubles the risk of stroke by causing "plaque to form in the skull, leading to narrowing arteries in the head" and "marijuana users suffer strokes at a younger age than those who don't."[51] It also disrupts hormones, increases the risk of addiction for harder drugs like cocaine and heroin as tolerance develops, and lowers IQ. Smoking it is associated with a higher risk of emphysema and other lung diseases and makes the user more susceptible to coughs, colds, and bronchitis. "Limited evidence suggests that a person's risk of heart attack during the first hour after smoking marijuana is nearly five times his or her usual risk."[52,53] It is also associated with lower education, less satisfaction in life, reduced employment and career-related achievements, and more interpersonal conflicts.[54]

In *End Your Addiction Now,* Dr. Charles Gant speculates, and I agree, one of the reasons why marijuana addiction is becoming so prevalent is because of the low-fat craze and the advice to avoid meat. He explains the body's natural cannabinoids are manufactured from arachidonic acid and lecithin. Arachidonic acid is an omega-6 fatty acid that is found in animal fat and butter, and lecithin is found in foods like eggs, organ meats, and sunflower seeds. Because many people now consume a low-fat, low-cholesterol, junk-food diet, including avoiding eggs and animal protein, these important substances are missing from their meals. Such a diet makes it harder for the brain to obtain the nutrients it needs to form dopamine and other neurotransmitters as well.

Marijuana temporarily provides relief from the symptoms of low endocannabinoid and dopamine production by stimulating the respective receptors. However, in the long run, it perpetuates the problem by causing even more disruption and depletion. Your brain doesn't need marijuana to feel better; it needs more fat and animal protein.

Five marijuana cigarettes per week contain as many cancer-causing agents as a pack of tobacco cigarettes per day for a week. One marijuana cigarette can exert the same harmful effects on the trachobronchial epithelium (lining of trachea and bronchi) as twenty tobacco cigarettes.[55] Tar content of marijuana cigarettes is 3.5 to 4.5 times greater than tar content of tobacco cigarettes.[56] That means smoking marijuana is potentially more harmful to the health of the lungs than smoking tobacco.[57,58] These toxins can damage tissue, making a person more vulnerable to candida and other microbes and harmfully impacting the immune system and detoxification system—which in the person with candida are already overloaded with candida toxins.

Although it is possible to avoid some of these issues such as exposure to tar by using a vaporizer, edible marijuana products, tinctures, tonics, or other forms of marijuana, the other problems remain. THC (and other cannabinoids), the primary active ingredient that is at the root of most of these effects, is present no matter what form is used.

Furthermore, some of the alternative versions, like wax and hash, contain an exceptionally high level of THC, making them even more harmful to the brain. Cannabis oil (even the kind with no psychotropic present) is still artificially tapping into the endocannabinoid system, which is going to lead to the problems we have discussed.

Heavy, long-term use of the various forms of marijuana is also associated with a condition known as cannabinoid hyperemesis syndrome, or CHS, which causes severe abdominal pain, nausea, and vomiting that can lead to dehydration and kidney failure. For reasons not yet understood, the symptoms of nausea and vomiting are relieved temporarily with a hot shower or bath. The syndrome usually resolves within days of stopping marijuana use. According to Dr. Kennon Heard, an emergency room physician at the University of Colorado Hospital in Aurora, Colorado, "When medical marijuana became widely available, emergency room visits diagnoses for CHS in two Colorado hospitals nearly doubled. In 2012, the state legalized recreational marijuana. It is certainly something that, before legalization, we almost never saw." Heard adds, "Now we are seeing it quite frequently." "Outside of Colorado, when patients do end up in an emergency room, the diagnosis is often missed. Partly because doctors don't know about CHS, and partly because patients don't want to admit to using a substance that's illegal."[59]

Recall that candida perpetuates addiction to alcohol and drugs. The occurrence of candida in marijuana users has been found to be higher than in those who smoke cigarettes. A study in the *International Journey of Dental Hygiene* urges health-care providers to be aware of cannabis-associated oral side effects, such as xerostomia (dry mouth), leukoedema (gray, blue, or white mucosa), and an increased prevalence and density of *Candida albicans*.[60] A study in the *Journal of Oral Pathology and Medicine* found an "increased prevalence and density of *C. albicans* in cannabis users."[61] A study from UCLA demonstrated that marijuana use decreases the ability of a particular type of white blood cell known as pulmonary alveolar macrophages to destroy *Candida albicans*.[62] Another study found that marijuana use inhibits neutrophil recruitment.[63] Neutrophils, white blood cells used by the immune system to protect the body from pathogenic invasion, are some of the most powerful weapons we have against candida. In a study that involved 1,248 women, one of the primary risk factors for vaginal yeast colonization was the use of marijuana in the previous four months.[64]

GET RID OF YOUR BRA

Women want to be aware that wearing a bra restricts lymph flow, which can allow toxins to build up. Typically lymph fluid carries toxins and wastes away from the breast, but bras inhibit this activity. The more restrictive the bra (underwire and push ups), the more it inhibits lymph flow.[65] Proper functioning of the lymph system is dependent on movement. Subtle bouncing of the breasts when we move, walk, exercise, make love, etc., is crucial to keep the lymph system functioning as it should. It gently massages and stimulates the lymph glands to move toxins out. The lymph system cannot function adequately when a bra is worn. As Dr. Ralph Reed points out, "women evolved under conditions where there was breast movement with every step that they took when they walked or ran."[66]

As a matter of fact bra wearing in general significantly increases your risk for breast cancer. In the work of medical researcher Sydney Singer and his wife, Soma Grismaijer, which is presented in their book, *Dressed to Kill: The Link Between Breast Cancer and Bras,* they found that women who wear a bra 24 hours a day are 125 times more likely to develop breast cancer than women who don't wear a bra at all. Women who wear a bra even 12 hours a day are 113 times more likely to develop breast cancer than women who wear their bra less than 12 hours a day. The correlation between breast cancer and bras is 4 to 12 times higher than the correlation between smoking and lung cancer. Singer and Grismaijer also found that 90 percent of women who have fibrocystic breast disease find relief by not wearing a bra. Restriction caused by bra wearing causes lymph fluid to create lumps, cysts, and fibrous tissue.

It has also been found that wearing a bra decreases the amount of melatonin one produces. Melatonin is a crucial hormone in the regulation of sleep, aging, and immune function and it slows the growth of breast cancer and other cancers. Wearing a bra causes a slight increase in the temperature of breast tissue and the levels of a hormone called prolactin, both of which may contribute to breast cancer.[67] Bra wearing restricts the circulatory system from distributing vital nutrients.[68]

Not only that, one study's data indicated "that the higher clothing pressures exerted by a conventional brassiere have a significant negative impact on the ANS (autonomic nervous system) activity, which is predominantly attributable to the significant decrease in the parasympathetic as well as the thermoregulatory sympathetic nerve activities. Since the ANS activity plays an important role in modulating the internal environment in the human body, excess clothing pressures caused by constricting types of foundation garments on the body would consequently undermine women's health."[69]

It is a myth that the breasts need support. Bras are not going to prevent the breasts from sagging. Sagging is going to happen regardless. It is an unavoidable and natural consequence of age, childbirth, and gravity. Bras may actually cause the breasts to sag more because they inhibit and destroy the breasts' natural ability to support themselves.[70]

The whole purpose of the breast is to provide nourishment for our children. That's it. Breasts are not supposed to remain perky, big, firm, sexy, etc. These definitions were created by society. Women have been brainwashed to believe that their breasts shouldn't sag and they should be kept restricted in a toxic undergarment. It is natural and normal for breasts to change shape and sag after pregnancy, breast-feeding, and as we age. Try to appreciate the beauty in their new look, knowing that they nurtured your beautiful child and performed such a life-affirming activity. Admire the stretch marks, elasticity, sagging, changes in shape, etc. They are beautiful symbols of motherhood and aging. They add character and uniqueness to who you are and should be embraced.

It is not immoral or an invitation for sex to go without a bra. There is not a commandment or rule somewhere that says women should wear bras. It is one of the many destructive, oppressive, and false messages that gets passed from generation to generation and has no real basis in truth. Respect your breasts and get rid of your bra. Dismiss any negative or disapproving looks or comments you may get. Take pride in going without a bra and comfort in knowing you're doing something good for your body. If you have situations in your life where bra wearing would be required because of a certain dress code, such as a work environment, then wear a camisole. Other better choices would be a shelf bra, tank top, cropped camisole, sleeveless T-shirt, or bra top.

SUPPORT THE GUT

The first step in helping to heal the enterocytes and brush border is to eliminate or reduce the presence of the microbe causing the inflammation. Next, all other factors that can contribute to inflammation and leaky gut need to be addressed as well, including parasites, *H. pylori*, sugar, grains, legumes, caffeine, chocolate, alcohol, food additives and preservatives, pesticides, herbicides, artificial sweeteners, heavy metals, birth control pills, too much omega-6, zinc deficiency, lack of sleep, casein, chronic stress, chlorinated drinking water, food sensitivities, steroids, antibiotics, soda pop, artificial sweeteners, NSAIDs, aspirin, ibuprofen, antacids, and other OTC or pharmaceutical drugs. Although each of these factors may cause damage in a different way, the bottom line is that they all cause inflammation in the gut, and inflammation, regardless of where it comes from, may encourage overgrowth of candida and other microbes. Leaky gut creates a vicious cycle, encouraging more overgrowth, which in turn exacerbates leaky gut.

A variety of nutrients may be used over the course of several months to help the epithelial to regenerate. Some of these include colostrum, lactoferrin, lecithin, glutamine, zinc carnosine, vitamins A, C, D, and E, fish oil, curcumin, resveratrol, glutathione, NAC, and digestive enzymes. Brush border enzymes may also be supplemented. As described on page 238, colostrum can decrease gut inflammation, produce antibodies that target candida and other organisms that contribute to leaky gut, and help heal the gut lining. Glutamine provides food for enterocytes, lecithin mends cell membranes, digestive enzymes improve breakdown of food, and fish oil decreases inflammation. Zinc strengthens the gut lining, has a natural antimicrobial effect, and stimulates antibodies. However, some of these nutrients can be problematic for other conditions; please refer to chapter 14 for more information. One of the best substances for healing the gut is colostrum, discussed in more detail on pages 237–239, and lactoferrin, discussed on pages 193–194; 239.

However, memory B cells can keep inflammation going. In chapter 9, you learned that memory B cells are a part of the immune system that are assigned the task of remembering invaders the body has encountered before. Memory B cells may continue to target foods and other substances that were problematic in the past.

REDUCE EXCESS OXALATES

As discussed on page 36, candida produces high levels of oxalates, which can result in excessive levels in the body. Many symptoms of overgrowth may be caused by oxalates, and reducing their levels may provide significant relief. Oxalates are not inherently bad; in most cases the body is equipped to get rid of them effectively. As with most things, it is about balance; oxalates cause problems when they are present in excess. A variety of factors may contribute to the imbalance.

Because certain kinds of kidney stones contain calcium, many people are under the impression that calcium should be avoided if they have kidney stones. According to the Great Plains Laboratory, the exact opposite is true.[71] When calcium is consumed with high-oxalate foods, it combines with the oxalic acid in the intestines to form insoluble calcium oxalate crystals, which are excreted in the stool. This form of oxalate is not absorbed by the body. On the other hand, if calcium levels in the body are low, then the oxalic acid in the gastrointestinal tract is soluble and is readily absorbed by the body. Therefore, adequate calcium levels are crucial for binding to and eliminating excess oxalate.

When yeast is present, elevation of the organic acid arabinose as shown by the organic acid test (OAT) often accompanies high oxalates. However, even if your candida markers are low when your oxalates are high, do not rule out a candida diagnosis. As mentioned previously, as far as lab tests go, the Great Plains OAT is the best tool available for diagnosing candida and the one I recommend. However, candida is a master at evading detection, so a negative lab test does not mean candida is absent. Candida has also been found surrounding the oxalates in kidney stones.

Inflammation in the gut results in increased absorption of oxalates. Inflammation, as discussed, may be caused by candida, bacteria, parasites, consumption of grains, legumes, sugar, or caffeine, and other factors. Vitamin B6 is a vital cofactor needed for one of the enzymes (AGXT) that break down oxalate. If B6 levels in the body are low, the enzyme will be unable to do its job adequately. As mentioned previously, deficiency in vitamin B6 is very common in the individual with candida. The organism binds to B6 and inhibits the vitamin's conversion into its active form, pyridoxal-5-phosphate.

When the healthy gut organisms lactobacillus and bifidus are low, more oxalate is absorbed. Normally the gut flora consume oxalate and turn it into a less harmful substance. Then it is eliminated through the stool. High levels of oxalate can kill *Lactobacillus acidophilus,* however, as well as altering pH and antioxidant levels. This means gut problems can cause high oxalates, and in turn high oxalates can degrade the gut. *Oxalobacter formigenes,* an organism that lives in the colon, relies solely on oxalate for its energy. One study found that adequate colonization of oxalobacter was associated with a 70 percent reduction in risk for developing a recurrent oxalate kidney stone.[72] Therefore, insufficient numbers of this organism may encourage elevated levels of oxalate. *Oxalobacter formigenes* can be found in some specialized forms of probiotics and may be used to reduce oxalate levels.

Other factors can contribute to excess oxalates. Leaky gut allows them to break through the gut barrier and be absorbed in higher numbers. Fructose is converted to oxalates, so high levels of fructose may contribute. Too much fat in the diet can contribute to elevated levels if the individual is not absorbing fatty acids properly—for example, if there is a bile salt deficiency. Unabsorbed fatty acids inhibit calcium's ability to bind with oxalates and move them out through the stool. Bile salt may be deficient for a variety of reasons, including taurine insufficiency, SIBO, reduced function of liver or gallbladder, antibiotics, insufficient gut bacteria, some pharmaceutical medications, low pH, and genetic impairments. Additionally, oxalates "encourage the oxidation of your fats, forming rancid fats in your body."[73] High levels of the omega-6 fatty acid arachidonic acid are also associated with elevated levels of oxalate deposition, another reason why maintaining balance between omega-3 and omega-6 fatty acids is important. The amino acid arginine can help prevent deposition.

Two different genetic variants can impair one's ability to metabolize oxalates: type 1 hyperoxaluria and type 2 hyperoxaluria. Both can be fatal. Type 1 hyperoxaluria involves a deficiency in the enzyme AGXT, and type 2 involves a deficiency in the enzyme GRHPR. If glycolic acid is elevated in addition to oxalate on the organic acids test, it may indicate the presence of the type 1 AGXT genetic variant. However, these can also be elevated by a B6 deficiency. Elevated levels of glyceric acid in addition to elevated levels of oxalates may indicate the presence of the type 2 GRHPR genetic variant. High oxalate in the absence of high levels of glycolic acid or glyceric acid typically rules out a genetic cause for the elevation.

Ethylene glycol, the main component in antifreeze, forms oxalates. As a matter of fact, it is the formation of oxalates in the body that makes antifreeze poisonous. Ethylene glycol is found in some foods, beverages, cosmetics, toothpaste, other personal-care products, and nutritional supplements. Oxalates are metabolites of a variety of other environmental pollutants as well.

In the body, decomposing vitamin C can cause formation of oxalate metabolites during transport and storage. However, this typically only occurs at very high doses of vitamin C (more than 4 grams per day in adults). In a study of eighty-five thousand women there was no correlation between kidney stones and vitamin C intake. An evaluation performed by Great Plains Laboratory on one hundred autistic children found nearly no correlation between vitamin C and oxalate levels in the urine. High doses of vitamin C have been found to significantly reduce the symptoms of autism. Since vitamin C can be highly beneficial for many of the conditions that may accompany high oxalate levels, one should not really be concerned about supplementing with vitamin C unless exceeding the 4 grams per day. That said, fungi like candida and aspergillus can produce vitamin C, which may cause elevated levels in the body. This is something to be aware of, but an elevation in vitamin C would show up on the OAT. It's also important to be aware that excess conversion of vitamin C to oxalates can occur if there are high levels of free copper in the body, so one should have one's copper levels assessed. High copper causes vitamin C breakdown. The same is true for excess iron.[74,75]

Surgery of the small intestine may contribute to high levels of oxalates. So may pancreatic insufficiency. It's also important to stay hydrated to help eliminate oxalates. A vegetarian diet (especially one containing spinach, nuts, and soy protein in many meals) is very high in oxalates, placing vegetarians at a much higher risk.

Many practitioners recommend taking calcium citrate supplements with meals to help reduce oxalate levels, because the calcium combines with and helps excrete the excess oxalates, and the citrate competes with the oxalates for absorption. However, please be aware that in an individual who has an excess glutamate problem in addition to elevated oxalate levels, this could be highly counterproductive. Calcium can increase glutamate levels, which is discussed in more detail in the next section. Magnesium citrate may be used instead, but too high a dose can produce diarrhea. Intravenous magnesium can dissolve oxalates.

Oxalates are also present in food; high-oxalate foods may need to be minimized or restricted (see page 350).

MANAGE GLUTAMATE LEVELS

In chapter 1, we learned that the toxins created by candida can stimulate surges of glutamate production, leading to an elevation in glutamate levels and low GABA levels. Although glutamate is a critical neurotransmitter, when present in excess it is toxic to the brain, impairs gut health, immunity, and detoxification, and encourages sympathetic dominance—all of which create an environment that perpetuates overgrowth of candida and other microbes and incites cravings for sugar and carbs. Many of the symptoms of candida overgrowth may be caused by excess glutamate; managing glutamate levels can significantly improve those symptoms and thus quality of life.

Glutamate is responsible for stimulating brain cells so that you can think, speak, pay attention, process and learn new information, and store that information in short- or long-term memory. Research implies that higher levels of intelligence and superior abilities in learning and memory are directly correlated to higher levels of glutamate receptors, but so are seizures and an increased risk for stroke, because of excess glutamate's toxicity to the brain.

Typically, glutamate is present in the brain in very modest concentrations. At increased concentrations it becomes an excitotoxin that overstimulates brain cells and nerves and leads to cell death and neurological inflammation. These actions can incite a wide variety of symptoms including excitability, restlessness, brain dysfunction, irritability, obsessive-compulsive behaviors, insomnia, anxiety, fear, panic, migraine headaches, self-stimulatory behaviors, and cravings for sugar, carbs, drugs, or alcohol. As you can see, many of these symptoms are associated with candida overgrowth.

Additionally, high glutamate depletes levels of glutathione, which among other actions is vital for managing inflammation, gut health, and detoxification. High glutamate increases the count of the white blood cell eosinophil, which creates inflammation; magnifies the toxicity of any mercury that may be present in the body; and fuels growth of cancer cells and tumors. Furthermore, microbes thrive in a glutamate-rich environment.

When glutamate is present in excess, GABA is deficient, because the two substances counterbalance one another. GABA (gamma-aminobutyric acid) has the exact opposite effect on the brain; it inhibits brain cells, calms and relaxes you, and helps regulate sleep, mood, appetite, sexual arousal, the endocrine system, and the autonomic nervous system. In the gastrointestinal tract, GABA is essential for contractions in the bowels, regulating the lower esophageal sphincter, and supporting adequate quantities of IgA, antibodies that defend the gut and other mucous linings from pathogens.

Hundreds of other toxins can produce this same surge in glutamate activity, including mold toxins, bacterial toxins, Lyme, pesticides, and organic solvents. The brain expert Dr. Sponaugle asserts that even the toxins released by bacteria in the mouth that cause gingivitis and periodontal disease can increase glutamate activity and lead to symptoms like anxiety.[76] I can attest to this personally. I have experienced high anxiety from a bout with gingivitis. Avoiding exposure to molds and environmental toxins as described on pages 385–387 and 380–383 is an important part of keeping glutamate levels in balance.

Glutamate is the precursor to GABA, and excess glutamate is supposed to be automatically converted into GABA. That is how the body maintains balance between the two. However, a variety of factors can inhibit this process, and many people get stuck with too much glutamate. The most common problem is inadequate levels of the enzyme GAD (glutamic acid decarboxylase), which is needed to convert glutamate into GABA. The ability of GAD to convert may be impaired, or its response time may be delayed—problems caused by a variety of potential factors, including some viruses and bacteria (e.g., rubella, streptococcus), impairment in the methylation system, heavy metals, type 1 diabetes, insufficient levels of taurine, or impairment in the pancreas (where GAD is produced). Vitamin B6 is a cofactor that works in conjunction with GAD to create GABA from glutamate, so insufficient levels of this nutrient can impair production as well. The genetic condition known as pyroluria, which can cause a depletion in B6, can indirectly lead to imbalance in GABA and glutamate. Production of GABA is dependent on the Krebs cycle, which can be impaired by heavy metals, deficiencies in key nutrients, or the toxins released by candida and bacteria.

Other excitatory substances besides glutamate can bind with glutamate receptors on cells, potentially contributing to the imbalance in GABA and glutamate. Such substances including the following:

- aspartate (can be converted into glutamate)

- aspartame

- aspartic acid

- glutamate

- glutamic acid

- glutamine

- monosodium glutamate (MSG)

- cysteine (but not N-acetylcysteine. NAC does, however, contain sulfur, which can be counterproductive in high amounts, so it should be used mindfully.)

- homocysteine

- citrate or citric acid (has the potential to be neurotoxic, because most citrate is derived from corn, which can result in trace amounts of glutamate or aspartate during processing)

The more glutamate receptors one has, the more excitatory substances that will be pulled in.

Many drugs target cells' GABA receptors because they have a similar chemical structure: Ativan, Xanax, Klonopin, Valium, Neurontin (gabapentin), and others. They artificially stimulate the receptors without actually increasing GABA production, so they do not address the underlying problem of insufficient production, because there must be some level of GABA present in order for the drugs to have an effect. Furthermore, as we learned previously, anytime a substance is used to artificially stimulate a neurotransmitter, the brain responds by reducing production or responsiveness, which results in greater depletion of the neurotransmitter. For these reasons, any drugs that target GABA receptors or manipulate GABA or glutamate inhibit the body's ability to acquire and maintain balance between the two neurotransmitters. I would put the natural substance phenibut in this category as well. Phenibut is an amino acid derivative that can function as a GABA agonist (binds to and activates GABA receptors). Because it is natural, people are under the false impression that this is a safe way to increase GABA, but it is not. The brain responds to this substance in a similar manner as it does to pharmaceutical benzodiazepines. Most people using this substance report that they develop tolerance and addiction and go through the same horrific withdrawal that is experienced during benzodiazepine withdrawal. As I see it, phenibut is an addictive mind-altering drug, no different than benzodiazepines and can do the same damage. It will perpetuate the imbalance and lead to even bigger problems.

GABA can be depleted or its transmission disrupted by a wide variety of foods and substances, including sugar, caffeine, chocolate, whole grains, high-starch foods, food additives and dyes, and artificial sweeteners and flavorings. GABA needs serotonin to work adequately, so insufficient levels of serotonin, a common complication of candida, can impair GABA function even if enough GABA is present in the system.

Chronic stress is a major contributing factor to depletion of GABA and other inhibitory neurotransmitters (including serotonin), which are needed to modulate the stress response system. They help the mind and body return to the parasympathetic state when the stressful event is over. If the stressful event never ends, these neurotransmitters are called upon repeatedly. As discussed, managing chronic stress and sympathetic dominance is vital for maintaining the balance between GABA and glutamate.

Glutamate and insulin also have a finely balanced reciprocal relationship. High levels of glutamate incite an insulin response, which promptly lowers blood glucose levels. However, glucose is required to manage glutamate levels at the synapses, so if glucose is too low, glutamate levels rise. Therefore, low blood sugar or hypoglycemia not only leads to higher levels of glutamate but also impedes the body's ability to reduce buildup. It is therefore critical to avoid foods that cause a spike in blood sugar and insulin in order to maintain balance between GABA and glutamate (demonstrating again the importance of the diet outlined in chapters 10 and 11). At the same time, controlling glutamate levels is equally as important for keeping insulin from spiking and for managing blood sugar and cravings for sugar and carbs. A ketogenic diet, discussed more in chapter 10, has been found to favor GABA production and to be exceptionally beneficial in the treatment of many conditions associated with excess glutamate, such as seizures and epilepsy.[77] Some people have a genetic mutation (VDR/Fok gene) that impairs the body's ability to regulate blood sugar levels. Dr. Amy Yasko recommends the use of a variety of pancreatic supplements to address this issue.[78]

To complicate things further, glutamate has the ability to bind with six other receptors in the brain—for example, the NMDA receptor, which assists in delivering calcium to the cells and plays a vital role in memory function and synaptic plasticity. Calcium is used by glutamate as the agent that actually inflicts harm on the cell. So if there is an excess of calcium in the body for any reason, it too will contribute to the GABA and glutamate imbalance. Glutamate and calcium together cause an ongoing firing of the neurons, which triggers the release of inflammatory mediators, leading to an increased influx of calcium. It becomes a vicious cycle that results in neural inflammation and cell death. Glutamate has been described as the gun and calcium as the bullet, says Dr. Mark Neveu, former president of the National Foundation of Alternative Medicine.[79] It's important to note that activation of the NMDA receptor also involves glycine, D-serine, and D-alanine; any one of them could allow for more influx of calcium.

Magnesium and zinc help regulate calcium levels. However, according to Dr. Amy Yasko, higher doses of zinc (more than 40 milligrams per day) can also activate the release of glutamate through non-NMDA glutamate receptors, so one must exercise caution with zinc.[80] If calcium is excessively high, other herbs or nutrients may be used to bring it down, including lithium orotate, boswellia, and wormwood. Lithium, as well as iodine and boron, can also assist in lowering glutamate. Calcium intake in food may need to be reduced or limited if calcium is too high. Magnesium is also able to bind to and activate GABA receptors.

Certain genetic polymorphisms can impede the ability to form GABA and some people are genetically predisposed to have a greater number of glutamate receptors than others. The more glutamate receptors one has, the higher the level will be. These people will always tend to lean toward excess glutamate activity, presenting them with a life-long need to monitor their glutamate levels to prevent overstimulation, cell damage, and neurological symptoms.

The amino acid taurine increases the enzyme GAD and consequently GABA levels. Taurine doubles as an inhibitory neurotransmitter and can bind directly to GABA receptors, so it can help to provide balance in that manner as well. High levels of any inhibitory neurotransmitter help lower high levels of any excitatory neurotransmitter. Taurine is found in high levels in the brain and cardiac tissue, indicating its importance in these areas. Taurine is found most abundantly in seafood and animal protein, so it is often deficient in one's diet.

If taurine is deficient, levels of GAD may be low as well; therefore, supplementing with taurine can be used to manage the GABA and glutamate balance and prevent neuron death. Certain genetic polymorphisms (particularly the CBS and SUOX gene mutations) can result in negative effects from taurine supplementation, because these mutations yield excess levels of sulfur in the body and taurine is sulfur based. An individual with either of these gene mutations may need to avoid other supplements that are high in sulfur and limit sulfur-based foods. These mutations can also impair ammonia detoxification. Vitamin B6 and SAMe increase the activity of these gene mutations, so supplementing with them may compound the problem. Candida produces a toxin called beta-alanine that competes with taurine for reabsorption in the kidney, causing taurine to be excreted through the urine. Candida patients, then, may have insufficient taurine levels, contributing to reduced GABA activity. Taurine can combine with magnesium to form magnesium taurate; the two of them may be eliminated together, which can lead to magnesium deficiency. Insufficient levels of magnesium result in excessive levels of calcium, which, as we established earlier, increases glutamate firing.

A diet that does not contain enough of the nutrients needed to make inhibitory neurotransmitters—specifically, animal protein and fat—contributes greatly to an imbalance between glutamate and GABA. Furthermore, proper transmission of any neurotransmitter can't happen without adequate levels of fat, and most people don't consume enough fat. Many foods and substances can deplete GABA levels or disrupt transmission; they should be removed from the diet. These include sugar, whole grains, any high-starch food, caffeine, chocolate, artificial sweeteners and flavorings, food additives, and dyes. Grains (including whole grains) can bring about an excitotoxic effect in some people by causing excessive glutamate formation. Caffeine disrupts normal metabolism of GABA and suppresses serotonin. A low-carb paleo diet as presented in chapters 10 and 11 is ideal for maintaining balance between GABA and glutamate. You may want to note that some fish (e.g., mackerel) have high levels of naturally occurring GABA.

Supplementing directly with GABA is effective for some people. However, I frequently work with clients who get a stimulating effect from supplementation with GABA. The same is true for me. Be sure to monitor your response. GABA can be converted back into glutamine, which is then converted back into glutamate through a metabolic pathway called the GABA shunt. This is how GABA supplementation can end up increasing glutamate in some people. According to brain expert Dr. Datis Kharrazian, if you have any effect from GABA (positive or negative), that means you probably have leaky brain.

In his book, *Why Isn't My Brain Working*, he explains that in a healthy brain, the junctions in the blood-brain barrier only permit nanoparticles to pass through. GABA "exceeds the nanoparticle size and does not have a blood-brain barrier transport protein." It should not be able to cross the blood-brain barrier. If it does, then this suggests there is leaky brain.

As a matter of fact, Dr. Kharrazian uses GABA supplementation as a screening tool to determine whether one has leaky brain or not, calling it the GABA Challenge Test. He also states you shouldn't take GABA supplementation, even if you have a positive effect, "because you risk shutting down your GABA receptor sites." If you have no effect from GABA, this is good sign, you most likely to do not have leaky brain. [81]

As I've highlighted repeatedly, environmental toxins like pesticides, air pollution, heavy metals, and chemicals found in everyday household and personal-care products all deplete and disrupt normal production and function of neurotransmitters. Therefore, another critical component for maintaining sufficient levels of GABA is to reduce exposure to these toxins by living an environmentally friendly lifestyle and eating organic.

One of the biggest contributors to an imbalance between GABA and glutamate is the presence of excitotoxins in the diet. Many foods and nutritional supplements contain excitotoxins (listed above), or they contain substances that can prompt the body to produce them. These foods and substances should be avoided by anyone trying to balance GABA and glutamate levels and anyone who leans toward excess glutamate. Other foods that may increase glutamate are discussed in chapter 11.

Many nutritional supplements can increase glutamate levels as well, including whey powder, amino acid formulas, protein powders, body-building formulas, anything with aspartate or aspartic acid, glutamic acid, L-cysteine, glutathione, glycine (in some people who already have excess glutamate), too much calcium, D-serine, pectin, D-alanine, citrate or citric acid derived from corn, zinc in excess of 40 mg per day, and, as mentioned, GABA itself. Many of these nutrients are discussed in more detail on pages 344–347. Two supplements that are commonly prescribed to increase GABA (glutamine and l-theanine) can actually cause an elevation in glutamate in some people due to the GABA shunt. Before glutamine is converted into GABA, it first becomes glutamate, and if you aren't converting your glutamate to GABA for any of the many reasons we listed above, then you end up with nothing but a bunch of excess glutamate. Additionally, glutamine and glutamate convert back and forth into one another. Anyone who has an issue with excess glutamate should probably avoid supplementation with glutamine. L-theanine is a glutamate analog, which means if you fall in the category of people who is having problems converting your glutamate to GABA, this could lead to excess glutamate rather than GABA. Additionally l-theanine is derived from tea or mushrooms; it is an artificial means of supplementing glutamate, not natural. Furthermore, it could have traces of caffeine or fungi from its original source, which could be problematic as well. Therefore, l-theanine may work for some, but have the opposite effect for others. I prefer to avoid it, unless I am working with someone who is detoxing from drugs and alcohol, in which case the need may outweigh the risks, but glutamine or lithium would be better choices.

Excess glutamate in the system that results from genetic mutations, methylation problems, and the like will also generate more glutamate receptors. As is true for all neurotransmitters, ensuring that you get adequate sleep is vital for normal functioning, because sleep deprivation causes neurons to lose sensitivity to neurotransmitters, thus impairing communication.

Vitamin K is important for GABA and glutamate balance as it is needed for healthy calcium metabolism. It reacts with glutamate and calcium to deliver calcium to the bones and teeth, and it prevents accumulation of excess calcium, which could contribute to cell death. Vitamin K is a fat-soluble vitamin; however, unlike other fat soluble vitamins, it is not stored in the body and must be consumed on a daily basis. Typically, vitamin K is produced when the friendly flora in the gut process leafy greens, but if dysbiosis is present, as it is with candida or SIBO, or if you're not eating leafy greens, then vitamin K is produced in insufficient quantities, and deficiency may develop.[82]

The pancreas uses vitamin K abundantly for sugar regulation. Like the brain, the pancreas is very vulnerable to accumulation of excessive glutamate or other excitotoxins, which impair regulation of sugar.[83] As discussed previously, too much or too little insulin or glucose can contribute to excess glutamate. As you can see, keeping glutamate and GABA in balance is critical for the health of the pancreas and all its functions, and the health of the pancreas is in turn vital for maintaining the balance.

One of the greatest aspects of GABA is that it also opposes norepinephrine, your other primary excitatory neurotransmitter, which is also important for stimulation, but it sets off the stress response system. Like glutamate, norepinephrine is also toxic to the brain when it is in excess. Excess norepinephrine can produce many of the same kinds of symptoms that excess glutamate produces and it can sometimes be hard to tell the difference between the two. Fortunately, when you focus on increasing your gamma-aminobutyric acid then you help reduce excess norepinephrine in addition to excess glutamate. It's also important to take note that it is not possible to eliminate every single source of glutamate, nor do you want to. Remember that glutamate is vital for proper brain function in small concentrations; the goal is to prevent excess.

BALANCE HISTAMINE

We've learned that overgrowth of candida and bacteria often results in elevated levels of histamine, which can be responsible for many of the symptoms one experiences with these conditions. Lowering histamine can eliminate many symptoms of candida overgrowth and improve the quality of life. Please review the applicable sections in chapters 1, 6, and 11 for detailed information about histamine.

To recap, histamine is a molecule produced in the body and is involved in the immune response, gastric acid production, vasodilation, cardiac stimulation, and most smooth-muscle contraction (in the ileum, bronchi, and uterus). It also acts as an excitatory neurotransmitter in the brain. It is derived from decarboxylation of the amino acid histidine via the enzyme L-histidine decarboxylase with vitamin B6 as a cofactor.

The majority of histamine is generated, stored, and released by mast cells or basophils as part of an immune response toward foreign invaders, but non mast cell histamine is found in the brain where it operates as a stimulatory neurotransmitter. As a neurotransmitter, it is involved in regulating aspects of the sleep/wake cycle, body temperature, appetite, mood, learning, memory, homeostasis of the endocrine system, pain sensitivity, libido, encoding and processing harmful stimuli in the nervous system, and regulating the release of serotonin, dopamine, and norepinephrine. It counterbalances dopamine levels. Histamine is also produced by enterochromaffin-like cells in mucosa underneath the epithelium, where it plays a role in the stimulation of hydrochloric acid and pepsinogen (pepsin) and it is also what causes tears to flow.[84,85,86]

Histamine exerts its effects by acting on H1, H2, H3, and H4 receptors. It is synthesized all over the body, but it is more highly concentrated in the lungs, gastrointestinal tract, and skin. The action exerted depends on which type of receptor histamine reacts with, and the receptor it interacts with depends on where histamine is released.

H1 receptors are located in most smooth muscle, endothelial cells (blood vessels), and the brain. They are critical for the sleep/wake cycle (e.g., sleepiness or insomnia) and are associated with motion sickness, vasodilation, hives, bronchoconstriction, hay fever, seasonal allergies, and possibly the increased peristalsis that accompanies food allergies.

H2 receptors are located in gastric parietal cells, heart, uterus, and vascular smooth muscle. They are associated with gastric acid production, heart rate, cardiac output, abdominal pain, nausea, gastroenteritis, and ulcers. H2 receptors are also found on neutrophils, where they can inhibit production of antibodies and cytokines.

H3 receptors are located in the central nervous system. They are involved in modulating neurotransmission and the synthesis of histamine.

H4 receptors are located in mast cells, thymus, spleen, bone marrow, colon, small intestine, and basophils. They are associated with the inflammatory response and with regulating the release of white blood cells from bone marrow.[87,88]

Problems with abnormally high levels of brain histamine (known as histadelia) were first identified by Dr. Carl Pfeiffer in his book *Nutrition and Mental Illness* many years ago. It can lead to headaches and migraines, insomnia or disrupted sleep, hyperactivity, attention deficit, depression, obsessive compulsive tendencies, high libido, sexual addiction, gambling addiction, abnormal fears, a racing brain, crying easily, aggressiveness, and schizophrenia. Alcohol, heroin, and other narcotics block histamine, providing some temporary relief from the high histamine symptoms, thus why many high histamine people become addicted to drugs and alcohol.[89]

Low levels of brain histamine (histapenia), also identified by Dr. Pfeiffer, may result in paranoia, ear ringing, visual or auditory hallucinations, fatigue, low libido, sensitivity to medications, irritability, and grandiose plans without the energy to see them through. If histamine is too low, then dopamine levels become elevated, which can produce many psychological disturbances. Histamine levels are found to be lower in the brains of people with Alzheimer's and elevated in people with Parkinson's.

High histamine in other parts of the body produce watery eyes, runny nose, congestion, sneezing, wheezing, itching, hives, inflammation, heart palpitations, fainting, changes in blood pressure (up or down), gastrointestinal disturbances (e.g., nausea or vomiting), and motion sickness to name a few. While too little could lead to insufficient gastric acid secretion that could contribute to microbial overgrowth and gastrointestinal problems, as with all things in the body, the key with histamine is balance; too much or too little will lead to negative effects. That said, it seems that excess histamine is a more common problem than low histamine, especially if we are dealing with candida and/or SIBO, so that is what we will primarily focus on in this discussion.

Many factors can contribute to elevated histamine. As discussed in chapter 1, it can be the result of candida antigens or leaky gut. However, some types of bacteria have the ability to convert the amino acid histidine into histamine as well, so when they are present on certain foods, they may generate histamine. If the level of histamine they create on the food is high, it can lead to excessive levels of histamine within the body in susceptible people when the food is eaten (a phenomenon known as histamine intolerance). A variety of different strains within the following genera and species of bacteria may produce histamine, lactobacillus, clostridium, *Escherichia coli,* staphylococcus, streptococcus, klebsiella, morganella, enterobacter, proteus, acinetobacter, pseudomonas, aeromonas, vibrio, plesiomonas, pediococcus, and micrococcus. Elevated levels of any of these bacteria in an individual's colon or small intestine may produce an excess of histamine.

It is believed that histamine intolerance is caused by insufficient levels of the enzyme diamine oxidase (DAO), which breaks down histamine. When too many high histamine foods are eaten, it causes an excess of histamine that may lead to a wide variety of symptoms like migraines or vascular headaches, gastrointestinal disturbances (constipation, diarrhea, flatulence, distention, heartburn, indigestion, acid reflux), fatigue, throat tightening, autonomic nervous system dysregulation, dizziness, restless leg syndrome, joint and muscle pain, hiccups, red flushing across the lower neck and upper chest known as histamine flush, low blood pressure, anxiety or panic attacks, heart racing, nasal congestion, runny nose, itching of eyes, ears, and nose, hives, watery and red eyes, tinnitus, and on rare occasion a loss of consciousness for brief periods and much more. Reducing consumption of foods that are high in histamine can provide significant relief from symptoms. However, diamine oxidase is produced by enterocytes (cells) in the small intestine. Therefore, one of the factors that can cause a deficiency in diamine oxidase is damage to the small intestine caused by bacterial overgrowth, candida, or other microbes. If the gut is damaged, then DAO may not be secreted in sufficient amounts. See chapter 6, on SIBO, for more information.

Furthermore, since some species of bacteria can convert histidine into histamine, the overgrowth of these types of bacteria in the gastrointestinal tract itself can contribute to higher levels of histamine within your body, as they will convert the histidine in your diet into histamine. So when you have bacterial overgrowth, your histamine levels may already be elevated, and then when foods that are high in histamine are eaten, then it becomes even more excessive. When that is the case, then histamine intolerance may improve, and possibly disappear, if one achieves some healing in the gut and reduces their level of microbial overgrowth.

After some healing has taken place, it may be possible to slowly reintroduce some high-histamine foods into the diet and see how you do. That said, however, until gut and bacteria issues are resolved, high-histamine foods will need to be limited. On the other hand, even if you do produce enough of the enzymes that break down histamine, if you have candida or bacterial overgrowth and eat a diet high in histamine foods, the enzymes may be unable to keep up, even if no other roadblocks are present. Intolerance develops when there is an imbalance between what's coming in and the body's ability to break it down. Furthermore, the pH of the gut is important in both high and low histamine; histamine release in the gastrointestinal tract is inhibited when gut pH is too low, leading to impaired production of hydrochloric acid.

Recall from chapter 6 that a deficiency in DAO can be caused by a variety of factors: a genetic polymorphism, low levels of certain nutrients (copper, vitamin C, vitamin B6), or impairment of the lymphatic system. That means in some cases histamine intolerance will be lifelong, requiring ongoing restriction of high-histamine foods. The bacteria *H. pylori* can also inhibit DAO.

Furthermore, DAO is not the only mechanism used by the body to break down histamine, it is also achieved by another enzyme called N-methyltransferase (HMT) and requires the methylation process to do so. In most tissue throughout the body, histamine is deactivated by DAO or N-methyltransferase. However, in the central nervous system, it is deactivated with N-methyltransferase only, because DAO is not found in the central nervous system.[90,91] Therefore, high brain histamine (histadelia) is generally a biochemical imbalance with this enzyme and the methylation process, particularly under-methylating. In people who have low brain histamine, then it is believed to be due to over-methylation. However, HMT is also produced by enterocytes in the small intestine, so bacteria or candida or anything contributing to a damaged gut could affect this enzyme as well. One may have a genetic polymorphism that impairs their ability to produce HMT as well.

Additionally, when leaky gut is present due to this damage to the gut, then histamine can get into the bloodstream without being acted upon by DAO or HMT. Furthermore, histamine is released when undigested food particles escape through the leaky gut into the bloodstream and the immune system goes after them, so leaky gut itself can generate higher levels of histamine. Plus, the toxins released by candida or bacteria can also incite the release of histamine, thus making the histamine load even higher. Each time the immune system launches an attack against the toxins, protein, or microbe then inflammation is generated, which then perpetuates the whole cycle. Additionally, Sarah Ballantyne, author of *The Paleo Approach*, explains that if basal cells are activated because of an autoimmune disorder or environmental allergy, then one's baseline level of histamine may be elevated, which would make the person more susceptible to histamine in his or her food.[92]

Since methylation can be impaired by candida, bacteria, and other microbes, then SIBO or candida overgrowth could potentially contribute to histadelia or histamine intolerance in this manner as well, but methylation is a very complex issue that can have many contributing factors like deficiencies in nutrients like folate, B12, B6, magnesium or SAMe, a mutation in the MTHFR gene or other polymorphisms in the HNMT gene (codes for the enzyme N-methyltransferase) itself. Therefore, histadelia (high brain histamine) may also require ongoing restriction of high histamine foods as well as a variety of other nutritional supplements like methionine to correct the imbalance in methylation.

Additionally, since both enzymes needed to break down histamine (DAO and HMT) are produced within enterocytes, then other things that damage the gut besides bacteria and candida could be potential contributors and should be avoided as well to promote healthy enterocytes, like caffeine, wheat and other grains, legumes, alcohol, NSAIDs, chlorinated drinking water, proton pump inhibitors, etc.

Other factors that can elevate histamine levels include the following:[93]

Drugs

There's an array of drugs that can inhibit the activity of DAO, which include some NSAIDs (e.g., ibuprofen and aspirin); antidepressants (e.g., Cymbalta, Zoloft, Effexor, Prozac); muscle relaxants; diuretics; histamine-2 blockers (e.g., Tagamet, Pepcid, Zantac); antihistamines (e.g., Allegra, Zyrtec, Benadryl); immune modulators; antiarrhythmics; local anesthetics; antihypertensives; the supplement N-acetylcysteine (NAC).

High-Intensity Exercise

High-intensity exercise, particularly when done in a warm environment, can trigger the release of histamine.

Sunshine

Ultraviolet light can stimulate the release of histamine. People who feel they are "allergic" to the sun are most likely having a histamine response. If you sneeze when you look toward the sun or get hives when exposed to the sun, it is a sign of a histamine reaction. Heat, with or without sunshine, stimulates release as well.

High Estrogen

People with elevated estrogen (estrogen dominance) may have a higher level of histamine response and, as we learned previously, many individuals with candida often have high levels of estrogen.

Stress

Stress increases histamine and decreases the body's ability to metabolize it.

A variety of nutritional supplements may be used to reduce histamine levels, depending on the underlying problems. Methionine, calcium, and magnesium are often used to address high histamine caused by undermethylation. Vitamin C has a mild antihistamine effect when used consistently, so it can be used to help alleviate symptoms. Flavonoids (molecules found in some plant foods) such as quercetin have been shown to inhibit the release of histamine and proinflammatory cytokines in mast cells.[94] There are DAO supplements on the market that replace the missing DAO enzyme and some people find helpful, but keep in mind that they only apply to the situation where DAO is the sole problem; this would not address all the other issues that can cause high histamine that we discussed. In the event of a severe histamine reaction, a pharmaceutical-based antihistamine may be effective, but avoid using it on a daily basis as it will perpetuate the problem.

And don't forget to pay attention to the numerous foods that are high in histamine (see pages 347–349) and probiotics on page 211. If you have high histamine, these foods and substances need moderated or eliminated.

If brain histamine is low, a high-protein diet is used to help restore levels. Additionally, low histamine is usually accompanied by high copper, one of the nutrients used in the breakdown of histamine. In turn, low histamine encourages a greater buildup of copper. Supplements that can help balance copper and increase histamine include zinc, manganese, niacin (vitamin B3), and vitamin C. Other steps may be needed to address high copper, you should discuss this issue with a knowledgeable practitioner, if it applies to you. Research suggests that people with blood type A are more prone to sequestering copper. Low histamine may result from a mutation in histidine decarboxylase, the gene that encodes for the enzyme L-histidine decarboxylase, which is needed to synthesize histamine. This mutation has been found to be associated with Tourette syndrome.

HISTAMINE TESTING

You can assess histamine levels through various tests. Which one to use depends on which factor you want to investigate. A genetic test can evaluate whether there are mutations in the genes associated with the enzymes DAO and HMT, in the MTHFR gene, or in other genes associated with methylation. There's a lab test that can analyze the ratio of histamine to DAO. A high ratio would indicate that the DAO level is insufficient for handling the histamine level. A blood histamine test can identify high or low levels. Testing copper levels may also be beneficial; if copper is high, then histamine is probably low.

The easiest, most affordable, and most effective way by far to assess whether your histamine is high is by observing your symptoms. A histamine challenge test can provide a very clear indication if you are high in histamine or intolerant. Simply consume high-histamine foods and monitor your response. Then try a low-histamine diet to see if it relieves some of your symptoms. Alternatively, you can do an elimination diet, in which you simply remove high-histamine foods and observe if symptoms improve, and then reintroduce them one at a time to see if symptoms reappear. You can also find a simple questionnaire for screening histamine levels, in the book *Depression Free Naturally* by Joan Mathews Larson.[95]

Both excess histamine and excess glutamate create an imbalance in the autonomic nervous system, which puts the body in a state of chronic sympathetic arousal—a condition with many negative consequences that I've discussed at length in this book—all of which encourages overgrowth of candida and other microbes, degradation of health, or exacerbation of conditions that already exist. As you can see, it is critical for your physical, emotional, and spiritual health to keep them both in balance, and it is important to understand all the interconnected factors that may be involved.

NEUROTRANSMITTER TESTING

Many of my clients come to me who have seen a practitioner who has tested their neurotransmitter levels with a blood or urine test. It is critical to be aware that this type of neurotransmitter testing is not a reliable or accurate method of assessment. Taking supplementation based on these results can be highly counterproductive and lead to a significant setback in health. I had a very negative experience with this type of testing myself before I knew better and so have a lot of my clients.

Cerebrospinal fluid (CSF) is the only method that can tell us the actual level of neurotransmitters in the brain. Blood platelet testing results correspond very closely to CSF, but only for dopamine, norepenephrine, and serotonin—not GABA or endorphins. Additionally, blood platelet testing isn't available at many labs besides Vitamin Diagnostics outside a research setting.

Mental health counselor Julia Ross writes in a *Townsend* article, testing performed at Vitamin Diagnostics, by Dr. Audhya's staff found that neither urine nor blood plasma results correspond to cerebrospinal fluid testing results. According to Dr. Audhya, "Levels of serotonin and the catecholamines are known to be stable and abundant in the blood platelets, but not in blood plasma, the levels of which are extremely reactive to stress (even the stress of the blood draw!)." Additionally, "levels of neurotransmitters in urine vary rapidly in reaction to both stress, chemistry and diet-related (especially pH) changes."[96]

Ross also writes, "Because neurotransmitter levels are so low in plasma, plasma testing is used primarily to track the dramatic increases in serotonin and catecholamines that can result from malignant tumors that secrete large amounts of one or the other of these neurotransmitters." So they can be beneficial in this capacity.

When I was studying under Dr. Charles Gant at the Academy of Functional Medicine, he also taught that urine and plasma testing did not tell us anything about neurotransmitter levels in the brain.[97]

Gant recommends testing for the neurotransmitter precursors (aminos, B vitamins, minerals, and fatty acids) and neurotransmitter metabolites through an organic acids test, an amino acid plasma, and an RBC mineral test. However, he also uses a written questionnaire that he designed as a screening tool as well. Ross also uses a written questionnaire that she designed. In my opinion, we can make a very good educated guess about what neurotransmitters are high or low simply by our symptoms, but I also use both Gant's and Ross's methods as well.

CANDIDA MAINTENANCE

Throughout the pages of this book we have learned that candida can mutate and develop resistance to just about any attempt at eradication. It can run and hide, lie dormant and repopulate later, adapt to just about any condition it finds itself in, create biofilms that protect it, manipulate the internal environment of its host to fit its needs, and disable the host's immune system. Additionally, it is commonly found in conjunction with bacteria, parasites, and viruses, which have similar characteristics that compound the issue even further. There is a high failure rate in the treatment of candida and other microbial overgrowth like SIBO. Therefore, the healing plan must be diverse, repeated, and ever changing to catch candida and its coconspirators off guard before they can adapt. It must also address in a holistic manner the many different factors usually present along with microbial overgrowth.

As discussed in the introduction, the process of healing chronic candida in most cases is lifelong, and changes in diet and lifestyle must be permanent. If one returns to old eating patterns and lifestyle choices, then not only will candida and other microbes return but so will the addiction to sugar and carbs and the many symptoms associated with each of these issues. Maintenance for candida and most other microbial issues must be ongoing to sustain any healing and improvement in symptoms and to manage sympathetic dominance.

Critics of my stance on chronic candida may say that the real problem lies in the gut and that the focus needs to be on eliminating dysbiosis. This is a valid point. They are absolutely right. However, the reality at this time is that we simply do not have the tools that enable us to do so. Due to all the factors presented in this book (biofilms, mutation, resistance, virulence, adaptation, disarming of the immune system, dormancy, manipulation of the environment to suit their needs, electromagnetic pollution, environmental toxins), microbes are able to outsmart us a lot of the time. Microbes have been around a lot longer than we have, and they have developed a multitude of ingenious ways to survive and advance their species. In order to improve complete remission rates and eliminate the need for strict dietary controls and the challenges of ongoing maintenance, future treatment needs to focus on how we can break down biofilms, prevent mutation, resistance, and adaptation, and outmaneuver the microbes at their own game. Many people are working diligently on these issues as I write, and new and exciting discoveries are made every day. Hopefully I will one day write a book that outlines these amazing findings, but until then it is management and damage control that will enable those of us with chronic candida to achieve the highest level of health possible and live our lives to the fullest.

CHAPTER 14

Choosing the Right Supplements and Dealing with Intolerance

C hronic candida (and other microbial overgrowth) frequently leads to nutritional deficiencies for a variety of reasons that I've discussed throughout this book. The microbes consume the host's nutrients for survival and development of the biofilm, and when the gut is compromised by candida and other microbes, the body's ability to absorb nutrients is impaired. Toxins can block nutrients from being utilized. The body needs lots of nutrients to eliminate those toxins and to deal with the stress of fighting a chronic condition, and after a while its nutritional resources can become drained—the demand for nutrients can exceed the supply.

Nutritional deficiencies may also exist prior to the presence of candida overgrowth as a result of chronic stress or a diet that is high in sugar, grains, legumes, and refined foods and lacking in animal protein and fat. Furthermore, modern farming practices have stripped the soil (and thus our food) of nutrients, which can weaken the adrenal glands, compromise the immune system, contribute to sympathetic dominance, degrade the health of the gut, and make one vulnerable to candida overgrowth.

It doesn't really matter which came first—the chronic candida or the nutritional deficiency. Either can perpetuate overgrowth, and to confuse matters, many of the symptoms of nutritional deficiencies overlap with the symptoms of candida (e.g., depression, anxiety, irritability, skin conditions, fatigue, headaches, muscle aches, chronic pain, and cravings for sugar, carbs, and other mind-altering substances). Sometimes it can be challenging to tease the two apart.

Careful supplementation can be beneficial in the healing journey for candida. The right nutrients can help alleviate many symptoms, improve detoxification, reduce sympathetic dominance, correct brain function and gut health, and strengthen the body's ability to fight off candida and other microbes. On the other hand, some nutritional supplements can be counterproductive and actually perpetuate candida overgrowth if they provide the microbes with fuel or contribute to sympathetic dominance. And a nutrient that helps support one health issue may aggravate another. So it's important to educate yourself before you begin supplementation.

Many people with candida have problems tolerating supplements that could otherwise be helpful; they have negative reactions to them or feel worse after taking them. The nutrients needed by each person will depend on what species and strains of yeast are involved, how well the detoxification system is working, and any other conditions that may accompany the yeast problem. We'll take a look at each of these issues in more detail.

BASIC SUPPLEMENTS

Vitamin C

In chapter 8 I wrote about the importance of vitamin C to help reduce die-off and keep the bowels moving, and in chapter 9 I mentioned that it helps boost the immune system and reduce the inflammation and oxidative stress associated with candida. Vitamin C is also needed in the production of acetylcholine, the primary neurotransmitter that regulates the autonomic nervous system. It is critical for supporting the adrenal glands, which are usually taxed in the individual with candida and which will perpetuate overgrowth if not supported. Vitamin C is used in the production of cortisol and other hormones produced by the adrenal glands, where it is found in high concentrations. As a matter of fact, the adrenal glands contain more vitamin C than any other part of the body.[1] Vitamin C also helps protect the body from the toxins that are created when these hormones are metabolized.[2] And unbuffered vitamin C can increase gut pH if you are too alkaline, which will help fight off candida.

Buffered vitamin C in the form of calcium ascorbate, magnesium ascorbate, and potassium ascorbate is more readily absorbed than straight ascorbic acid and is easier on the gastrointestinal tract. Plus, those forms provide calcium, magnesium, and potassium, which can become imbalanced when taking high-dose vitamin C. Be sure your vitamin C does not contain any form of sugar; many tablets and lozenges do. Ascorbyl palmitate is another highly absorbable form and is fat soluble, so unlike most forms of vitamin C it can be stored in the body for use at a later date, but it can be hard on the stomach. Ascorbic acid is water soluble, so it will be utilized at consumption and any extra will be flushed through the urine. Liposomal vitamin C can enhance absorption even more. A combination of the different forms can be used to achieve each of their desired effects.

High-dose vitamin C may provide other benefits—for example, reducing excess LDL and increasing HDL, preventing plaque buildup, reducing carcinogens, and increasing the formation of collagen. It can also kill bacteria directly and neutralize their toxins. Vitamin C when used consistently has an antihistamine effect, so it can be used to lower histamine levels and to alleviate allergic reactions to yeasts, foods, and other antigens. It must be taken daily to get an antihistamine effect, as it must first reach a particular level of concentration in the body. Vitamin C is also a mild chelator, so it can be used in this capacity as well.

High doses of buffered vitamin C powder taken on a daily basis can be used to keep the bowels loose and moving. Magnesium can be used in the short term for this purpose, but it should not be utilized long term without supplementation of calcium; it can cause an imbalance in the important calcium/magnesium ratio.

Vitamin C can also be found abundantly in a variety of foods: Brussels sprouts, kale, cauliflower, broccoli, and strawberries.

It can significantly reduce symptoms of withdrawal from giving up sugar, carbs, nicotine, caffeine, and even alcohol and drugs, enabling a person to remain committed to the candida diet with more comfort. In combination with a high-protein diet (like the one presented in chapters 10 and 11), very high doses of vitamin C have been shown to be effective for eliminating withdrawal symptoms associated with heroin addiction. In higher dosages, it is more effective than methadone in eliminating cravings for the drug.[3]

According to some doctors, like the late Dr. Robert Atkins, healthy people need at least 1,000 mg of vitamin C a day, and those dealing with a chronic health condition require more. As is the case when taking vitamin C for microbe die-off and bowel regularity, supplement to bowel tolerance—that is, take as much as your body can handle comfortably without producing diarrhea. According to Dr. Robert Cathcart, who developed the bowel tolerance system, the more vitamin C your body can take without producing diarrhea, the more serious the health issue.[4] If one needs higher doses of vitamin C than their bowels allow, then intravenous vitamin C can circumvent this problem.

Pantethine

I've talked about the importance of pantethine (the active form of vitamin B5) for reducing die-off because of its ability to improve detoxification and increase production of the aldehyde dehydrogenase enzymes. This group of enzymes eliminates candida's primary byproducts, acetaldehyde and alcohol, which are responsible for many of the symptoms of candida: brain fog, headaches, fatigue, memory problems, chronic pain, and more. Pantethine is also the most critical nutrient for the adrenal glands to produce cortisol and other hormones. Pantethine increases levels of coenzyme A (CoA), which, you may recall, is a cofactor in numerous enzymatic pathways. It is the foundation for the formation of hormones produced by the adrenal glands, as well as sex hormones, cholesterol, hemoglobin, bile, and the neurotransmitter acetylcholine that is so vital for the autonomic nervous system. It is pivotal in the breakdown of protein, fats, and carbohydrates and in energy production. It also helps increase our level of omega-3 fatty acids (EPA and DHA). In Dr. Atkins's book, *Vita Nutrient Solution,* he states that pantethine is so effective at improving the production of cortisone and increasing omega-3, thereby reducing inflammation, that it is often used for autoimmune disorders, arthritis, colitis, Crohn's, and other inflammatory conditions. The dosage of pantethine as support for the adrenal glands may be as high as 1,200 to 1,800 mg, depending on the severity of the damage and how the adrenal glands respond. It should be combined with vitamin C, as discussed above. The two nutrients together provide the support needed for the adrenals to function more effectively.

Pantethine also decreases LDL and increases HDL, strengthens metabolism in the heart muscle, strengthens the heart's contractions, and helps increase the growth of *Lactobacillus bulgaricus,* bifidobacterium, and other friendly bacteria that can help fight off candida. For this reason, pantethine can be used when taking an antibiotic to minimize the killing off of good bacteria. Cardiologist Robert Atkins found that pantethine was more effective than any cholesterol-lowering drug and yielded no side effects, and it also rebalanced levels of triglycerides and other fats in the blood.[5]

Pantothenic acid is converted into pantethine, which is then converted into coenzyme A. However, many people don't make the conversion from pantothenic acid to pantethine very well. Taking pantethine eliminates this problem. It makes twice as much coenzyme A as pantothenic acid. On the other hand, Dr. Atkins points out that pantothenic acid offers additional benefits for some conditions, like acne, gout, surgical wound healing, and burning feet caused by inflammation, so some practitioners recommend a combination of pantethine and pantothenic acid in a one-to-one ratio.[6]

Dosages: Pantethine and Vitamin C

For both vitamin C and pantethine, dosage should be started low and gradually increased. Moving too quickly or taking too much can cause the adrenal glands to crash. Furthermore, they should be taken in divided doses, throughout the day, not all at once, and should not be taken too late in the afternoon (after dinner) or they could have a stimulating effect that disrupts sleep.[7]

Dosage of both is dependent on the stage of adrenal fatigue. As discussed on pages 395–396, adrenal fatigue occurs on a spectrum. Someone in an earlier stage will most likely need lower doses of these nutrients than someone in a more advanced stage. Dosage may need to be adjusted as the adrenal glands strengthen or if a setback occurs. Taking the correct dose is important: not enough may fail to improve symptoms, but too much can be too stimulating. The right dosage for one person could be counterproductive for another; your dose should be individualized for your biochemical needs depending on how your body responds.

Molybdenum

In chapter 8, we learned that the mineral molybdenum helps the body increase production of the enzymes aldehyde dehydrogenase and aldehyde oxidase, both of which help eliminate the acetaldehyde and alcohol that are produced by candida overgrowth. It is critical for dealing with die-off. It should be taken in conjunction with pantethine to increase this activity even more. Molybdenum also helps form an enzyme in the mitochondria known as sulfite oxidase, which is needed to break down sulfite and eliminate it from the body. It is needed to metabolize the sulfur compounds that occur naturally in food. Many people with candida overgrowth are intolerant of sulfur, possibly due to insufficient levels of molybdenum. (Some genetic polymorphisms can cause an increase in bodily sulfur levels—for example, the CBS and SUOX gene mutations. To learn how to address these mutations, take a look at Dr. Amy Yasko's book, *Autism: Pathways to Recovery.*) Molybdenum also plays a role in ATP production, which means it can help boost low energy.

Molybdenum, in combination with pantethine, can be highly beneficial for the individual with chemical sensitivities, which commonly occur in people with candida overgrowth. Many toxins in the environment, particularly fragrances and other formaldehyde-based chemicals, are eliminated from the body with the help of the enzymes aldehyde dehydrogenase and aldehyde oxidase. These toxins are similar in structure to acetaldehyde, and if the body is overloaded with acetaldehyde from candida overgrowth, it can have a hard time handling environmental toxins. Acetaldehyde also inhibits phase 1 detoxification. By reducing acetaldehyde, molybdenum decongests the liver and enables it to handle the environmental toxins more effectively, reducing sensitivity to them.

Next to the changes I made in my diet and lifestyle, supplementing with a combination of molybdenum and pantethine has helped me more than anything else in my healing journey. They significantly improved my quality of life by lowering my sensitivity to fragrances, improving brain fog and cognitive function, eliminating widespread chronic pain, and enabling me to tolerate sulfur. Later, when I was going through menopause and had a serious adrenal crash, a higher dose of pantethine in combination with vitamin C was central to strengthening my adrenal glands and restoring my ability to produce cortisol and DHEA.

Prior to the use of molybdenum and pantethine, I was so sensitive to perfume and other fragrances that it was almost impossible for me to go into public places. I was so sensitive to sulfur that I couldn't eat sulfur-based foods like cruciferous vegetables, and I endured frequent bouts of chronic, widespread pain. After beginning supplementation with these nutrients, I could go into public places with minimal discomfort, could eat cruciferous vegetables freely, and experienced relief from the chronic pain. When my adrenal glands crashed during menopause, my cortisol and DHEA levels flatlined, as demonstrated by the adrenal cortisol saliva test. After supplementing with high-dose pantethine and vitamin C for a couple of years, my production returned to normal. Prior to molybdenum I frequently smelled sulfur in the air, and it significantly impaired my brain function; after supplementation, I rarely smell it, and when I do my tolerance for it is much higher.

It is important to be aware that taking molybdenum long term can cause a decrease in copper, so be sure to monitor your copper levels, as insufficient levels of copper can lead to numerous problems as well, including overgrowth of yeast. This is usually an issue with high-dose molybdenum, but be cautious anyhow. It may be necessary to supplement with copper, but be careful because too much copper is toxic and can contribute to overgrowth as well.

Vitamin A

As discussed in other chapters, vitamin A is essential for the immune system and for repairing the lining of the gut. It is also vital for preventing adrenal fatigue because cholesterol cannot be converted into cortisol and the other adrenal hormones without vitamin A. Additionally, it must be true vitamin A, from animal sources, because it is more easily metabolized than beta-carotene, which comes from plant sources. Beta-carotene must be converted to vitamin A, and many people (especially those with adrenal fatigue) do not make this conversion very well. The richest sources of true vitamin A include liver (from pastured beef, buffalo, chicken, duck), cod liver oil, egg yolks, butter from grass-fed animals, and heavy cream. It is best acquired through your diet, but if you can't eat enough of these sources for one reason or another, desiccated liver or vitamin A palmitate may be useful as supplements. However, beta-carotene is a powerful antioxidant.

Vitamin D

As described in chapter 9, vitamin D is critical for the health of the immune system. It also creates antimicrobial peptides that directly kill candida, bacteria, and other microbes and help break down biofilms. Vitamin D is needed for the body to utilize vitamin A properly and to prevent toxicity of vitamin A. In *Grain Brain*, Dr. David Perlmutter makes the case that vitamin D is critical for proper brain function because it helps control enzymes in the brain and cerebrospinal fluid that are associated with creating neurotransmitters and activating nerve growth. It also shields neurons from the harmful effects of free radicals, and it decreases inflammation. Vitamin D can boost serotonin production anywhere from twofold to thirtyfold.[8]

Vitamin D plays a critical role in insulin sensitivity and blood sugar regulation. It is needed for production of insulin and increases glycogen production and storage. In *Your Best Health Under the Sun,* Dr. Al Sears, reveals that some studies have shown that type 1 diabetes, which is caused by a genetic mutation in the gene that produces insulin, is connected to a vitamin D deficiency in the infant's mother. In another study researchers in Australia "found that low vitamin D levels predispose people to adult diabetes. They discovered that as vitamin D levels decreased, blood sugar and insulin levels increased. This increase is what eventually leads to insulin resistance. A prediabetic condition follows and sometimes diabetes. The researchers concluded that the epidemic of diabetes is in part due to the modern day sun avoidance that leads to vitamin D deficiency." In a study in the *American Journal of Clinical Nutrition*, researchers found that "increasing a person's blood concentration of vitamin D from 25 nmol/l to about 75 nmol/l would improve insulin sensitivity by 60 percent. This is a much greater improvement than the current best anti-diabetic drug, metformin, which only gives about a 13 percent improvement in insulin sensitivity. In another study "using 1,332 IU of vitamin D per day for only 30 days improved insulin sensitivity by 21 percent in 10 women with adult diabetes." Vitamin D also makes the GI tract more receptive to calcium absorption and mobilizes the minerals in other areas of the body to direct them to the bones. All of this means that maintaining adequate vitamin D levels is vital for reducing sympathetic dominance, managing cravings for sugar and carbs, and remaining committed to the candida diet.

The best way to get your vitamin D is through sun exposure, which is discussed in more detail in chapter 13. If you're unable to obtain this amount of sun exposure, then supplementation with vitamin D3 (cholecalciferol) may be useful. Dr. Sears says supplementation with D3 should be accompanied by supplementation with vitamin K because vitamin K helps "activate and improve absorption of D3."[9]

Vitamin D is created in the skin when the sun interacts with cho-lesterol in the body, so if you don't have sufficient levels of cholesterol you won't produce vitamin D. As discussed in chapter 10, maintaining adequate levels of cholesterol in the body is critical for this reason and many others. You should also know that your body can store vitamin D for later use, so if you can only get out in the sun once in a while, aim for more sun exposure at one time to manufacture vitamin D for storage. Additionally, you can get lots of sun during the summer months to build up reserves of vitamin D for the winter. Vitamin D can also be acquired to some degree by consuming cold-water fish (e.g., salmon), butter, egg yolks, and mushrooms. Sun-dried mushrooms contain three times the amount of vitamin D as fresh mushrooms; eating them can easily supply your daily requirements.[10] However, people with candida often do not tolerate mushrooms, because they are a fungi. Also, it's important to be aware that high doses of vitamin D can increase calcium levels, which could increase glutamate levels in those with excess glutamate.

Vitamin B6

Vitamin B6 (pyridoxine) participates in more than one hundred enzyme pathways in the body, including those involved with hemoglobin syn-thesis, making antibodies, producing prostaglandins, regulating blood sugar, breaking down protein, metabolism, and methylation. B6 is a cofactor in the production of all the key neurotransmitters (serotonin, dopamine, etc.), which, as you know by now, regulate mood, thought, cognitive functions, appetite, and sympathetic dominance. It also helps moderate the action of glucocorticoid hormones (steroid hormones produced by the adrenal glands) and is needed in the production of hydrochloric acid in the stomach. Therefore, it plays a critical role in many aspects of candida overgrowth, including stabilizing blood sugar, managing cravings for sugar and carbs, and supporting the adrenal glands.

B6 is a cofactor needed for the enzyme AGXT to break down oxalates (see page 433). It is also a cofactor for the DAO enzyme, which breaks down histamine (see page 148), and is required for glutamate to be converted into GABA (see page 347).

Vitamin B6 is converted into its active form, pyridoxal-5-phosphate, in the body, but many people don't make this conversion very well. Additionally, candida depletes B6 and prevents it from being converted into pyridoxal-5-phosphate. Arabinose, one of candida's byproducts, can bind with lysine and arginine and form pentosidines, which can block B6. For these reasons, B6 deficiency is very common in people with candida. To bypass these issues B6 is best supplemented with pyridoxal-5-phosphate rather than pyridoxine. That said, be aware that *Candida glabrata* and a variety of other species use B6 for its survival, so if one of these species is involved in your overgrowth, supplementation with B6 could make your candida proliferate.

Digestive Enzymes and HCl

A good digestive enzyme can help the body break down food more efficiently, enhancing absorption of nutrients and enabling the body to acquire more of the nutrients before yeast and other microbes get to them. Reducing microbes' access to nutrients will inhibit their growth. Digestive enzymes may also help alleviate gastrointestinal symptoms like gas, bloating, and abdominal pain, improve food sensitivities, and reduce inflammation.

Many different opinions exist about what constitutes a good digestive enzyme. I advocate taking pancreatic enzymes; select a brand that is labeled as being ten times (10X) in strength. Plant-based enzymes are very popular in the natural health world because some practitioners believe they are effective at a wider range of pH levels. However, plant-based enzymes are typically derived from the fungi aspergillus, usually making them problematic for people with candida. (This does not include papain, which is derived from papaya, and bromelain, which comes from pineapple.)

Additionally, an insufficiency of pancreatic enzymes may contribute to overgrowth of candida and other microbes, because one of the roles of these enzymes is to help degrade candida, bacteria, and parasites in the small intestine. Pancreatic enzymes are typically taken with the meal for digestive benefits and between meals for anti-inflammatory effects. Taking them between meals can also help reduce levels of candida and other microbes.

If you did the betaine challenge test (see pages 89–91) and discovered that you are in need of HCl, then it should be supplemented as well. Dosage should be based on your response to the test.

Both low stomach acid and insufficient pancreatic enzyme output can result in the failure of amino acids to break down sufficiently, rendering them unavailable for production of neurotransmitters.

Chromium

The mineral chromium is commonly depleted in the individual with candida because this nutrient is typically void in a diet that is high in sugar and carbs. Chromium is vital for keeping blood sugar stable, alleviating fatigue, managing weight gain, and controlling cravings for sugar and carbs. It is needed for insulin to carry glucose out of the blood and into the cell, where it is burned for energy. Without enough chromium, you are likely to crave sugar and carbs, experience low energy, store more fat, gain weight, and be more prone to develop diabetes. It is also needed for the mood, gut, appetite, and sympathetic nervous system–regulating neurotransmitter serotonin to work properly. According to Dr. Al Sears, chromium needs to be combined with niacin to be effective; any supplement purchased should be niacin-bound chromium or chromium polynicotinate.[11]

L-Carnitine

L-carnitine is a derivative of amino acid metabolism that assists in energy conversion by carrying fat into the mitochondria so it can be burned for energy. If you're burning fat for energy, then there will be less need for energy from carbohydrates. According to Nora Gedgaudas, author of *Primal Body, Primal Mind*, very high doses of L-carnitine may be required—as much as 2 to 5 grams per day. Supplementing with L-carnitine can make the transition to the paleo for candida diet a little smoother and more comfortable by helping to alleviate some of the energy loss that typically occurs when one first lowers carb intake.

SUPPLEMENTS FOR OTHER PURPOSES

Methylation

Recall that methylation converts one substance to another. It takes place when one molecule passes a chemical unit called a methyl group to another molecule. Methylation plays a critical role in numerous bodily processes—for example, converting serotonin to melatonin, eliminating estrogens, detoxification, energy production, breaking down histamine, production and function of neurotransmitters, and regulating the autonomic nervous system, to name a few.

Methylation requires adequate levels of vitamin B12, folic acid, vitamin B6, magnesium, copper, and SAMe. Betaine or TMG (trimethylglycine) can improve methylation. Methylation problems are abundant in the population and can be caused by a wide variety of factors besides nutrient deficiencies, including a genetic polymorphism, toxins, and candida.

As mentioned previously, one should work with a practitioner who has a great deal of expertise in this area, if they are focusing on this issue. A great deal of negative effects can occur if not done correctly.

Healing the Enterocytes and Brush Border

As discussed in earlier chapters, enterocytes (cells that line the intestines) and the brush border of the small intestine are often damaged in the individual with candida or other microbial overgrowth. Once overgrowth is reduced, then a variety of nutritional supplements may be used to help heal the gut lining, including colostrum, lactoferrin, glutamine, zinc carnosine, vitamins A, C, D, and E, fish oil, curcumin, resveratrol, glutathione, and NAC. Colostrum and lactoferrin are very effective for this purpose; see pages 237–239 for more detail. Brush border enzymes may be used as well. At the same time, however, some of the nutrients listed above (particularly zinc, glutamine, and NAC) can be problematic for other conditions. Be sure to take a look at the section further below "Supplements That Are Double-Edged Swords."

Supporting the Liver

The liver is the primary organ involved in detoxification, which means it has the responsibility of eliminating candida and its toxic byproducts. It needs to function as well as possible to perform these roles adequately. Liver function in individuals with candida is often compromised because it has become overwhelmed with candida toxins, so it may need some additional support.

As discussed in earlier chapters, the liver can be supported with molybdenum, pantethine, dandelion root, burdock root, artichoke, milk thistle (also known as silymarin), vitamin C, enemas or colon cleansing, vitamin B6, lecithin, alpha-lipoic acid, glutathione, N-acetylcysteine (NAC), and exercise. Supplementation with NAC should be accompanied by vitamin C, at two to three times the dosage of NAC. Be sure to read about each of these nutrients as presented individually in this chapter, especially for any contraindications. I found a combination of silymarin, artichoke, dandelion, molybdenum, and pantethine to provide excellent liver support.

Addressing Inflammation

Vitamins A, C, and E, CoQ10, curcumin, zinc, omega-3s, and colostrum can be highly beneficial for reducing inflammation.

Treating Pyroluria

Many people with candida or other microbial issues may have a condition called pyroluria, a genetic problem in heme production that leads to deficiencies in vitamin B6 and zinc. Since zinc and B6 are so critical for numerous functions that may contribute to overgrowth of candida and other microbes (e.g., immune function, intestinal permeability, and production of neurotransmitters), pyroluria can lead to or perpetuate overgrowth. Common symptoms of pyroluria include anxiety, depression, and social withdrawal. Many people with pyroluria are addicted to sugar and carbs or other psychotropic substances, which are used to self-medicate the associated symptoms, and which can contribute to candida overgrowth. A test called the Kryptopyrrole test can identify pyroluria. The condition is treated with high-dose B6 and zinc and possibly with other nutrients that have become deficient, for example, manganese and biotin. It's important to work with a health-care provider who has expertise in pyroluria because the dosage of B6 and zinc is extremely important. If you take too much, it can be toxic; if you take too little, it will be ineffective.

SUPPLEMENTS THAT ARE DOUBLE-EDGED SWORDS

The nutrients listed in this section may produce potential complications along with their benefits. Be aware of both before using them.

Magnesium

Magnesium is essential for more than three hundred biochemical reactions in the body, including energy production, helping insulin work more effectively, regulating blood sugar, neurotransmitter production and function, bone strength, methylation, lowering cortisol levels, and cardiovascular health, to name just a few. Magnesium is also critical for elimination and maintaining balance between GABA and glutamate as it prevents excess calcium and can bind to and activate GABA receptors. As mentioned earlier, candida can contribute to magnesium deficiency. The use of magnesium for improving a variety of conditions is well documented, including fibromyalgia, muscle pain and spasms, insomnia, depression, anxiety, addiction, and fatigue.

However, candida needs magnesium for survival and morphogenesis, and magnesium is used in the formation of biofilms by candida and other microbes. Studies have demonstrated that magnesium concentrate makes candida proliferate.[12] When supplementing with oral magnesium, many people report an increase in itching around the anus, brain fog, headaches, sinusitis, depression, irritability, and fatigue. One of these studies also showed that calcium inhibited the growth of candida.[13] On the flip side, work by scientist George Eby, who is a strong advocate for the use of magnesium, reports that high doses of oral magnesium concentrate without calcium significantly worsened candida, rhinovirus, and herpes virus.[14] It's possible that taking calcium with magnesium could help balance out this issue.

Magnesium is needed to create aldehyde dehydrogenase, the enzyme that helps to eliminate candida's primary byproduct, acetaldehyde; therefore, a magnesium deficiency could lead to accumulation of acetaldehyde.

These various effects explain why some people report feeling better and others worse when supplementing with magnesium; in some cases it is facilitating removal of acetaldehyde, and in others it is causing candida to proliferate. One's response is likely dependent on factors such as the extent of overgrowth, how depleted the nutrient is, how well the body is eliminating acetaldehyde, and whether calcium is also being supplemented.

Response may also be influenced by what form of magnesium a person takes. Some people report negative symptoms from one form of magnesium but not another. Additionally, some people report that if they are able to bypass the gut by using sprays, creams, or Epsom salt baths to supplement with magnesium, they can avoid or significantly reduce negative symptoms. Using a non-oral route for taking magnesium allows the body to absorb it before candida or other microbes can access it.

Biotin and other B Vitamins

Biotin is often prescribed to individuals with candida because they are frequently deficient in this nutrient, and it is thought to inhibit candida's ability to morph into mycelial form. Biotin is a very important B vitamin that plays a critical role in metabolism, blood sugar balance, the nervous system, and growth of skin, hair, and nails. Many are unaware that one of the reasons biotin deficiency is so common in candida overgrowth is because it is one of the basic nutrients that candida needs for growth and metabolite production. This is also true of a variety of other fungi, yeasts, and bacteria.[15] Therefore, supplementation with biotin may encourage overgrowth of candida in the plankton form and frequently results in an increase in brain fog, pain, urinary tract infections, anxiety, and other symptoms. On the other hand, some practitioners use biotin to draw candida out, and then they slam it with a potent antifungal.

The formation of pentosidines by candida's byproduct arabinose can also block biotin from being utilized. Biotin is manufactured by the friendly bacteria in the gastrointestinal tract. If you lack sufficient levels of friendly microbes, which is commonly the case in individuals with candida, your ability to produce biotin may be impaired. Some genetic disorders can lead to biotin deficiency as well.

It appears that most species of candida require biotin for existence, not just *C. albicans*. That said, remember from chapter 1 that thiamine is "stimulatory or essential for some strains." Some strains and species, especially the *C. krusei* family, need thiamine, B6, or nicotinic acid (B3) either singly or in combination in addition to biotin. Pantothenic acid stimulates some strains of *C. pseudotropicalis* and *Candida glabrata* requires niacin and vitamin B6—which means supplementing those nutrients could potentially contribute to overgrowth if these organisms are involved. And yet, another study discovered that niacin could help reduce overgrowth of *C. albicans* and aspergillus.[16] This really demonstrates how determining which nutrients will be beneficial can largely depend on the species of candida you are dealing with. It also shows how easy it is to inadvertently worsen your condition.

Antioxidants

As mentioned in previous chapters, vitamins C and E, beta carotene, CoQ10, and herbs like turmeric can be used to help manage the inflammation that occurs from overgrowth of candida, bacteria, or parasites. Be aware, too, that if you're trying to kill candida or other microbes with a substance that achieves its goal by increasing oxidative stress, you must be careful to avoid taking your antioxidants at the same time. Doing so will reduce the oxidative stress and inhibit the supplements' ability to kill the microbe.

Glutamine

Glutamine is another nutrient that is frequently prescribed to people with candida. Glutamine is the preferred source of fuel and of nitrogen needed for the epithelial cells that line the gut; it therefore promotes regeneration and repair of leaky gut. It also stops insulin from being released and can be used as an alternative source of fuel when glucose levels are low, thereby helping to balance blood sugar and reduce cravings for sugar and carbs. Pouring glutamine directly on the tongue when cravings feel overwhelming or blood sugar has dropped can eliminate the cravings and restore blood sugar almost instantly. I'd also like to make you aware that butter can have this same effect, so if you can't take glutamine, butter will do the trick.

Recall from chapter 13 that glutamine increases production of GABA, the primary inhibitory and calming neurotransmitter. However, first, glutamine is converted into glutamate, which is the primary excitatory neurotransmitter and is toxic at excessive levels. Supplementing with glutamine may increase glutamate levels in individuals who have problems converting their glutamate to GABA, and thus contribute to the wide array of negative symptoms associated with excess glutamate (see pages 440–442 for more detail). Candida can create glutamate storms, leading to elevation of glutamate. The individual with candida is exceptionally vulnerable to elevated glutamate. People with high glutamate issues should generally avoid supplementing with glutamine.

GABA

As discussed in chapter 13, a metabolic pathway called the GABA shunt can convert GABA back into glutamine, which is then converted back into glutamate. So GABA supplementation can end up increasing glutamate in some people. In addition, according Dr. Datis Kharrazian GABA should not be able to cross the blood-brain barrier; it will only do so in the presence of leaky brain. And Kharrazian warns that the use of GABA, regardless of whether one experiences a positive or negative effect, may shut down GABA receptors.

Glutathione

Supplementing too heavily with glutathione may contribute to excess glutamate. According to Dr. Nathan, in some people glutathione supplementation can impair methylation and should be done with caution.[17] Please read additional information about glutathione on pages 213–214.

NAC

The antioxidant NAC (N-acetylcysteine) is frequently used to increase glutathione levels to reduce oxidative stress and improve detoxification. It provides support for elements of the immune system that control mucosal surfaces, and it can be used to bind with acetaldehyde, which neutralizes acetaldehyde's ability to exert its negative effects. As mentioned in chapter 3, NAC is also effective in breaking down some biofilms, and it has an inhibiting effect on the ability of gliotoxins (a type of mycotoxin) to kill cells. NAC is commonly used for heavy metal detoxification. However, some practitioners like Dr. Charles Gant warn that supplementation with NAC too early in the process can move mercury and other metals to the brain. NAC should not be used in high doses until later in the process, after heavy metals have been eliminated through the skin and the gut via baths, minerals, and chlorella as described in chapter 13.[18] It can be used in smaller doses earlier in the process. This is also true of cilantro and alpha-lipoic acid. Additionally, it can be counterproductive to increase cysteine levels if one's levels are sufficient or too high. Furthermore, some practitioners believe that NAC, as well as alpha lipoic acid, cysteine, and other sulfur-based supplements may increase candida overgrowth when taken orally.[19] You may be able to resolve this by using transdermal supplementation.

Tyrosine

Tyrosine is often prescribed to people with candida to increase depleted dopamine levels or support the thyroid. However, tyrosine also increases norepinephrine, and if the body is unable to methylate norepinephrine into epinephrine, it may build up in excess. As mentioned before, norepinephrine is an important excitatory neurotransmitter, but it is toxic to the brain at excessive levels. It sets off the stress response system, and when it is elevated it keeps the sympathetic nervous system dominant. Some people can take tyrosine with no problems while others can't tolerate it at all. If you experience symptoms like anxiety, agitation, insomnia, restlessness, hyperactivity, fear, panic, or other mental health disturbance when supplementing with tyrosine, then most likely your norepinephrine levels are too high.

You should note that any supplement you have a sensitivity to can increase norepinephrine and set off the stress response system. Many herbal supplements may increase norepinephrine as well—for example, St. John's wort, olive leaf, and others.

Calcium

As mentioned previously, too much calcium can increase glutamate levels. If an individual needs calcium but has excess glutamate, Dr. Amy Yasko recommends using nettle or chamomile to increase calcium levels rather than supplementing directly with calcium.[20] In other situations, it may be the dosage that prompts a negative response. You may be able to tolerate a little bit of a nutrient that causes symptoms in larger doses. It may also be tolerated if accompanied by magnesium, but not always.

Glycine

Glycine can be inhibitory or excitatory, and in people who tend to lean toward excess glutamate it typically becomes excitatory, so it may need to be avoided.

5-HTP

5-HTP is another commonly recommended supplement for people with candida; it is used to increase serotonin levels, which are often depleted. However, 5-HTP can increase cortisol levels, which is highly counterproductive for the individual with adrenal fatigue. Again, some people do fine with this supplement, and some get worse. It has the potential to cause a significant adrenal crash.

Manganese

If you have Lyme disease, you should be aware that Lyme bacteria need manganese for survival. Therefore, supplementation with this nutrient may exacerbate the condition.

Beta-Glucans and D-Mannose

As discussed elsewhere in the book, beta-glucans can be used in the battle against candida. D-mannose is often prescribed for urinary tract infections that commonly occur with candida or SIBO. Both of these substances can feed SIBO.[21]

Other Notes on Minerals

The minerals calcium, magnesium, selenium, zinc, and iron play an extremely critical role in mental and physical health. Adequate levels are vital for many factors related to candida overgrowth, such as managing cravings for sugar and carbs, blood sugar balance, adrenal function, brain health, neurotransmitters, eliminating toxins from the body, gut health, and immune function. However, candida and other microbes use many minerals (e.g., zinc, calcium, magnesium, and iron) in the formation of biofilms. Many of them are essential for the pathogens' survival.

For these reasons, supplementation with minerals may encourage proliferation and increase symptoms. As mentioned in the chapter on biofilms (chapter 3), when a person is actively trying to break down the biofilm, he or she should typically avoid supplementing with minerals. When one is breaking down the biofilm, minerals are typically chelated and then replenished after chelation. So supplementation with minerals should be done at the right time. Additionally, according to Dr. Amy Yasko, zinc supplementation in excess of 40 mg a day can increase glutamate levels.[22]

Colostrum

In chapter 7 and chapter 9, we learned that colostrum can be highly beneficial for repairing the gut, supporting immune function, and directly killing candida and other microbes. However, be aware that if you have a negative reaction to dairy exorphins (discussed in more detail on pages 265–267), you could have a problem with colostrum.

Inositol and Monolaurin

Inositol is frequently prescribed to people with OCD, a condition that is also very common in individuals with candida or bacterial overgrowth. Monolaurin is often used as an antimicrobial and it contains glycerol. Know that inositol and glycerol are an alcohol sugar, which can be very inflammatory to the gut and can exacerbate symptoms of both candida and SIBO.

D-Ribose and Other
Adrenal-Support Supplements

D-ribose, which is frequently used for the adrenal glands, can feed candida and possibly SIBO, and it may be too stimulating for the adrenal glands in the individual who has advanced-stage adrenal fatigue. Other substances commonly used for the adrenal glands (e.g., glandulars, adaptogens, ginseng, and licorice) can also be stimulating for the person with advanced-stage adrenal fatigue and may worsen their condition. As mentioned previously, ginseng is an amphetamine that shouldn't be considered.

FOS

Fructooligosaccharides (FOS) are naturally occurring substances found in a variety of plants. They are often extracted for use as prebiotics and put in a probiotic, but they can feed candida and SIBO.

Omega-3 and Omega-6 Fatty Acids

Both omega-3 and omega-6 fatty acids are critical for many aspects of our health, including brain function, neurotransmission, gut, and immunity. However, too much omega-6 can lead to inflammation, which can perpetuate candida overgrowth. Therefore, keeping the omega fatty acids in balance is an important component of healing. If omega-6 is high, then supplementation with omega-3 can be beneficial. Other good sources of omega-3 include cold-water fish such as salmon and grass-fed beef. However, even too much omega-3 is associated with an increased risk in colitis and changes in immune function that may inhibit the body's ability to fight off microbes like candida and bacteria, so don't go overboard.

Miscellaneous Herbs

A variety of herbs may be prescribed for sympathetic dominance and many of its associated symptoms like anxiety, insomnia, or depression. Some of the more popular include valerian root, kava kava, holy basil, olive leaf, and St. John's wort, but there are others. Any herb that is used to manipulate mood, energy, pain, or cognitive function, or to induce relaxation has a similar impact on the brain as antidepressants, anti-anxiety medication, or other psychotropic drugs, meaning it provides artificial or excessive stimulation to the neurotransmitter receptors in the brain, which may prompt the brain to reduce responsiveness to or production of the neurotransmitter. Tolerance develops and then more of said herb is needed, and then more tolerance, and so on and so on. It is only a matter of time before they are no longer effective and then they have made the condition worse by depleting neurotransmitters even further and promoting dependence on the herb. If these herbs are used at all, it should be short term. But, be aware tolerance to them can develop quickly. I developed tolerance to valerian root (acts on the brain like a benzodiazepine similar to Valium) and noticed an addictive cycle developing within a couple weeks of use. Other clients have reported the same. I had a similar experience with olive leaf. I was using olive leaf for killing bacteria and candida and it was pretty effective. Initially I noticed a boost in mood and energy, but in a few weeks I noticed a lowering of serotonin and an elevation in norepinephrine, which put great stress on my adrenals. So much so, that I began to pant. However, if I take the olive leaf for just a few days to a week every now and then I can get around this and utilize its microbe-killing abilities for a short period of time.

Melatonin

Melatonin, often prescribed to help with sleep, can be habit forming and increase norepinephrine. If used, it should be short-term.

Resistant Starch

As discussed in several places in this book, starch feeds candida yeast and other microbes. It also contributes greatly to sugar and carb addiction, compulsive overeating, depression, anxiety, autonomic nervous system dysfunction, low blood sugar problems, obesity, and unwanted weight gain. It's hard on the adrenal glands and may contribute to insulin resistance, type 2 diabetes, heart disease, dementia, cancer, and more.

There are two types of starch: digestible and resistant. Digestible starch is what causes the rise in blood sugar, the inevitable insulin response, and the spike in neurotransmitters that are responsible for all the negative health effects. Resistant starch, by contrast, is a type of carbohydrate that cannot be broken down into glucose. It resists digestion in the small intestine and travels on to the large intestine, where it becomes a food source for the bacteria that reside there. The rationale for supplementing with resistant starch is to feed and cross-feed the healthy flora that live in the colon so they will multiply in numbers.

Recall that the healthy microbes in the gastrointestinal tract play a vital role in many bodily functions. Consequently, there has been a movement in the natural health field to encourage people with candida to supplement with resistant starch. Proponents of supplementing with resistant starch report a variety of health benefits, including deeper sleep with more vivid dreams, less body fat, improved insulin sensitivity and blood sugar control, lower blood cholesterol and triglyceride levels, better digestion and bowel movements, higher energy, enhanced mood and feelings of well-being, and increased satiation with meals. So it seems that consuming a lot of resistant starch could be nothing but good, right? Well, not necessarily so.

As you learned in chapter 7, your gut biome (the community of commensal, symbiotic, and pathogenic microorganisms that share space within your gut) is incredibly complex, and the microbes that reside there vary greatly from individual to individual. Some people have more pathogenic microbes than others. If a lot of unfriendly microbes are present, or if certain microbes live in the small intestine that don't belong there, or if there are too many of a particular microbe, they, too, will feed on the resistant starch, which can lead to a host of problems. Additionally, even the good guys become pathogenic when they are out of balance.

If you visit online forums that discuss the topic of resistant starch, you will notice that people report a range of responses. Some report miraculous improvements, while others report significant setbacks and a decline in health (including diarrhea, abdominal pain, gas, constipation, nausea, bloating, cramps, acid reflux, fatigue, anxiety, psychological disturbances, and intestinal blockage). One's response depends on what microbes they have in their gut biome and where these fellas are located.

Norm Robillard, PhD, microbiologist and author of *Fast Tract Digestion,* helps shed some light on why. He explains that if many of the microbes that typically live in the colon are also present in the small intestine—as is the case in SIBO and related conditions like IBS and GERD—then the organisms in the small intestine will feed on the resistant starch, thus aggravating the condition. Furthermore, according to research by Robillard, people with IBS tend to have an overabundance of a particular group of bacteria called firmicutes and an overall decrease in microbial diversity. Firmicutes feed primarily on carbs, sugar, fiber, and starches.

A healthy gut houses an array of bacterial species competing for space and nutrients. An unhealthy gut has less diversity, and one particular group of bacteria may become dominant. Robillard explains that a disproportionate number of a particular type of bacteria that feeds on resistant starch (e.g., firmicutes) may lead to an increase in symptoms. Therefore, in response to a high intake of resistant starch, people with IBS, SIBO, acid reflux, autoimmune conditions (e.g., multiple sclerosis, lupus, rheumatoid arthritis, Grave's and Hashimoto's thyroiditis, psoriasis, inflammatory bowel disease, Crohn's, ulcerative colitis, and celiac disease), allergies, and asthma—all of which are related to microbial overgrowth or imbalances—are likely to have an increase in symptoms.

Robillard cites studies indicating that a diet rich in complex polysaccharides leads to an increase in firmicutes, actinobacteria, and certain species of clostridia, and to a decrease in bacteroidetes and other species of clostridia—which results in less diversity, the same circumstances that are associated with IBS. As described in chapter 6, by limiting the food source for the "polysaccharide-loving microbes," we put them on a diet. Eating a diet that is rich in animal-based foods combined with a limited amount of fermentable carbs promotes an environment wherein species of bacteria that metabolize amino acids and other animal-based macronutrients can compete with the firmicutes and clostridia that prefer carbs, without allowing one or the other to become dominant.

Robillard explains that too much resistant starch—like any other indigestible carb that can be fermented by our microbes—can lead to SIBO, infection with pathogens, excess toxin and gas production, and an increase in "microbe-mediated formation of carcinogenic compounds." "A lean diet for our gut microbes fosters healthy competition in the gut that will favor the survival of well adapted organisms best suited to be our partners in digestion and health." My personal experience with resistant starch, which I share in more detail further ahead, supports these findings.

Dr. Grace Liu, a medical pharmacist who has a great deal of knowledge on this topic, also cautions that anyone with IBS, SIBO, or an autoimmune condition, or who is precancerous or cancerous for colorectal cancer, should avoid resistant starch for the same reasons: rogue bacteria, pathogens, or microbes inhabiting places they shouldn't. She also cites research suggesting that people with IBS have too many short-chain fatty acids, which can lead to symptoms of depression, anxiety, and migraines. Increasing fermentable and indigestible carbs will further increase short-chain fatty acids.[23]

Additionally, Dr. Allison Siebecker, medical director of the SIBO Center for Digestive Health at the NCNM Clinic in Portland, Oregon, lists resistant starch as one of the food sources for the bacteria that fuel SIBO.[24]

For all these reasons, people with candida often fall under the category of those whose symptoms worsen in response to resistant starch—but not always. It depends on many factors: age, the severity of yeast overgrowth, how long the person has lived with the illness, the presence of other conditions, and, primarily, the individual's gut biome.

I have read accounts of people with candida who felt that resistant starch was beneficial, but it is my opinion that they are the exception and not the rule. If you have a simple, clear-cut case of candida (and candida only), then benefits may be possible. Resistant starch should not feed candida. However, few people fit this criteria, because candida rarely is simple or occurs alone. Although resistant starch may increase bacteria that deter candida, it will also increase those that fuel SIBO, IBS, GERD, and autoimmunity, potentially causing an exacerbation of symptoms that perpetuate candida. I would encourage anyone with candida to exercise extreme caution if they want to experiment with resistant starch. As I describe below, the side effects can be very disruptive and produce a significant setback in health that is not easily reversed. If you have SIBO, IBS, or GERD, I wouldn't even consider it. It's also critical to note that you may not be aware that you have SIBO, because many of its symptoms overlap with candida and other conditions, and it is often overlooked. (Review the chapter on SIBO for more information.)

If you do decide to experiment with resistant starch against my advice, be aware of the following points.

There are four different types of resistant starch:

- RS1: found in seeds, legumes, and unprocessed whole grains. It is resistant because the substances are coated with a protective matrix.

- RS2: occurs naturally in some foods, including uncooked potato, green bananas, and plantains.

- RS3: forms when foods that contain starch are cooked and then cooled (e.g., potatoes, legumes, sushi rice), which causes the starch to become less soluble.

- RS4: produced by chemically modifying a starch to resist digestion.

Since legumes and grains contain a variety of antinutrients and are unhealthy for the reasons described earlier in the book, we won't consider using them. Nor do we want to consume the manmade version. In the paleo world, people using resistant starch select from the RS2 and RS3 categories, primarily uncooked potato starch, green bananas (including green banana flour), plantain flour, or by cooking and cooling potatoes (although potatoes are not truly paleo). Lesser amounts are contained in other starchy foods, including yams, sweet potatoes, squash, tubers, roots, and nuts.

The most popular method for supplementing with resistant starch is to take 2 to 4 tablespoons of Bob's Red Mill unmodified potato starch, green banana flour, or plantain flour. If you choose the potato starch, be sure that it is unmodified. Potatoes eaten raw are poisonous; the starch in Bob's Red Mill has been processed in a manner that removes the toxins. Additionally, you don't want potato flour; it must be pure potato starch.

However, according to Dr. Grace Liu, "whole food resistant starch trumps potato starch" for effectiveness because it feeds the whole village of microbes, not just the ones that eat RS2, thus promoting more microbial diversity and preventing overfeeding of one particular species. So make sure to include whole-food sources with any of the supplemental starches or flours.[25]

Herein lies another problem for people with candida. Any of the foods that are high in resistant starch are also high in digestible starch, which feeds candida, spikes blood sugar and insulin, and overstimulates neurotransmitters in the brain, resulting in cravings for sugar and carbs.

Additionally, most people with candida have an addiction to sugar and carbs, which means they have metabolic damage. As discussed in chapter 10, people with metabolic damage do not handle foods that are high in glucose (starch) very well. Consuming them leads to cravings and to bingeing on sugar and carbs, which feeds candida.

If you stick with the raw starch from potatoes, banana flour, or plantain flour, you will avoid consuming very much digestible starch. However, if you add starchy foods like cooked and cooled potatoes, yams, sweet potatoes, or squash, you will boost your intake of digestible carbs. In order to address candida overgrowth and prevent cravings for sugar and carbs, total carbohydrate levels (including the foods high in resistant starch) must be minimized. As discussed in the chapters on diet, in most cases total carbohydrate intake should be kept below 50 grams per day, an impossible goal if you eat a lot of resistant starch.

I'd like to share my experiences with resistant starch. A couple of sources that I trust touted its benefits, and clients were asking my opinion on the topic, so I decided to try supplementing to observe. I like to have firsthand experience with a regimen before advising clients whether they should engage or abstain. I've had a lifelong issue with candida and IBS and more recently with *H. pylori*, all of which I managed very well with a strict low-carb, low-starch, low-FODMAPs, paleo diet and a variety of other strategies presented in this book. I had begun to suspect I had a mild SIBO problem, but I wasn't completely sure until I did this experiment.

I started out taking a teaspoon of potato starch per day. Nothing happened, so I slowly increased my intake. When I reached the recommended 4 tablespoons per day, I developed severe acid reflux, indigestion, heartburn, pain in my stomach and small intestine, and foul-smelling gas and stool. I discontinued for two days. After two days I felt better, so I tried a lower dose of 2 tablespoons per day. For about four days I didn't notice much of anything except a mild increase in gas, and then I was hit hard with the following symptoms, none of which I had prior to taking resistant starch:

- extremely excessive gas

- foul-smelling gas and stool (smelled like sulfur)

- disturbed sleep

- an increase in migraines

- severe inflammation, swelling, burning, and pain in the small intestine

- severe acid reflux, indigestion, and heartburn that woke me in the middle of the night with intense belching

- achy sore spots all over my body

- increased adrenal stress

- pain and burning in my bladder and right kidney

- gallbladder inflammation

- mild depression and loss of feelings of well-being

- high levels of unexplained and irrational fear

- brain fog

- other unusual brain symptoms

Symptoms continued to snowball for several days after I stopped taking the resistant starch. The pain, burning, and inflammation traveled to the large intestine. There was so much swelling that I looked like I was six months pregnant. The pain in my colon radiated into my right shoulder blade and spine. I found it difficult to move.

At this point I was freaking out because I knew I had fed a microbe I shouldn't have fed, and it was spreading like a wildfire even though I'd cut off its food source. I started drinking food-grade hydrogen peroxide to kill some of the microbes. That helped for a bit, but soon stopped. Two weeks after I discontinued the resistant starch I was still not completely back to normal. I experienced severe GI distress if I ate more than 30 grams of carbs per day, and even that restriction did not provide complete relief.

I searched the Internet to find out what had happened to me and that is when I discovered the information compiled by Norm Robillard, Grace Liu, and Allison Siebecker that I presented to you above. I reviewed my bacteria levels from the GI Effects Comprehensive Stool Profile I'd undergone a few months earlier, and sure enough my results reflected the profile that Norm predicted would produce negative effects: I had high levels of firmicutes and little diversity.

Prior to this experiment I had tried consuming cooked and cooled potatoes, but after only one meal I experienced intense diarrhea, cramping, pain, burning and inflammation in my small intestine, disturbed sleep, acid reflux, and more, so I discontinued immediately and didn't consider trying again. I don't eat potatoes very often, because they trigger sugar addiction and feed candida, but I'd done so for this experiment. I wasn't sure if it was the resistant starch or the fermentable carbs that were the problem, and that is why for my second experiment I tried pure potato starch.

Three months after the second experiment, I continued to endure severe GI distress. I'd lost the ability to consume any fruit or nuts, and I had to keep my carb intake at 30 grams per day. Even that didn't provide complete relief, and if I went above that amount, most of my symptoms returned. Prior to my experiment with resistant starch I could eat a half cup of fruit and 2 tablespoons of nut butter three times a week with very few symptoms, and I had no pain with protein or fat.

Three months after my experiment, I still had quite a bit of belching from consuming protein and fat. I had less gas when I stayed off the carbs, but I still had more than usual. If I ate carbs, the gas smelled like sulfur, but when I ate protein and fat, it smelled like ammonia, which indicated that my bacteria were eating my protein and fat. I had severe abdominal pain all the time. I believe I had several bouts of pancreatitis, but I didn't have it confirmed by a doctor. My pancreas, duodenum, gallbladder, and bile duct consistently hurt.

I started on a regimen of herbal antibiotics to kill the bacteria and reduce inflammation. It provided quite a bit of relief, but not complete. After starting the herbals, most of the pain in my pancreas stopped, but it moved down toward the cecum area. Apparently the bacteria had relocated to that area, and the herbs were less effective at killing them there. I was forced to take a pharmaceutical-based antibiotic, which helped significantly, but I have never returned to the level of health I had prior to supplementing with resistant starch. Even today I must keep my daily carb consumption below 25 grams to prevent SIBO symptoms from returning in full force. I must continue to use herbal antibiotics on a regular basis and take a pharmaceutical-based antibiotic a couple times a year to keep levels minimized. Clearly, the resistant starch increased the bacteria in my small intestine to an outrageous level, and once that happens it is not easy to reduce the population.

I share this with you because I want others to know how serious the side effects and aftermath can be from resistant starch if you have SIBO. I would never have experimented with resistant starch had I known what I know now. It is truly the worst thing I have ever done for myself. I never imagined that the consequences could be so severe or so difficult to turn around. I assumed the worst that could happen was an increase in symptoms that would resolve once I stopped consumption, but that was not the case. So, once again, I urge you to exercise extreme caution with resistant starch. After I posted this story on my blog, other people shared with me that they have had similar experiences. Resistant starch can be downright dangerous for a person with SIBO.

I can sum up my experience by saying that resistant starch resulted in a very significant setback in my health. I have never experienced such severe GI distress in my life. However, the good thing to come out of the situation is that I learned something very valuable about my gut biome, and now I know where I need to direct my efforts to make more improvements. Prior to this experiment I had attributed all my upper GI symptoms to *H. pylori*, but I discovered that SIBO was causing many of them.

I have arrived at the same conclusion as Robillard, and I couldn't say it any better than he has:

"Clearly there is evidence that we, and our resident microbes, derive benefit from some level of resistant starch and/or other indigestible fibers in our diet. Whether or not we need to supplement our diet beyond what we receive from simply eating some fiber rich green leafy vegetables, avocados, nuts, and some fruit . . . is an open question."[26]

RECONCILING THE PROS AND CONS OF SUPPLEMENTATION

First, be aware that just because a nutrient is in the double-edged sword section doesn't necessarily mean it *must* be avoided. Again, a person's response to a nutrient depends on many different factors. You may or may not have the same negative reactions as another individual. I simply want to call attention to the fact that the potential for contraindications exists, and you should watch out for these issues. I have had bad experiences with many of the nutrients described above in that section, and so have the majority of my clients with candida or SIBO. They are very common. The people who experience the most problems are those who have severe sympathetic dominance and adrenal fatigue. Furthermore, toxicity in the body from environmental toxins can interfere in the ability of nutritional supplements to perform their job by hindering their absorption or utilization.

Even in the event of a negative response to a nutrient, one must still weigh the benefits against the risks and against the symptoms. For example, if you have a severe magnesium, zinc, or iron deficiency, you may need to take supplements for a period of time despite the fact that these minerals can reinforce the biofilm and encourage overgrowth. You'll address those issues later. Or if you're looking at the possibility of a heart attack versus an increase in candida overgrowth, then obviously dealing with the heart attack takes precedence. If, on the other hand, taking a nutrient incapacitates you, then clearly avoiding it is the right course of action. These decisions should be made on a case-by-case basis because the right direction for one person could be the wrong direction for another.

Sometimes the issue can be resolved by taking a different form of the supplement. As mentioned in the section on magnesium, it may be possible to bypass problems by using transdermal nutrients rather than oral ones, which takes the gut out of the picture. Other options for delivery include creams, sprays, and inhalers. These may eliminate all negative responses to the nutrient or reduce them enough to make it tolerable.

I'd like to emphasize that in no way am I saying you should eliminate these nutrients from your diet by avoiding foods that contain them. You cannot restrict consumption of all foods that contain these critical nutrients even if they do feed the microbe or biofilm. Nutrient deficiency is a much worse problem. I am saying that *supplementation* should perhaps be avoided. Rather than supplementing, in fact, you may be able to boost your intake of a particular nutrient by eating more of the foods that contain this nutrient. Supplementation can provoke a negative response because the nutrient is being delivered in a very large and concentrated dose at one time. Consumption of the nutrient in food delivers it in a less concentrated form. You can't completely restrict nutrients that are needed for survival, but you can avoid the megadoses provided by supplements.

This chapter has outlined some of the most common supplements used by people who have candida overgrowth, but it is not complete. There are others we will not discuss. Again, however, keep in mind that everyone is unique biochemically, so what constitutes a good supplement plan for one person may not for another. Undertake nutritional testing whenever possible to identify the nutrients your body needs. Furthermore, to avoid negative reactions and achieve optimal benefits, you must do your homework and discuss the issue with your healthcare provider before using any form of supplementation. Always use your body as a guide for the supplements you take by observing how it responds. Adjust accordingly. There are discussions on other supplements that may be helpful in chapters 8 and 9, so be sure to read those as well. You'll find details on contraindications for probiotics and antifungals in chapter 7.

TROUBLESHOOTING SUPPLEMENT INTOLERANCE

Many people with candida and associated conditions (e.g., adrenal fatigue, sympathetic dominance, SIBO) have problems tolerating supplements. Some people may be limited in what they can take, and others may be unable to take any supplements at all. Let's take a look at some of the factors that may be at play here and some possible steps to resolve them.

Unfortunately, there is no easy solution to the problem of supplement intolerance. Many possible issues may lie at the root of the matter, and, again, what is true for one person may not be true for another. However, the most common underlying cause by far is an overactive sympathetic nervous system, which, as you know, is often in overdrive in people with candida or other chronic health conditions. When that is the case, the body can become hypersensitive to seemingly everything, including foods, pharmaceuticals, chemicals, sounds, and nutrients. The more severe the sympathetic stress, the more hypersensitive they will become. The body starts perceiving everything as a threat, including nutritional supplements. Essentially, your brain thinks that the nutritional supplements are harmful, which sets off an alarm, producing a variety of negative physical and psychological symptoms. These can range from anxiety and depression, to heart palpitations, dizziness, and nausea, to insomnia, trembling, headaches, gastrointestinal distress, and so on. The list of symptoms that one may experience is endless and one can feel stuck in a catch-22.

The solution is to focus on restoring parasympathetic nervous system activity. Eat the right diet, eliminate environmental toxins from your living space, engage in deep-breathing exercises, practice mindfulness and meditation, smile more often, do exercises to rewire the brain—in general, follow the steps laid out in great detail in chapters 10 through 13. As mentioned in chapter 12, sometimes a person needs to spend a notable amount of time working on reducing sympathetic dominance before becoming capable of taking nutritional supplements or engaging in treatment strategies. The sicker you are, the more likely it is that your sympathetic nervous system is in overdrive and the more severe it is likely to be. It can take a long time to restore balance so it may be awhile before you can take supplements successfully. Sometimes an overactive sympathetic nervous system will accept nutrients in small dosages. Then you can wait a day or so to let symptoms subside, and take a little bit more and wait again for symptoms to subside—continuing until the nervous system settles down and produces no symptoms. Be aware that when the body is in sympathetic stress mode, it does not absorb nutrients very effectively, so they won't benefit you much if you don't work on this fundamental issue.

Another common underlying cause of feeling worse on nutritional supplements is that there are too many problems occurring within different organs and systems. When you try to jump-start one organ or system with a nutrient while missing nutrients that are needed for other organs and systems, it backfires. For example, a problem can develop if you take a supplement to detox your body while being deficient in other nutrients that are needed to eliminate the toxins you have mobilized. Before mobilizing toxins, you must be capable of moving them out. All organs and systems are interconnected; if one of them starts working better because of a nutrient you are taking, but others remain impaired, then you can run into a roadblock that triggers symptoms. To address these two issues, one must replenish all depleted nutrients and try to get all organs and systems on board. This, too, takes time and can be quite tricky to achieve in complex conditions.

In other cases, the body is simply too toxic from exposure to environmental toxins or internal toxins produced by bacteria, candida, or parasites. Supplements can overwhelm the body even more, requiring that the person proceed slowly with replenishing nutrients. As discussed above, some supplements may feed the pathogenic organisms, resulting in proliferation and ultimately more symptoms. Supplementation use may need to be suspended for a while until candida and other microbes are under better control.

Identifying and addressing one of your core problems may enable you to take supplements for other issues. For example, I used to have a great deal of problems taking nutritional supplements, but after I took high doses of pantethine and vitamin C to support my adrenal glands, and molybdenum to remove acetaldehyde, I became tolerant of a lot more supplements. Additionally, using some limbic system retraining techniques that turn off the sympathetic nervous system (see chapter 13) enabled me to take more supplements.

The third most common cause for an exacerbation of symptoms when taking nutritional supplements is taking too many too fast. If you are quite sick or you have a very overactive sympathetic nervous system, it is usually best to proceed quite slowly with nutritional supplementation. Don't start by taking everything you've learned may be beneficial all at once. Start out with one, and give your body time to adjust before adding another. Observe how your body reacts, and if all is okay proceed with another, and so on. Again, the sicker you are, the more important this is, and the slower you need to go.

Sometimes the dosage is the problem. People who are really sick, or very nutrient deficient, often do best with very small dosages of supplements rather than large ones. Then you can work your way up to larger doses. Alternatively, Dr. Amy Yasko states that it may be about taking the right nutrients in the right sequence.[27] It may be necessary to introduce a particular supplement after taking another supplement to correct a different issue. If you or your practitioner doesn't know what that sequence is, then you can get into trouble. Unfortunately, very few practitioners have the level of expertise needed to address these complex issues.

Certain genetic polymorphisms can have a profound impact on how someone responds to a particular nutrient. For example, maybe you have a mutation in a gene that causes one condition to get worse when you take vitamin B6, cysteine, or taurine to help with another condition. In this case, another nutrient is needed to support the genetic mutation before taking other types of nutrients that may make the mutation worse. To understand this issue further, read Dr. Yasko's book *Autism: Pathways for Recovery*, even if you don't have autism. The information it contains applies to most other chronic health conditions as well. A test called Nutrigenomics can help you identify any genetic mutations that may affect nutrients. It also provides a snapshot of overall nutrient status and an abundance of information on other issues such as methylation and neurotransmitters. The book will open your eyes to exactly how complex it can be to use nutritional supplements and to the depth of these conditions.

Taking a nutrient that you don't really need can produce negative side effects. Too much of a nutrient can be just as bad as too little. On the other side of this coin is taking only one nutrient when the body requires three or four others to address a particular problem. For example, many people take tryptophan to increase serotonin. However, tryptophan cannot be converted into serotonin unless there are sufficient levels of B6, B3, iron, and folic acid. If you are deficient in any of these nutrients, the tryptophan is not going to be able to do the job.

Deficiency in minerals can cause reactions to other supplements. Minerals are like the spark plugs in the body. They are needed for all other nutrients to do their jobs. If you supplement with a vitamin but are missing its mineral cofactors, then you may feel worse. Spending a few months replenishing minerals before taking anything else sometimes enables a person to tolerate other nutrients. Minerals will also help drive out heavy metals, which may lie at the root of many symptoms. Heavy metals destroy friendly gut bacteria, interfere with absorption, and may affect the way the body processes nutrients. They also interfere in neurotransmitter production and function, disrupt the endocrine system, and overstimulate the sympathetic nervous system. Minerals can be a good place to start for someone who is very toxic.

Taking supplements of inferior quality may contribute to problems. Be sure to take a high-quality brand. Some of my favorites are Thorne and Douglas Labs. Before giving up and assuming that your symptoms are caused by the nutrient itself, try several different brands. It may be something in the additives or processing that causes the problem and not the nutrient itself.

Another issue, especially for those with a sympathetic nervous system in overdrive, is the presence of something in the supplement (e.g., the nutrient itself or an additive) that increases the excitatory neurotransmitters norepinephrine or glutamate, or that is too stimulating for other reasons. Sometimes supplements with this effect may be tolerated by alternating them every other week or every other day. Some nutrients may increase cortisol. Additionally, the body's failure to methylate properly can affect one's ability to take supplements.

Some people simply do not respond well to certain supplements. For example, I cannot take any of the amino acid precursors for neurotransmitters, or any supplements that manipulate my neurotransmitters or hormones. They all have the opposite effect on me and produce unbearable symptoms. My brain and body will just not have it. This is true for many people I work with. If that is the case, you simply must avoid these nutrients.

Many health practitioners explain negative responses to nutritional supplements by saying that the body is undergoing a "healing crisis." Although this may be partially true some of the time, in my experience it is not the case the majority of the time. Since many practitioners really don't know why their patients are having a negative response, this becomes their "go-to" response.

With that being said, it does take the body a while to "reorganize" itself when depleted nutrients are presented or when biochemistry is being corrected. This reorganization can result in making you feel worse before you feel better. Healing crises occur most often with supplementation that is killing off some kind of unfriendly organism. It can be difficult to know if one is truly having a "healing crisis" or if one of the other issues I have discussed in this chapter may be at play.

It's important to note that if a healing crisis is so severe that it impairs your ability to function, it is counterproductive. Overwhelming the detoxification system or the sympathetic nervous system will only perpetuate the problem. You can try reducing the dosage and going at a slower pace. Another option is to try a different form of the supplement—for example, a liquid, a spray, an inhaler, a transdermal delivery system, or an IV. As mentioned, if you can bypass the gut, perhaps you can eliminate the negative symptoms. And, as mentioned previously, try different regimens like one week on and one week off, or two days on and two days off, etc.

Some practitioners will blame or shame their client when they are not able to take the prescribed supplements or have an unexpected response. They often claim that nobody else has these problems and act like you are unique. That is not true. Don't let them put this on you. Intolerance of nutritional supplements is very common. Almost everyone I work with (including myself) has problems to one extent or another taking nutritional supplements. Don't beat yourself up for it or feel like you are an oddball.

As discussed in chapter 7, there is a difference between nutritional supplements and herbs. Vitamins, minerals, amino acids, and fatty acids are essential components for the body. We need them to function. Herbs are basically natural drugs that the body does not need. Although herbs can be helpful for a variety of health conditions, I am not in favor of using them for insomnia, addiction, depression, anxiety, or other mental health issues because they do not correct the underlying issue. In some cases they perpetuate the problem. As mentioned, many herbs, such as St. John's wort and valerian, work like addictive drugs; they provide artificial stimulation, which results in tolerance and addiction.

A common misconception is the notion that nutritional supplements don't produce any side effects because they are natural. It's vital to be aware that natural therapies can be just as powerful as prescription drugs and should be taken seriously. This is especially true of supplements that affect neurotransmitters and hormones, which are typically the ones that people have the most trouble with. It really is best to work with a knowledgeable health-care provider rather than tackling the issue by yourself.

It's also important to note that nutritional supplements are not the be-all and end-all. Yes, they play an important role in most treatment plans, and replenishing depleted nutrients is vital for many ailments, but for some people less is more. As the name implies, nutritional supplements are designed to *supplement* the diet, not replace nutrients obtained from food. Many people put way too much focus on supplements while failing to address other, more important issues such as diet, managing stress, reducing sympathetic dominance, and being mindful of environmental toxins. No matter how you look at it, we are a pill-popping society. In traditional medicine it is pharmaceuticals, and in the natural health industry it's supplements and herbs.

The first step in addressing depleted nutrients is to fix your diet by eating organic, consuming adequate animal protein and fat and low-starch vegetables, eliminating sugars, grains, and legumes, and avoiding caffeine, alcohol, and refined foods. Strive to get most of your nutrients from the food you eat. Furthermore, if you do not change your diet you are unlikely to see significant or long-term results from nutritional supplements, no matter how many you take. You cannot fix a poor diet with nutritional supplements.

If you can't tolerate any nutritional supplements, eat the foods that are richest in the nutrients you are trying to replenish—while staying within paleo guidelines, of course. A simple Google search for any food will provide you with its nutrient content. Put more focus on the things you can do: eating healthy, getting proper exercise, communing with nature, getting adequate sunshine and sufficient sleep, doing deep breathing exercises, living green, meditating, and practicing positive thinking. Don't lose sight of the fact that the most profound improvements in health are typically made by eating the right foods and living a healthier lifestyle, and don't underestimate their power to do so.

CHAPTER 15

Acquiring a Competent Doctor

I t is very difficult to find a practitioner who has knowledge about everything we've covered in this book. Even most practitioners specializing in candida do not understand the true nature of this fascinating beast, fully appreciate the magnitude of the issues, or have the level of expertise that is needed to help their patients achieve the highest level of healing. While many practitioners may be very skilled at their craft in general, few have mastered the complete picture when it comes to chronic candida. In many cases, this is not really the fault of the practitioner; it is simply due to the complexity of the disorder, the adaptability and virulence of microbes, and the lack of data available on the topic. Additionally, there is a level of knowledge and understanding that can only be acquired through experiencing a condition firsthand. But, even then, the knowledge and experience acquired can vary widely from one practitioner to another. As you have learned, candida and other microbes are masters at survival. And unless a person has an astute knowledge of all the issues that come into play, his or her health may be compromised further. It is critical for the individual with chronic candida to become thoroughly educated so he or she can guide recovery in the right direction.

Although the focus of this book is on self-care, acquiring a competent physician is a necessary step on the path. The right practitioner can enhance the process. The best candida healing plan involves a combination of self-care strategies mixed with the knowledge of a competent health-care provider. Even when taking the natural approach, you may need prescriptions and assistance with conditions that develop as a result of candida, such as disorders related to the thyroid, hormones, or autoimmunity. Your relationship with your doctor can play a very important role in your healing journey, but many people are unaware that achieving quality care requires them to be active participants in the treatment process. You should be the one guiding the direction of the healing plan and what takes place in your appointments with the doctor.

Communication is vital in making any relationship satisfying and productive, and the first step in communicating effectively with your doctor is to examine and rearrange the dynamics of power. Dr. Stephen Katz, internist and professor of medicine and health management and policy at the University of Michigan, teaches that you should view your doctor as your employee.[1] You should be the supervisor overseeing everything, directing, organizing, and making final decisions about the care you will receive. You are paying the doctor for a service, and as with any other service you purchase you should be getting what you want. If you don't, you should go elsewhere.

I frequently hear statements like the following from my clients:

"My doctor put me on drug X, Y, or Z."

"My doctor won't support the paleo diet or a low-carb diet."

"My doctor says there is no value in natural medicine."

"My doctor doesn't believe in candida overgrowth."

These are signs of an unhealthy doctor/patient relationship.

Your doctor should not "have you" on anything. He or she should present you with treatment options, but whether you try them should be your choice, not your doctor's. Drugs should always be a last resort and only taken when absolutely necessary. The potential benefits should greatly outweigh the risks. The decision about whether to take a drug or follow any advice from the doctor should be yours alone, and that decision should be made only after doing thorough research and understanding everything involved. You should never do anything because your doctor "told you to." Any treatment options you put into action should be done because you chose to do them with your eyes wide open. You and your doctor should work together as a team.

Develop an intimate relationship with your body as explained on pages 336–338, and use it as your guide throughout your recovery process. Learn to listen to what it has to say about the food you eat and about its responses to treatment options, and adjust accordingly. It will tell you what is beneficial and what isn't, what it needs, and what direction to go. You are the expert when it comes to your body, and an enlightened physician will know this.

Don't make hasty, on-the-spot decisions about your medical care. Go home, think about it, and do some research. Better yet, educate yourself on every facet of your health condition, and present your doctor with the treatment options you would like to try. Learn everything you possibly can about candida, and know your options. You cannot assume that your doctor knows best, because in many cases they do not, especially on issues around candida, sugar and carb addiction, sympathetic dominance, and a low-carb diet. Many drugs are prescribed, lab tests carried out, and surgeries performed each day that are completely unnecessary and put people's health and lives at risk.

For example, medical errors are now the third leading cause of death.[2] In October 2009, Otis Brawley, the chief medical officer of the American Cancer Society, made a stunning and controversial announcement that we are over-screening for breast and prostate cancer, which results in a large number of people being treated for cancer when it really isn't needed. Screening the healthy population results in identifying and treating a large number of false positives and tumors that will never actually become cancerous. He also states that the American Cancer Society may have exaggerated the health benefits of screening.[3] According to Dr. Jonathan Wright, "each mammogram (which delivers 1 rad of ionizing radiation) increases risk of breast cancer by 1%. So if you follow the 'expert' recommendation to get a mammogram every year after you turn 40, by the time you are 50, you'll already have increased your chance of getting breast cancer by 10%."[4] Additionally, compression of the breast tissue during a mammogram can result in spreading of cancer cells if cancer is present.

The same can be said for nutritional supplements and natural remedies. They are often over prescribed or done so without educating the patient about possible contraindications or ramifications. Their benefits are often over-exaggerated and health conditions are over-simplified. It is your responsibility to make sure you are not one of the people put at needless risk.

Do not be afraid to speak up, challenge your doctor, and stand up for yourself. If you feel wobbly in the knees at the thought of doing this, then take someone with you who can step up for you, nudge you, or stand behind you. Be assertive and ask for what you want. Be aware that you have the right to obtain copies of your medical records, your lab test results, and anything else related to the care you receive. Get a folder to put them in, and keep notes of things you have tried, things you want to try, responses to treatment, results, and the like so you can refer back to them as needed. You must be your own best advocate.

If your doctor does not believe that chronic candida exists, then you need a different doctor. Healing cannot take place in this type of an environment and it will grate away at your self-esteem and quality of life. It's a waste of time and money, and it's demeaning and disrespectful to you. There is absolutely no reason why you should subject yourself to this type of treatment. Could you imagine that someone with cancer or heart disease would work with a physician who claims the conditions don't exist? No, absolutely not. That would be completely unacceptable. Chronic candida is no different, and you deserve to be treated with the same level of care as you would if you had any other health issue. You deserve to expect your practitioner to have at least a basic working knowledge of your condition. There is no point in banging your head against the wall to try and convince a nonbeliever, or in wasting valuable time and money that can be spent better elsewhere.

Along the same lines, your doctor should keep up-to-date with the latest medical practices and research. What we know about candida and other microbes grows and expands regularly, and the best treatment path may change accordingly. If your doctor is still approaching the issue with nothing but the knowledge he or she acquired ten or twenty years ago, then you are not going to get the best possible care. They should remain interested in and passionate about learning.

Additionally, you are free to eat whatever diet you feel best supports your health; you don't need your doctor's permission. If your doctor does not understand that mental and physical health are profoundly affected by diet, and that many health conditions can be improved with changes in diet, or if he or she still believes that high cholesterol, obesity, heart disease, cancer, high blood pressure, and other chronic conditions are caused by eating meat and thinks that whole grains or a vegetarian diet is healthy, it is time to find someone who is more up-to-date and advanced.

You are under no obligation to remain tethered to a doctor who gives you bad dietary advice or whose treatment suggestions keep you stuck or cause more harm than good. There are many other doctors to choose from—find another one. If you need that doctor for something specific you can't get elsewhere, then go ahead and keep them on board, but bring someone else on board who can help you accomplish the changes you want to make and who is more enlightened about diet, nutrition, and pharmaceuticals. Go to the former physician only for that specific need, not for anything else.

If your mechanic, hairdresser, plumber, or housekeeper didn't do the job you expected or treat you in the manner you desired, you would fire them and find someone else. The same applies to your doctor. We don't give our money to someone who does not provide the service we want. You should expect the same quality of service from your doctor that you would require from any other service provider. If they do not fulfill the criteria, then you find someone who does. It is your health and your life that are at risk.

You want a doctor who values and welcomes your input, who expects you to play an active role in the process, who has beliefs similar to yours when it comes to diet and healing, who views you as an equal partner, and who listens to you and welcomes questions. You should not feel unheard, afraid, demeaned, or intimidated by your doctor, and they should not feel threatened by your involvement or contributions.

Finding a health-care provider who can deal effectively with the complex cases that frequently develop with this condition is even more difficult. Complex patients can become a forgotten, pushed-aside, and neglected group of people. Many practitioners would rather not deal with them and often blame them. Choose a practitioner who is not afraid of complex cases, who does not dismiss you, and who is willing to try even if they don't have all the answers.

Yes, doctors with this mind-set are rare, but they do exist. You may have to travel a good distance to find one. I currently drive two and a half hours to see my doctor. At other times in my life, I have driven as long as five hours to access the doctor I preferred. You have to be willing to go the extra mile to get better care. Many doctors provide service through the telephone once you have become an established patient, and many practitioners offer their services online or over the phone without ever seeing you in person as long as they are not writing prescriptions. Some services even provide prescriptions. Accessing a doctor who can provide the best care is possible with additional effort. The Internet has made this process so much easier and opened new doors. All you need to do is look. I have clients who come to me from all over the world—including the UK, Australia, and South Africa.

Doctors in this category usually have titles such as doctor of environmental medicine, integrative medicine doctor, functional medicine doctor, doctor of orthomolecular medicine, or naturopathic doctor. They can be found through organizations like the American Holistic Medical Association, the American Academy of Environmental Medicine, the Institute for Functional Medicine, or the American Association of Naturopathic Physicians.

You can begin your search for a more enlightened physician at the websites listed below, all of which have a database broken down by state and, in some cases, country. Remember that everyone, even a doctor, is at a different place in the learning process, and just because they are on this list doesn't mean they have the level of expertise you desire. Additionally, nobody knows everything. It will be necessary to ask a lot of questions and basically interview a candidate to see if they are a right fit for you. If they are not, then continue the search until you find someone who is. In order to get your needs met adequately you may end up seeing more than one practitioner and possibly several, as each one may have something to offer that the others do not.

Primal doctors (a doctor who already practices primal/paleo principles is always preferred): www.primaldocs.com

Functional medicine doctors: www.functionalmedicine.org

Naturopaths: www.naturopathic.org

Doctors of environmental medicine: www.aaemonline.org/

American Holistic Medical Association: www.holisticmedicine.org

Orthomolecular doctors: www.orthomolecular.org

Do not put the responsibility for your health or your healing path in the hands of your doctor. The quality of care you receive is largely dependent on how proactive and well-versed you are on your condition. Choose your doctor wisely, be informed, and lead the way. You are the one in control of your medical care.

CHAPTER 16

Healing Chronic Candida: A Snapshot

We've covered a lot of material in this book. Assimilating it all can feel a bit daunting and take some time. Here is a brief summary that highlights the most important points in the healing journey:

Understand that healing is a long-term (often life-long) journey, not a one-time event. Chapter 1.

Educate yourself thoroughly on all aspects of your condition, know what you are dealing with inside and out, and be your own best advocate.

Choose a practitioner who keeps up-to-date with current medical advances, who is unafraid of complex cases, who values and welcomes your input, who expects you to play an active role in the healing process, who has beliefs similar to yours about diet and healing, who views you as an equal partner, and who listens to you and welcomes questions. Chapter 15.

Insist that you and your doctor work together as a team.

Take responsibility for your healing. It lies in your hands, not your doctor's.

Adhere to the paleo for candida diet (sugar-free, grain-free, legume-free, starch-free, low-carb, and rich in animal protein and fat) to cut off the food source for candida and other microbes, reduce biofilm formation, support optimal gut health and immune function, prevent inflammation, overcome cravings for sugar and carbs, and encourage parasympathetic nervous system activity. Chapters 10 and 11.

Reduce exposure to everyday environmental toxins by living an eco-friendly lifestyle that fosters an internal environment that is unfriendly to candida and other microbes, discourages cravings for sugar and carbs, promotes strong immunity, and reduces sympathetic nervous system activity. Use personal-care products, household cleaning supplies, cosmetics, etc., that are nontoxic and environmentally friendly and minimize exposure to electromagnetic radiation. Chapter 13.

Assess whether probiotics will be beneficial for your situation and, if so, which ones will best support gut and immune health, weaken biofilms, and crowd out yeast and other pathogens. Chapter 7.

Support the immune system. Consider taking vitamin D, lactoferrin, and colostrum; get adequate sleep, sun exposure, and appropriate exercise; decrease stress. Chapter 9.

Utilize agents that break down biofilms (e.g., EDTA, lactoferrin, NAC, garlic, silver, etc.). Chapter 3.

Utilize agents to penetrate the cell wall of candida (e.g., amylase, protease, cellulase, etc.). Chapters 3 and 7.

Utilize agents to kill candida, parasites, and bacteria (e.g., antifungals, antibacterials, antiparasiticals, etc.). Combine and rotate use of these agents to optimize eradication and reduce mutation and resistance. Chapters 5, 6 and 7.

Utilize a medium or engage in a practice to absorb or increase elimination of microbial toxins and to reduce die-off (e.g., activated charcoal, bentonite clay, sauna, enemas, etc.). Chapter 8.

Use agents for gut health (e.g., zinc, colostrum, lactoferrin, fish oil, etc.). Chapters 13 and 14.

Keep bowels in good working order (e.g., vitamin C, enemas, adequate fat and water intake, colonics, sufficient magnesium intake, mild exercise). Chapters 8 and 13.

Control inflammation through supplementation (e.g., vitamin C, vitamin E, CoQ10, selenium, omega-3 fatty acids, curcumin) and by avoiding other substances and circumstances that tend to promote inflammation (e.g., sugar, grains, legumes, caffeine, chocolate, food additives and preservatives, insecticides, herbicides, artificial sweeteners, heavy metals, birth control pills, too much omega-6, zinc deficiency, lack of sleep, casein, stress, chlorinated water, alcohol, foods that trigger sensitivities, steroids, NSAIDs).

Support the liver and improve detoxification (e.g., silymarin, dandelion, artichoke, molybdenum, pantethine). Chapter 8.

Reduce stress and sympathetic dominance (e.g., deep-breathing exercises, mindfulness meditation, smiling, communing with nature, green living, diet). Chapters 12 and 13.

Get emotional support if needed. (e.g., mental health counselor, life coach, clergy, support group, trusted advisor). Chapter 13.

Keep physically active, but avoid overdoing it (e.g., walking, qigong, tai chi, yoga). Chapter 13.

Identify and confront any other issues that frequently occur with, contribute to, or perpetuate overgrowth of candida (e.g., adrenal fatigue, sugar and carb addiction, excess oxalates, high glutamate, elevated histamine, chronic stress, heavy metal toxicity, nicotine use, food sensitivities, hypothyroidism, psychotropic drug use, low blood sugar, etc.).

Commit to lifelong maintenance. Be aware that changes in diet and lifestyle should be permanent to maintain improvements, and treatment remedies almost always need to be repeated periodically.

And finally, know that each of these steps must be done simultaneously.

Please be aware, although I am very knowledgeable on this topic, I do not know everything. I am always learning. Our collective understanding of candida and other microbes is continuously evolving. The path to healing may change. It is critical that you keep up-to-date on the information base by continuing to educate yourself periodically.

Making the changes required to manage yeast overgrowth and the many accompanying conditions is challenging initially. However, once the transition is complete, it will feel normal and right. You will question how you ever lived any other way and going back will seem unfathomable. Your life will be more aligned with your native roots and primal wisdom, which promotes more optimal health physically, emotionally, and spiritually, as it did for our ancestors for millions of years. I wish you an abundance of inner peace and strength on your journey and leave you with the following thought.

"Life's not about waiting for the storm to pass.
It's about learning to dance in the rain."

—VIVIAN GREEN

References

All web pages were last accessed September 2016 unless noted otherwise.

Chapter 1

1. William Shaw. *Biological Treatments for Autism and PDD Online.* Chapter Two. The microorganisms in the gastrointestinal tract. http://www.greatplainslaboratory.com/book/bk4sect1.html (Accessed 2013. Page no longer exists.)

2. W. L. Chaffin et al. "Cell Wall and Secreted Proteins of Candida Albicans: Identification, Function, and Expression." *Microbiology and Molecular Biology Reviews* 62.1 (1998). http://www.ncbi.nlm.nih.gov/pmc/articles/PMC98909/.

3. M. D. Lenardon, Carol A Munro, and Neil A.R. Gow. "Chitin Synthesis and Fungal Pathogenesis." *Current Opinion in Microbiology* 13.4 (2010). http://www.ncbi.nlm.nih.gov/pmc/articles/PMC2923753/.

4. Ingrid E. Frohner, et al. "Candida Albicans Cell Surface Superoxide Dismutases Degrade Host-Derived Reactive Oxygen Species to Escape Innate Immune Surveillance." *Molecular Microbiology* 71.1 (2009). https://www.ncbi.nlm.nih.gov/pmc/articles/PMC2713856/.

5. S. Hida et al. "Effect of Candida Albicans Cell Wall Glucan as Adjuvant for induction of Autoimmune Arthritis in Mice." *Journal of Autoimmunity* 25.2 (2005). http://www.ncbi.nlm.nih.gov/pubmed/16242302.

6. R. J. Marijnissen, et al. "Exposure to Candida Albicans Polarizes a T-cell Driven Arthritis Model Towards Th17 Responses, Resulting in a More Destructive Arthritis." *PLoS One* 7.6 (2012). http://www.ncbi.nlm.nih.gov/pubmed/22719976.

7. M. K. Lin, et al. "Secretory phospholipase A2 as an index of disease activity in rheumatoid arthritis. Prospective double blind study of 212 patients." *Journal of Rheumatology* 23.7 (1996). http://www.ncbi.nlm.nih.gov/pubmed/8823686.

8. Stephen Olmstead, et al. "Candida, Fungal-Type Dysbiosis and Chronic Disease—Exploring the Nature of the Yeast Connection." *Townsend Letter* June 2012. http://www.townsendletter.com/June2012/candida0612.html.

9. A. Bertling, et al. "Candida Albicans and its Metabolite Gliotoxin Inhibit Platelet Function via Interaction with Thiols." *Thrombosis and Haemostosis* 104.2 (2010). http://www.ncbi.nlm.nih.gov/pubmed/20431851.

10. M. R. Yeaman, et al. "Thrombin-induced Rabbit Platelet Microbicidal Protein is Fungicidal in Vitro."*Antimicrobial Agents and Chemotherapy* 37.3 (1993). http://www.ncbi.nlm.nih.gov/pubmed/8460923.

11. D. T. Shah and B. Larsen. "Clinical Isolates of Yeast Produce a Gliotoxin-like Substance." *Mycopathologia* 116.3 (1991). http://www.ncbi.nlm.nih.gov/pubmed/1724551.

12. D. T. Shah, D. D. Glover, and B. Larsen. "In Situ Mycotoxin Production by Candida Albicans in Women with Vaginitis." *Gynecologic and Obstetric Investigation* 39.1 (1995). http://www.ncbi.nlm.nih.gov/pubmed/7534255.

13. C. Kupfahl, et al. "Candida species fail to produce the immunosuppressive secondary metabolite gliotoxin in vitro." *FEMS Yeast Research* 7(6) (2007). http://www.ncbi.nlm.nih .gov/pubmed/17537180.

14. S. Bruns, et al. "Functional Genomic Profiling of Aspergillus Fumigatus Biofilm Reveals Enhanced Production of the Mycotoxin Gliotoxin." *Proteomics* 10.17 (2010). http://www.ncbi.nlm.nih.gov/pubmed/20645385.

15. C. A. Kumamoto. "Inflammation and Gastrointestinal Candida Colonization." *Current Opinion in Microbiology* 14.4 (2011). http://www.ncbi.nlm.nih.gov/pmc/articles/PMC 3163673/.

16. David Perlmutter, *Grain Brain: The Surprising Truth About Wheat, Carbs, and Sugar —Your Brain's Silent Killers.* New York, NY: Little, Brown and Company (2013).

17. S. Polákováa, et al. "Formation of New Chromosomes as a Virulence Mechanism in Yeast Candida Glabrata." *PNAS* 106.8 (2009). http://www.pnas.org/content/106/8/2688 .full?sid=e1d75c59-1e52-471b-9647-f83d9b54e5b1.

18. Michael Biamonte, C.C.N. "Confessions of a Candida Killer." http://www.examiner .com/article/confessions-of-a-candida-killer-michael-biamonte-c-c-n (Accessed 2013. Page no longer exists.)

19. William Shaw. *Biological Treatments for Autism and PDD Online.* Chapter Two. The microorganisms in the gastrointestinal tract. http://www.greatplainslaboratory.com/book/ bk4sect1.html (Accessed 2013. Page no longer exists.)

20. Datis Kharrazian. *Why Isn't My Brain Working?: A Revolutionary Understanding of Brain Decline and Effective Strategies to Recover Your Brain's Health.* Carlsbad, California: Elephant Press (2013).

21. J. Borg, et al. "The Serotonin System and Spiritual Experiences." *American Journal of Psychiatry* 160.11 (2003). https://ils.unc.edu/bmh/neoref/nrschizophrenia/jsp/review /tmp/490.pdf.

22. O. C. Truss. "Metabolic Abnormalities in Patients with Chronic Candidiasis: The Acetaldehyde Hypothesis." *Journal of Orthomolecular Psychiatry* 13.2 (1984). http:// orthomolecular.org/library/jom/1984/pdf/1984-v13n02-p066.pdf.

23. L. M. Epp and B. Mravec. "Chronic Polysystemic Candidiasis as a Possible Contributor to Onset of Idiopathic Parkinson's Disease." *Bratislava Medical Journal* 107.6–7 (2006). http://www.ncbi.nlm.nih.gov/pubmed/17051898.

24. Intelegen, Inc. "Acetaldehyde: A Common and Potent Neurotoxin How to Prevent the Damaging Effects of Smoking, Alcohol Consumption, and Air Pollution." http:// intelegen.com/nutrients/prevent_the_damaging_effects_of_.htm.

Referencing. O. C. Truss. "Metabolic Abnormalities in Patients with Chronic Candidiasis: The Acetaldehyde Hypothesis." *Journal of Orthomolecular Psychiatry*. 13.2 (1984). http://orthomolecular.org/library/jom/1984/pdf/1984-v13n02-p066.pdf.

25. Joan Mathews Larson. *Depression Free Naturally*. New York, NY: Ballantine (2001).

26. Rick Sponaugle. "Anxiety Disorder Causes." http://sponauglewellness.com/wellness-programs/anxiety/anxiety-panic-disorder-causes/ (Accessed 2013. Page no longer exists.)

27. Amy Yasko. *Autism: Pathways to Recovery*. Bethel, ME: Neurological Research Institute, LLC (2004, 2007, 2009).

28. Charles Gant. Endocrine Stress Webinar. http://www.cegant.com/.

29. James L. Wilson. AdrenalFatigue.org http://www.adrenalfatigue.org/.

30. Michael Lam. "Adrenal Fatigue vs Hypothyroidism." https://www.drlam.com/blog/adrenal-fatigue-versus-hypothyroidism-part-1/3643/.

31. Chris Kresser. "Five Ways that Stress Causes Hypothyroid Symptoms." http://chriskresser.com/5-ways-that-stress-causes-hypothyroid-symptoms/.

32. Charles Gant. Endocrine Stress Webinar. http://www.cegant.com/.

33. Chris Kresser. "Five Ways that Stress Causes Hypothyroid Symptoms." August 2, 2010. http://chriskresser.com/5-ways-that-stress-causes-hypothyroid-symptoms/.

34. William Shaw. "The Role of Oxalates in Autism and Chronic Disorders." The Weston A. Price Foundation. March 26, 2010. http://www.westonaprice.org/health-topics/the-role-of-oxalates-in-autism-and-chronic-disorders/.

35. William Shaw. "Oxalates: Test Implications for Yeast and Heavy Metals." http://www.greatplainslaboratory.com/home/eng/oxalates.asp (Accessed 2013. Page no longer exists.)

36. Great Plains Laboratory - OAT Test. http://www.greatplainslaboratory.com.

37. William Shaw. "Oxalates: Test Implications for Yeast and Heavy Metals." http://www.greatplainslaboratory.com/home/eng/oxalates.asp (Accessed 2013. Page no longer exists.)

38. Marjorie Crandall. "Yeast Infections, Candida Allergy, and Vulvodynia." http://www.empowher.com/yeast-infection/content/dr-marjorie-crandall-yeast-infections-candida-allergy-and-vulvodynia.

39. William Shaw. "The Role of Oxalates in Autism and Chronic Disorders." The Weston A. Price Foundation. March 26, 2010. http://www.westonaprice.org/health-topics/the-role-of-oxalates-in-autism-and-chronic-disorders/.

40. B. Y. Firestone and Stewart A. Koser. "Growth Promoting Effect of Some Biotin Analogues for Candida Albicans." *Journal of Bacteriology* 79.5 (1960). http://www.ncbi.nlm.nih.gov/pmc/articles/PMC278756/?page=1.

41. Ibid.

42. Robert C. Atkins. *Vita-Nutrient Solution: Nature's Answers to Drugs*. New York, NY: Fireside (1998).

43. Ma Biao, et al. "High-Affinity Transporters for NAD+ Precursors in *Candida Glabrata* Are Regulated by Hst1 and Induced in Response to Niacin Limitation." *Molecular and Cellular Biology* 29.15 (2009). http://www.ncbi.nlm.nih.gov/pmc/articles/PMC2715804/.

Orian C. Truss. *The Missing Diagnosis.* Birmingham, AL: Missing Diagnosis (1983).

Warren M. Levin and Fran Gare. *Beyond the Yeast Connection: A How-To Guide to Curing Candida and Other Yeast-Related Conditions.* Laguna Beach, CA: Basic Health Publications (2013).

John P. Trowbridge and Morton Walker. *The Yeast Syndrome: How to Help Your Doctor Identify and Treat the Real Cause of Your Yeast-Related Illness.* New York, NY: Bantam (1986).

Chapter 2

1. K. E. Fujimura, et al. "Role of the Gut Microbiota in Defining Human Health." *Expert Review of Anti-infective Therapy* 8.4 (2010). http://www.ncbi.nlm.nih.gov/pmc/articles PMC2881665/.

2. E. A. Grice and J. A. Segre. "The Human Microbiome: Our Second Genome." *Annual Review of Genomics and Human Genetics* 13 (2012). http://www.ncbi.nlm.nih.gov/pmc /articles/PMC3518434/.

3. B. Zhu, X. Li L.Wang. "Human Gut Microbiome: the second genome of human body." *Protein Cell* 1.8 (2010). http://www.ncbi.nlm.nih.gov/pubmed/21203913.

4. Joseph Mercola. "How your Gut Flora Influences Your Health." June 27, 2012. http:// articles.mercola.com/sites/articles/archive/2012/06/27/probiotics-gut-health-impact.aspx.

5. Joseph Mercola. "100 Trillion Bacteria in Your Gut: Learn How to Keep the Good Kind There." October 18, 2003. http://articles.mercola.com/sites/articles/archive/2003/10/18/ bacteria-gut.aspx.

6. David Perlmutter. "How Gut Bacteria Protect the Brain." http://www.drperlmutter .com/gut-bacteria-protects-brain/ (accessed September 2016).

7. William Shaw. *Biological Treatments for Autism and PDD Online.* Chapter Two. The microorganisms in the gastrointestinal tract. http://www.greatplainslaboratory.com/book /bk4sect1.html (Accessed 2013. Page no longer exists.).

8. Ibid.

9. Josh Kendall. "How Child Abuse and Neglect Damage the Brain." *The Boston Globe* 2002.

10. Madhusree Mukerjee. "Hidden Scars: Sexual and Other Abuse May Alter a Brain Region." *Scientific American* Issue: October 1995, vol 273.

11. Douglas J. Bremner. *Does Stress Damage the Brain: Understanding Trauma-Related Disorders from a Neurological Perspective.* W.W. Norton & Company, 2002.

12. Bruce Perry, "Neurobiological Sequelae of Childhood Trauma: Post-traumatic Stress Disorders in Children." Child Trauma Academy. http://www.childtrauma.org/.

13. Emeran A. Mayer, et al. "V. Stress and Irritable Bowel Syndrome." *American Journal of Physiology -Gastrointestinal and Liver Physiology* 280.4 (2001). http://ajpgi.physiol-ogy .org/content/280/4/G519.

14. Charles Gant. Endocrine Stress Webinar. www.cegant.com.

15. Dana Davis. "Adaptation to Environmental pH in Candida Albicans and its Relation to Pathogenesis." *Current Genetics* 44.1 (2003). http://link.springer.com/article/10.1007/s00294-003-0415-2.

16. N. Konno, et al. "Mechanism of Candida Albicans Transformation in Response to Changes of pH." *Biological and Pharmaceutical Bulletin* 29.5 (2006). http://www.ncbi.nlm.nih.gov/pubmed/16651720.

17. Slavena Vylkova, et al. "The Fungal Pathogen Candida Albicans Autoinduces Hyphal Morphogenesis by Raising Extracellular pH." *American Society for Microbiology* 2.3 (2011). http://www.ncbi.nlm.nih.gov/pmc/articles/PMC3101780/.

18. Chris Kresser. "What Everybody Ought to Know (but Doesn't) About Heartburn & Gerd." March 29, 2010. https://chriskresser.com/what-everybody-ought-to-know-but-doesnt-about-heartburn-gerd/.

19. Warren M. Levin and Fran Gare. *Beyond the Yeast Connection: A How-To Guide to Curing Candida and Other Yeast-Related Conditions.* Laguna Beach, CA: Basic Health Publications (2013).

20. Joseph Mercola. "'Extreme' Levels of Roundup Detected in Food—Are You Eating This Toxic Contaminant?" May 20, 2014. http://articles.mercola.com/sites/articles/archive/2014/05/20/glyphosate-roundup-levels.aspx.

21. Stephen C. Frantz. "Glyphosate . . . Misery in a Bottle." LA Progressive. https://www.laprogressive.com/glyphosate/.

22. Ibid.

23. Joseph Mercola. "New Research Fuels Roundup Weed Killer Toxicity Concerns." February 4, 2014. http://articles.mercola.com/sites/articles/archive/2014/02/04/roundup-glyphosate-toxicity.aspx.

24. Stephen C Frantz. "Glyphosate . . . Misery in a Bottle." LA Progressive. https://www.laprogressive.com/glyphosate/.

25. Charles Gant. Glyphosate Dangers webinar. www.cegant.com.

26. Terezia Farkas. "Why Farmer Suicide Rates are the Highest of Any Occupation." *The Huffington Post.* July 23, 2014. http://www.huffingtonpost.com/terezia-farkas/why-farmer-suicide-rates-_1_b_5610279.html.

27. Tom Philpott. "No GMOs Didn't Create India's Farmer Suicide Problem, But." Mother Jones. September 30, 2015. http://www.motherjones.com/tom-philpott/2015/09/no-gmos-didnt-create-indias-farmer-suicide-problem.

28. S. Thongprakaisang, et al. "Glyphosate Induces Human Breast Cancer Cells Growth via Estrogen Receptors." *Food and Chemical Toxicology* 59 (2013). http://www.ncbi.nlm.nih.gov/pubmed/23756170.

29. Joseph Mercola. "The Horrific Truth About Monsanto's Roundup Herbicide." June 9, 2013. http://articles.mercola.com/sites/articles/archive/2013/06/09/monsanto-roundup-herbicide.aspx.

30. Joseph Mercola. "New Research Fuels Roundup Weed Killer Toxicity Concerns." February 4, 2014. http://articles.mercola.com/sites/articles/archive/2014/02/04/roundup-glyphosate-toxicity.aspx.

31. Stephanie Seneff, PhD. "Roundup the Nontoxic Chemical That May be Destroying Our Health." The Weston A. Price Foundation. October 30, 2013. http://www.westona price.org/environmental-toxins/roundup-the-nontoxic-chemical-that-may-be-destroying-our-health.

32. Pesticide Action Network Asia and the Pacific. "An in-depth and comprehensive report of independent research on impacts and effects of Glyphosate and Roundup." November 2009.

33. Andre Leu. "Monsanto's Toxic Herbicide Glyphosate: A Review of its Health and Environmental Effects." Organic Producers Association of Queensland, May 15, 2007. https://www.organicconsumers.org/news/monsantos-toxic-herbicide-glyphosate-review-its-health-and-environmental-effects.

34. Charles Gant. Glyphosate Dangers webinar. www.cegant.com.

35. Joseph Mercola. "Toxic Herbicides Now Common in Pregnant Women's Breast Milk, Placentas and Umbilical Cords." April 22, 2014. http://articles.mercola.com/sites/articles/archive/2014/04/22/glyphosate-herbicide.aspx.

36. B.K. Binukumar, et al. "Nigrostriatal Neuronal Death Following Chronic Dichlorvos Exposure: Crosstalk between Mitochondrial Impairments, Synuclein Aggregation, Oxidative Damage and Behavioral Changes." *Molecular Brain* 3.35 (2010). http://www.ncbi.nlm.nih.gov/pmc/articles/PMC2996378/.

37. Northwest Coalition for Alternatives to Pesticides. "Insecticide Factsheet - Naled." *Journal of Pesticide Reform* Fall 22.3 (2002). https://d3n8a8pro7vhmx.cloudfront.net/ncap/pages/26/attachments/original/1428423409/naled.pdf?1428423409.

38. Naled Insecticide Fact Sheet. No Spray Coalition. http://nospray.org/naled-insecticide-fact-sheet/.

39. Kenneth D. Katz, et al. "Organophosphate Toxicity." Medscape. http://emedicine.medscape.com/article/167726-overview.

40. Sherry Rogers. *Depression: Cured at Last.* Syracuse, NY: Prestige Publishing (1997).

41. Naled Insecticide Fact Sheet. No Spray Coalition. http://nospray.org/naled-insecticide-fact-sheet/.

42. Janie F. Shelton, et al. "Neurodevelopmental Disorders and Prenatal Proximity to Agricultural Pesticides: The CHARGE Study." Environmental Health Perspectives. 122.10 (2014). http://www.drperlmutter.com/wp-content/uploads/2016/02/ehp.1307044.alt_1.pdf.

43. Diabetes and the Environment. Pesticides. http://www.diabetesandenvironment.org/home/contam/pesticides.

44. Sarah Myhill. http://www.drmyhill.co.uk/.

45. C. Nasuti, et al. "Changes on Fecal Microbiota in Rats Exposed to Permethrin During Postnatal Development." *Environmental Science and Pollution Research* 23.11 (2016). http://www.ncbi.nlm.nih.gov/pubmed/26898931.

46. J. Kim, et al. "Permethrin Alters Adipogenesis in 3T3-L1 Adipocytes and Causes Insulin Resistance in C2C12 Myotubes." *Journal of Biochemical and Molecular Toxicology* 28.9 (2014). http://www.ncbi.nlm.nih.gov/pubmed/24911977.

47. National Pesticide Information Center. "Pyrethrins General Fact Sheet." http://npic .orst.edu/factsheets/pyrethrins.pdf.

48. National Pesticide Information Center. "Permethrin." http://npic.orst.edu/factsheets /PermGen.html.

49. Liz Szabo. "Exposure to Pesticides in Womb Linked to Learning Disabilities." February 7, 2011. Organic Consumers Association. https://www.organicconsumers.org/news /exposure-pesticides-womb-linked-learning-disabilities.

50. A. V. Krebs. "Buzz Off: L.L. Bean's New Line of Sportswear Coated with a Likely Carcinogenic Bug Repellent." Organic Consumers Association. https://www. organicconsumers.org/old_articles/clothes/llbean20805.php.

51. Nikita Naik. "Tea Steeped in Toxics." Pesticides and You. 2015; 35 (3). http:// beyondpesticides.org/assets/media/documents/ToxicTea.pdf.

52. Beyond Pesticides. "Chemical Watch Fact Sheet. Permethrin." http://beyondpesticides .org/assets/media/documents/pesticides/factsheets/permethrin.pdf.

53. Beyond Pesticides. "Chemical Watch Fact Sheet. Synthetic Pyrethroids." http:// beyondpesticides.org/assets/media/documents/pesticides/factsheets/Synthetic%20 Pyrethroids.pdf.

54. Al Sears. "How I Keep the Critters Out." http://www.alsearsmd.com/2011/04/ how-i-keep-the-critters-out/.

55. Beyond Pesticides. "Chemical Watch Fact Sheet. Piperonyl Butoxide." https://www .beyondpesticides.org/assets/media/documents/pesticides/factsheets/Piperonyl%20 Butoxide.pdf.

56. Al Sears. "How I Keep the Critters Out." http://www.alsearsmd.com/2011/04/how-i -keep-the-critters-out/.

57. Michael. "Care what You Wear: Facts on Cotton and Clothing." Organic Consumers Association. July 29, 2007. https://www.organicconsumers.org/news /care-what-you-wear-facts-cotton-clothing-production.

58. Bruce Perry. "Aggression and Violence: The Neurobiology of Experience." http:// teacher.scholastic.com/professional/bruceperry/aggression_violence.htm.

59. Jeffrey McCombs. "Myth #6 Mercury Feeds Candida." https://www.youtube.com /watch?v=kZ7c0wpGsxw.

60. Charles Gant. Endocrine Stress webinar. Detoxification webinar. www.cegant.com.

61. Ibid.

62. M. T. Sutter-Dub. "Effects of Pregnancy and Progesterone and/or Oestradiol on the Insulin Secretion and Pancreatic Insulin Content in the Perfused Rat Pancreas." Diabetes & Metabolism 15.1 (1979). http://www.ncbi.nlm.nih.gov/pubmed/446833.

63. Nahdid D. Madani, et al. "Candida Albicans Estrogen-binding Protein Gene Encodes an Oxidoreductase that is Inhibited by Estradiol." Microbiology. Proceedings of the National Academy of Science. USA 91 (1994). http://www.pnas.org/content/91/3/922.full. pdf.

64. S. White, et al. "Candida Albicans Morphogenesis is Influenced by Estrogen."

Cellular and Molecular Life Sciences 53.9 (1997). https://www.researchgate.net/publication /13860576_Candida_albicans_morphogenesis_is_influenced_by_estogen.

65. P. L. Fidel, et al. "Effects of Reproductive Hormones on Experimental Vaginal Candidiasis." *Infection and Immunity* 68.2 (2000). http://www.ncbi.nlm.nih.gov/pmc/articles/ PMC97188/.

66. Women's International. "A Connection with Yeast." https://www.womensinternational .com/connections/yeast.html.

67. Michael Biamonte. C.C.N. "Confessions of a Candida Killer." http://www.examiner .com/article/confessions-of-a-candida-killer-michael-biamonte-c-c-n (Accessed 2013. Page no longer exists.)

S. A. Meyer, D. G. Ahearn, and D. Yarrow. Candida Berkhout. In N. J. W. Kreger-van Rij (ed.), *The Yeasts: A Taxonomic Study*. Elsevier Science Publishers, Amsterdam. 1984.

Chapter 3

1. Center for Biofilm Engineering. Montana State University. http://www.biofilm .montana.edu/biofilm-basics.html.

2. M. A. Al-Fattani and L. J. Douglas. "Biofilm Matrix of Candida Albicans and Candida Tropicalis: Chemical Composition and Role in Drug Resistance." *Journal of Medical Microbiology* 55.8 (2006). http://www.ncbi.nlm.nih.gov/pubmed/16849719.

3. Gordon Ramage, et al. "Candida Biofilms: An Update." *Eukaryotic Cell* 4.4 (2005). http://ec.asm.org/content/4/4/633.full.

4. Heather T. Taff, et al. "Mechanisms of Candida Biofilm Drug Resistance." *Future Microbiology* 8.10 (2013). http://www.ncbi.nlm.nih.gov/pmc/articles/PMC3859465/.

5. C. Potera. "Antibiotic Resistance: Biofilm Dispersing Agent Rejuvenates Older Antibiotics." *Environmental Health Perspectives* 118.7 (2010). http://www.ncbi.nlm.nih.gov /pmc/articles/PMC2920928/.

6. Jyotsna Chandra, et al. "Biofilm Formation by the Fungal Pathogen Candida Albicans: Development, Architecture, and Drug Resistance." *Journal of Bacteriology* 183.18 (2001). http://www.ncbi.nlm.nih.gov/pmc/articles/PMC95423/?report=reader.

7. D. M. Kuhn, et al. "Antifungal Susceptibility of Candida Biofilms: Unique Efficacy of Amphotericin B Lipid Formulations and Echinocandins." *Antimicrobial Agents and Chemotherapy* 46.6 (2002). http://www.ncbi.nlm.nih.gov/pmc/articles/PMC127206/.

8. C. Potera. "Antibiotic Resistance: Biofilm Dispersing Agent Rejuvenates Older Antibiotics." *Environmental Health Perspectives* 118.7 (2010). http://www.ncbi.nlm.nih.gov /pmc/articles/PMC2920928/.

9. Gordon Ramage, et al. "Candida Biofilms: An Update." *Eukaryotic Cell* 4.4 (2005). http://ec.asm.org/content/4/4/633.full.

10. Center for Biofilm Engineering. Montana State University. http://www.biofilm .montana.edu/biofilm-basics.html.

11. M. A. Al-Fattani and L. J. Douglas. "Biofilm Matrix of Candida Albicans and Candida Tropicalis: Chemical Composition and Role in Drug Resistance." *Journal of Medical Microbiology* 55.8 (2006). http://www.ncbi.nlm.nih.gov/pubmed/16849719.

12. Stephanie Pappas. "Weird Way Lyme Disease Bugs Avoid Immune System." Live Science. March 22, 2013. http://www.livescience.com/28120-lyme-disease-manganese.html.

13. Anju Usman. http://www.autismpedia.org/wiki/index.php?title=Protocols/Usman (Accessed 2013. Page no longer exists.).

14. D. M. Kuhn, et al. "Antifungal Susceptibility of Candida Biofilms: Unique Efficacy of Amphotericin B Lipid Formulations and Echinocandins." *Antimicrobial Agents and Chemotherapy* 46.6 (2002). http://www.ncbi.nlm.nih.gov/pmc/articles/PMC127206/.

15. M. A. El-Feky, et al. "Effect of Ciprofloxacin and N-acetylcysteine on Bacterial Adherence and Biofilm Formation on Ureteral Stent Surfaces." *Polish Journal of Microbiology* 58.3 (2009). https://www.ncbi.nlm.nih.gov/pubmed/19899620.

16. Prothera. "Interfase Plus." Integrated Nutraceuticals for Healthcare Professionals. https://www.protherainc.com/prod/proddetail.asp?ID=K-INTP (Accessed 2013. Page no longer exists.).

17. National Institutes of Health. "Research on Microbial Biofilms." December 20, 2002. https://grants.nih.gov/grants/guide/pa-files/PA-03-047.html.

18. Anju Usman. http://www.autismpedia.org/wiki/index.php?title=Protocols/Usman (Accessed 2013. Information no longer exists.).

Chapter 4

1. Jeffrey McCombs. "The Candida Spit Test." https://www.youtube.com/watch?v=o6 iryzPoBow.

2. Mary Budinger. "Dispatches from the Front Lines of Autism and Lyme Disease." *Townsend Letter* October 2009. http://www.townsendletter.com/Oct2009/dispatch1009 .html.

3. Warren M. Levin and Fran Gare. *Beyond the Yeast Connection: A How-to Guide to Curing Candida and Other Yeast-Related Conditions*. Laguna Beach, CA: Basic Health Publications (2013).

William G. Crook. *The Yeast Connection: A Medical Breakthrough*. Revised ed. New York, NY: Vintage Books (1986).

Jonathan V. Wright. *Why Stomach Acid is Good for You: Natural Relief from Heartburn, Indigestion, Reflux and Gerd*. Lanham, MD: M. Evans & Company (2001).

Chapter 5

1. Ingrid Kohlstadt. "Klinghardt Academy's Biological Medicine 2012: Conference Highlights." *Townsend Letter* 2012. http://www.townsendletter.com/June2012/ klinghardt0612.html.

2. Telegraph Reporter. "Parasite in Cats Linked to Learning Difficulties in Children." *The Telegraph* June 1 2015. http://www.telegraph.co.uk/news/science/science-news/11644581 /Cats-make-children-stupid-study-suggests.html.

3. A. L. Sutterland, et al. "Beyond the Association. Toxoplasma gondii in Schizophrenia, Bipolar disorder, and Addiction: Systematic Review and Meta-analysis." *Acta Psychiatrica Scandinavica* 132.3 (2015). http://onlinelibrary.wiley.com/doi/10.1111/acps.12423 /abstract.

4. Christof Koch. "Protozoa Could Be Controlling Your Brain." *Scientific American* May 1 2011. https://www.scientificamerican.com/article/fatal-attraction/.

5. Ibid.

6. Kathleen Mcauliffe. "How Your Cat Is Making You Crazy." *The Atlantic* March 2012. http://www.theatlantic.com/magazine/archive/2012/03/how-your-cat-is-making -you-crazy/308873/.

7. Carl Zimmer. "Hidden Epidemic: Tapeworms Living Inside People's Brains. *Discover Magazine* June 2012. http://www.theatlantic.com/magazine/archive/2012/03/how-your -cat-is-making-you-crazy/308873/.

8. Leo Galland. "Dysbiotic Relationships in the Bowel." American College of Advancement in Medicine Conference, Spring 1992.

9. Ingrid Kohlstadt. "Klinghardt Academy's Biological Medicine 2012: Conference Highlights." *Townsend Letter* 2012. http://www.townsendletter.com/June2012/ klinghardt0612.html.

10. Charles Gant. "Parasite Protocol." 2012 Class Webinar from the Academy of Functional Medicine & Genomics.

11. Ibid. The remainder of quotations and statistics from Dr. Gant in this chapter were obtained from this source.

12. Better Health Guy. "A Deep Look Beyond Lyme." April 27, 2013. http://www. betterhealthguy.com/a-deep-look-beyond-lyme.

13. Larry M. Bush. "Overview of Bacteria." *Merck Manual.* Consumer Version. http:// www.merckmanuals.com/home/infections/bacterial-infections/overview-of-bacteria.

14. Judith Romero-Gallo, et. al. "Effect of Helicobacter pylori Eradication on Gastric Carcinogenesis." *Laboratory Investigation* 88.3 (2008). http://www.ncbi.nlm.nih.gov /pmc/articles/PMC2833422/.

15. Qi-Jun Wu, et al. "Cruciferous Vegetable Consumption and Gastric Cancer Risk: A Meta-Analysis of Epidemiological Studies."*Cancer Science* 104.8 (2013). http://online library.wiley.com/doi/10.1111/cas.12195/pdf.

16. L. E. Wroblewski, R. M. Peek, and K.T. Wilson. "Helicobacter pylori and Gastric Cancer: Factors That Modulate Disease Risk." *Clinical Microbiology Reviews* 23.4 (2010). http://www.ncbi.nlm.nih.gov/pmc/articles/PMC2952980/.

17. N. F. Azevedo, et al. "Coccoid Form of Helicobacter pylori as a Morphological Manifestation of Cell Adaptation to the Environment." *Applied and Environmental Microbiology* 73.10 (2007). http://www.ncbi.nlm.nih.gov/pmc/articles/PMC1907093/.

18. News Medical. "H. Pylori Bacterium produces Urease to Neutralize Gastric Acid." December 8, 2011. http://www.news-medical.net/news/20111208/H-pylori-bacterium -produces-urease-to-neutralize-gastric-acid.aspx.

19. H. Suzuki, T. Nishizawa, and T. Hibi. "Helicobacter Pylori Eradication Therapy." *Future Microbiology* 5.4 (2010). http://www.ncbi.nlm.nih.gov/pubmed/20353303.

20. Mary Budinger. "Dispatches from the Front Lines of Autism and Lyme Disease." *Townsend Letter* October 2009. http://www.townsendletter.com/Oct2009/dispatch1009. html.

21. Warren M. Levin and Fran Gare. *Beyond the Yeast Connection: A How-to Guide to Curing Candida and Other Yeast-Related Conditions*. Laguna Beach, CA: Basic Health Publications (2013).

22. Ben Tufft. "Virus that Makes Humans More Stupid Discovered." *Independent*. November 9, 2014. http://www.independent.co.uk/news/science/virus-that-makes-humans -more-stupid-discovered-9849920.html.

23. Robert H. Yolkena, et al. "Chlorovirus ATCV-1 is Part of the Human Oropharyngeal Virome and is Associated with Changes in Cognitive functions in Humans and Mice." *PNAS* 111.45 (2014). http://www.pnas.org/content/early/2014/10/23/1418895111 .abstract.

John P. Trowbridge and Morton Walker. *The Yeast Syndrome: How to Help Your Doctor Identify and Treat the Real Cause of Your Yeast-Related Illness*. New York, NY: Bantam (1986).

World Health Organization. www.who.int.

Chapter 6

1. Chris Kresser. "SIBO - What Causes it and why it's so hard to treat." November 4, 2014. http://chriskresser.com/sibo-what-causes-it-and-why-its-so-hard-to-treat.

2. Allison Siebecker and Steven Sandberg-Lewis. "Small Intestine Bacterial Overgrowth: Often-Ignored Cause of Irritable Bowel Syndrome." *Townsend Letter* February / March 2013. http://www.townsendletter.com/FebMarch2013/ibs0213_2.html.

3. A. Fasano. "Leaky gut and Autoimmune Diseases." *Clinical Reviews in Allergy and Immunology* 42.1 (2012). http://www.ncbi.nlm.nih.gov/pubmed/22109896.

4. Adam Hadhazy. "Think Twice. How the Guts 'Second Brain' Influences Mood and Well Being." February 12, 2010. http://www.scientificamerican.com/article/gut-second-brain/.

5. William Shaw. "Inhibition of Dopamine Conversion to Norepinephrine by Clostridia Metabolites Appears to be a (the) Major cause of Autism, Schizophrenia, and Other Neuropsychiatric Disorders." http://www.greatplainslaboratory.com/home/eng/articles /Interference%20in%20dopamine%20conversion%20to%20norepinephrine%20 FINAL.pdf (Accessed 2013. Page no longer exists.)

6. Debora MacKenzie. "Bacteria Could be Significant Cause of OCD." *New Scientist*. March 28, 2012. http://www.newscientist.com/article/dn21635-bacteria-could-be -significant-cause-of-ocd.

7. Rob Stein. "Gut Bacteria Might Guide the Workings of Our Minds." National Public Radio. November 18, 2013. http://www.npr.org/sections/health-shots/2013/11/18/244526773 /gut-bacteria-might-guide-the-workings-of-our-minds.

8. Ibid.

9. Ibid.

10. Jeffrey Norris. "Do Gut Bacteria Rule Our Minds." University of California San Francisco. August 15, 2014. https://www.ucsf.edu/news/2014/08/116526 /do-gut-bacteria-rule-our-minds.

11. Grace Liu. "Don't Take Resistant Starch If You Have Moderate to Severe Irritable

Bowel Syndrome (IBS) Temporarily" (Part 3) October 2, 2014. http://drbganimalpharm .blogspot.com/2014/10/dont-take-raw-resistant-starch-if-you.html.

12. C. Tana, et al. "Altered profiles of intestinal microbiota and organic acids may be the origin of symptoms in irritable bowel syndrome." *Journal of Neurogastroenterology & Motility* 22.5 (2010). http://onlinelibrary.wiley.com/doi/10.1111/j.1365–2982.2009.01427.x /full.

13. Katsunari Nishihara. "Disclosure of the Major Causes of Mental Illness— Mitochondrial Deterioration in Brain Neurons via Opportunistic Infection." *Journal of Biological Physics and Chemistry* 12.1 (2012). https://www.researchgate.net/ publication /270937404_Disclosure_of_the_major_causes_of_mental_illness-mitochondrial_ deterioration_in_brain_neurons_via_opportunistic_infection.

14. Uday C. Ghoshal, et al. "The Gut Microbiota and Irritable Bowel Syndrome: Friend or Foe?" *International Journal of Inflammation,* vol. 2012, Article ID 151085 (2012). http://www.hindawi.com/journals/iji/2012/151085/.

15. M. Pimentel, et al. "A Link between Irritable Bowel Syndrome and Fibromyalgia may be Related to Findings on Lactulose Breath Testing." *Annals of the Rheumatic Diseases* 63.4 (2004). http://www.ncbi.nlm.nih.gov/pubmed/15020342.

16. Michael Eades. "GERD: Treat it with a low or high carb diet." September 23, 2013. http://www.proteinpower.com/drmike/gerdacid-reflux/gerd-treat-low-high-carb-diet/.

17. Andrew C. Dukowicz, Brian E. Lacy, and Gary M. Levine. "Small Intestinal Bacterial Overgrowth: A Comprehensive Review." *Gastroenterology & Hepatology* 3.2 (2007). http://www.ncbi.nlm.nih.gov/pmc/articles/PMC3099351/.

18. Toku Takahashi. "Mechanism of Interdigestive Migrating Motor Complex." *Journal of Neurogastroenterology and Motility* 18.3 (2012). http://www.ncbi.nlm.nih.gov/pmc /articles/PMC3400812/.

19. Mark Pimentel. *A New IBS Solution: Bacteria—The Missing Link in Treating Irritable Bowel.* Sherman Oaks, CA: Health Point Press (2008).

20. T. Hauge, J. Persson, and D. Danielsson. "Mucosal Bacterial Growth in the Upper Gastrointestinal Tract in Alcoholics (Heavy Drinkers)." *Digestion* 58.6 (1997). http:// www.karger.com/Article/Abstract/201507.

21. S. L. Gabbard, et al. "The Impact of Alcohol Consumption and Cholecystectomy on Small Intestinal Bacterial Overgrowth." *Digestive Diseases and Sciences* 59.3 (2014). http://www.ncbi.nlm.nih.gov/pubmed/24323179.

22. I. Levin, et al. "The Ternary Complex of Pseudomonas Aeruginosa Alcohol Dehydrogenase with NADH and Ethylene Glycol." *Protein Science* 13.6 (2004). http://online library.wiley.com/doi/10.1110/ps.03531404/full.

23. Chris Kresser. "SIBO and Methane - What's the Connection." September 18, 2014. http://chriskresser.com/sibo-and-methane-whats-the-connection.

24. Marian Dix Lemle. "Hypothesis: Is ME/CFS Caused by Dysregulation of Hydrogen Sulfide Metabolism." *Medical Hypotheses* 72.1 (2009). http://www.mecfswa.org.au /News_and_Media/News_Details/Hypothesis_Is_ME-CFS_caused_by_dysregulation_of _hydrogen_sulfide_metabolism/Default.aspx12.

25. Allison Siebecker and Steven Sandberg-Lewis. "Small Intestine Bacterial Overgrowth:

Often-Ignored Cause of Irritable Bowel Syndrome." *Townsend Letter* February / March 2013. http://www.townsendletter.com/FebMarch2013/ibs0213_2.html.

26. Chris Kresser. "SIBO and Methane - What's the Connection." September 18, 2014. http://chriskresser.com/sibo-and-methane-whats-the-connection.

27. Ibid.

28. Ibid.

29. M. Simrén and P. O. Stotzer. "Use and Abuse of Hydrogen Breath Tests." *Gut* 55.3 (2006). http://www.ncbi.nlm.nih.gov/pmc/articles/PMC1856094/.

30. Allison Siebecker and Steven Sandberg-Lewis. "Small Intestine Bacterial Overgrowth: Often-Ignored Cause of Irritable Bowel Syndrome." *Townsend Letter* February / March 2013. http://www.townsendletter.com/FebMarch2013/ibs0213_2.html.

31. M. Simrén and P. O. Stotzer. "Use and Abuse of Hydrogen Breath Tests." *Gut* 55.3 (2006). http://www.ncbi.nlm.nih.gov/pmc/articles/PMC1856094/.

32. Allison Siebecker. "Key Indicators of Small Intestinal Bacterial Overgrowth." https://www.youtube.com/watch?v=GXGJNsDAGi8&feature=youtu.be.

33. Chris Kresser. "SIBO and Methane - What's the Connection." September 18, 2014. http://chriskresser.com/sibo-and-methane-whats-the-connection.

34. Allison Siebecker and Steven Sandberg-Lewis. "Small Intestine Bacterial Overgrowth: Often-Ignored Cause of Irritable Bowel Syndrome." *Townsend Letter* February / March 2013. http://www.townsendletter.com/FebMarch2013/ibs0213_2.html.

35. Jill Carnahan. "6 Signs that SIBO might be the Root Cause of Your IBS." Primal Docs. http://primaldocs.com/opinion/6-signs-that-sibo-might-be-the-root-cause-of-your-ibs/.

36. V. Chedid, et al. "Herbal Therapy is Equivalent to Rifaximin for the Treatment of Small Intestinal Bacterial Overgrowth." *Global Advances in Health and Medicine* 3.3 (2014). http://www.ncbi.nlm.nih.gov/pubmed/24891990.

37. A. C. Logan and T.M. Beaulne. "The Treatment of Small Intestinal Bacterial Overgrowth with Enteric-Coated Peppermint Oil: a Case Report." *Alternative Medicine Review* 7.5 (2002). http://www.ncbi.nlm.nih.gov/pubmed/12410625.

38. Amlan K. Patra and Zhongtang Yu. "Effects of Essential Oils on Methane Production and Fermentation by, and Abundance and Diversity of, Rumen Microbial Populations." *Applied and Environmental Microbiology* 78.12 (2012). http://aem.asm.org/content/78/12/4271.full.

39. R. Snowden, et al. "A Comparison of the Anti-Staphylococcus Aureus Activity of Extracts from Commonly Used Medicinal Plants." *Journal of Alternative and Complementary Medicine* 20.5 (2014). http://www.ncbi.nlm.nih.gov/pubmed/24635487.

40. University of Maryland Medical Center. Complimentary and Alternative Medicine Guide. "Uva ursi." http://umm.edu/health/medical/altmed/herb/uva-ursi.

41. D. A. Mahmoud, et al. "Antifungal Activity of Different Neem Leaf Extracts and the Nimonol against Some Important Human Pathogens." *Brazilian Journal of Microbiology* 42.3 (2011). http://www.ncbi.nlm.nih.gov/pmc/articles/PMC3768785/.

42. Allison Siebecker and Steven Sandberg-Lewis. "Small Intestine Bacterial Overgrowth:

Often-Ignored Cause of Irritable Bowel Syndrome." *Townsend Letter* February / March 2013. http://www.townsendletter.com/FebMarch2013/ibs0213_2.html.

43. Chris Kresser. "SIBO and Methane - What's the Connection." September 18, 2014. http://chriskresser.com/sibo-and-methane-whats-the-connection.

44. Allison Siebecker and Steven Sandberg-Lewis. "Small Intestine Bacterial Overgrowth: Often-Ignored Cause of Irritable Bowel Syndrome." *Townsend Letter* February / March 2013. http://www.townsendletter.com/FebMarch2013/ibs0213_2.html.

45. Norm Robillard. *Heartburn: Fast Tract Digestion.* Watertown, MA: Self Health Publishing (2012).

IBS: Fast Tract Digestion. Watertown, MA: Self Health Publishing (2013).

46. Allison Siebecker and Steven Sandberg-Lewis. "Small Intestine Bacterial Overgrowth: Often-Ignored Cause of Irritable Bowel Syndrome." *Townsend Letter* February / March 2013. http://www.townsendletter.com/FebMarch2013/ibs0213_2.html.

47. Larry M. Bush. "Overview of Bacteria." *Merck Manual.* Consumer Version. http://www.merckmanuals.com/home/infections/bacterial-infections/overview-of-bacteria.

48. Kate Ruder. Genome News Network. "Got a Toxic Mess? Call in the Microbes." April 2, 2004. http://www.genomenewsnetwork.org/articles/2004/04/02/toxic_microbe.php.

49. Allison Siebecker and Steven Sandberg-Lewis. "Small Intestine Bacterial Overgrowth: Often-Ignored Cause of Irritable Bowel Syndrome." *Townsend Letter* February / March 2013. http://www.townsendletter.com/FebMarch2013/ibs0213_2.html.

50. Joseph Mercola. "New Research Fuels Roundup Weed Killer Toxicity Concerns." February 4, 2014. http://articles.mercola.com/sites/articles/archive/2014/02/04/roundup--glyphosate-toxicity.aspx.

51. D. A. Gorard. "Is the Cyclic Nature of Migrating Motor Complex Dependent on the Sleep Cycle?" *Primary Motility Disorders of the Esophagus* 1998. http://www.hon.ch/OESO/books/Vol_5_Eso_Junction/Articles/art014.html.

52. Chris Kresser. "SIBO and Methane - What's the Connection." Sept 18, 2014. http://chriskresser.com/sibo-and-methane-whats-the-connection.

53. Y. Wang, et al. "Vagal Nerve Regulation is Essential for the Increase in Gastric Motility in Response to Mild Exercise." *The Tohoku Journal of Experimental Medicine* 222.2 (2010). http://www.ncbi.nlm.nih.gov/pubmed/20948179.

54. Andrew C. Dukowicz, Brian E. Lacy, and Gary M. Levine. "Small Intestinal Bacterial Overgrowth: A Comprehensive Review." *Gastroenterology & Hepatology* 3.2 (2007). http://www.ncbi.nlm.nih.gov/pmc/articles/PMC3099351/.

55. Allison Siebecker and Steven Sandberg-Lewis. "Small Intestine Bacterial Overgrowth: Often-Ignored Cause of Irritable Bowel Syndrome." *Townsend Letter* February / March 2013. http://www.townsendletter.com/FebMarch2013/ibs0213_2.html.

56. Ibid.

57. James Schaller. *Combating Biofilms: The Reason Many Diseases Do Not Respond to Treatment.* Naples, FL: International Infectious Disease Press (2014). Kindle Version.

58. U.S. Food and Drug Administration. Zelnorm (tegaserod maleate) Information.

http://www.fda.gov/Drugs/DrugSafety/PostmarketDrugSafetyInformationforPatientsand
Providers/ucm103223.htm.

59. Muhammad Nabeel Ghayur and Anwarul Hassan Gilani. "Pharmacological Basis for the Medicinal Use of Ginger in Gastrointestinal Disorders." *Digestive Diseases and Sciences* 50.10 (2005). http://link.springer.com/article/10.1007%2Fs10620-005-2957-2.

Chapter 7

1. William Shaw. "Candida and Yeast Overgrowth. The Yeast Problem and Bacteria By-products." http://www.greatplainslaboratory.com/home/eng/candida.asp (Accessed 2013. Page no longer exists.).

2. M.A. Pfaller, et al. "Candida Krusei, a Multidrug-Resistant Opportunistic Fungal Pathogen: Geographic and Temporal Trends from the ARTEMIS DISK Antifungal Surveillance Program, 2001 to 2005." *Journal of Clinical Microbiology* 46.2 (2008). http://www.ncbi.nlm.nih.gov/pmc/articles/PMC2238087/.

3. Carol A Kauffman. "Treatment of Candidemia and Invasive Candidiasis in Adults." Up to Date. Literature review current through: August 2016. http://www.uptodate.com/contents/treatment-of-candidemia-and-invasive-candidiasis-in-adults.

4. Thomas J. Walsh, et al. "Amphotericin B Lipid Complex for Invasive Fungal Infections: Analysis of Safety and Efficacy in 556 Cases." *Clinical Infectious Diseases* 26.6 (1998). http://cid.oxfordjournals.org/content/26/6/1383.full.pdf.

5. William Shaw. *Biological Treatments for Autism and PDD Online*. Chapter Four. Yeasts and Fungi: How to Control Them. http://www.greatplainslaboratory.com/book/bk6sect1.html (Accessed 2013. Page no longer exists.).

6. Warren M. Levin and Fran Gare. *Beyond the Yeast Connection: A How-To Guide to Curing Candida and Other Yeast-Related Conditions*. Laguna Beach, CA: Basic Health Publications (2013).

7. Gary A. Dykes, Ryszard Amarowicz, and Ronald B. Pegg. "Enhancement of Nisin Antibacterial Activity by a Bearberry (Arctostaphylos uva-ursi) Leaf Extract." *Food Microbiology* 20.2 (2003). http://www.researchgate.net/publication/248565236_Enhancement_of_nisin_antibacterial_activity_by_a_bearberry_%28_Arctostaphylos_uva-ursi%29_leaf_extract.

8. V. Manohar, et al. "Antifungal Activities of Origanum Oil Against Candida Albicans." *Molecular and Cellular Biochemistry* 228.(1–2) (2001). http://www.ncbi.nlm.nih.gov/pubmed/11855736.

9. Georgetown University Medical Center. "Oregano Oil May Protect Against Drug-Resistant Bacteria, Georgetown Researcher Finds." ScienceDaily. October 11, 2001. http://www.sciencedaily.com/releases/2001/10/011011065609.htm.

10. H. J. D. Dorman and S. G. Deans. "Antimicrobial Agents from Plants: Antibacterial Activity of Plant Volatile Oils." *Journal Applied Microbiology* 88.2 (2000). http://onlinelibrary.wiley.com/doi/10.1046/j.1365-2672.2000.00969.x/full.

11. M. Ponce-Macotela, et al. "Oregano (Lippia spp.) Kills Giardia Intestinalis Trophozoites in Vitro: Antigiardiasic Activity and Ultrastructural Damage." *Parasitology Research* 98.6 (2006). https://www.ncbi.nlm.nih.gov/pubmed/16425064.

12. K. Bright, et al. "Antiviral Efficacy and Mechanisms of Action of Oregano Essential Oil and its Primary Component Carvacrol Against Murine Norovirus." *Journal of Applied Microbiology* 116.5 (2014). http://onlinelibrary.wiley.com/doi/10.1111/jam.12453/abstract.

13. Catherine Paddock. "Himalayan Oregano Effective Against MRSA." November 24, 2008. http://www.medicalnewstoday.com/articles/130620.php.

14. Y. Omura, et al. "Caprylic Acid in the Effective Treatment of Intractable Medical Problems of Frequent Urination, Incontinence, Chronic Upper Respiratory Infection, Root Canalled Tooth Infection, ALS, etc., Caused by Asbestos & Mixed Infections of Candida Albicans, Helicobacter Pylori & Cytomegalovirus with or without other Microorganisms & Mercury." *Acupuncture and Electro-therapeutics Research* 36.(1–2) (2011). http://www.ncbi.nlm.nih.gov/pubmed/21830350.

15. M. Takahashi, et al. "Inhibition of Candida Mycelia Growth by a Medium Chain Fatty Acids, Capric Acid in Vitro and its Therapeutic Efficacy in Murine Oral Candidiasis." *Medical Mycology Journal* 53.4 (2012). http://www.ncbi.nlm.nih.gov/pubmed/23257726.

16. G. Bergsson, et al. "In Vitro Killing of Candida Albicans by Fatty Acids and Monoglycerides." *Antimicrobial Agents and Chemotherapy* 45.11 (2001) http://www.ncbi.nlm.nih.gov/pmc/articles/PMC90807/?tool=pubmed.

17. B. G. Carpo, V. M. Verallo-Rowell, and J. Kabara. "Novel Antibacterial Activity of Monolaurin Compared with Conventional Antibiotics Against Organisms from Skin infections: an in Vitro Study." *Journal of Drugs in Dermatology* 6.10 (2007) http://www.ncbi.nlm.nih.gov/pubmed/17966176.

18. G. Bergsson, O. Steingrímsson, and H. Thormar. "Bactericidal Effects of Fatty Acids and Monoglyccrides on Helicobacter Pylori." *International Journal of Antimicrobial Agents* 20.4 (2002). http://www.ncbi.nlm.nih.gov/pubmed/12385681.

19. William Shaw. *Biological Treatments for Autism and PDD Online.* Chapter Four. Yeasts and Fungi: How to Control Them. http://www.greatplainslaboratory.com/book/bk6sect1.html (Accessed 2013. Page no longer exists.).

20. Thorne Research Inc. "Undecylenic acid. (Monograph: undecylenic acid)." *Alternative Medicine Review* 7.1 (2002). http://www.altmedrev.com/publications/7/1/68.pdf.

21. L. M. Gonçalves, et. al. "Effects of Undecylenic Acid Released from Denture Liner on Candida Biofilms." *Journal of Dental Research* 91.10 (2012). http://www.ncbi.nlm.nih.gov/pubmed/22904206.

22. L. N. Nguyen, et al. "Sodium Butyrate Inhibits Pathogenic Yeast Growth and Enhances the Functions of Macrophages." *Journal of Antimicrobial Chemotherapy* 66.11 (2011). http://www.ncbi.nlm.nih.gov/pubmed/21911344.

23. Mahmoud A. Ghannoum. "Studies on the Anticandidal Mode of Action of Allium satioum (Garlic)." *Journal of General Microbiology* 134 (1988). http://mic.sgmjournals.org/content/134/11/2917.full.pdf.

24. Joseph Mercola. "Raw Garlic for Parasites and Viral Infections." March 17, 2001. http://articles.mercola.com/sites/articles/archive/2001/03/17/garlic-infections.aspx.

25. T. H. Jakobsen, et al. "Ajoene, a Sulfur-Rich Molecule from Garlic, Inhibits Genes

Controlled by Quorum Sensing." *Antimicrobial Agents and Chemotherapy* 56.5 (2012). http://www.ncbi.nlm.nih.gov/pubmed/22314537.

26. National Center for Complementary and Integrative Health. "Garlic." https://nccih.nih.gov/health/garlic/ataglance.htm.

27. S. H. Lee, et al. "In Vitro Antifungal Susceptibilities of Candida albicans and Other Fungal Pathogens to Polygodial, a Sesquiterpene Dialdehyde." *Planta Medica* 65.3 (1999). http://www.ncbi.nlm.nih.gov/pubmed/10232062.

28. V. Chopra, et al. "Prophylactic Strategies in Recurrent Vulvovaginal Candidiasis: A Two Year Study Testing a Phytonutrient vs Itraconazole." *Journal of Biological Regulators & Homeostatic Agents* 27.3 (2013). http://www.kolorex.com/wp-content/uploads/2013/12/Chopra-2013.pdf.

29. Regenera Research Group of Milan. University of Milan Italy. "The Kolorex Horopito Difference -Fighting Candida Overgrowth the Natural Way." http://www.kolorex.com/the-kolorex-difference.

30. K. Fujita, T. Fujita, and I Kubo. "Anethole, a Potential Antimicrobial Synergist, Converts a Fungistatic Dodecanol to a Fungicidal Agent." *Phytotherapy Research* 21.1 (2007). http://www.ncbi.nlm.nih.gov/pubmed/17078111.

31. Y. Metugriachuk, et al. "In View of an Optimal Gut Antifungal Therapeutic Strategy: an in Vitro Susceptibility and Toxicity Study Testing a Novel Phyto-compound." *Chinese Journal of Digestive Diseases* 6.2 (2005). http://www.ncbi.nlm.nih.gov/pubmed/15904429.

32. B. C. Nzeako, Z.S.N. Al-Kharousi, and Z. Al-Mahrooqui. "Antimicrobial Activities of Clove and Thyme Extracts." *Sultan Qaboos University Medical Journal* 6.1 (2006). http://www.ncbi.nlm.nih.gov/pmc/articles/PMC3074903/.

33. P. Pozzatti, et al. "In Vitro Activity of Essential Oils Extracted from Plants Used as Spices Against Fluconazole-Resistant and Fluconazole-Susceptible Candida spp." *Canadian Journal of Microbiology* 54.11 (2008). http://www.ncbi.nlm.nih.gov/pubmed/18997851.

34. Saeid Mahdavi Omran and Seddighe Esmailzadeh. "Comparison of Anti-Candida Activity of Thyme, Pennyroyal, and Lemon Essential Oils versus Antifungal Drugs against Candida Species." *Jundishapur Journal of Microbiology* 2.2 (2009). http://jjmicrobiol.com/?page=article&article_id=3772.

35. G. X. Wei, X. Xu, and C. D. Wu. "In Vitro Synergism between Berberine and Miconazole against Planktonic and Biofilm Candida Cultures." *Archives of Oral Biology* 56.6 (2011). http://www.ncbi.nlm.nih.gov/pubmed/21272859.

36. Y. Xu, et. al. "Proteomic Analysis Reveals a Synergistic Mechanism of Fluconazole and Berberine Against Fluconazole-Resistant Candida Albicans: Endogenous ROS Augmentation." *Journal of Proteome Research* 8.11 (2009). http://www.ncbi.nlm.nih.gov/pubmed/19754040.

37. C. Chen, Y. Zhang, and C. Huang. "Berberine Inhibits PTP1B Activity and Mimics Insulin Action." *Biochemical and Biophysical Research Communications* 397.3 (2010). http://www.ncbi.nlm.nih.gov/pubmed/20515652.

38. J. Yin, X. H. Xing, and J. Ye. "Efficacy of Berberine in Patients with Type 2 Diabetes."

Metabolism: Clinical and Experimental 57.5 (2008). http://www.ncbi.nlm.nih.gov /pmc/articles/PMC2410097/.

39. B. Lee, et al. "Inhibitory Effects of Coptidis rhizoma and Berberine on Cocaine-induced Sensitization." *Evidence Based Complementary and Alternative Medicine* 6.1 (2009). http://www.ncbi.nlm.nih.gov/pubmed/18955248.

40. W. H. Peng, et al. "Berberine Produces Antidepressant-Like Effects in the Forced Swim Test and in the Tail Suspension Test in Mice." *Life Sciences* 81.11 (2007). http:// www.ncbi.nlm.nih.gov/pubmed/17804020.

41. L. Huang, et al. "Synthesis, Biological Valuation, and Molecular Modeling of Berberine Derivatives as Potent Acetylcholinesterase Inhibitors." *Bioorganic and Medicinal Chemistry* 18.3 (2010). http://www.ncbi.nlm.nih.gov/pubmed/20056426.

42. H .B. Singh, et al. "Cinnamon Bark Oil, a Potent Fungitoxicant Against Fungi Causing Respiratory Tract Mycoses."*Allergy* 50.12 (1995). http://www.ncbi.nlm.nih.gov /pubmed/8834832.

43. J. M. Quale, et al. "In Vitro Activity of Cinnamomum Zeylanicum against Azole Resistant and Sensitive Candida Species and a Pilot Study of Cinnamon for Oral Candidiasis." *The American Journal of Chinese Medicine* 24.2 (1996). http://www.ncbi.nlm.nih .gov/pubmed/8874667.

44. L. S. Ooi, et al. "Antimicrobial Activities of Cinnamon Oil and Cinnamaldehyde from the Chinese Medicinal Herb Cinnamomum Cassia Blume." *The American Journal of Chinese Medicine* 34.3 (2006). http://www.ncbi.nlm.nih.gov/pubmed/16710900.

45. Allison Siebecker and Steven Sandberg-Lewis. "Small Intestine Bacterial Overgrowth: Often-Ignored Cause of Irritable Bowel Syndrome." *Townsend Letter* February / March 2013. http://www.townsendletter.com/FebMarch2013/ibs0213_2.html and www .siboinfo.com.

46. Christian Nordqvist. "Coumarin in Cinnamon Causes Liver Damage in Some People." Medical News Today. May 13, 2013. http://www.medicalnewstoday.com/ articles/260430.php.

47. Hidayat Hussain, et al. "Lapachol: an Overview." Special Issue Reviews and Accounts. *ARKIVOC* 2007 (ii) 145–171 ARKAT USA, Inc. https://www.arkat-usa.org /get-file/23192/.

48. Ibid.

49. American Cancer Society. Complementary and Alternative Medicine. http://www .cancer.org/treatment/treatmentsandsideeffects/complementaryandalternativemedicine /herbsvitaminsandminerals/pau-d-arco (Accessed 2014. Page no longer exists.)

50. Inder Singh Rana, Aarti Singh Rana, and Ram Charan Rajak. "Evaluation of Antifungal Activity in Essential Oil of the Syzygium Aromaticum (L.) by Extraction, Purification and Analysis of Its Main Component Eugenol." *Brazilian Journal of Microbiology* 42.4 (2011). http://www.ncbi.nlm.nih.gov/pmc/articles/PMC3768706/.

51. E. Pinto, et al. "Antifungal Activity of the Clove Essential Oil from Syzygium Aromaticum on Candida, Aspergillus and Dermatophyte Species." *Journal of Medical Microbiology* 58.11 (2009). http://www.ncbi.nlm.nih.gov/pubmed/19589904.

52. GreenMed Info. "Clove Appears Interfere with Quorum Sensing Activity in Bacteria,

Reducing Their Drug Resistant Virulence and Pathogenicity." http://www.greenmedin-fo .com/article/clove-appears-interfere-quorum-sensing-activity-bacteria-reducing-their-drug-resistant.

53. B. C. Nzeako, Zahra S. N. Al-Kharousi, and Zahra Al-Mahrooqui. "Antimicrobial Activities of Clove and Thyme Extracts." *Sultan Qaboos University Medical Journal* 6.1 (2006). http://www.ncbi.nlm.nih.gov/pmc/articles/PMC3074903/.

54. R. Shapiro. "Prevention of Vector Transmitted Diseases with Clove Oil Insect Repellent." *Journal of Pediatric Nursing* 27.4 (2012). http://www.ncbi.nlm.nih.gov /pubmed/22703681 mosquitos.

55. James Schaller. *Combating Biofilms: The Reason Many Diseases Do Not Respond to Treatment*. Naples, FL: International Infectious Disease Press (2014). Kindle Version.

56. American Cancer Society. Complementary and Alternative Medicine. http://www .cancer.org/treatment/treatmentsandsideeffects/complementaryandalternativemedicine /herbsvitaminsandminerals/cloves (Accessed 2014. Page no longer exists.).

57. Medline Plus. "Clove." http://www.nlm.nih.gov/medlineplus/druginfo/natural/251 .html.

58. S. R. Reis, et al. "Immunomodulating and Antiviral Activities of Uncaria Tomentosa on Human Monocytes Infected with Dengue Virus-2." *International Immunopharmacology* 8.3 (2008). http://www.ncbi.nlm.nih.gov/pubmed/18279801.

59. GreenMed Info. "Cats Claw has Anti-inflammatroy and Immunomodulatory Activity via Suppression of TNFalpha Synthesis." http://www.greenmedinfo.com/article/cats-claw-has-anti-inflammatory-and-immunomodulatory-activity-suppression-tnfalpha-synthesis.

60. D. R. Herrera, et al. "In Vitro Antimicrobial Activity of Phytotherapic Uncaria Tomentosa against Endodontic Pathogens." *Journal of Oral Science* 52.3 (2010) http:// www.ncbi.nlm.nih.gov/pubmed/20881342.

61. National Center for Complementary and Integrative Health. "Cat's Claw." https:// nccih.nih.gov/health/catclaw.

62. B. Lal, et al. "Efficacy of Curcumin in the Management of Chronic Anterior Uveitis." *Phytotherapy Research* 13.4 (1999). http://www.ncbi.nlm.nih.gov/pubmed/10404539.

63. Y. Takada, et al. "Nonsteroidal anti-inflammatory agents differ in their ability to suppress NF-kappaB activation, inhibition of expression of cyclooxygenase-2 and cyclin D1, and abrogation of tumor cell proliferation." *Oncogene* 23.57 (2004). http://www.ncbi .nlm.nih.gov/pubmed/15489888.

64. R. Agarwal, S. K. Goel, and J.R. Behari. "Detoxification and antioxidant effects of curcumin in rats experimentally exposed to mercury." *Journal of Applied Toxicology* 30.5 (2010). http://onlinelibrary.wiley.com/doi/10.1002/jat.1517/abstract.

65. Soheil Zorofchian Moghadamtousi, et al. "A Review on Antibacterial, Antiviral, and Antifungal Activity of Curcumin," *BioMed Research International* vol. 2014, Article ID 186864. http://www.hindawi.com/journals/bmri/2014/186864/.

66. C. V. B. Martins, et al. "Curcumin as a Promising Antifungal of Clinical Interest." *Journal of Antimicrobial Chemotherapy* 63.2 (2009). http://jac.oxfordjournals.org/ content/63/2/337.long.

67. Soheil Zorofchian Moghadamtousi, et al. "A Review on Antibacterial, Antiviral, and Antifungal Activity of Curcumin." *BioMed Research International,* vol. 2014, Article ID 186864. http://www.hindawi.com/journals/bmri/2014/186864/.

68. Ibid.

69. Arafat Kdudsi Khalil, et al. "Curcumin Antifungal and Antioxidant Activities are Increased in the Presence of Ascorbic Acid." *Food Chemistry* 133.3 (2012). http://www.sciencedirect.com/science/article/pii/S0308814612001744.

70. Soheil Zorofchian Moghadamtousi, et al. "A Review on Antibacterial, Antiviral, and Antifungal Activity of Curcumin." *BioMed Research International,* vol. 2014, Article ID 186864. http://www.hindawi.com/journals/bmri/2014/186864/.

71. Laura L. Hurley, et al. "Antidepressant-like Effects of Curcumin in WKY Rat Model of Depression is Associated with an Increase in Hippocampal BDNF." *Behavioural Brain Research* 239 (2013). http://www.sciencedirect.com/science/article/pii/S0166432812006997.

72. Xu Ying, et al. "Curcumin Reverses the Effects of Chronic Stress on Behavior, the HPA axis, BDNF Expression and Phosphorylation of CREB." *Brain Research* 1122.1 (2006). http://www.sciencedirect.com/science/article/pii/S0006899306027144.

73. G. Shoba, et al. "Influence of Piperine on the Pharmacokinetics of Curcumin in Animals and Human Volunteers." *Planta Medica* 64.4 (1998). http://www.ncbi.nlm.nih.gov/pubmed/9619120.

74. A. M. Clark, T. M. Jurgens, and C. D. Hufford. "Antimicrobial Activity of Juglone." *Phytotherapy Research* 4.1 (1990). http://onlinelibrary.wiley.com/doi/10.1002/ptr.2650040104/abstract.

75. Y. H. Kong, et al. "Natural Product Juglone Targets Three Key Enzymes from Helicobacter Pylori: Inhibition Assay with Crystal Structure Characterization." *Acta Pharmacologica Sinica* 29.7 (2008). http://www.ncbi.nlm.nih.gov/pubmed/18565285.

76. G. Ionescu, et al. "Oral Citrus Seed Extract in Atopic Eczema: In Vitro and In Vivo Studies on Intestinal Microflora." *Journal of Orthomolecular Medicine* 5.3 (1990). http://orthomolecular.org/library/jom/1990/pdf/1990-v05n03-p155.pdf.

77. Stephanie Greenwood. "The Truth About Grapefruit Seed Extract." Organic Consumers Association. January 27, 2010. https://www.organicconsumers.org/news/truth-about-grapefruit-seed-extract.

78. Environmental Working Group. "Benzalkonium Chloride." http://www.ewg.org/skindeep/ingredient/700674/BENZALKONIUM_CHLORIDE/.

79. Stephanie Greenwood. "The Truth About Grapefruit Seed Extract." Organic Consumers Association. January 27, 2010. https://www.organicconsumers.org/news/truth-about-grapefruit-seed-extract.

80. N. Zoric, et al. "Hydroxytyrosol Expresses Antifungal Activity in Vitro." *Current Drug Targets* 14.9 (2013). http://www.ncbi.nlm.nih.gov/pubmed/23721186.

81. D. Markin, L. Duek, and I. Berdicevsky. "In Vitro Antimicrobial Activity of Olive Leaves." *Mycoses* 46.3–4 (2003). http://www.ncbi.nlm.nih.gov/pubmed/12870202.

82. Syed Haris Omar. "Oleuropein in Olive and Its Pharmacological Effects." *Scientia Pharmaceutica* 78.2 (2010). http://www.ncbi.nlm.nih.gov/pmc/articles/PMC3002804/.

83. W. Lajean Chaffin, et al. "Cell Wall and Secreted Proteins of Candida Albicans: Identification, Function, and Expression." *Microbiology and Molecular Biology Reviews* 62.1 (1998). http://www.ncbi.nlm.nih.gov/pmc/articles/PMC98909/.

84. Y. Ben-Ziony and B. Arzi. "Use of Lufenuron for Treating Fungal Infections of Dogs and Cats: 297 cases (1997–1999)." *Journal of the American Veterinary Medical Association* 217.10 (2000). http://www.ncbi.nlm.nih.gov/pubmed/11128542.

85. E. Dubuis and D. Lucas. "Control of Cutaneous Mycosis in Five Chimpanzees (Pan troglodytes) with Lufenuron." *The Veterinary Record* 152.21 (2003). http://www.ncbi.nlm.nih.gov/pubmed/12790235.

86. R. F. Hector, A. P. Davidson, and S. M. Johnson. "Comparison of Susceptibility of Fungal Isolates to Lufenuron and Nikkomycin Z Alone or in Combination with Itraconazole." *American Journal of Veterinary Research* 66.6 (2005). http://www.ncbi.nlm.nih.gov/pubmed/16008236.

87. S. R. Dean, et al. "Mode of Action of Lufenuron in Adult Ctenocephalides felis (Siphonaptera: Pulicidae)." *Journal of Medical Entomology* 36.4 (1999). http://www.ncbi.nlm.nih.gov/pubmed/10467778.

88. Juliana F. Mansur, et al. "The Effect of Lufenuron, a Chitin Synthesis Inhibitor, on Oogenesis of Rhodnius Prolixus." *Pesticide Biochemistry and Physiology* 98.1 (2010). http://www.sciencedirect.com/science/article/pii/S0048357510000702.

89. European Food Safety Authority. "Conclusion on the peer review of Lufenuron." *EFSA Journal* 7.6 (2009). http://www.efsa.europa.eu/en/scdocs/doc/189r.pdf.

90. R. Hamid, et al. "Chitinases: An Update." *Journal of Pharmacy & Bioallied Sciences* 5.1 (2013). http://www.ncbi.nlm.nih.gov/pmc/articles/PMC3612335/.

91. D. L. Danley, A. E. Hilger, and C. A. Winkel. "Generation of Hydrogen Peroxide by Candida Albicans and Influence on Murine Polymorphonuclear Leukocyte Activity." *Infection and Immunity* 40.1 (1983). http://www.ncbi.nlm.nih.gov/pmc/articles/PMC264822/.

92. N. Orsi. "The Antimicrobial Activity of Lactoferrin: Current Status and Perspectives." *Biometals* 17.3 (2004). http://link.springer.com/article/10.1023/B:BIOM.0000027691.86757.e2.

93. A. S. Naidu, et al. "Activated Lactoferrin's Ability to Inhibit Candida Growth and Block Yeast Adhesion to the Vaginal Epithelial Monolayer." *The Journal of Reproductive Medicine* 49.11 (2004). http://www.ncbi.nlm.nih.gov/pubmed/15603095.

94. H. Wakabayashi, et al. "Inhibition of Hyphal Growth of Azole-Resistant Strains of Candida Albicans by Triazole Antifungal Agents in the Presence of Lactoferrin-related Compounds." *Antimicrobial Agents and Chemotherapy* 42.7 (1998). http://www.ncbi.nlm.nih.gov/pubmed/9660988.

95. M. P. Venkatesh and L. Rong. "Human Recombinant Lactoferrin Acts Synergistically with Antimicrobials Commonly Used in Neonatal Practice Against Coagulase-Negative Staphylococci and Candida Albicans Causing Neonatal Sepsis." *Journal of Medical Microbiology* 57.9 (2008). http://www.ncbi.nlm.nih.gov/pubmed/18719181.

96. Cell Press. "In Decision To Grow, Bacteria Follow The Crowd." ScienceDaily. October 31, 2008. http://www.sciencedaily.com/releases/2008/10/081030123827.htm.

97. Prothera and Klaire Labs. "Should Probiotics be Taken with Food or on an Empty Stomach?" Update. Summer 2011. http://www.klaire.com/images/Probiotics_Update_Summer_2011_3.pdf.

98. Leonard Smith. "Is it Possible to Get Too Much Fermented Food in Your Diet." http://bodyecology.com/articles/too_much_fermented_food.php.

99. Anna Krasowska, et al. "The Antagonistic Effect of Saccharomyces Boulardii on Candida Albicans Filamentation, Adhesion and Biofilm Formation." *FEMS Yeast Research* 9.8 (2009). Sacchromyces Boulardii http://www.ncbi.nlm.nih.gov/pubmed/19732158.

100. Theodoros Kelesidis and Charalabos Pothoulakis. "Efficacy and Safety of the Probiotic Saccharomyces Boulardii for the Prevention and Therapy of Gastrointestinal Disorders." *Therapeutic Advances in Gastroenterology* 5.2 (2012). http://www.ncbi.nlm.nih.gov/pmc/articles/PMC3296087/.

101. R. Herbrecht and Y. Nivoix. "Saccharomyces cerevisiae Fungemia: An Adverse Effect of Saccharomyces boulardii Probiotic Administration." *Clinical Infectious Diseases* 40.11 (2005). http://cid.oxfordjournals.org/content/40/11/1635.long.

102. A. Enache-Angoulvant and C. Hennequin. "Invasive Saccharomyces Infection: a Comprehensive Review." *Clinical Infectious Diseases* 41.11 (2005). http://www.ncbi.nlm.nih.gov/pubmed/16267727.

103. Marco Rinaldo Oggioni, et al. "Recurrent Septicemia in an Immunocompromised Patient Due to Probiotic Strains of Bacillus Subtilis." *Journal of Clinical Microbiology* 36.1 (1998). http://jcm.asm.org/content/36/1/325.full.

104. H. A. Hong, et al. "Bacillus subtilis isolated from the human gastrointestinal tract." *Research in Microbiology* 160.2 (2009). http://www.ncbi.nlm.nih.gov/pubmed/19068230.

105. Melissa R. Cruz, et al. "Enterococcus Faecalis Inhibits Hyphal Morphogenesis and Virulence of Candida Albicans." *Infection and Immunity* 81.1 (2013). https://www.ncbi.nlm.nih.gov/pubmed/23115035

106. R. Sreedhar, et al. "Endocarditis and Biofilm-Associated Pili of Enterococcus Faecalis." *The Journal of Clinical Investigation* 116.10 (2006). http://www.jci.org/articles/view/29021.

107. David M. Phillips. "Enterococcus Faecalis." *The New England Journal of Medicine* (1995). http://www.nejm.org/doi/full/10.1056/NEJM199501053320105.

108. Public Health Agency of Canada. "Enterococcus Faecalis." Pathogen Safety Data Sheet. http://www.phac-aspc.gc.ca/lab-bio/res/psds-ftss/enterococcus-eng.php.

Amy Yasko. *Autism: Pathways to Recovery.* Bethel, ME: Neurological Research Institute, LLC (2004, 2007, 2009).

Chapter 8

1. Scott Forsgren, Neil Nathan, and Wayne Anderson. "Mold and Mycotoxins: Often Overlooked Factors in Chronic Lyme Disease." *Townsend Letter* July 2014. http://www.townsendletter.com/July2014/mold0714_2.html.

2. A. Watanabe, et al. "Lowering of Blood Acetaldehyde but not Ethanol Concentrations by Pantethine Following Alcohol Ingestion: Different Effects in Flushing and Nonflushing Subjects." *Alcohol Clinical and Experimental Research* 9.3 (1985). http://www.ncbi.nlm.nih.gov/pubmed/3893199.

3. Stephan Cooter. *Beating Chronic Illness*. Chapter 11. San Francisco, CA: ProMotion Publishing. http://www.mall-net.com/cooter/moly.html.

4. Mary Budinger. "Dispatches from the Front Lines of Autism and Lyme Disease." *Townsend Letter* October 2009. http://www.townsendletter.com/Oct2009/dispatch1009.html.

Chapter 9

1. Joseph Mercola. "7 Reasons to Eat More Saturated Fat." September 22, 2009. http://articles.mercola.com/sites/articles/archive/2009/09/22/7-reasons-to-eat-more-saturated-fat.aspx.

2. Will Dubois. "High Blood Sugar Symptoms." *Diabetes Self-Management* January 11, 2013. http://www.diabetesselfmanagement.com/managing-diabetes/blood-glucose-management/high-blood-glucose/3/.

3. Mark Sisson. *The Primal Blueprint: Reprogram Your Genes for Effortless Weight Loss, Vibrant Health and Boundless Energy*. Malibu, CA: Primal Nutrition, Inc.; paperback 2nd edition (2012).

4. G. C. Sturniolo, et al. "Zinc Supplementation Tightens "leaky gut" in Crohn's Disease." *Inflammatory Bowel Diseases* 7.2 (2001). http://www.ncbi.nlm.nih.gov/pubmed/11383597.

5. Krishna Ramanujan-Cornell. "Gut bacteria Differ when Zinc Goes Missing." Futurity. December 31, 2015. http://www.futurity.org/zinc-gut-microbes-1082552-2/.

6. Robert C. Atkins. *Vita-Nutrient Solution: Nature's Answers to Drugs*. New York, NY: Fireside (2011). Kindle version.

7. Joseph Mercola. "Up to 70 Percent of Americans May be Deficient in Vitamin D—Find Out Why You Don't Want to be One of Them." December 24, 2003. http://articles.mercola.com/sites/articles/archive/2003/12/24/vitamin-d-deficiency.aspx.

8. Robert C. Atkins. *Vita-Nutrient Solution: Nature's Answers to Drugs*. New York, NY: Fireside (2011). Kindle version.

9. M. Irwin, et al. "Partial Night Sleep Deprivation Reduces Natural Killer and Cellular Immune Response in Humans." *FASEB Journal* 10.5 (1996). http://www.ncbi.nlm.nih.gov/pubmed/8621064.

10. Christian Nordqvist. "Severe Sleep Loss Affects Immune System Like Physical Stress Does." *Medical News Today*. http://www.medicalnewstoday.com/articles/247320.php.

11. Chris Kresser. "5 Steps to Personalizing Your Autoimmune Paleo Protocol." January 23, 2015. http://chriskresser.com/5-steps-to-personalizing-your-autoimmune-paleo-protocol/.

12 . Leonid Ber. "Yeast Derived Beta-1,3-D-Glucan: An Adjuvant Concept." *Townsend Letter*. http://www.tldp.com/issue/184/Yeast%20Derived%20Beta.htm.

13. Life Extension Vitamins. "Beta 1, 3-Glucan: Extraordinary Support." http://www.lifeextensionvitamins.com/beta13glucan.html.

14. P. W. Mansell, et al. "Macrophage Mediated Destruction of Human Malignant Cells in Vivo." *Journal of the National Cancer Institute* 54.3 (1975). http://www.ncbi.nlm.nih.gov/pubmed/1123850.

15. Vaclav Vetvicka, et al. "Pilot Study: Orally-Administered Yeast 1,3-glucan Prophylactically Protects Against Anthrax Infection and Cancer in Mice." *JANA* 5.1 (2002). http://alternativecancer.us/betaglucan.pdf.

16. Douglas A. Wyatt. "Leaky Gut Syndrome: A modern Epidemic with an Ancient Solution?" *Townsend Letter* June 2014. http://www.townsendletter.com/June2014/leaky0614_2.html.

17. C. R. Markus, et. al. "The Bovine Protein Alpha-lactalbumin Increases the Plasma Ratio of Tryptophan to the other Large Neutral Amino Acids, and in Vulnerable Subjects Raises Brain Serotonin Activity, Reduces Cortisol Concentration, and Improves Mood Under Stress." *The American Journal of Clinical Nutrition* 71.6 (2000). http://www.ncbi.nlm.nih.gov/pubmed/10837296.

18. Calvin W. McCausland and Emma Oganova. "Effect of Transfer Factor Advanced Formulas Containing E-XF Blends on Natural Killer (NK) Cell Activity." A 4Life Summary of an Independent NK Cell Study Report. http://www.4vidas.com/4life.htm.

19. H. Aso, et al. "Induction of Interferon and Activation of NK Cells and Macrophages in Mice by Oral Administration of Ge-132, an Organic Germanium Compound." *Microbiology and Immunology* 29.1 (1985). http://www.ncbi.nlm.nih.gov/pubmed/2581116.

20. Scott Forsgren, Neil Nathan, and Wayne Anderson. "Mold and Mycotoxins: Often Overlooked Factors in Chronic Lyme Disease." *Townsend Letter* July 2014. http://www.townsendletter.com/July2014/mold0714_2.html.

James Schaller. *Combating Biofilms: The Reason Many Diseases Do Not Respond to Treatment*. Naples, FL. International Infectious Disease Press (2014) Kindle Version.

Chapter 10

1. University of Cambridge. "From Athletes to Couch Potatoes: Humans Through 6,000 Years of Farming." Science Daily. April 7, 2014. www.sciencedaily.com/releases/2014/04/140407214904.htm.

2. Barry Groves. "Vegetarians Have Smaller Brains." Second Opinions. http://www.second-opinions.co.uk/vegetarians-have-smaller-brains.html#.V-acSYWjRyQ.

3. University of Cambridge. "From Athletes to Couch Potatoes: Humans Through 6,000 Years of Farming." Science Daily. April 7, 2014. www.sciencedaily.com/releases/2014/04/140407214904.htm.

4. Will Dubois. "High Blood Sugar Symptoms." *Diabetes Self-Management.* January 11, 2013. http://www.diabetesselfmanagement.com/managing-diabetes/blood-glucose-management/high-blood-glucose/3/.

5. Mark Sisson. *The Primal Blueprint: Reprogram Your Genes for Effortless Weight Loss, Vibrant Health and Boundless Energy.* Malibu, CA: Primal Nutrition, Inc.; paperback 2nd edition (2012).

6. Ibid.

7. Mark Hyman. "5 Clues You are Addicted to Sugar." http://drhyman.com/blog /2013/06/27/5-clues-you-are-addicted-to-sugar/.

8. American Diabetes Association. http://www.diabetes.org/ (Accessed 2013.).

9. Jeffrey Norris. "Do Gut Bacteria Rule Our Minds." University of California San Francisco. August 15, 2014. https://www.ucsf.edu/news/2014/08/116526/do-gut -bacteria-rule-our-minds.

10. Charles Gant. Webinars. www.cegant.com.

11. David Perlmutter. *Grain Brain: The Surprising Truth About Wheat, Carbs, and Sugar -Your Brain's Silent Killers.* New York, NY: Little, Brown and Company (2013).

12. R. M. Wilson and W. G. Reeves. "Neutrophil Phagocytosis and Killing in Insulin-Dependent Diabetes." *Clinical and Experimental Immunology* 63.2 (1986). http://www .ncbi.nlm.nih.gov/pubmed/3084140.

13. F. A. Saeed. "Production of Pyruvate by Candida Albicans: Proposed Role in Virulence." *FEMS Microbiology Letters* 190.1 (2000). http://onlinelibrary.wiley.com /doi/10.1111/j.1574-6968.2000.tb09258.x/pdf.

14. R. Calderone, et al. "Candida Albicans: Adherence, Signaling and Virulence." *Medical Mycology* 38.1 (2000). http://www.ncbi.nlm.nih.gov/pubmed/11204138.

15. Neal D. Barnard. *Breaking the Food Seduction: The Hidden Reasons Behind Food Cravings.* New York, NY: St. Martin's Griffin (2004). Kindle version.

16. James Greenblatt. "Neuroactive Peptides from Common Foods Contribute to Psychiatric Disorders." Great Plains Laboratory. https://vimeo.com/19231456.

17. Ibid.

18. Mueen Aslam and Walter L. Hurley. "Biological Activities of Peptides Derived from Milk Proteins." Illinois DairyNet. University of Illinois. August 5, 1998. http://www .livestocktrail.illinois.edu/dairynet/paperDisplay.cfm?ContentID=249.

19. Loren Cordain. *The Paleo Diet: Lose Weight and Get Healthy by Eating the Foods You Were Designed to Eat.* Hoboken, NJ: Wiley (2001).

20. Chris Masterjohn. "Does Milk Cause Cancer?" April 30, 2007. http://www.realmilk .com/health/does-milk-cause-cancer/.

21. Neal D. Barnard. *Breaking the Food Seduction: The Hidden Reasons Behind Food Cravings.* New York, NY: St. Martin's Griffin (2004). Kindle version.

22. Al Sears. "Some Shrooms for Your Brain." http://www.alsearsmd.com/2014/10 /some-shrooms-for-your-brain-2/.

23. Michelle Klampe. "Excess omega-3 fatty acids could lead to negative health effects." October 28, 2013. Oregon State University. http://oregonstate.edu/ua/ncs/archives/2013 /oct/excess-omega-3-fatty-acids-could-lead-negative-health-effects.

24. Mark Sisson. "The Definitive Guide to Nuts." http://www.marksdailyapple.com /the-definitive-guide-to-nuts/.

25. Loren Cordain. *The Paleo Diet: Lose Weight and Get Healthy by Eating the Foods You Were Designed to Eat.* Hoboken, NJ: Wiley (2001).

26. Joseph Mercola. "America's Deadliest Sweetener Betrays Millions, Then Hoodwinks

You With Name Change." *The Huffington Post*. July 6, 2010. http://www.huffingtonpost
.com/dr-mercola/americas-deadliest-sweete_b_630549.html.

27. M. B. Abou-Donia, et al. "Splenda Alters Gut Microflora and Increases Intestinal
P-glycoprotein and Cytochrome p-450 in Male rats." *Journal of Toxicology and Environmental Health* 71.21 (2008). http://www.ncbi.nlm.nih.gov/pubmed/18800291.

28. Marcelle Pick. "Sugar Substitutes and the Potential Danger of Splenda." https://www
.womentowomen.com/healthy-weight/sugar-substitutes-and-the-potential-danger-of
-splenda/.

29. G. H. Zhang, et al. "Effects of Mother's Dietary Exposure to Acesulfame-K in Pregnancy or Lactation on the Adult Offspring's Sweet Preference." *Chemical Senses* 36.9
(2011). http://www.ncbi.nlm.nih.gov/pubmed/21653241.

30. W. N. Cong, et al. "Long-Term Artificial Sweetener Acesulfame Potassium Treatment
Alters Neurometabolic Functions in C57BL/6J Mice." *PLoS ONE* 8.8 (2013). http://
www.ncbi.nlm.nih.gov/pubmed/23950916.

31. M. M. Andreatta, et al. "Artificial Sweetener Consumption and Urinary Tract Tumors
in Cordoba, Argentina." *Preventive Medicine* 47.1 (2008). http://www.ncbi.nlm.nih.gov/
pubmed/18495230.

32. Mike Adams. "Truvia Sweetener a Powerful Pesticide: Scientists Shocked as Fruit
Flies Die in Less than a Week from Eating GMO-derived Erythritol." June 5, 2014. http://
www.naturalnews.com/045450_Truvia_erythritol_natural_pesticide.html.

33. H. M. Staudacher, et al. "Comparison of Symptom Response Following Advice for a
Diet Low in Fermentable Carbohydrates (FODMAPs) Versus Standard Dietary Advice in
Patients with Irritable Bowel Syndrome." *Journal of Human Nutrition and Dietetics* 24.5
(2011). http://www.ncbi.nlm.nih.gov/pubmed/?term=21615553.

34. Kate Scarlata. "The FODMAPs Approach—Minimize Consumption of Fermentable
Carbs to Manage Functional Gut Disorder Symptoms." *Today's Dietitian* 12.8 (2010).
http://www.todaysdietitian.com/newarchives/072710p30.shtml.

35. Jasvinder Chawla, et al. "Neurologic Effects of Caffeine." Medscape. November 11,
2015. http://emedicine.medscape.com/article/1182710-overview.

36. Sandra Blakeslee. "Yes, People are Right. Caffeine is Addictive." October 5, 1994.
http://www.nytimes.com/1994/10/05/us/yes-people-are-right-caffeine-is-addictive.html.

37. National Institute on Drug Abuse (NIDA). "Adolescent Caffeine Use and Cocaine
Sensitivity." https://www.drugabuse.gov/news-events/latest-science/adolescent-caffeine
-use-cocaine-sensitivity.

38. Joseph Stromberg. "This is How Your Brain Becomes Addicted to Caffeine."
Smithsonian.com August 9, 2013. http://www.smithsonianmag.com/science-nature
/this-is-how-your-brain-becomes-addicted-to-caffeine-26861037/?no-ist.

39. Steven E. Meredith, et al. "Caffeine Use Disorder: A Comprehensive Review and Research Agenda." *Journal of Caffeine Research* 3.3 (2013). https://www.ncbi.nlm.nih.gov
/pmc/articles/PMC3777290/.

40. Maggie Barrett. "Caffeine Use Disorder Needs More Attention." American University. Washington D.C. http://www.american.edu/media/news/20140203_Caffeine-Use-
-Disorder-Needs-Attention.cfm.

41. National Institute on Drug Abuse (NIDA). "Adolescent Caffeine Use and Cocaine Sensitivity." https://www.drugabuse.gov/news-events/latest-science/adolescent-caffeine-use-cocaine-sensitivity.

42. Al Sears. "One Cup Away From Destroying Your Brain." Email Newsletter June 28, 2012.

43. Mayo Clinic Staff. "Caffeine content for coffee, tea, soda and more." Mayo Clinic. http://www.mayoclinic.org/healthy-lifestyle/nutrition-and-healthy-eating/in-depth/caffeine/art-20049372.

44. L. S. Guzzo, et al. "Cafestol, a Coffee-Specific Diterpene, Induces Peripheral Antinociception Mediated by Endogenous Opioid Oeptides." *Clinical and Experimental Pharmacology and Physiology* 39.5 (2012). https://www.ncbi.nlm.nih.gov/pubmed/22332877.

45. Steven E. Meredith, et al. "Caffeine Use Disorder: A Comprehensive Review and Research Agenda." *Journal of Caffeine Research* 3.3 (2013). https://www.ncbi.nlm.nih.gov/pmc/articles/PMC3777290/.

46. Karen Fernau. "Coffee Grinds Fuel the Nation." *USA Today* April 9, 2013. http://www.usatoday.com/story/money/business/2013/04/09/coffee-mania/2069335/.

47. Melinda Wenner Moyer. "It's Time to End the War on Salt." *Scientific American* July 8, 2011. http://www.scientificamerican.com/article/its-time-to-end-the-war-on-salt/.

48. Mark Sisson. "Salt and Blood Pressure." Mark's Daily Apple. http://www.marksdailyapple.com/salt-and-blood-pressure/.

49. Al Sears. "Cardiologists Bungle Blood Pressure." http://www.alsearsmd.com/2014/09/cardiologists-bungle-blood-pressure/.

50. Mark Sisson. "Salt: What is it Good For?" Mark's Daily Apple. http://www.marksdailyapple.com/salt-what-is-it-good-for/.

51. Joseph Mercola. "Low Salt is Bad for Heart Health." June 8, 2016. http://articles.mercola.com/sites/articles/archive/2016/06/08/consuming-right-amount-of-salt.aspx.

52. M. Panneerselvam, et al. "Dark Chocolate Receptors: Epicatechin-induced Cardiac Protection is Dependent on Delta-opioid Receptor Stimulation." *American Journal of Physiology Heart and Circulatory Physiology* 299.5 (2010). https://www.ncbi.nlm.nih.gov/pubmed/20833967.

53. Neal D. Barnard. *Breaking the Food Seduction: The Hidden Reasons Behind Food Cravings.* New York, NY: St. Martin's Griffin (2004). Kindle version.

54. K. Bruinsma and D. L. Taren. "Chocolate: Food or Drug?" *The Journal of the American Dietetic Association* 99.10 (1999). http://www.ncbi.nlm.nih.gov/pubmed/10524390.

55. Neal D. Barnard. *Breaking the Food Seduction: The Hidden Reasons Behind Food Cravings.* New York, NY: St. Martin's Griffin (2004). Kindle version.

56. Jeff Volek and Stephen Phinney. *The Art and Science of Low Carbohydrate Living.* Beyond Obesity, LLC. May 2011.

57. Al Sears. Health Confidential. Issue No 35. January 22, 2009. http://www.alsearsmd.com/healthconfidentials/HCE35.html.

58. Ibid.

59. Mark Sisson. "The Importance of Cooking the Evolution of the Human Brain." http://www .marksdailyapple.com/the-importance-of-cooking-in-the-evolution-of-the-human-brain/.

60. Loren Cordain, et al. "Plant-animal subsistence ratios and macronutrient energy estimations in worldwide hunter-gatherer diets." *American Journal of Clinical Nutrition* 71.3 (2000). https://www.ncbi.nlm.nih.gov/pubmed/10702160.

61. Jeff Volek and Stephen Phinney. *The Art and Science of Low Carbohydrate Living.* Beyond Obesity, LLC. May 2011.

62. Amber O'Hearn. Ketogenic Diets and Stress Part 1. http://www.ketotic.org/2012/07 /ketogenic-diets-and-stress-part-i.html.

63. P. K. Elias, et al. "Serum Cholesterol and Cognitive Performance in the Framingham Heart Study." *Psychosomatic Medicine* 67.1 (2005). http://www.ncbi.nlm.nih.gov /pubmed/15673620.

64. T. Partonen, et al. "Association of Low Serum Total Cholesterol with Major Depression and Suicide." *The British Journal of Psychiatry* 175.3 (1999). https://www.ncbi.nlm .nih.gov/pubmed/10645328.

65. B. A. Golomb, H. Stattin, and S. Mednick. "Low Cholesterol and Violent Crime." *Journal of Psychiatric Research* 34.4–5 (2000). https://www.ncbi.nlm.nih.gov/ pubmed/11104842.

66. H. Kunugi, et al. "Low Serum Cholesterol in Suicide Attempters." *Biological Psychiatry* 41.2 (1997). https://www.ncbi.nlm.nih.gov/pubmed/9018390.

67. Al Sears. "Vitamin D3 is Better than Drugs for Depression." http://www.alsearsmd .com/2015/09/vitamin-d3-better than-drugs-for-depression/.

68. David Perlmutter, *Grain Brain: The Surprising Truth About Wheat, Carbs, and Sugar —Your Brain's Silent Killers.* New York, NY: Little, Brown and Company (2013).

69. Great Plains Laboratory. Tourettes, TICS and OCD. http://www.greatplainslaboratory .com/home/eng/tourettetics.asp (Accessed 2014. Page no longer exists.).

70. Charles Gant. "Endocrine Stress" webinar. www.cegant.com.

71. Mark Sisson. "Fun with Fiber: The Real Scoop." http://www.marksdailyapple.com /fiber/.

(this is inaccurate number in content before renumbering)

72. Allison Siebecker and Steven Sandberg-Lewis. "Small Intestine Bacterial Overgrowth: Often-Ignored Cause of Irritable Bowel Syndrome." *Townsend Letter* February / March 2013. http://www.townsendletter.com/FebMarch2013/ibs0213_2.html.

David Perlmutter. *Grain Brain: The Surprising Truth About Wheat, Carbs, and Sugar -Your Brain's Silent Killers.* New York, NY: Little, Brown and Company (2013).

Neal D. Barnard. *Breaking the Food Seduction: The Hidden Reasons Behind Food Cravings.* New York, NY: St. Martin's Griffin (2004). Kindle version.

Stephen Cherniske. *Caffeine Blues: Wake Up to the Hidden Dangers of Americas #1 Drug.* New York, NY. Warner Books (1998). Kindle version.316.

Charles Gant, M.D. *End Your Addiction Now*. Garden City Park, NY: Square One Publishers (2009).

Nora T. Gedgaudas, *Primal Body Primal Mind: Beyond the Paleo Diet for Total Health and a Longer Life*. Rochester, VT: Healing Arts Press (2011).

William Davis. *Wheat Belly: Lose the Wheat, Lose the Weight, and Find Your Path Back to Health*. Emmaus, PA: Rodale Books; Reprint edition (2014).

Jimmy Moore and Dr. Eric Westman. *Keto Clarity*. Las Vegas: Victory Belt Publishing, Inc. (2014).

Mark Sisson. *The Primal Blueprint: Reprogram Your Genes for Effortless Weight Loss, Vibrant Health and Boundless Energy*. Malibu, CA: Primal Nutrition, Inc.; paperback 2nd edition (2012).

Chapter 11

1. Mary G. Enig and Sally Fallon. "The Skinny on Fats." The Weston A Price Foundation. January 2000. http://www.westonaprice.org/know-your-fats/skinny-on-fats http://www.westonaprice.org/health-topics/the-skinny-on-fats/.

2. Medical News Today. "Organic Foods in Relation to Nutrition and Health Key Facts." July 11, 2004. http://www.medicalnewstoday.com/releases/10587.php.

3. Mark Sisson. *The Primal Blueprint: Reprogram Your Genes for Effortless Weight Loss, Vibrant Health and Boundless Energy*. Malibu, CA: Primal Nutrition, Inc.; paperback 2nd edition (2012).

4. Arjun Walia. "Science Sheds Light on Why Heating Your Food with Microwave Radiation Might be a Bad Idea." Collective Evolution. January 20, 2016. http://www.collective-evolution.com/2016/01/20/science-sheds-light-why-heating-your-food-with-microwave-radiation-might-be-a-bad-idea/.

5. S. Kyrylenko, et al. "Long-term Exposure to Microwave Radiation Provokes Cancer Growth: Evidence from Radars and Mobile Communication Systems." *Experimental Oncology* 33.2 (2011). http://exp-oncology.com.ua/article/1845/long-term-exposure-to-microwave-radiation-provokes-cancer-growth-evidences-from-radars-and-mobile-communication-systems.

6. Marin Plumb. "Undergraduate researcher evaluates frozen blueberries." South Dakota State University. http://www.sdstate.edu/news/articles/undergraduate-researcher-evaluates-frozen-blueberries.cfm.

7. Andrea L. Jones. "Consumer Alert: Toxic Hormone-Disrupting Chemical BPA is Leaching from Food Can Liners." Organic Consumers Association. http://www.organicconsumers.org/articles/article_6472.cfm.

8. ABC7 News, Lori Corbin, Health Coach Segment, 2010.

9. Sushma Subramanian. "Fact or Fiction: Raw Veggies are Healthier than Cooked Ones." *Scientific American* March 31, 2009. http://www.scientificamerican.com/article/raw-veggies-are-healthier/.

10. The American Association for the Advancement of Science. "What's Cooking? The evolutionary role of cookery." *The Economist*. February 19, 2009. http://www.economist.com/node/13139619.

11. Ann Gibbons. "Raw Food Not Enough to Feed Big Brains." *Science Now*. October 23, 2012. http://www.wired.com/2012/10/raw-food-big-brains/.

12. The American Association for the Advancement of Science. "What's Cooking? The evolutionary role of cookery." *The Economist*. February 19, 2009. http://www.economist .com/node/13139619.

13. Charles Gant, "Endocrine Stress" webinar. www.cegant.com.

14. Jeff Volek and Stephen Phinney. Jimmy Moore Interviews. http://livinlavidalowcarb .com/blog/.

15. Charles Gant, Detoxification Webinar. www.cegant.com.

16. William Shaw. "The Role of Oxalates in Autism and Chronic Disorders." http://www .westonaprice.org/health-topics/the-role-of-oxalates-in-autism-and-chronic-disorders/.

17. W. Chai and M. Liebman. "Effect of Different Cooking Methods on Vegetable Oxalate Content." *Journal of Agricultural and Food Chemistry* 53.8 (2005). http://www.ncbi .nlm.nih.gov/pubmed/15826055.

Nora T. Gedgaudas, *Primal Body Primal Mind: Beyond the Paleo Diet for Total Health and a Longer Life*. Rochester, VT: Healing Arts Press (2011).

Loren Cordain. *The Paleo Diet: Lose Weight and Get Healthy by Eating the Foods You Were Designed to Eat*. Hoboken, NJ: Wiley (2001).

Mark Sisson. *The Primal Blueprint: Reprogram Your Genes for Effortless Weight Loss, Vibrant Health and Boundless Energy*. Malibu, CA: Primal Nutrition, Inc.; paperback 2nd edition (2012).

Loren Cordain and Stephenson Nell. *The Paleo Diet Cookbook: More Than 150 Recipes for Paleo Breakfasts, Lunches, Dinners, Snacks and Beverages*. Boston, MA: Houghton Mifflin Harcourt (2010).

Chapter 12

1. Ashok Gupta. *Gupta Amygdala Retraining*. Harley Street Solutions. 2011. Learned from the Art of Living Foundation. www.artofliving.org.

2. Sue McGreevey. "Eight Weeks to a Better Brain." *Harvard Gazette* January 21, 2011. http://news.harvard.edu/gazette/story/2011/01/eight-weeks-to-a-better-brain/.

3. Jon Kabat-Zinn, et al. "Four Year Follow-Up of a Meditation-Based Program for the Self-Regulation of Chronic Pain: Treatment Outcomes and Compliance." *Clinical Journal of Pain* 2.3 (1986). http://journals.lww.com/clinicalpain/Abstract/1986/02030 /Four_Year_Follow_Up_of_a_Meditation_Based_Program.4.aspx.

4. Jon Kabat-Zinn, J. Lipworth, and R. Burney. "The Clinical Use of Mindfulness Meditation for Self-Regulation of Chronic Pain." *Journal of Behavioral Medicine* 8.2 (1985). https://www.ncbi.nlm.nih.gov/pubmed/3897551.

5. Susan Gaylord, et al. "Mindfulness Training Reduces the Severity of Irritable Bowel Syndrome in Women: Results of a Randomized Controlled Trial." *The American Journal of Gastroenterology* 106 (2011). http://www.nature.com/ajg/journal/v106/n9/full /ajg2011184a.html Was first presented as "Mindfulness vs. Support Groups for Irritable

Bowel Syndrome." Presented at University of North Carolina at Chapel Hill during Digestive Disease Week, May 7, 2011.

6. C. Mahagita. "Roles of Meditation on Alleviation of Oxidative Stress and Improvement of Antioxidant System." *Journal of the Medical Association of Thailand* 93.6 (2010). http://www.ncbi.nlm.nih.gov/pubmed/21280542.

7. Catherine Guthrie. "Mind Over Matters through Meditation." Oprah.com. http://www.oprah.com/health/A-3-Minute-Dose-of-Meditation.

8. Jon Kabat-Zinn, J. Lipworth, and R. Burney. "The Clinical Use of Mindfulness Meditation for Self-Regulation of Chronic Pain." *Journal of Behavioral Medicine* 8.2 (1985). https://www.ncbi.nlm.nih.gov/pubmed/3897551.

9. Charles Gant. "Mindfulness" webinar. http://www.cegant.com/ and "Endocrine Stress" webinar. http://www.cegant.com/.

10. Ron Gutman. "The Hidden Power of Smiling." YouTube. TEDtalksDirector, May 11, 2011. Web. 24 July 2012. https://www.youtube.com/watch?v=U9cGdRNMdQQ.

11. Video Medicine. "Science Proves that Smiling Makes us Happy." https://videomedicine.com/blog/science-proves-the-smiling-makes-us-happy/.

12. Ron Gutman. "The Hidden Power of Smiling." YouTube. TEDtalksDirector, May 11, 2011. Web. 24 July 2012. https://www.youtube.com/watch?v=U9cGdRNMdQQ.

13. Mark Sisson. "The Rich and Measurable Benefits to Spending more Time in Nature." http://www.marksdailyapple.com/the-rich-and-measurable-benefits-to-spending-more-time-in-nature/.

14. Rob Kanter. "Trees, Green Space, and Human Well-being." Environmental Almanac radio show. Thursday, July 7, 2005 http://lhhl.illinois.edu/media/2005.07_kanter.htm.

15. Bum Jin Park, et al. "The Physiological Effects of Shinrin-Yoku (taking in the Forest Atmosphere or Forest Bathing): Evidence from Field Experiments in 24 Forests across Japan." *Environmental Health and Preventive Medicine* 15.1 (2010). https://www.ncbi.nlm .nih.gov/pmc/articles/PMC2793346/.

16. Richard Louv. "Health Benefits of Being Outdoors." *AARP Bulletin,* July 23, 2012. http://www.aarp.org/politics-society/advocacy/info-07-2012/health-benefits-of-nature .html.

17. Andrew Weil. "Is Forest Therapy for Real." Q & A Library. http://www.drweil.com/drw/u/QAA401159/Is-Forest-Therapy-for-Real.html.

18. Koga Kazuko, and Yutaka Iwasaki. "Psychological and Physiological Effect in Humans of Touching Plant Foliage - Using the Semantic Differential Method and Cerebral Activity as Indicators." *Journal of Physiological Anthropology* 32.1 (2013). https://www .ncbi.nlm.nih.gov/pubmed/23587233.

19. Richard Louv. "Health Benefits of Being Outdoors." *AARP Bulletin,* July 23, 2012. http://www.aarp.org/politics-society/advocacy/info-07-2012/health-benefits-of-nature .html.

20. John Lennon and Yoko Ono. *Double Fantasy.* November 17, 1980. "Watching the Wheels."

21. Lauren Ware. Interview. "Herbert Benson: The Mind's Healing Power."

Massachusetts General Hospital. Proto. Fall 2010. http://archive.protomag.com/assets /herbert-benson-the-minds-healing-power.

Andrew Weil. *Breathing: The Master Key to Self Healing* (CD). Louisville, CO: Sounds True Incorporated. (2001).

Chapter 13

1. T. G. Randolph and Ralph W. Moss. *An Alternative Approach to Allergies*. New York: Lippincott & Crowell Publishers (1980).

2. Californians for Pesticide Reform. "Kids at Risk: Pesticides & Children's Health." http://www.pesticidereform.org/article.php?id=139.

3. Vincent Corbel, et al. "Evidence for Inhibition of cholinesterases in insect and mammalian nervous systems by the insect repellent DEET." *BMC Biology* 2009. http://bmcbiol .biomedcentral.com/articles/10.1186/1741-7007-7-47.

4. Beyond Pesticides. "DEET. Chemical Watch Factsheet." http://www.beyondpesticides .org/assets/media/documents/pesticides/factsheets/deet.pdf.

5. Beyond Pesticides. "DEET and Permethrin a Dangerous Combination." http://www .beyondpesticides.org/programs/mosquitos-and-insect-borne-diseases/publications/deet -and-permethrin-a-dangerous-combination.

6. Michael. "Care What You Wear: Facts on Cotton Clothing Production." Organic Consumers Association. July 29, 2007. https://www.organicconsumers.org/news /care-what-you-wear-facts-cotton-clothing-production.

7. EcoChoices. "Conventional Cotton Statistics." From Agricultural Chemical Usage, 1992 Field Crops Summary, USDA National Agricultural Statistics Service. http://www .ecochoices.com/1/cotton_statistics.html.

8. Scott Forsgren, Neil Nathan, and Wayne Anderson. "Mold and Mycotoxins: Often Overlooked Factors in Chronic Lyme Disease." *Townsend Letter* July 2014. http://www .townsendletter.com/July2014/mold0714_2.html.

9. Sandy Ross. "Smart Meters are Dangerous to Your Health." *Our Toxic Times* September 2010.

10. EMF Safety Network. http://emfsafetynetwork.org/?page_id=2292.

11. Maine's Smart Meter Safety Coalition. "Interview with Dr. David Carpenter. Public Health Physician Warns of Smart Meter Dangers. Stresses Need for Analog Option." https://youtu.be/n7L21XOC2wA.

12. Scott Forsgren, Neil Nathan, and Wayne Anderson. "Mold and Mycotoxins: Often Overlooked Factors in Chronic Lyme Disease." *Townsend Letter* July 2014. http://www .townsendletter.com/July2014/mold0714_2.html.

13. Warren M. Levin and Fran Gare. *Beyond the Yeast Connection: A How-To Guide to Curing Candida and Other Yeast-Related Conditions*. Laguna Beach, CA: Basic Health Publications (2013).

14. Scott Forsgren, Neil Nathan, and Wayne Anderson. "Mold and Mycotoxins: Often Overlooked Factors in Chronic Lyme Disease." *Townsend Letter* July 2014. http://www .townsendletter.com/July2014/mold0714_2.html.

15. David Rainoshek. "How Facebook is Altering Your Mind." June 12, 2013. http://davidrainoshek.com/2013/06/how-facebook-fb-is-altering-your-mind-2/.

16. Mark Sisson. *The Primal Blueprint: Reprogram Your Genes for Effortless Weight Loss, Vibrant Health and Boundless Energy.* Malibu, CA: Primal Nutrition, Inc.; paperback 2nd edition (2012).

17. Elena Santos. "Coloring Isn't Just For Kids. It Can Actually Help Adults Combat Stress." *The Huffington Post.* October 13, 2014. http://www.huffingtonpost.com/2014/10/13/coloring-for-stress_n_5975832.html.

18. Amber O'Hearn. "Ketogenic Diets and Stress Part 1." http://www.ketotic.org/2012/07/ketogenic-diets-and-stress-part-i.html.

19. Jerome W. Conn. "The Advantage of a High Protein Diet in the Treatment of Spontaneous Hypoglycemia: Preliminary Report." *Journal of Clinical Investigation* 15.6 (1936). http://www.jci.org/articles/view/100819/pdf.

20. Michael Lam. "Adrenal Fatigue vs. Hypothyroidism." http://www.drlam.com/articles/adrenalfatiguevshypothyroidism.asp.

21. Ibid.

22. Ibid.

23. C. Orian Truss. *The Missing Diagnosis.* Missing Diagnosis (1983).

24. Laurel Finn. "Chronic Insomnia Increases Mortality." SLEEP 2010: Associated Professional Sleep Societies 24th Annual Meeting: Abstract 0607. Presented June 7, 2010. http://www.medscape.com/viewarticle/725126.

25. ABC News - Stanford University. "Lack of Sleep is as Dangerous as Being Drunk."

26. Christopher Bergland. "Insomnia Increases Junk Food Cravings." *Psychology Today* August 7, 2013. http://www.psychologytoday.com/blog/the-athletes-way/201308/insomnia-increases-junk-food-cravings.

27. Mark Sisson. *The Primal Blueprint: Reprogram Your Genes for Effortless Weight Loss, Vibrant Health and Boundless Energy.* Malibu, CA: Primal Nutrition, Inc.; paperback 2nd edition (2012).

28. Joseph Mercola. "Up to 70 Percent of Americans May be Deficient in Vitamin D." December 24, 2003. http://articles.mercola.com/sites/articles/archive/2003/12/24/vitamin-d-deficiency.aspx.

29. Al Sears. *Your Best Health Under the Sun.* Wellington, FL: Wellness Research & Consulting, Inc. (2007).

30. Charles Gant. Quit Smoking Webinar. www.cegant.com.

31. Al Sears. *Your Best Health Under the Sun.* Wellington, FL: Wellness Research & Consulting, Inc. (2007).

32. Ibid.

33. N.A. Mischel, et al. "Physical (in)activity-dependent Structural Plasticity in Bulbospinal Catecholaminergic Neurons of Rat Rostral Ventrolateral Medulla." *The Journal of Comparative Neurology* 522.3 (2014). https://www.ncbi.nlm.nih.gov/pubmed/24114875.

34. Madelyn Fernstrom. "The Biggest Loser Contestants Gain Again." May 3, 2016.

http://www.today.com/health/biggest-loser-contestants-gain-again-why-weight-keeps
-coming-back-t90261.

35. Al Sears. *PACE: The 12 Minute Fitness Revolution*. Royal Palm Beach, FL: Wellness Research & Consulting, Inc. (2010).

36. Loren Cordain. *The Paleo Diet: Lose Weight and Get Healthy by Eating the Foods You Were Designed to Eat*. Hoboken, NJ: Wiley (2001).

37. Al Sears. *PACE: The 12 Minute Fitness Revolution*. Royal Palm Beach, FL: Wellness Research & Consulting, Inc. (2010).

38. Mark Sisson. *The Primal Blueprint: Reprogram Your Genes for Effortless Weight Loss, Vibrant Health and Boundless Energy*. Malibu, CA: Primal Nutrition, Inc.; paperback 2nd edition (2012).

39. A. Biswas, et. al. "Sedentary Time and Its Association With Risk for Disease Incidence, Mortality, and Hospitalization in Adults: A Systematic Review and Meta-analysis." *Annals of Internal Medicine* 162.2 (2015). http://annals.org/aim/article/2091327/sedentary-time-its-association-risk-disease-incidence-mortality-hospitalization-adults.

40. C. Matthews, et al. "Amount of Time Spent in Sedentary Behaviors and Cause-Specific Mortality in US Adults." *The American Journal of Clinical Nutrition* 95.2 (2012). https://www.ncbi.nlm.nih.gov/pubmed/22218159.

41. Joseph Mercola. "Intermittent Movement Benefits Your Health. Here's How to Get More of It into Your Work Day." April 11, 2014. http://fitness.mercola.com/sites/fitness/archive/2014/04/11/intermittent-movement.aspx.

42. Al Sears. "Moving Day is Every Day." http://www.alsearsmd.com/2015/02/moving-day-is-every-day/.

43. Joseph Mercola. "Sitting Kills, Moving Heals." June 23, 2013. http://articles.mercola.com/sites/articles/archive/2013/06/23/vernikos-sitting-kills.aspx.

44. Charles Gant. "Detoxification" webinar. http://www.cegant.com/.

45. Joan Mathews Larson. *Seven Weeks to Sobriety: The Proven Program to Fight Alcoholism through Nutrition*. Revised ed. New York, NY. (Fawcett Columbine, 1992; Ballantine Books, 1997).

46. Ibid.

47. Alanazi Humidah, et al. "Cigarette Smoke-Exposed Candida albicans Increased Chitin Production and Modulated Human Fibroblast Cell Responses." *BioMed Research International* 2014, Article ID 963156. https://www.hindawi.com/journals/bmri/2014/963156/.

48. Joseph Mercola. "Electronic Cigarettes Contain Higher Levels of Toxic Metal Nanoparticles than Tobacco Smoke." April 10, 2013. http://articles.mercola.com/sites/articles/archive/2013/04/10/electronic-cigarette.aspx.

49. S. D. Wells. "Electronic Cigarette Explodes in Man's Mouth, Blows Out his Teeth." Natural News. February 21, 2012. http://www.naturalnews.com/035026_e-cigarettes_explode_teeth.html.

50. Charles Gant. "Psychotropics" webinar. www.cegant.com.

51. Colin Fernandez. "How Smoking Cannabis Raises the Risk for Stroke." Daily Mail.

October 26, 2015. http://www.dailymail.co.uk/health/article-3290223/How-smoking cannabis-raises-risk-STROKE-Drug-significantly-narrows-blood-vessels-head.html.

52. National Institute on Drug Abuse (NIDA). "Marijuana. What Are Marijuana's Effects on General Health?" https://www.drugabuse.gov/publications/research-reports/marijuana/what-are-marijuanas-effects-general-physical-health.

53. Frontline. "A Fact Sheet on the Effects of Marijuana." Reprint from Partnership for a Drug-Free America. http://www.pbs.org/wgbh/pages/frontline/shows/dope/body/effects.html.

54. National Institute on Drug Abuse (NIDA). "DrugFacts: Marijuana. What is Marijuana?" https://www.drugabuse.gov/publications/drugfacts/marijuana.

55. Nancy Burkhart. "Marijuana." *Registered Dental Hygienist* 30.8. http://www.rdhmag.com/articles/print/volume-30/issue-8/columns/marijuana.html.

56. DrugScience.org "The Effects of Marijuana Smoke." http://www.drugscience.org/Petition/C2B.html.

57. National Institute on Drug Abuse (NIDA). "Marijuana. What Are Marijuana's Effects on General Health?" https://www.drugabuse.gov/publications/research-reports/marijuana/what-are-marijuanas-effects-general-physical-health.

58. Frontline. "A Fact Sheet on the Effects of Marijuana." Reprint from Partnership for a Drug-Free America. http://www.pbs.org/wgbh/pages/frontline/shows/dope/body/effects.html.

59. Jonathan Lapook. "Mysterious Illness Tied to Marijuana Use on the Rise in States with Legal Weed." CBS News. December 28, 2016. http://www.cbsnews.com/news/mysterious-illness-tied-to-marijuana-use-on-the-rise-in-states-with-legal-weed/.

60. P. A. Versteeg, et al. "Effect of Cannabis Usage on the Oral Environment: a Review." *International Journal of Dental Hygiene* 6.4 (2008). http://www.ncbi.nlm.nih.gov/pubmed/19138182.

61. M. R. Darling, T. M. Arendorf, and N. A. Coldrey. "Effect of Cannabis Use on Oral Candidal Carriage." *Journal of Oral Pathology & Medicine* 19.7 (1990). http://www.ncbi.nlm.nih.gov/pubmed/2231436.

62. M. P. Sherman, et al. "Antimicrobial and Respiratory Burst Characteristics of Pulmonary Alveolar Macrophages Recovered from Smokers of Marijuana Alone, Smokers of Tobacco Alone, Smokers of Marijuana and Tobacco, and Nonsmokers." *The American Review of Respiratory Disease* 144.6 (1991). http://www.ncbi.nlm.nih.gov/pubmed/1660230.

63. S. Murikinati, et al. "Activation of Cannabinoid 2 Receptors Protects Against Cerebral Ischemia by Inhibiting Neutrophil Recruitment." *FASEB Journal* 24.3 (2010). http://www.ncbi.nlm.nih.gov/pubmed/19884325.

64. R. H. Beigi, et al. "Vaginal Yeast Colonization in non-pregnant Women: A longitudinal study." *Obstetrics and Gynecology* 104.5 (Pt 1) (2004). https://www.ncbi.nlm.nih.gov/pubmed/15516380

65. Gayane Dolyan Descornet. "Bras and Breast Cancer." *Women Health & Lifestyle*. http://www.women-info.com/en/bras-breast-cancer/.

66. Ralph L. Reed. "Bras and Breast Cancer: Women Who Wear Bras Versus Those That Do Not." http://all-natural.com/womens-health/bras/.

67. Gayane Dolyan Descornet. "Bras and Breast Cancer." *Women Health & Lifestyle*. http://www.women-info.com/en/bras-breast-cancer/.

68. Sydney Ross Singer and Soma Grismaijer. *Dressed to Kill: The Link Between Breast Cancer and Bras*. Pahoa, Hawaii: I.S.C.D. Press (1995). Kindle version.

69. A. Miyatsuji, et al. "Effects of Clothing Pressure Caused by Different Types of Brassieres on Autonomic Nervous System Activity Evaluated by Heart Rate Variability Power Spectral Analysis." *Journal of Physiological Anthropology and Applied Human Science* 21.1 (2002). https://www.ncbi.nlm.nih.gov/pubmed/11938611.

70. Gayane Dolyan Descornet. "Wearing a Bra." *Women Health & Lifestyle*. http://www.women-info.com/en/wearing-bra/.

71. Great Plains Laboratory -OAT Test.

72. David W. Kaufman, et al. "Oxalobacter Formigenes May Reduce the Risk of Calcium Oxalate Kidney Stones." *Journal of the American Society of Nephrology: JASN* 19.6 (2008). https://www.ncbi.nlm.nih.gov/pmc/articles/PMC2396938/.

73. William Shaw. "The Role of Oxalates in Autism and Chronic Disorders." The Weston A. Price Foundation. March 26, 2010. http://www.westonaprice.org/health-topics/the-role-of-oxalates-in-autism-and-chronic-disorders/.

74. Ibid.

75. William Shaw. "Oxalates: Test Implications for Yeast and Heavy Metals." (Accessed 2014. Page no longer exists.) http://www.greatplainslaboratory.com/home/eng/oxalates.asp.

76. Rick Sponaugle. "Anxiety Disorder Causes." http://sponauglewellness.com/wellness-programs/anxiety/anxiety-panic-disorder-causes/ (Accessed 2013. Page no longer exists.)

77. Emily Deans. "Your Brain on Ketones." August 30, 2010. http://evolutionarypsychiatry.blogspot.com/2010/08/your-brain-on-ketones.html.

78. Amy Yasko. *Autism: Pathways to Recovery*. Bethel, ME: Neurological Research Institute, LLC (2004, 2007, 2009).

79. Ibid.

80. Ibid.

81. Datis Kharazzian. "The Gut Brain Axis." http://digestionsessions.com/dr-datis-kharrazian/ (Accessed 2013. Page no longer available.)

82. Amy Yasko. *Autism: Pathways to Recovery*. Bethel, ME: Neurological Research Institute, LLC (2004, 2007, 2009).

83. Ibid.

84. Laura Maintz and Natalija Novak. "Histamine and Histamine Intolerance." *The American Journal of Clinical Nutrition* 85.5 (2007). https://www.ncbi.nlm.nih.gov/pubmed/17490952.

85. Janice Joneja. "Histamine Intolerance." Foods Matter. http://www.foodsmatter.com/allergy_intolerance/histamine/articles/histamine_joneja.html.

86. R. Bowen. "Enterochromaffin-Like (ECL) Cells." Coloroda State University. January 31, 2003. http://www.vivo.colostate.edu/hbooks/pathphys/digestion/stomach/ecl_cells .html.

87. R. Bowen. "Histamine and Histamine Receptors." Colorado State University. http:// arbl.cvmbs.colostate.edu/hbooks/pathphys/endocrine/otherendo/histamine.html.

88. "Histamine Receptors." University of Bristol. http://www.chm.bris.ac.uk/motm /histamine/jm/receptors.htm.

89. Joan Mathews Larson. *Depression Free Naturally: 7 Weeks to Eliminating Anxiety, Despair, Fatigue and Anger from Your Life.* New York, NY: Ballantine (2001).

90. HNMT histamine N-methyltransferase [Homo sapiens (human)]. http://www.ncbi .nlm.nih.gov/gene/3176.

91. D. D. Brown, R. Tomchick, and J. Axelrod "The Distribution and Properties of a His-tamine-methylating Enzyme" (pdf). *The Journal of Biological Chemistry* 234.11 (1959). http://www.jbc.org/content/234/11/2948.full.pdf.

92. Sarah Ballantyne. "Teaser Excerpt from The Paleo Approach: Histamine Intol-erance." June 2013. https://www.thepaleomom.com/teaser-excerpt-from-the-paleo -approach-histamine-intolerance/.

93. David Jockers. "Are You Suffering from Histamine Intolerance." May 2014. http:// www.organiclifestylemagazine.com/are-you-suffering-from-histamine-intolerance/.

94. H. H. Park, et al. "Flavonoids Inhibit Histamine Release and Expression of Proinflam-matory Cytokines in Mast Cells." *Archives of Pharmacal Research* 31.10 (2008). https:// www.ncbi.nlm.nih.gov/pubmed/18958421.

95. Joan Mathews Larson. *Depression Free Naturally.* New York, NY: Ballantine (2001)

96. Julia Ross. "Urinary Neurotransmitter Testing: Problems and Alternatives." *Townsend Letter* October 2006. https://www.moodcure.com/pdfs/urinetesting.pdf.

97. Charles Gant. Addiction Webinar. www.cegant.com.

Al Sears. *PACE: The 12-Minute Fitness Revolution.* Royal Palm Beach, FL: Wellness Research & Consulting, Inc. (2010).

Charles Gant. *End Your Addiction Now.* Garden City Park, NY: Square One Publishers (2009).

Ashok Gupta. *Gupta Amygdala Retraining.* Harley Street Solutions (2011).

Annie Hopper. *Dynamic Neural Retraining System.* Annie Hopper (2011).

David Berceli. *Trauma Releasing Exercises: A Revolutionary New Method for Stress/ Trauma Recovery.* North Charleston, SC: Booksurge (2005).

Nora T. Gedgaudas, *Primal Body Primal Mind: Beyond the Paleo Diet for Total Health and a Longer Life.* Rochester, VT: Healing Arts Press (2011).

Chapter 14

1. Robert C. Atkins. *Vita-Nutrient Solution: Nature's Answers to Drugs.* New York, NY: Fireside (2011). Kindle version.

2. Ibid.

3. Ibid.

4. Ibid.

5. lbid.

6. lbid.

7. Personal consult, Dr. Lam's office with his wife.

8. Al Sears. "Vitamin D3 is Better than Drugs for Depression." http://www.alsearsmd .com/2015/09/vitamin-d3-better-than-drugs-for-depression/.

9. lbid.

10. Al Sears. "Some Shrooms for Your Brain." http://www.alsearsmd.com/2014/10/some -shrooms-for-your-brain-2/.

11. Al Sears. "Stop wasting money on vitamin and mineral supplements. (Is he joking?)" http://www.alsearsmd.com/2014/07/is-he-joking.

12. A. R. Holmes, R. D. Cannon, and M.G. Shepherd. "Effect of Calcium Ion Uptake on Candida Albicans Morphology." *FEMS Microbiology Letter* 61.2-3 (1991). http://www .ncbi.nlm.nih.gov/pubmed/2037228.

13. lbid.

14. G. A. Eby. "Rescue Treatment and Prevention of Asthma Using Magnesium Throat Lozenges: Hypothesis for a Mouth-lung Biologically Closed Electric Circuit." *Medical Hypotheses* 67.5 (2006). http://www.ncbi.nlm.nih.gov/pubmed/16797866.

15. Gaby Tiemi Suzukii, Juliana Alves Macedo, and Gabriela Alves Macedo. "Medium Composition Influence on Biotin and Riboflavin Production by Newly Isolated Candida Sp." *Brazilian Journal of Microbiology* 42.3 (2011). http://www.ncbi.nlm.nih.gov/pmc /articles/PMC3768789/.

16. Hugo Wurtele, et al. "Modulation of Histone H3 Lysine 56 Acetylation as an Antifungal Therapeutic Strategy." *Nature Medicine* 16 (2010). http://www.nature.com /nm/journal/v16/n7/abs/nm.2175.html.

17. Scott Forsgren, Neil Nathan, and Wayne Anderson. "Mold and Mycotoxins: Often Overlooked Factors in Chronic Lyme Disease." *Townsend Letter* July 2014. http://www .townsendletter.com/July2014/mold0714_2.html.

18. Charles Gant. "Heavy Metals" webinar. www.cegant.com.

19. Jon Pangborn and Sidney MacDonald Baker. *Autism: Effective Biomedical Treatments*. Autism Research Institute. Second Edition. 2005.

20. Amy Yasko. *Autism: Pathways to Recovery.* Bethel, ME: Neurological Research Institute, LLC (2004, 2007, 2009).

21. Allison Siebecker and Steven Sandberg-Lewis. "Small Intestine Bacterial Overgrowth: Often-Ignored Cause of Irritable Bowel Syndrome." *Townsend Letter* February / March 2013. http://www.townsendletter.com/FebMarch2013/ibs0213_2.html.

22. Amy Yasko. *Autism: Pathways to Recovery.* Bethel, ME: Neurological Research Institute, LLC (2004, 2007, 2009).

23. Grace Liu. "Don't Take Resistant Starch If You Have Moderate to Severe

Irritable Bowel Syndrome (IBS) Temporarily (Part 3)." Thursday, October 2, 2014. http://drbganimalpharm.blogspot.com/2014/10/dont-take-raw-resistant-starch-if-you.html.

24. Allison Siebecker and Steven Sandberg-Lewis. "Small Intestine Bacterial Overgrowth: Often-Ignored Cause of Irritable Bowel Syndrome." *Townsend Letter* February / March 2013. http://www.townsendletter.com/FebMarch2013/ibs0213_2.html.

25. Grace Liu. "Don't Take Resistant Starch Alone: Whole Real Food RS3 Expands Lean Core Microbiota Whereas High-Dose Raw Potato Starch Doesn't Appear To, N=1 (Part 2)." http://drbganimalpharm.blogspot.com/2014/09/dont-take-resistant-starch-alone-part-2.html.

26. Norm Robillard. "Resistant Starch—Friend or Foe?" http://digestivehealthinstitute.org/2013/05/10/resistant-starch-friend-or-foe/.

27. Amy Yasko. *Autism: Pathways to Recovery.* Bethel, ME: Neurological Research Institute, LLC (2004, 2007, 2009).

28. Al Sears. *Your Best Health Under the Sun.* Wellington, FL. Wellness Research & Consulting, Inc. (2007).

David Perlmutter. *Grain Brain: The Surprising Truth About Wheat, Carbs, and Sugar— Your Brain's Silent Killers.* New York, NY. Little, Brown and Company (2013).

Chapter 15

1. Catherine Guthrie. "How to Train Your Doctor." Oprah.com. http://www.oprah.com/omagazine/How-to-Get-the-Best-Medical-Care-from-Your-Doctor.

2. Ariana Eunjung Cha. "Researchers: Medical Errors Now Third Leading Cause of Death in United States." *The Washington Post.* https://www.washingtonpost.com/news/to-your-health/wp/2016/05/03/researchers-medical-errors-now-third-leading-cause-of-death-in-united-states/.

3. ABC Nightly News. October 2009.

4. Jonathan Wright. http://tahomaclinic.com/.

Additional Resources

Salil A. Lachke, et al. "Phenotypic switching and filamentation in Candida glabrata." Microbiology 148.9 (2002). http://mic.sgmjournals.org/content/148/9/2661.full.pdf.

X. Zhang, et al. "Estrogen Effects on Candida albicans: a Potential Virulence-regulating Mechanism." *Journal of Infectious Diseases* 18.14 (2000). https://www.ncbi.nlm.nih.gov/pubmed/10762574.

X. Zhao, et al. "Oestrogen-binding protein in Candida albicans: antibody development and cellular localization by electron immunocytochemistry." *Microbiology* 141.10 (1995). https://eurekamag.com/research/002/910/002910359.php.

Endocrine Society. "Diverse Gut Bacteria Associated with Favorable Ratio of Estrogen Metabolites." ScienceDaily, September 11, 2014. http://www.sciencedaily.com/releases/2014/09/140911135316.htm.

H. Santelmann and J. M. Howard. "Yeast Metabolic Products, Yeast Antigens and Yeasts as Possible Triggers for Irritable Bowel Syndrome." *European Journal of Gastroenterology and Hepatology* 17.1 (2005). https://www.ncbi.nlm.nih.gov/pubmed/15647635.

K. Lewis. "Persister Cells." *Annual Review of Microbiology* 64 (2010). 134306. http://www.ncbi.nlm.nih.gov/pubmed/20528688.

R. J. Blinkhorn, D. Adelstein, and P. J. Spagnuolo. "Emergence of a New Opportunistic Pathogen, Candida Lusitaniae." *Journal of Clinical Microbiology* 27.2 (1989). http://www.ncbi.nlm.nih.gov/pmc/articles/PMC267283/.

D. Abi-Said, et al. "The Epidemiology of Hematogenous Candidiasis Caused by Different Candida Species." *Clinical Infectious Diseases* 24.6 (1997).

J. Aisner, et al. "Torulopsis Glabrata Infections in Patients with Cancer: Increasing Incidence and Relationship to Colonization." *American Journal of Medicine* 61.1 (1976)

S. Arif, et al. "Techniques for Investigation of an Apparent Outbreak of Infections with Candida Glabrata." *Journal of Clinical Microbiology* 34.9 (1996).

G. G. Baily, et al. "Candida Inconspicua, a Fluconazole-resistant Pathogen in Patients Infected with Human Immunodeficiency Virus." *Clinical Infectious Diseases* 25.1 (1997).

Margaret Borg-von Zepelin, et al. "Changes in the Spectrum of Fungal Isolates: Results from Clinical Specimens Gathered in 1987/88 Compared with those in 1991/92 in the University Hospital Göttingen, Germany." *Mycoses* 36.7–8 (1993).

F. Barchiesi, et al. 1993. Emergence of Oropharyngeal Candidiasis caused by Non-albicans Species of Candida in HIV-infected Patients (letter). *European Journal of Epidemiology* 9.4 (1993).

David Kadosh and Alexander D. Johnson. "Induction of the *Candida Albicans* Filamentous Growth Program by Relief of Transcriptional Repression: A Genome-Wide Analysis." Ed. Thomas Fox. *Molecular Biology of the Cell* 16.6 (2005).

Cletus Kurtzman, J.W. Fell and Teun Boekhout. *The Yeasts: A Taxonomic Study.* Elsevier Science; 5 edition (2011).

Candida Genome Database. http://www.candidagenome.org/.

Sam K. Bashar and Amal K. Mitra. "Effect of Smoking on Vitamin A, Vitamin E, and Other Trace Elements in Patients with Cardiovascular Disease in Bangladesh: A Cross-Sectional Study." *Nutrition Journal* 3 (2004). https://www.ncbi.nlm.nih.gov/pmc/articles/PMC524516/.

E. A. Krall and B. Dawson-Hughes. "Smoking Increases Bone Loss and Decrease Calcium Absorption." *Journal of Bone and Mineral Research* 14.2 (1999). http://www.ncbi.nlm.nih.gov/pubmed/9933475.

S. Malhotra, et al. "Yeast Infection and Psychiatric Disorders." *Delhi Psychiatry Journal* 13.2 (2010). http://medind.nic.in/daa/t10/i2/daat10i2p345.pdf.

R. E. Cater. "Chronic Intestinal Candidiasis as a Possible Etiological Factor in the Chronic Fatigue Syndrome." *Medical Hypotheses* 44.6 (1995). http://www.ncbi.nlm.nih.gov/pubmed/7476598.

Jill Carnahan. "Zonulin & Leaky Gut: A Discovery that Changed the way we View Inflammation, Autoimmune disease and Cancer!" Primal Docs. http://primaldocs.com/members-blog/zonulin-leaky-gut/.

C. Monteagudo, et al. "Tissue Invasiveness and Non-Acidic pH in Human Candidiasis Correlate with 'in Vivo' Expression by *Candida Albicans* of the Carbohydrate Epitope Recognized by New Monoclonal Antibody 1H4." *Journal of Clinical Pathology* 57.6 (2004). http://www.ncbi.nlm.nih.gov/pmc/articles/PMC1770313/.

Andrea Walther and Jürgen Wendland. "Hyphal Growth and Virulence in Candida albicans." *The Mycota: Human and Animal Relationships.* Volume 6 of the series. Springer Berlin Heidelberg (2008). http://link.springer.com/chapter/10.1007%2F978-3-540-79307-6_6.

K. E. Elkind-Hirsch, L. D. Sherman, R. Malinak. "Hormone Replacement Therapy Alters Insulin Sensitivity in Young Women with Premature Ovarian Failure." *Journal of Clinical Endocrinology and Metabolism* 76.2 (1993). https://www.ncbi.nlm.nih.gov/pubmed/8432792.

Chris Kresser. "How Stress Wreaks Havoc on Your Gut." March 23, 2012. http://chriskresser.com/how-stress-wreaks-havoc-on-your-gut.

T. L. Han, R. D. Cannon, S. G. Villas-Bôas. "The Metabolic Basis of Candida Albicans Morphogenesis and Quorum Sensing." *Fungal Genetics and Biology* 48.8 (2011). http://www.ncbi.nlm.nih.gov/pubmed/21513811.

Anna Dongari-Bagtzoglou. "Pathogenesis of Mucosal Biofilm Infections: Challenges and Progress." *Expert Review of Anti-infective Therapy* 6.2 (2008). http://www.ncbi.nlm.nih.gov/pmc/articles/PMC2712878/.

M. Martins, et al. "Presence of Extracellular DNA in the *Candida Albicans* Biofilm Matrix and Its Contribution to Biofilms." *Mycopathologia* 169.5 (2010): 323–331. PMC. Web. October 30, 2016. https://www.ncbi.nlm.nih.gov/pmc/articles/PMC3973130/.

Salil A. Lachke, et al. "Phenotypic Switching and Filamentation in Candida Glabrata." *Microbiology* 148.9 (2002). https://www.ncbi.nlm.nih.gov/pubmed/12213913.

David G. Davies and Cláudia N. H. Marques. "A Fatty Acid Messenger Is Responsible for Inducing Dispersion in Microbial Biofilms." *Journal of Bacteriology* 191.5 (2009). https://www.ncbi.nlm.nih.gov/pmc/articles/PMC2648214/.

Rawya S. Al-Dhaheri and L. Julia Douglas. "Apoptosis in Candida Biofilms Exposed to Amphotericin B." *Journal of Medical Microbiology* 59.2 (2010). https://www.ncbi.nlm.nih.gov/pubmed/19892857.

Y. Nakagawa, N. Ohno, and T Murai. "Suppression by Candida albicans β-Glucan of Cytokine Release from Activated Human Monocytes and from T Cells in the Presence of Monocytes." *Journal of Infectious Diseases* 187.4 (2003). http://jid.oxfordjournals.org/content/187/4/710.full.

Anju Usman. G.I. Biology, Pathology and Treatment Strategies. True Health Medical Center. 2011. http://www.autismone.org/sites/default/files/usman-bugs.pdf.

M. Matsushima, et al. "Growth Inhibitory Action of Cranberry on Helicobacter Pylori." *Journal of Gastroenterology and Hepatology* 23 (2008). http://www.ncbi.nlm.nih.gov/pubmed/19120894.

M. V. Galan, A. A. Kishan and A. L. Silverman. "Oral Broccoli Sprouts for the Treatment of Helicobacter Pylori Infection: a Preliminary Report." *Digestive Diseases and Sciences* 49.7–9 (2004). http://www.ncbi.nlm.nih.gov/pubmed/15387326.

A. Yanaka, et al. "Dietary Sulforaphane-rich Broccoli Sprouts Reduce Colonization and Attenuate Gastritis in Helicobacter Pylori-Infected Mice and Humans." *Cancer Prevention and Research* 2.4 (2009). http://www.ncbi.nlm.nih.gov/pubmed/19349290.

G. B. Mahady, et al. "Turmeric (Curcuma longa) and Curcumin Inhibit the Growth of Helicobacter Pylori, a Group 1 Carcinogen." *Anticancer Research* 22.6C (2002). http://www.ncbi.nlm.nih.gov/pubmed/12553052.

J.W. Olson, R.J. Maier. "Molecular Hydrogen as an Energy Source for Helicobacter Pylori." *Science* 29.298 (2002) http://www.ncbi.nlm.nih.gov/pubmed/12459589.

J. G. Kusters, et al. "Coccoid Forms of Helicobacter Pylori Are the Morphologic Manifestation of Cell Death." *Infection and Immunity* 65.9 (1997). http://www.ncbi.nlm.nih.gov/pmc/articles/PMC175523/.

P. Saniee, et al. "Localization of H.pylori Within the Vacuole of Candida Yeast by Direct Immunofluorescence Technique." *Archives of Iranian Medicine* 16.12 (2013). http://www.ncbi.nlm.nih.gov/pubmed/24329143.

Y. Bourbonnais, David Bolin, and Dennis Shields. "Secretion of Somatostatin by Saccharomyces Cerevisiae." *The Journal of Biological Chemistry* 263.30 (1988). https://www.ncbi.nlm.nih.gov/pubmed/2902090.

H. S. Ormsbee III, S. L. Koehler Jr., G. L. Telford. "Somatostatin Inhibits Motilin-Induced Interdigestive Contractile Activity in the Dog." *The American Journal of Digestive Diseases* 23.9 (1978). http://www.ncbi.nlm.nih.gov/pubmed/707449.

R. Guillemin. "Somatostatin Inhibits the Release of Acetylcholine Induced Electrically in the Myenteric Plexus." *Endocrinology* 99.6 (1976). https://www.ncbi.nlm.nih.gov/pubmed/187417.

Jen Broyles. "The Link Between Food Poisoning IBS and SIBO." Primal Docs. http://primaldocs.com/opinion/the-link-between-food-poisoning-ibs-and-sibo/.

H. Mönnikes, et. al. "Role of Stress in Functional Gastrointestinal Disorders. Evidence for Stress-Induced Alterations in Gastrointestinal Motility and Sensitivity." *Digestive Diseases* 19.3 (2001). http://www.ncbi.nlm.nih.gov/pubmed/11752838.

Siri Carpenter. "That Gut Feeling." *American Psychological Association* September 43.8 (2012). http://www.apa.org/monitor/2012/09/gut-feeling.aspx.

Phillip Low. "Overview of the Autonomic Nervous System." Merck Manual Online. http://www.merckmanuals.com/home/brain,-spinal-cord,-and-nerve-disorders/autonomic-nervous-system-disorders/overview-of-the-autonomic-nervous-system.

Jan Bures, et al. "Small Intestinal Bacterial Overgrowth Syndrome." *World Journal of Gastroenterology: WJG* 16.24 (2010). https://www.ncbi.nlm.nih.gov/pmc/articles/PMC2890937/.

Peter Ott, Otto Clemmesen, and Fin Stolze Larsen. "Cerebral Metabolic Disturbances in the Brain During Acute Liver Failure: From Hyperammonemia to Energy Failure and Proteolysis." *Neurochemistry International* 47.1–2 (2005). https://www.ncbi.nlm.nih.gov/pubmed/15921824.

R. Todd Frederick. "Current Concepts in the Pathophysiology and Management of Hepatic Encephalopathy." *Gastroenterology & Hepatology* 7.4 (2011). http://www.ncbi.nlm .nih.gov/pmc/articles/PMC3127024/.

A. J. Vince and S. M. Burridge. "Ammonia Production by Intestinal Bacteria: the Effects of Lactose, Lactulose and Glucose." *Journal of Medical Microbiology* 13.2 (1980). http://www.ncbi.nlm.nih.gov/pubmed/7381915.

Irena Ciećko-Michalska, et al. "Pathogenesis of Hepatic Encephalopathy," *Gastroenterology Research and Practice* vol. 2012, Article ID 642108, (2012). http://www.hindawi .com/journals/grp/2012/642108/.

Christopher Bergland. "The Neurobiology of Grace Under Pressure." Psychology Today. February 2, 2013. https://www.psychologytoday.com/blog/the-athletes-way/201302/the-neurobiology-grace-under-pressure.

Caroline Westwater, Edward Balish, and David A. Schofield. "Candida Albicans-Conditioned Medium Protects Yeast Cells from Oxidative Stress: A Possible Link between Quorum Sensing and Oxidative Stress Resistance." *Eukaryotic Cell* 4.10 (2005). https://www.ncbi.nlm.nih.gov/pmc/articles/PMC1265892/.

Ingrid E. Frohner, et al. "Candida Albicans Cell Surface Superoxide Dismutases Degrade Host-Derived Reactive Oxygen Species to Escape Innate Immune Surveillance." *Molecular Microbiology* 71.1 (2009). https://www.ncbi.nlm.nih.gov/pmc/articles/PMC2713856/.

A. Kropec, et al. "In vitro Assessment of the Host Response against Enterococcus faecalis Used in Probiotic Preparations." *Infection* 33.5–6 (2005). https://www.ncbi.nlm.nih.gov/pubmed/16258871.

W. M. Deepika Priyadarshani and W. K. Rakshit. "Screening Selected Strains of Probiotic Lactic Acid Bacteria for their Ability to Produce Biogenic Amines (histamine and tyramine)." *International Journal of Food Science & Technology* 46.10 (2011). http://onlinelibrary.wiley.com/doi/10.1111/j.1365-2621.2011.02717.x/abstract.

R. Bowen. "Enterochromaffin-Like (ECL) Cells." Colorado State University http://www.vivo.colostate.edu/hbooks/pathphys/digestion/stomach/ecl_cells.html.

University of Bristol. Histamine Receptors. Molecule of the Month. http://www.chm.bris.ac.uk/motm/histamine/jm/receptors.htm.

R. Bowen. "Histamine and Histamine Receptors." Colorado State University. http://arbl.cvmbs.colostate.edu/hbooks/pathphys/endocrine/otherendo/histamine.html.

Janice Joneja. "Histamine Intolerance." Foods Matter. http://www.foodsmatter.com/allergy_intolerance/histamine/articles/histamine_joneja.html.

J. R. Sheedy, et al. "Increased D-lactic Acid Intestinal Bacteria in Patients with Chronic Fatigue Syndrome. *In Vivo* 23.4 (2009). https://www.ncbi.nlm.nih.gov/pubmed/19567398.

Elaine Gottschall. "Probiotics." Breaking the Vicious Cycle. http://www.breakingthe viciouscycle.info/knowledge_base/detail/probiotics/.

P. Valenti and G. Antonini. "Lactoferrin: an Important Host Defence Against Microbial and Viral Attack." *Cellular and Molecular Life Sciences* 62.22 (2005). http://www.ncbi.nlm.nih.gov/pubmed/16261253.

A. Lupetti, et al. "Human Lactoferrin-derived Peptide's Antifungal Activities against Disseminated Candida Albicans Infection." *The Journal of Infectious Diseases* 196.9 (2007). http://www.ncbi.nlm.nih.gov/pubmed/17922408.

K. P. Latté and H. Kolodziej. "Antifungal Effects of Hydrolysable Tannins and Related Compounds on Dermatophytes, Mould Fungi and Yeasts." *Zeitschrift fur Naturforschung* 55.5–6 (2000). http://www.ncbi.nlm.nih.gov/pubmed/10928561.

I. Ahmad and A. Z. Beg. "Antimicrobial and Phytochemical Studies on 45 Indian Medicinal Plants against Multi-drug Resistant Human Pathogens." *Journal of Ethnopharmacology* 74.2 (2001). http://www.ncbi.nlm.nih.gov/pubmed/11167029.

Akiyama Hisanori et al. "Antibacterial Action of Several Tannins against Staphylococcus Aureus." *Journal of Antimicrobial Chemotherapy* 48.4 (2001). http://jac.oxfordjournals.org/content/48/4/487.long.

Y. Xu, et al. "The Effects of Curcumin on Depressive-like Behaviors in Mice." *European Journal of Pharmacology* 518.1 (2005). https://www.ncbi.nlm.nih.gov/pubmed/15987635.

Shrinivas K. Kulkarni, Mohit Kumar Bhutani, and Mahendra Bishnoi. "Antidepressant Activity of Curcumin: Involvement of Serotonin and Dopamine System." *Psychopharmacology* 201.3 (2008).

L. Panizzi, et al. "Composition and Antimicrobial Properties of Essential Oils of Four Mediterranean Lamiaceae." *Journal of Ethnopharmacology* 39.3 (1993). http://www.ncbi.nlm.nih.gov/pubmed/8258973.

S. Carrero, H. Romero and R. Apitz-Castro. "In Vitro Inhibitory Effect of Ajoene on Candida Isolates Recovered from Vaginal Discharges." *Revista Iberoamericana de Micologia* 26.3 (2009). http://www.ncbi.nlm.nih.gov/pubmed/19635444.

E. Ledezma and R. Apitz-Castro. "Ajoene the Main Active Compound of Garlic (Allium sativum): a New Antifungal Agent." *Revista Iberoamericana de Micologia* 23.2 (2006). http://www.ncbi.nlm.nih.gov/pubmed/16854181.

Rawya S. Al-Dhaheri and L. Julia Douglas. "Apoptosis in Candida Biofilms Exposed to Amphotericin B." *Journal of Medical Microbiology* 59.2 (2010). https://www.ncbi.nlm .nih.gov/pubmed/19892857.

D. O. Ogbolu, et al. "In Vitro Antimicrobial Properties of Coconut Oil on Candida Species in Ibadan, Nigeria." *Journal of Medicinal Food* 10.2 (2007). http://www.ncbi.nlm. nih .gov/pubmed/17651080.

G. Bergsson, et al. "In Vitro Killing of *Candida Albicans* by Fatty Acids and Monoglycerides." *Antimicrobial Agents and Chemotherapy* 45.11 (2001). https://www.ncbi. nlm.nih .gov/pmc/articles/PMC90807/.

M. Baginski and J. Czub. "Amphotericin B and its New Derivatives - Mode of Action." *Current Drug Metabolism* 10.5 (2009). http://www.ncbi.nlm.nih.gov/pubmed/19689243.

C. Petersen. "D-lactic Acidosis." *Nutrition in Clinical Practice* 20.6 (2005). http://www .ncbi.nlm.nih.gov/pubmed/16306301.

J. Uribarri, M. S. Oh, and H. J. Carroll. "D-lactic Acidosis. A Review of Clinical Presentation, Biochemical Features, and Pathophysiologic Mechanisms." *Medicine* 77.2 (1998). http://www.ncbi.nlm.nih.gov/pubmed/9556700.

A. Forche, et al. "Stress Alters Rates and Types of Loss of Heterozygosity in *Candida Albicans*." *mBio* 2.4 (2011). https://www.ncbi.nlm.nih.gov/pmc/articles/PMC3143845/.

National Cancer Institute. Complimentary & Alternative Medicine. "Milk Thistle -Health Professional Version." http://www.cancer.gov/about-cancer/treatment/cam/hp/ milk-thistle-pdq#section/_7.

Y. Adachi, et al. "Enhancement of Cytokine Production by Macrophages tSimulated with 1,3 beta D glucan, Grifolan, Isolated from Grifola Frondosa." *Biological & Pharmaceutical Bulletin* 17.12 (1994).

Intelegen. "Beta-Glucan Enhances Action of Immune Cells." http://intelegen.com/ ImmuneSystem/betaglucan_enhances_action_of_i.htm.

A. Nicoletti, et al. "Preliminary Evaluation of Immunoadjuvant Activity of an Orally Administered Glucan Extracted from Candida Albicans." Arzneimittel-Forschung. 42:10 (1992).

Heike Stier, Veronika Ebbeskotte, and Joerg Gruenwald. "Immune-Modulatory Effects of Dietary Yeast Beta-1,3/1,6-D-Glucan." *Nutrition Journal* 13 (2014). http://www.ncbi .nlm.nih.gov/pmc/articles/PMC4012169/.

E. Vivier, et al. "Functions of Natural Killer Cells." *Nature Immunology* 9.5 (2008). http://www.ncbi.nlm.nih.gov/pubmed/18425107.

A. W. Segal. "How Neutrophils Kill Microbes." *Annual Review of Immunology* 23 (2005). https://www.ncbi.nlm.nih.gov/pmc/articles/PMC2092448/.

R. J. Smialowicz, et al. "In Vitro Augmentation of Natural Killer Cell Activity by Manganese Chloride." *Journal of Toxicology and Environmental Health* 19.2 (1986).

Albert Sanchez, et al. "Role of Sugars in Human Neutrophilic Phagocytosis." *The American Journal of Clinical Nutrition* 26.11 (1973).

V. Snoeck, B. Goddeeris, and E. Cox. "The Role of Enterocytes in the Intestinal Barrier Function and Antigen Uptake." *Microbes and Infection* 7.7–8 (2005). https://www.ncbi .nlm.nih.gov/pubmed/15925533.

D. D. Kilpatrick. "Mechanisms and Assessment of Lectin-mediated Mitogenesis." Molecular Biotechnology 11.1 (1999). https://www.ncbi.nlm.nih.gov/labs/articles/10367282/.

Sayer Ji. "Do Hidden Opiates In Our Food Explain Food Addictions?" May 2012. http://www.greenmedinfo.com/blog/do-hidden-opiates-our-food-explain-food-addictions1.

M. Y. Pepino, et al. "Sucralose Affects Glycemic and Hormonal Responses to an Oral Glucose Load." Diabetes Care 36.9 (2013). https://www.ncbi.nlm.nih.gov/pmc/articles/PMC3747933/.

Ferris Jabr. "The Food Fight in Your Gut: Why Bacteria Will Change the Way You Think About Calories." Scientific American. September 12, 2012. http://blogs.scientific american.com/brainwaves/2012/09/12/the-food-fight-in-your-guts-why-bacteria-will-change-the-way-you-think-about-calories/.

University of Pittsburgh. Low Oxalate Diet. http://www.upmc.com/patients-visitors/education/nutrition/pages/low-oxalate-diet.aspx.

Kelly Herring. "Can a Raw Diet Make You Sick?" The Wellness Blog. Grassland Beef. http://blog.grasslandbeef.com/bid/86873/Can-a-Raw-Diet-Make-You-Sick.

Corinna Koebnick, et al. "Long-Term Consumption of a Raw Food Diet Is Associated with Favorable Serum LDL Cholesterol and Triglycerides but Also with Elevated Plasma Homocysteine and Low Serum HDL Cholesterol in Humans." The Journal of Nutrition 135.10 (2005). https://www.ncbi.nlm.nih.gov/pubmed/16177198.

Charles Q. Choi. "Eating Meat Made us Human." Live Science. October 3, 2012 http://www.livescience.com/2367-eating-meat-made-us-human.html.

R. B. Gearry, et al. "Reduction of Dietary Poorly Absorbed Short-Chain Carbohydrates (FODMAPs) Improves Abdominal Symptoms in Patients with Inflammatory Bowel Disease: a Pilot Study." Journal of Crohns and Colitis 3.1 (2009). http://www.ncbi.nlm.nih.gov/pubmed/21172242.

Al Sears. "Why I Prescribe Meat to My Patients." http://www.alsearsmd.com/why-i-prescribe-meat-to-my-patients/.

C. A. Daley, et al. "A Review of Fatty Acid Profiles and Antioxidant Content in Grass-fed and Grain-fed Beef." Nutrition Journal 9 (2010). https://www.ncbi.nlm.nih.gov/pmc/articles/PMC2846864/.

University of Alberta. "Natural Trans Fats Have Health Benefits, New Study Shows." ScienceDaily, April 5, 2008. https://www.sciencedaily.com/releases/2008/04/080402152140.htm.

Stephen Byrnes. "Myths & Truths about Vegetarianism." The Weston A. Price Foundation, December 31, 2002. http://www.westonaprice.org/health-topics/abcs-of-nutrition/myths-of-vegetarianism/.

E. J. Shepherd, et al. "Stress and Glucocorticoid Inhibit Apical GLUT2-Trafficking and Intestinal Glucose Absorption in Rat Small Intestine." The Journal of Physiology 560.1 (2004). https://www.ncbi.nlm.nih.gov/pmc/articles/PMC1665211/.

D. K. Ong, et al. "Manipulation of Dietary Short Chain Carbohydrates Alters the Pattern of Gas Production and Genesis of Symptoms in Irritable Bowel Syndrome." Journal of Gastroenterology and Hepatology 25.8 (2010). https://www.ncbi.nlm.nih.gov/pubmed/20659225.

Qing Yang. "Gain Weight by 'going Diet?' Artificial Sweeteners and the Neurobiology of Sugar Cravings." *Yale Journal of Biology and Medicine* 83.2 (2010). https://www.ncbi.nlm.nih.gov/pmc/articles/PMC2892765/.

M. Yanina Pepino, PHD, Courtney D. Tiemann, MPH, MS, RD, Bruce W. Patterson, et al. "Sucralose Affects Glycemic and Hormonal Responses to an Oral Glucose Load." Published online before print April 30, 2013, doi: 10.2337/dc12-2221 *Diabetes Care* April 30, 2013. http://care.diabetesjournals.org/content/early/2013/04/30/dc12-2221.

M. Yanina Pepino, et al. "Sucralose Affects Glycemic and Hormonal Responses to an Oral Glucose Load." *Diabetes Care* 36.9 (2013). https://www.ncbi.nlm.nih.gov/pmc/articles/PMC3747933/.

Loren Cordain, et al. "Plant-animal Subsistence Ratios and Macronutrient Energy Estimations in Worldwide Hunter-gatherer Diets." *American Journal of Clinical Nutrition* 71.3 (2000). https://www.ncbi.nlm.nih.gov/pubmed/10702160.

A. Paoli, et al. "Beyond Weight Loss: A Review of the Therapeutic Uses of Very-Low-Carbohydrate (ketogenic) Diets." *European Journal of Clinical Nutrition* 67.8 (2013). https://www.ncbi.nlm.nih.gov/pmc/articles/PMC3826507/.

Peter Attia. "Is Ketosis Dangerous?" The Eating Academy. http://eatingacademy.com/nutrition/is-ketosis-dangerous.

M. Guzman and C. Blazquez. "Ketone Body Synthesis in the Brain: Possible Neuroprotective Effects." *Prostaglandins, Leukotrienes, and Essential Fatty Acids* 70.3 (2004). https://www.ncbi.nlm.nih.gov/pubmed/14769487.

J. Alcock, C. C. Maley and C.A. Aktipis. "Is Eating Behavior Manipulated by the Gastrointestinal Microbiota? Evolutionary Pressures and Potential Mechanisms." *Bioessays* 36.10 (2014). http://onlinelibrary.wiley.com/doi/10.1002/bies.201400071/full.

Al Sears. "Addicted to Nature." http://www.alsearsmd.com/2011/06/addicted-to-nature-2/.

Sue McGreevey. "Relaxation Response Proves Positive." *Harvard Gazette*. October 13, 2015. http://news.harvard.edu/gazette/story/2015/10/relaxation-response-proves-positive/.

Sarah McKay. "27 Minutes of Mindfulness Meditation a Day Changes Brain Structure." http://yourbrainhealth.com.au/27-minutes-mindfulness-meditation-day-changes-brain-structure/.

Connie Strasheim. "Eliminate Electromagnetic Pollution to Eliminate Disease." Townsend Letter. November 2014. http://townsendletter.com/Nov2014/elimelectro1114.html.

Laura Maintz and Natalija Novak. "Histamine and Histamine Intolerance." *The American Journal of Clinical Nutrition* 85.5 (2007). https://www.ncbi.nlm.nih.gov/pubmed/17490952.

D. D. Brown, R. Tomchick, and J Axelrod. "The Distribution and Properties of a Histamine-methylating Enzyme." *The Journal of Biological Chemistry* 234.11 (1959). http://www.jbc.org/content/234/11/2948.full.pdf.

NCBI. "HNMT – histamine N-methyltransferase." http://www.ncbi.nlm.nih.gov/gene/3176.

L. C. Baldan, et al. "Histidine Decarboxylase Deficiency Causes Tourette Syndrome: Parallel Findings in Humans and Mice." *Neuron* 81.1 (2014). https://www.ncbi.nlm.nih.gov/pmc/articles/PMC3894588/.

H. H. Park, et al. "Flavonoids Inhibit Histamine Release and Expression of Proinflammatory Cytokines in Mast Cells." Archives of Pharmacal Research 31.10 (2008). http://www.ncbi.nlm.nih.gov/pubmed/18958421.

V. M. Abshire, et al. "Injection of L-allylglycine into the Posterior Hypothalamus in Rats Causes Decreases in local GABA which Correlate with Increases in Heart Rate." Neuropharmacology 27.11 (1988). https://www.ncbi.nlm.nih.gov/pubmed/3205383.

William J. L'Amoreaux, Alexandra Marsillo, and Abdeslem El Idrissi. "Pharmacological Characterization of GABA(A) Receptors in Taurine-Fed Mice." Journal of Biomedical Science 17.1 (2010). https://www.ncbi.nlm.nih.gov/pmc/articles/PMC2994404/.

A. El Idrissi and W.J. L'Amoreaux. "Selective Resistance of Taurine-fed Mice to Isoniazide-potentiated Seizures: in Vivo Functional Test for the Activity of Glutamic Acid Decarboxylase." Neuroscience 156.3 (2008).

Richard W. Olsen and Timothy M. DeLorey. "GABA Synthesis, Uptake and Release." Basic Neurochemistry: Molecular, Cellular and Medical Aspects 6th edition. Philadelphia: Lippincott-Raven; 1999. http://www.ncbi.nlm.nih.gov/books/NBK27979/.

Todd D. Prickett and Yardena Samuels. "Molecular Pathways: Dysregulated Glutamatergic Signaling Pathways in Cancer." Clinical Cancer Research: An Official Journal of the American Association for Cancer Research 18.16 (2012). https://www.ncbi.nlm.nih.gov/pmc/articles/PMC3421042/.

T. Möykkynen, et al. "Magnesium Potentiation of the Function of Native and Recombinant GABA(A) receptors." Neuroreport 12.10 (2001). https://www.ncbi.nlm.nih.gov/pubmed/11447329.

TA. Medicolegal.tripod.com, "Prevent Alcoholism." http://medicolegal.tripod.com/preventalcoholism.htm.

Carol Pierce-Davis. "The Biochemistry and Physiology of Smoking." Texas Department of Health Bulletin (2005). http://www.carolpiercedavisphd.com/files/The_Biochemistry_and_Physiology_of_Smoking.pdf.

University of California - San Francisco. "Smoking Interferes With Brain's Recovery From Alcoholism." ScienceDaily, March 16, 2006. https://www.sciencedaily.com/releases/2006/03/060316093333.htm.

Nicole M. Avena, Pedro Rada, and Bartley G. Hoebel. "Evidence for Sugar Addiction: Behavioral and Neurochemical Effects of Intermittent, Excessive Sugar Intake." Neuroscience and Biobehavioral Reviews 32.1 (2008). http://www.ncbi.nlm.nih.gov/pmc/articles/PMC2235907/.

Joseph Mercola. "Please Don't Visit this Type of Doctor Unless You Absolutely Have To." March 7, 2011. http://articles.mercola.com/sites/articles/archive/2011/03/07/reversing-depression-without-antidepressants.aspx.

S. Sinha, et al. "Improvement of Glutathione and Total Antioxidant Status with Yoga." Journal of Alternative and Complementary Medicine 13.10 (2007). http://www.ncbi.nlm.nih.gov/pubmed/18166119.

F. Zeidan, et al. "Brain Mechanisms Supporting Modulation of Pain by Mindfulness Meditation." The Journal of Neuroscience: The Official Journal of the Society for Neuroscience 31.14 (2011). https://www.ncbi.nlm.nih.gov/pmc/articles/PMC3090218/.

A. B. Wachholtz and K. I. Pargament. "Migraines & Meditation: Does Spirituality Matter." *Journal of Behavioral Medicine* 31.4 (2008). https://www.ncbi.nlm.nih.gov/pubmed/18551362.

S. Rosenzweig, et al. "Mindfulness-Based Stress Reduction for Chronic Pain Conditions: Variation in Treatment Outcomes and Role of Home Meditation Practice." *Journal of Psychosomatic Research* 68.1 (2010). https://www.ncbi.nlm.nih.gov/pubmed/20004298.

L. E. Carlson and S. N. Garland. "Impact of Mindfulness-Based Stress Reduction (MBSR) on Sleep, Mood, Stress and Fatigue Symptoms in Cancer Outpatients." *International Journal of Behavioral Medicine* 12.4 (2005). https://www.ncbi.nlm.nih.gov/pubmed/16262547.

R. Davidson, et al. "Alterations in Brain and Immune Function Produced by Mindfulness Meditation." *Psychosomatic Medicine* 65.4 (2003). https://www.ncbi.nlm.nih.gov/pubmed/12883106.

S. Vasdev, et al. "N-acetyl cysteine Attenuates Ethanol Induced Hypertension in Rats." *Artery* 21.6 (1995). http://www.ncbi.nlm.nih.gov/pubmed/8833231.

E. Poleszak. "Benzodiazepine/GABA(A) Receptors are Involved in Magnesium-induced Anxiolytic-Like Behavior in Mice." *Pharmacological Reports* 60.4 (2008). http://www.ncbi.nlm.nih.gov/pubmed/18799816.

George A. Eby and K. L. Eby. George Eby Research Institute. "Treatment of side effects induced by oral, high-dose magnesium therapy of mental illnesses." Abstracts of 12th International Magnesium Symposium A16. http://www.researchgate.net/profile/Naomi_Cook/publication/260084388_Characterisation_of_TRPM_channel_mRNA_levels_in_Parkinsons_disease/links/0f31752f6cec0a42b5000000.pdf.

Cletus Kurtzman (Editor), J.W. Fell (Editor), Teun Boekhout (Editor). *The Yeasts: A Taxonomic Study*. April 2011. Elsevier Science; 5 edition (April 15, 2011).

D. Fedeli, et al. "Early Life Permethrin Exposure Leads to Hypervitaminosis D, Nitric Oxide and Catecholamines Impairment." *Pesticide Biochemistry and Physiology* 107.1 (2013). http://www.ncbi.nlm.nih.gov/pubmed/25149241.

Mark Sisson. "The Definitive Guide to Dairy." http://www.marksdailyapple.com/dairy-intolerance/.

Emanuel Abrahamson. *Body, Mind & Sugar*. New York, NY: Avon Books, 1977.

Margarida Martins, et al. "Presence of Extracellular DNA in the Candida Albicans Biofilm Matrix and Its Contribution to Biofilms." *Mycopathologia* 169.5 (2010). https://www.ncbi.nlm.nih.gov/pmc/articles/PMC3973130/.

Steven Sandberg-Lewis and Allison Siebecker. "SIBO: Dysbiosis Has A New Name." *Townsend Letter* February/March 2015.

R. Picton, et al. "Mucosal Protection against Sulphide: Importance of the Enzyme Rhodanese." *Gut* 50.2 (2002). https://www.ncbi.nlm.nih.gov/pmc/articles/PMC1773108/.

G. M. Walker et al. "Magnesium and the regulation of germ-tube formation in Candida albicans." *Journal of General Microbiology* 130.8 (1984). https://www.ncbi.nlm.nih.gov/pubmed/6432954.

Index

CPSIA information can be obtained
at www.ICGtesting.com
Printed in the USA
JSHW020225051120
9325JS00001B/1